Forthcoming Monographs

Travis and Brouhard
Diabetes Mellitus in Children

Bluestone and Klein
Otitis Media in Infants and Children

Dworkin
Learning and Behavior Problems of School Children

Viral Diseases of the Fetus and Newborn

SECOND EDITION

James Barry Hanshaw, M.D.

Professor and Chairman, Department of Pediatrics,
University of Massachusetts Medical School
Pediatrician-in-Chief, University of Massachusetts
    Medical Center, Worcester, Massachusetts
Lecturer, Department of Pediatrics,
Harvard Medical School, Boston, Massachusetts

John Alastair Dudgeon, C.B.E., M.A., M.D. (Cantab.), F.R.C.P., F.R.C.Path.

Professor Emeritus in Microbiology,
The University of London
Consulting Microbiologist, The Hospital for Sick Children,
Great Ormond Street, London, England

William Courtenay Marshall, M.D., Ph.D., M.R.A.C.P., D.C.H. (Deceased)

Formerly Consultant Physician, The Hospital
    for Sick Children, Great Ormond Street, London
Senior Lecturer in Infectious Diseases,
The Institute of Child Health, London, England

Volume 17 in the Series
MAJOR PROBLEMS IN CLINICAL PEDIATRICS

1985   W.B. SAUNDERS COMPANY
Philadelphia London Toronto Mexico City Rio de Janeiro Sydney Tokyo

W. B. Saunders Company: West Washington Square
                            Philadelphia, PA   19105

                            1 St. Anne's Road
                            Eastbourne, East Sussex BN21 3UN, England

                            1 Goldthorne Avenue
                            Toronto, Ontario M8Z 5T9, Canada

                            Apartado 26370—Cedro 512
                            Mexico 4, D.F., Mexico

                            Rua Coronel Cabrita, 8
                            Sao Cristovao Caixa Postal 21176
                            Rio de Janeiro, Brazil

                            9 Waltham Street
                            Artarmon, N.S.W. 2064, Australia

                            Ichibancho, Central Bldg., 22-1 Ichibancho
                            Chiyoda-Ku, Tokyo 102, Japan

Library of Congress Cataloging in Publication Data

Hanshaw, James Barry, 1928–
    Viral diseases of the fetus and newborn.

    (Major problems in clinical pediatrics; 17)

1. Virus diseases in children.   2. Fetus—Diseases.
    3. Infants (Newborn)—Diseases.   4. Virus diseases in preg-
    nancy.   I. Dudgeon, John Alastair.   II. Marshall, William
    C.   III. Title.   IV. Series: Major problems in clinical
    pediatrics; v. 17. [DNLM: 1. Virus diseases—In infancy and
    childhood. W1 MA492N v. 17/WC 500 H249v]

RG629.V57H36 1985   618.3′2   84–5397

ISBN 0–7216–4501–1

Viral Diseases of the Fetus and Newborn   ISBN   0–7216–4501–1

Last digit is the print number: 9   8   7   6   5   4   3   2   1

Dedication

Dr. William C Marshall, our co-author, died suddenly at his home in London on October 24, 1983, just as the final stages of the rewriting were being completed. The sudden and tragic death of this paediatrician at the height of his career will be mourned by his colleagues all over the world. We wish to dedicate this new edition, to which he had made important contributions, to his memory.

Foreword

It is a pleasure to present the second edition of *Viral Diseases of the Fetus and Newborn*. The first edition, published in 1978, was a well received monograph containing a wealth of information written with style and clarity. In this edition, the original outline has been retained and each chapter has been completely revised to include recent major advances in virology pertinent to the developing fetus and the newborn infant.

Dr. William C. Marshall joined Drs. Hanshaw and Dudgeon in the preparation of this volume, and it is with sadness and regret that we note that Dr. Marshall died unexpectedly just about the time the manuscript was completed. He graduated from Sydney University in 1954 with the degrees of M.B. and B.S., received his D.C.H. (London) in 1959, Ph.D. in 1972 and M.D. in 1976. He was Registrar in Pediatrics at the Hospital for Sick Children, Great Ormond Street, where he spent much of his prematurely shortened medical career. He was highly regarded as a consultant in infectious disease, and at the time of his death in 1983, Dr. Marshall had approximately 60 publications to his credit.

Dr. James Barry Hanshaw continues as Professor and Chairman of the Department of Pediatrics at the University of Massachusetts Medical Center, a position he assumed in 1975. His list of publications has grown as has his stature as a teacher and world authority on cytomegalovirus infections. Professor John Alastair Dudgeon has retired as Dean and from full-time appointments at the Hospital for Sick Children, Great Ormond Street. He has had a distinguished career as a teacher and researcher and now holds honorary appointments at that famous institution.

Dr. Duncan McEwan Gould and Professor Arie Jeremy Zuckerman have contributed special sections to this volume. Dr. Gould qualified at the University of Edinburgh for his M.B., Ch.B. in 1970 and his M.R.C.P. in 1975. He worked closely with Dr. Marshall in testing new anti-viral compounds. Dr. Zuckerman is Professor of Microbiology in the University of London at the London School of Hygiene and Tropical Medicine. He is one of the leading authorities in the world on viral hepatitis, and he is the Medical Director of the W.H.O. Collaboration Centre for Reference and Research on Viral Hepatitis.

MILTON MARKOWITZ

Preface to the Second Edition

The aims of this edition remain substantially the same as those of the first. However, in the intervening five years more information has accumulated as to the effects of viral infections on the fetus and newborn, so an updating seems warranted. In part this may be the result of clinicians, especially pediatricians and obstetricians, being more aware of the serious consequences these infections may often have—at least we hope that this is a reasonable assumption. Another factor has been the rapid development of new and improved laboratory techniques for the diagnosis and investigation of these infections. We do not contend that any major change has taken place that would alter our previously stated view on the overall impact of infectious agents as a cause of congenital defects. Although the number of children born each year with defects is large and shows little likelihood of changing in the immediate future, the proportion of these defects caused by infectious agents in general and viruses in particular is small. Nevertheless, they remain important for the reasons we have previously given. We have decided therefore to bring this volume up to date, concentrating in the main on those areas where there have been significant advances.

When the first edition was published the prospects of controlling congenital rubella defects were promising—and they still are. However, difficulties in the implementation of immunization programs may have been underestimated, and congenital rubella continues to occur, although there has been a decline in its incidence in some countries, especially the United States. We reiterate what we said before—that congenital rubella is a preventable disease—and therefore this edition examines closely vaccination programs currently in use.

In the case of cytomegalovirus infections, two issues predominate. First is the recognition that reactivation may be more important as a cause of fetal infection that was hitherto thought to be the case. Reactivation may affect the overall impact of cytomegalovirus as a cause of fetal damage and subsequent disability, but this has yet to be established. Second, we discuss the current difficulties in preventing this common fetal infection by immunization.

The importance of herpes simplex infection in the newborn may have been overestimated. Current thinking on the management of women with genital herpes at the time of delivery is changing. Important advances have been made in the treatment of herpetic infections with new antiviral drugs; these developments emphasize the need for prompt diagnosis by sensitive laboratory tests.

Opinion is also changing about the impact of varicella-zoster virus infections acquired in pregnancy. A few more cases of congenital varicella syndrome have been reported since the first edition was published, but there is still no discernible reason why such cases appear to be so rare, as chickenpox in women of child-bearing age is not uncommon. The management of neonatal varicella also needs reappraisal, as this condition is more common than previously envisaged and can be fatal.

We have retained the chapter on smallpox and vaccinia not only because of its historical interest but because the scientific material contained in it reflects upon the pathogenesis of fetal infections in general.

A major advance in our knowledge of hepatitis B infection in pregnancy has taken place. Fetal infection occurs more commonly as a result of maternal infection than was thought five years ago. This has important implications for management and prevention and raises once again the important issue of the relationship between an *infected* fetus and an *affected* fetus and infant.

Major advances have taken place in the development of laboratory techniques; these can only improve our understanding of the effect of viral infections upon the fetus and newborn and lead to improved methods of prevention. The development of a number of antiviral drugs for treatment of some of the herpesviruses has been considerable, and there is now hope that in the future treatment as well as prevention of some virus infections will be possible.

These are some of the changes which we have made in this second edition and which we hope will be of interest to our readers.

J. B. HANSHAW
J. A. DUDGEON
W. C. MARSHALL

Acknowledgments

I am grateful to Dr. T. H. Weller of Harvard University, who introduced me to virology during an exciting age of discovery. He is unquestionably one of the great clinical scientists of modern medicine. The late Dr. W. L. Bradford of the University of Rochester taught me pediatrics and a type of interaction with patients and parents that has not been surpassed in my experience. There have been many other people who took time along the way to teach by their example, especially Dr. G. B. Forbes. To many co-workers—Drs. A. P. Scheiner, R. F. Betts, G. Simon, M. M. Melish, the late L. A. Glasgow, H. Steinfeld, and V. Abel—I am especially grateful. The National Institutes of Health provided generous support through Career Research Development Awards (1962 to 1972) as well as through project grants (NICH & HD, NIAID) from 1960 to 1975. My debt to the National Foundation began in 1958 with a postdoctoral fellowship to the Harvard University School of Public Health. In addition, I am grateful to the Board of Governors of the Hospital for Sick Children, Great Ormond Street, and the Institute of Child Health in London, for providing me the opportunity to serve as a Visiting Professor in Professor J. A. Dudgeon's Department of Microbiology during the 1971–1972 academic year. It is this opportunity that made the present monograph possible. Last, I wish to thank Mrs. Janetta Petkus for her excellent assistance in the preparation of the manuscript and Mr. Christopher Duggan for bringing extraordinary competence and efficiency to the completion of this effort.

We are extremely grateful to Professor A. J. Zuckerman, Professor of Microbiology, the London School of Hygiene and Tropical Medicine, University of London, for his helpful comments and suggestions in the re-drafting of the chapter on hepatitis. Dr. J. D. M. Gould, the Hospital for Sick Children, Great Ormond Street, London, undertook to update the section on antiviral chemotherapy following Dr. Marshall's untimely death. For this we are also very grateful.

J.B.H.

Acknowledgments

I am grateful to a number of my former teachers who gave me great encouragement in the early days of virology. My interest in the subject was first aroused by the late Dr. Marius van den Ende, Head of the Scrub Typhus Research Team, and later by Dr. Christopher Andrewes, F.R.S. (now Sir Christopher Andrewes), at the National Institute for Medical Research in Hampstead. I owe a great deal to the training enjoyed under Sir Macfarlane Burnet, O.M., F.R.S., at the Walter and Eliza Hall Institute, the Royal Melbourne Hospital, Victoria, and to his continuing friendship. I have been especially fortunate during my time on the staff of the Hospital for Sick Children, Great Ormond Street, in meeting many pediatricians who not only became great personal friends, but whose help and interest in virus infections of children has done so much to promote the development of virological research. I was particularly fortunate in the support and encouragement I received from the late Sir Alan Aird Moncrieff, the first Nuffield Professor of Child Health and Honorary Consultant Physician to the Hospital. In his quiet, persuasive way he did much to help young consultants in many branches of pediatrics, and he was a great advocate of preventive medicine. Like so many others of my generation, I owe him a great deal.

I also want to express my thanks to the nursing staff of the Hospital, who have never failed in their help and have always risen to the occasion when special investigations were underway. Throughout my time at the Hospital, I have received constant help from members of the Board of Governors. To them I am grateful for their permission to include details of the case material from patients at the Hospital in this monograph. In expressing my thanks to my colleagues at the Hospital, I wish to make special reference to Dr. Olga Stark and to Dr. Catherine S. Peckham for their help and advice in our joint research efforts. I wish to record my special appreciation to the technical and scientific staff in the Department of Microbiology and in particular to my Chief Assistant, Mr. George Hawkins, F.I.M.L.T. He has assisted me for over 30 years and has played a major part in the development of virological techniques, in particular those used in the diagnosis of infections of the fetus and newborn. Many of the excellent illustrations in Chapter 14 are the result of his labors.

Much of the research into congenital defects has been supported by research grants from the Medical Research Council in London, Action Research for the Crippled Child, the Wellcome Trust, and the Board of Governors; to all of these bodies I am much indebted. I also want to record my appreciation to the members of the Department of Medical Illustration for the preparation of the figures, tables, and clinical photographs, to the library staff of the Hospital and to successive research secretaries, Mrs. Elizabeth Ryan, Mrs. Mary Whelan, and Miss Ann Milton, who took much trouble in preparing the details of the National Congenital Rubella Surveillance Programme. Finally, I want to express my great gratitude to my former secretary, Mrs. Sandra Hyder, who once again has given most valuable assistance and advice in the preparation of this new edition. This has required skill and patience in the preparation of the typescripts, checking bibliographies, and a mass of other details which are so often taken for granted. I know that both Dr. Hanshaw and Dr. Marshall were as pleased as I was that she felt able to undertake this onerous task.

I also wish to thank Mr. D. J. Rumsey, librarian, and the staff of the William Harvey Hospital, Ashford, Kent, for their help in checking references for me.

Writing a monograph with a co-author on the other side of the Atlantic is no easy task. This could never have been accomplished without the forebearance of Dr. Barry Hanshaw.

J.A.D.

Preface to the First Edition

This book is about the effects of viruses on the fetus and the newborn. It is concerned with the short-term as well as the long-term effects of viral infections upon normal fetal development and upon the child after birth. It is concerned with identifying the causes of these infections and with methods of diagnosis without which little progress can be made toward the final and most important aspect of the subject—that of management, treatment, and prevention.

Textbooks of pediatrics published prior to the Second World War contained virtually no reference to intrauterine infections, with the exception of congenital syphilis. The reasons for this are self-evident. At the time, pediatricians and family doctors were concerned with treating the severe communicable diseases—whooping cough, diphtheria, tuberculosis, measles, poliomyelitis, and gastroenteritis. As a result of improved health care and specific measures directed toward treatment and prevention in many countries, these previously serious problems have markedly declined in importance. The effect of these measures is reflected not only in a progressive fall in the childhood mortality rates but also in the order of disease conditions of children requiring admission to hospital. Whereas in the 1930's the communicable diseases were the predominant causes of death and ill health, their place has now been taken by neoplasms, congenital malformations, and accidents of all types. For example, a comparison of the causes of death among children at The Hospital for Sick Children, Great Ormond Street, London, during the period from 1914 to 1954 showed a fall of 52 per cent in deaths from environmental causes and an increase in deaths from congenital malformations and neoplasms, or from conditions that were due wholly or in part to genetic causes (Carter, 1956).

The discovery in 1941 that such a mild disease as rubella contracted in pregnancy could lead to severe congenital defects in the offspring led inevitably to the expectation that many other viruses would have the same effect. This has not proved to be the case, and although comparatively few viruses appear to play a significant part as a cause of congenital defects in terms of actual numbers of children involved, they are important in other respects. The damage they cause is extremely variable; it may be severe, even fatal; the fetus may be infected without obvious sign of damage or may escape infection altogether. The outcome is unpredictable, but the investigations that have led to the identification of these viruses have also led to a better understanding of the mechanisms responsible for the damage they cause. And so in the ensuing chapters of this monograph we shall seek to bring together for the clinician and pediatrician the information they must have in order to diagnose and manage the case and to advise the families of patients exposed to infections from conception throughout pregnancy into the first few weeks of life.

The study of intrauterine infections is yet another example of the way in which modern pediatrics has had to adapt to the changing pattern of medicine and an example of the need for those who practice to think in terms of events that occur before birth and that may be harmful to subsequent development.

Carter, C. O.: Changing patterns in the causes of death at The Hospital for Sick Children. Great Ormond Street Journal *11*:65–68, 1956.

J. B. HANSHAW
J. A. DUDGEON

Contents

1

Introduction 1

2

Evidence for the Viral Etiology of Congenital Defects 7

3

Rubella 13

4

Congenital Cytomegalovirus 92

5

Herpes Simplex Infection of the Fetus and Newborn 132

6

Enteroviral Infections 154

7

Varicella Zoster Infections 161

8

Smallpox and Vaccinia 175

9

Viral Hepatitis 182

10

Other Viruses as Potential Pathogens of the Fetus and Newborn 200

11

Pathology of the Placenta and Cord in Some Viral Infections 213

12

The Development of Immune Mechanisms in the Fetus and Newborn 230

13

Differential Diagnosis on the Basis of Physical Findings 243

14

Laboratory Diagnosis 258

Appendix—Principal Tests Used in the Diagnosis of Viral Diseases:
A Glossary of Terms 268

15

Prevention and Treatment 272

Index 297

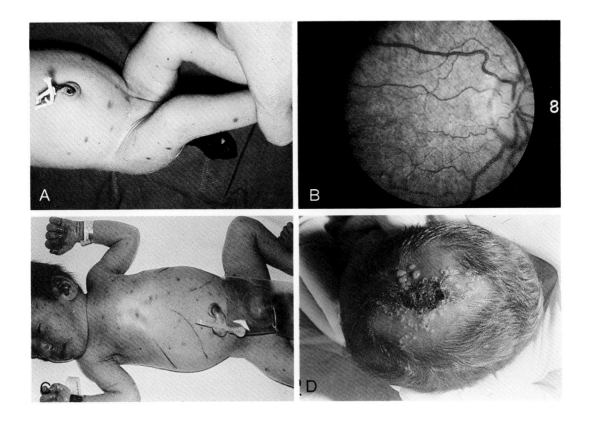

Figure A. Two day old infant with severe neonatal pupura, enlarged anterior fontanelle, bilateral corneal edema with increased ocular tension, osteopathy, and persistent ductus arteriosus. Platelets fell to 17,000/cu mm. She weighed 3 lb at birth. There was a history of maternal rubella at eight weeks' gestation. The infant died at six weeks of age from heart failure and severe hepatic involvement due to hepatitis. The infant's case was diagnosed by virus isolation and persistence of rubella antibody. (See Chapter 3.) (By permission of the Board of Governors, the Hospital for Sick Children, Great Ormond Street, London.)

Figure B. Generalized purpura and hepatosplenomegaly in a newborn infant with cytomegalic inclusion disease. (See Chapter 4.) (Courtesy of Dr. Joseph L. Butterfield, Denver, Colorado.)

Figure C. Pigmentary retinopathy. (See Chapter 3.) (By permission of the Board of Governors, the Hospital for Sick Children, Great Ormond Street, London.)

Figure D. Herpes simplex vesicles of the scalp of the newborn infant. (See Chapter 5.)

Introduction

One of the major unsolved problems in medicine today involves the great number of children born each year with congenital defects. The problem is a serious one because many defects affect organs and tissues, such as those of the central nervous system (including the organs responsible for vision and hearing), the cardiovascular system, and others, the integrity of which is vital to normal bodily function. Congenital defects frequently occur in combination and thus lead to severe dysfunction and to a permanent handicap for those who survive.

Many children with congenital defects are born with limited potential into a society whose members are increasingly expected to be intellectually, as well as physically, productive. Many are destined to live with significantly less than the average intellectual capacity, suffering from major defects in vision and hearing, sometimes with loss of motor function as well, and with a myriad of other disabilities that profoundly affect their lives and those of family members. An even greater number of children are born who will never reach their full potential because of more subtle and perhaps more poorly understood prenatal influences that culminate in failure to thrive and lead to failure at school for a variety of reasons not clearly identifiable with motivation or cultural determinants.

The crucial fact is that so little is known about the causation of congenital defects. Once a cause is established prevention is much easier. Because prevention of congenital defects is of such importance, we adjudge it to be essential to look in the first instance at the causes of congenital defects in general, because doing so may help to elucidate the specific role played by infectious agents and by viruses in particular.

The causes of congenital defects can be broadly classified under three main headings: (1) purely genetic causes, due to chromosomal anomalies and mutant gene defects; (2) purely environmental causes, in which the defect can be directly related to some agent, such as an infection, a drug, or ionizing radiation; and (3) mixed genetic and environmental causes, which probably account for the majority of congenital defects. It seems probable that the genetic predisposition in this large group of congenital disorders, possibly accounting for 70 to 80 per cent of the total, is polygenic (Carter, 1968).

This classification is convenient for a general approach to the study of congenital defects, but it would be a mistake to regard it in too rigid a fashion. There is some evidence from the work of Menser and co-workers (1974) that there may be a genetic susceptibility to rubella infection, and although there is as yet no proof that the cause of the more common defects can be explained on the basis of an interaction between genetic factors and infectious agents, this possibility should be borne in mind.

The incidence of the more common malformations is shown in Table 1–1; there is an overall incidence of approximately 25 per 1000 total births (the number varies according to the definition of "malformation" used) (Carter, 1968). These disorders, by virtue of the organs involved, should be recognizable at or soon after birth. They are, in the strict sense of the term, "malformations," or defects of the structural type; this list does not

Table 1–1. **INCIDENCE OF MALFORMATIONS (PER 1000 TOTAL BIRTHS): ESTIMATES BASED ON OBSERVATIONS BEYOND THE NEONATAL PERIOD**

	Birmingham (U.K.)	New York (U.S.)	Japan
Period of observation	(to 5 years)	(to 1 year)	(to 9 months)
Total births	56,760	5749	16,144
Anencephalus	2.0	1.6	0.6
Spina bifida	3.0	1.6	0.3
Hydrocephalus	2.6	0.9	0.5
Cardiac malformation	4.2	8.5	7.0
Cleft lip and palate	1.9	1.6	3.0
Dislocation of the hip	0.7	1.2	7.1
Talipes equinovarus	4.4	5.2	1.4
Down's syndrome	1.7	1.9	0.9
All individuals with major malformations	23.1	(not given) total malformed 75.3	24.5

From McKeown, T., and Record, R. G.: Malformations in a population observed for five years after birth. Ciba Foundation Symposium on Congenital Malformations. London, J. and A. Churchill, 1960.

include defects caused by destruction of anatomically normal organs, which is a recognized feature of some intrauterine virus infections. Other important defects such as mental retardation and congenital deafness are also not included, mainly because they can be difficult to diagnose at birth or in the early months of life.

The question of definition or terminology is of relevance to the subject of this book. The matter was discussed at the First International Conference on Congenital Malformations held in 1960 in London. Speaking then on the role of environmental teratogenic factors, Dr. Joseph Warkany said,

A remark about terminology may be in order here. It has been suggested that the anomalies produced by prenatal rubella are not congenital malformations but embryopathies. Similarly, some have recommended that the defects produced by toxoplasmosis should not be considered as congenital malformations because they are due to secondary destruction of originally normal organs. There is little justification for such hair- or term-splitting. The term congenital malformations should be applied to gross, structural anomalies *present at birth*, irrespective of their etiology or morphogenesis. It would lead to needless confusion if we were to call a septal defect due to rubella an embryopathy, and a septal defect of unknown origin a congenital malformation. Similarly, a hydrocephalus present at birth should be considered a congenital malformation whether it is of genetic, toxoplasmic, or unknown origin.

Since that time much more information has come to light concerning the role of infectious agents such as rubella and cytomegalovirus (CMV) as causes of a wide spectrum of fetal damage. It would seem inappropriate to classify conditions such as neonatal hepatitis, thrombocytopenia with or without purpura, low birth weight, mental retardation, and failure to thrive under the same heading as persistent ductus arteriosus or a cardiac septal defect. The preferred term, therefore, is "congenital defect," which will be taken to mean any abnormality, including those that can be correctly classified as malformations, present at or detectable after birth, *that have been caused by an environmental insult before birth.* As far as viral infections of the fetus, the main topic of this book, are concerned, the prime insult is deemed to be the result of an infection contracted by the mother during pregnancy or immediately prior to conception. It will, however, become apparent that the damage caused to the fetus by a virus such as rubella, in contrast to that caused by some other teratogenic agent, may not all occur at the time of the initial infection. Although the time of infection is of great importance to the outcome, it is now established that fetal infections may result in an ongoing process of damage that occurs throughout fetal life and even after birth. Moreover, the nature of the lesions encountered in fetal virus infections points to complex and multifactorial pathological processes, in contrast to those encountered in defects of genetic origin or those induced by a drug such as thalidomide.

Although the total number of children born each year with congenital defects is large, the proportion of these defects due directly to infections is only a small fraction of the total. They are important, however, because they may be preventable. This applies to all environmental or nongenetic causes of congenital defects; once the cause can be clearly identified, whether it is a drug, an infection, or some other cause, steps can be taken to prevent further occurrences.

Prevention of congenital defects may be achieved by several methods. It is important to distinguish between *primary* prevention and *secondary* prevention: the former is directed toward preventing a defect from occurring in the first place and the latter toward preventing the birth of a seriously defective infant after the event has occurred. The administration of the drug thalidomide (Distaval, Contergan) to pregnant women as a tranquilizer resulted in the birth of many children with phocomelia and associated limb deformities. Withdrawal of the drug from the market resulted in a marked decline in the number of such cases from the epidemic numbers of the 1960's, but not in the total disappearance of defects of a similar kind, which suggested that some other factor was causing those defects. Prevention of thalidomide defects by prohibition of the sale and distribution of potentially teratogenic drugs comes under the category of primary prevention.

Both genetic and environmental influences are almost certainly responsible for neural tube defects. Amniocentesis, together with other techniques, now permits considerable accuracy in prediction of a neural tube defect in the fetus, especially with defects of the major type. In such cases, the option to terminate a pregnancy can be offered if this is considered appropriate. But such a secondary prevention procedure is, for obvious reasons, far less satisfactory than primary prevention. Recent work by Smithells and his colleagues (1981) in England on the "apparent prevention of neural tube defects by periconceptional vitamin supplementation" to mothers who had already given birth to one or more infants with neural tube defects illustrates the importance of primary prevention. This report also emphasizes the need for a careful scrutiny of all possible contributory causes of defects. Although there are important scientific data to support the hypothesis of a causal relationship between vitamin deficiency and birth defects in animals, the evidence of such a relationship in humans is by no means clear. Vitamin supplementation appears to have prevented some neural tube defects, but whether this is the final answer to the problem has not yet been fully established.

Finally, the prevention of congenital rubella by immunization of susceptible women before they become pregnant is another example of primary prevention, and one which could serve as a model for the elucidation of the cause and prevention of other viral infections contracted in pregnancy.

Despite important advances in our understanding of the pathogenesis of many inborn errors of metabolism, as well as of the teratogenic effects of certain drugs and a few infectious agents, including viruses, we cannot yet claim to have made any significant advance in the prevention and control of the great majority of prenatally determined conditions, and until more is known about the details of their causation progress is likely to be slow.

In the nineteenth century, inflammation was regarded as the cause of all ills, including congenital defects. Kreysig (ca.1814) attributed many forms of congenital heart disease to fetal endocarditis, a view that was seldom substantiated by morbid anatomists of the day. At the time when congenital syphilis was prevalent, many children were also born with congenital defects, and when it was found that congenital syphilis was associated with mental retardation and other neurological diseases, it was not unnatural to assume that *Treponema pallidum* was an important teratogenic agent. As the incidence of congenital syphilis declined with modern medical treatment and the incidence of congenital malformations did not change, this theory had to be abandoned.

The concept of an infectious origin of congenital defects was first established with absolute certainty in 1941 by the late Sir Norman Gregg following his observations on congenital cataracts and other congenital defects in children whose mothers had had German measles during pregnancy (Gregg, 1941). On this occasion the observations were proved to be correct as confirmation of the same defects came from countries all over the world, and it was confidently expected that other viruses would be found to be the cause of other birth defects. Measles, mumps, chickenpox, poliomyelitis, hepatitis, and influenza were all considered as potential teratogenic agents. Could they behave as teratogens in a like manner to rubella, and if so, what was the evidence that this was the case? Many observers have incriminated these viruses as causes of congenital defects (see the review by Rhodes [1960]), but mainly on the basis of isolated observations that cannot be distinguished from purely coincidental associations. Originally it was thought that all children whose mothers had had rubella at any stage in pregnancy were born with defects, so the fact that most children born after maternal mumps, chickenpox, or influenza were normal appeared to rule out these infections as causes of fetal damage. Later, when it was found that only a proportion of fetuses exposed to rubella were affected, it was clearly difficult to say with certainty that an association between other viral infections of the mother and congenital defects in the offspring could be more than a coincidence. In any case, these early studies on rubella embryopathy raised important questions, such as why some embryos or fetuses were affected and others not, and by what mechanism a virus could cause the varied types of congenital defects affecting many different organ systems, which are different from those encountered in other types of congenital defects.

The surprising and rather unexpected finding is that some 35 years after Gregg's discovery concerning the relationship between maternal rubella and congenital rubella, few viruses other than rubella and CMV have been found to affect the fetus with the same consistency. Evidence is accruing to indicate that maternal varicella-zoster may lead to a congenital varicella syndrome, but only very rarely. On the other hand, there has been a change in our concept of the "effect" of a virus infection upon the fetus or newborn. No longer do we think solely in terms of a teratogenic agent leading to a malformation. The effect is now assessed in relation to the total impact upon the fetus—fetal death and spontaneous abortion, stillbirth, congenital defects, and other forms of fetal damage.

The viruses listed in Table 1–2 have been incriminated as causes of prenatal disease leading to spontaneous abortion, stillbirth, congenital defects, or other forms of fetal damage. It can further be posited that these viruses, or others not yet known to be associated with fetal infection, may play a significant part in the long-term development of the individual. This is especially true when we realize that most of the information available today concerns viruses and other infectious agents that produce disease after birth. The recognition of the importance of a given infectious agent is based on an assumption that one agent behaves in a fashion similar *in vitro* and *in vivo* to other agents and that it produces infection and thereby disease and

is capable of stimulating an immune response. It is now clear that not all viruses behave in a like manner and that what applies to one may well not apply to another.

The thalidomide disaster of the early 1960's and the rubella pandemic of 1964–65 focused attention yet again on the need to be constantly on the alert for environmental factors that may interfere with organogenesis. The number of drugs that are known to be teratogenic is small (Smithells, 1976) compared with the vast number that may be administered for one reason or another in pregnancy (Sutherland and Light, 1965), yet the fact that some can cause damage is the reason why many countries have set up national organizations to examine and scrutinize all drugs and biological products from the point of view of safety.

The effect of maternal influenza upon the fetus is still not known for certain. At present there is no firm evidence that influenza in pregnancy causes fetal damage, but the difficulty lies in establishing a cause-and-effect relationship that distinguishes the potentially harmful effect of the virus from the potentially harmful effect of any medicament that may be prescribed for patients suffering from influenza. It also has to be recognized that some of the clinical entities that may present as congenital defects are not always due solely to genetic causes. The etiology of congenital heart disease and deafness is a case in point. A significant proportion of cases of congenital sensorineural deafness can be related solely to intrauterine infections, especially rubella and CMV. Possibly 50 per cent of such cases are genetically determined, and the remainder are probably of mixed genetic and environmental origin. It is conceivable that a virus infection, leading to an infection either clinical or subclinical at precisely the crucial time before, during, or after fertilization of the ovum, could damage the chromosomes in such a way as to affect normal organogenesis.

A great deal of work has been carried out in the past 30 years on the induction of malformations in developing chick embryos and in certain mammalian species. The relevance of much of this work to human malformations is difficult to interpret, yet it would be advantageous if an animal model were available in the study of some potentially damaging infections. One of the main difficulties in interpreting the significance of results obtained from experimental studies in animals lies in the structure and function

Table 1–2. **VIRUSES AFFECTING THE FETUS AND NEWBORN**

Agent	Abortion	Still-Birth	Low Birth Weight	Main Congenital Defect	Other Defects
Rubella	+	+	+	Cataract, deafness, congenital heart defects (others less frequent)	Inapparent to severe infection with disease manifested by hepatosplenomegaly, thrombocytopenia, psychomotor retardation, bone lesions, etc.
Cytomegalovirus	?	+	+	Microcephaly, deafness (others less frequent)	Chronic infection may be inapparent. Also associated with hepatosplenomegaly, thrombocytopenia, psychomotor retardation, purpura, cerebral calcification, chorioretinitis
Herpesvirus hominis	–	–	+	Microcephaly	Chorioretinitis, hepatitis, psychomotor retardation, fulminant disease common in intrapartum infection
Varicella-zoster	?	?	+	Hypoplasia of limb, rudimentary digits, cutaneous scars	Convulsions, retardation, cataracts, chorioretinitis, microphthalmos
Mumps	+	+	–	–	Relationship between maternal mumps and endocardial fibroelastosis is unproven
Influenza	+	+	–	?	Conflicting evidence on increased risk of malformation following first trimester illness
Vaccinia	+	+	+	–	Generalized fetal vaccinia
Smallpox	+	+	?	?	Fetal smallpox
Hepatitis B (HBV)	–	–	–	–	Rarely, hepatosplenomegaly, hepatitis, jaundice, active fulminant neonatal hepatitis, chronic cirrhosis
Hepatitis A (HAV)	+	–	+	–	–
Measles	+	+	–	?	Nil proven
Poliovirus	+	+	+	–	Occasionally infants born with paralysis
Coxsackie B	?	?	–	–	Myocarditis meningoencephalitis, and pneumonitis during neonatal period

of the placenta. The placental membrane differs so greatly among mammalian species that it is extremely difficult to extrapolate data from one species to another, and species also vary greatly in their susceptibility to infection with animal viruses (Mims, 1976). In the case of congenital rubella, all our knowledge concerning the production of defects has been gleaned from a detailed study of human cases. Initial hopes that animal models could be found for the study of the pathogenesis of rubella infection have not been realized. There are many gaps in our knowledge concerning the pathogenesis of congenital CMV infection, but a study of CMV in certain strains of mice may be rewarding in relation to the human situation.

A study of comparative medicine is frequently helpful, but it cannot be relied upon to produce the answers to all unsolved problems. The possibility also has to be considered that diseases that appear to be familial may be transmitted to the offspring through the mother's milk. The Bittner agent, which is associated with a high incidence of mammary carcinomas in certain strains of mice, may be transmitted in this way. The animal leukemia viruses infect the ovum directly and can be passed to the offspring, with the onset of disease occurring several months after birth. Human CMV may also be passed on to the newborn child with the mother's milk. If baby hamsters can develop hydrocephalus and aqueductal stenosis secondary to congenital mumps infection (Johnson, 1968; Johnson and Johnson, 1969), then it is reasonable to assume that similar phenomena may occur in humans, although account must be taken of the artificial route by which infection was established in these experimental procedures. The same applies in general principle to other induced congenital defects in animals, such as cerebellar hypoplasia associated with intrauterine feline panleukopenia virus (Herndon et al., 1971) and the cerebellar degeneration produced by the rat virus in newborn hamsters (Kilham and Margolis, 1964). Account also has to be taken of the well-documented evidence that leukemias, lymphomas, sarcomas, and other solid tumors are induced in lower mammalian species by viruses that become established in the host during intrauterine life, but one must be exceedingly cautious in projecting these findings to the human situation and concluding that congenital leukemia in humans represents an example of the same pathological process as occurs in lower animals.

We are so accustomed to thinking of viruses in terms of their cytocidal effect on cells *in vitro* in the laboratory that we at times forget that the majority of viral infections are more often asymptomatic than symptomatic. It is well known that congenital rubella can follow subclinical maternal infection, and it is very rare for the mother of an infant with cytomegalic inclusion disease to have had a clinically recognizable illness. Eventually it may be found that defects in organogenesis or subsequent damage may occur with greater frequency than is at present known, without any evidence of an unusual illness during the pregnancy. Catalano and Sever (1971) have concluded with some justification that "in terms of the potential number of individuals affected, inapparent and latent viral infections may prove to be the most important group of deleterious agents which are congenitally acquired."

These are some of the facts that have come to light in recent years and that should be taken into account in studies aimed at defining the etiological role of viruses in the fetus and the newborn.

Bibliography

Carter, C. O.: Incidence and etiology. In Norman, A. P. (ed.): Congenital Abnormalities in Infancy. 2nd ed. Oxford, Blackwell Scientific Publications, 1968, pp. 1–24.

Catalano, L. W., and Sever, J. L.: The role of viruses as causes of congenital defects. Annu. Rev. Microbiol. 25:255–282, 1971.

Gregg, N. M.: Congenital cataract following German measles in the mother. Trans. Ophthalmol. Soc. Aust. 3:35–46, 1941.

Herndon, R. M., Margolis, G., and Kilham, L.: The synaptic organization of the malformed cerebellum induced by perinatal infection with the feline panleukopenia virus. J. Neuropathol. Exp. Neurol. 30:196–205, 557–570, 1971.

Johnson, R. T.: Hydrocephalus following viral infection. The pathology of aqueductal stenosis developing after experimental mumps infection. J. Neuropathol. Exp. Neurol. 27:591–606, 1968.

Johnson, R. T., and Johnson, K. P.: Hydrocephalus as a sequela of experimental myxovirus infections. Exp. Mol. Pathol. 10:68–80, 1969.

Kilham, L., and Margolis, G.: Cerebellar ataxia in hamsters inoculated with rat virus. Science 143:1047–1048, 1964.

Kreysig, F. L.: Krankheiten des Herzens systematisch bearbeitet. Berlin, circa 1814–17.

McKeown, T., and Record, R. G.: Malformations in a population observed for five years after birth. Ciba Foundation Symposium on Congenital Malformations. London, J. and A. Churchill, 1960.

Menser, M. A., Forrest, J. M., Honeyman, M. C., and Burgess, J. A.: Diabetes, HL-A antigens and congenital rubella. Lancet 2:1508–1509, 1974.

Mims, C.: Comparative aspects of infective malformations. In Human malformations. Br. Med. Bull. 32:84–88, 1976.

Rhodes, A. J.: Virus infections and congenital malformations. In Congenital Malformations. Papers and Discussions Presented at the 1st International Conference on Congenital Malformations, London. Philadelphia, J. B. Lippincott Company, 1960, pp. 106–116.

Smithells, R. W.: Environmental teratogens of man. In Human malformations. Br. Med. Bull. 32:27–33, 1976.

Smithells, R. W., Shepherd, S., Schorak, C. J., Seller, M. J., Nevin, N. C., Harris, R., Read, A. P., and Fielding, D. W.: Apparent prevention of neural tube defects by periconceptional vitamin supplementation. Arch. Dis. Child. 56:911–918, 1981.

Sutherland, J. M., and Light, I. J.: The effect of drugs on the developing fetus. Pediatr. Clin. North Am. 12:781–806, 1965.

Warkany, J.: Environmental teratogenic factors. In Congenital Malformations. Papers and Discussions Presented at the 1st International Conference on Congenital Malformations, London. Philadelphia, J. B. Lippincott Company, 1960, pp. 99–105.

Evidence for the Viral Etiology of Congenital Defects

There are two main reasons why it is important to identify those viral infections which, if they occur in pregnancy, may lead to congenital defects or other forms of fetal damage. In the first place, proof of an etiological relationship is an essential prerequisite if preventive measures are to be considered. In addition to proof of causation, some estimate of the size of the problem is also necessary. In the past few years, methods of cost-benefit analysis have been introduced to determine the efficacy of vaccination procedures against infectious diseases such as smallpox, measles, and poliomyelitis. In the case of rubella the total costs, direct and indirect, of the treatment of thousands of multiply handicapped congenital rubella children born in the United States as a result of the 1964–65 pandemic has been estimated at $2.2 billion (Cooper et al., 1969). The cost of a rubella immunization program to prevent such a disaster from occurring at the present time would be a fraction of the sum required for long-term care and rehabilitation of the surviving affected children (Koplan and Axnick, 1982).

The second reason is of a more immediate practical nature. Advice is frequently sought from physicians about the possible risk to a woman who is or may be pregnant and who has either been in contact with or contracted an infectious disease, not necessarily rubella. What is the risk of damage to the fetus and birth of a child with a congenital defect? Now that a number of countries have introduced legislation to make the termination of a pregnancy legal under certain conditions, such inquiries have increased, as have the number of requests for advice as to the risk in a given circumstance and for laboratory tests to make a precise diagnosis. In the United Kingdom it is legal under statute law to terminate a pregnancy, among other reasons, "if there is a *substantial* risk that if the child were born it would suffer from such physical or mental abnormalities as to be *seriously* handicapped" (Abortion Act, 1966).* Legislation in some other countries is similar in general intent; elsewhere, the laws are more precise in laying down conditions under which termination can legally be performed and place the onus of determining whether the conditions are met on those whose opinion is sought as to relative risks. In addition to rubella, the most frequent requests for advice concern contact or clinical infection with mumps, varicella,

---

*Italics added for emphasis.

7

hepatitis, cytomegalovirus (CMV), and influenza or "influenza-like illness" at some stage in pregnancy. Inquiries used to be made about the risk from smallpox vaccine inadvertently administered in pregnancy, but this is no longer a problem following the worldwide eradication of smallpox. On the other hand, advice concerning other live vaccines—in particular, rubella vaccine—administered in pregnancy is frequently sought.

The manner in which the evidence incriminating maternal rubella as a cause of congenital defects has been gradually accumulated, from initial clinical impressions to established facts, provides a model that can be used for collating evidence about the risk from other infectious agents. In the case of rubella, the first evidence came from clinical observations of a syndrome, that is, a repetitive pattern of similar clinical features, consisting, in the main, of cataracts, heart disease, and, later, deafness. The clinical impression was followed by the epidemiological association, made retrospectively, linking the noted defects with a history of the mothers' having contracted German measles (rubella) in pregnancy. The finding of the same repetitive pattern of defects not only throughout the continent of Australia, where the first observations were made, but in countries all over the world, established a cause-and-effect relationship. Some 20 years later, following the isolation of rubella virus, it was found that laboratory tests could be used to make a retrospective diagnosis of intrauterine infection, either by isolation of the infecting agent or by immunological tests (Dudgeon et al., 1964), or by both (Alford, et al., 1964).

If the evidence concerning the association between maternal rubella and congenital defects is accepted, then it is reasonable to suggest that four main criteria should be satisfied before an illness contracted in pregnancy is accepted as the cause of a congenital defect (Dudgeon, 1976). These criteria, set out in Table 2–1, are intended as guidelines and cannot be satisfied in every situation. It will also be clear that cases of congenital defects due to inapparent or subclinical infections in pregnancy will probably not be recognized. Thus, in such cases the supporting laboratory tests are dependent upon the fetus being *infected* for results of diagnostic value to be obtained. Fetal infection appears to be a prerequisite because otherwise the virus cannot be isolated nor the immunological response determined. Maternal infections with rubella and CMV undoubtedly cause fetal damage as a direct result of maternal-fetal infection, but in the case of influenza in pregnancy there is no evidence that fetal infection occurs; this is not surprising, since viremia is not a feature of influenza infection.

In order to establish this evidence of a causal relationship, account should also be taken of the nature of fetal damage following a maternal infection. This will depend on a number of factors—the virus, the gestational age at which infection occurs, and the route by which the virus is transmitted from the mother to the fetus or ways in which it may indirectly cause damage. The summary of the effects of viruses upon the fetus and newborn shown in Table 2–2 draws attention to the varied manifestations of fetal damage that have been established. Any prospective clinical and epidemiological study designed to establish a viral etiology of fetal damage should take these into account.

Table 2–1. CRITERIA FOR ESTABLISHING A CAUSAL RELATIONSHIP BETWEEN A MATERNAL INFECTION AND CONGENITAL DEFECTS OR FETAL DAMAGE

(1) *Clinical*: each infection tends to produce a syndrome or repetitive pattern of clinical manifestations

(2) *Epidemiological*: the same manifestations should be observed with the same agent following maternal illness in different countries

(3) *Virological*: persistence of the infective agent in fetal tissues and a chronic infective state after birth

(4) *Immunological*: persistence of antibody in the child after the normal decline of maternal antibody; presence of antibody in the IgM fraction

Table 2–2. **EFFECTS OF MATERNAL INFECTIONS UPON THE FETUS**

Fetal death
Intrauterine growth retardation resulting in low birth weight for gestational age
Stillbirth
Death in infancy
Congenital defects
Late onset of congenital disease or defects
Subclinical infection without evidence of damage
No evidence of fetal infection or damage

The evidence linking maternal rubella and CMV infection with congenital infection has been clearly established on all four criteria. The clinical and epidemiological data are also supported by laboratory tests for evidence of intrauterine infection, and the same applies to other congenital infections—toxoplasmosis and syphilis. Infection with herpes simplex virus occurring late in pregnancy may cause severe neonatal disease (Nahmias et al., 1975) and is similar in some respects to varicella-zoster infection occurring at the same stage in pregnancy.

No such clear evidence is available with respect to congenital defects or disease in the case of mumps, measles, poliomyelitis, or viral hepatitis A, but opinion regarding the effect of maternal hepatitis B infection on the fetus and newborn is changing. The evidence with varicella-zoster (V-Z) infections was less clear until recently. This was the general conclusion of several large-scale prospective studies carried out to examine the effect of a number of viral infections when contracted in pregnancy. Manson and colleagues (1960), in their prospective study of rubella and other viral infections during pregnancy, concluded that there was no harmful effect to the child following chickenpox or mumps in pregnancy, but in the case of measles there was a higher infant death rate and a higher rate of malformed children than would have been expected, compared with the control group (Table 2–3). It is difficult to explain these findings as purely fortuitous, but the few malformations that were encountered in the measles group were not confined to any particular period of pregnancy, and there is also the possibility of a mistaken diagnosis of the maternal infection, since one of the children had a rubella-type defect. These investigators also found that the outcome of the pregnancy was remarkably poor in the six cases in which poliomyelitis was contracted between the ninth and twelfth weeks of pregnancy (one

spontaneous abortion, two stillbirths, one malformation, and two surviving children). However, the adverse effect of maternal poliomyelitis on the fetus, whatever its extent, is now of lesser significance, since poliomyelitis is preventable by immunization in most parts of the world.

These findings were confirmed by Bradford Hill and co-workers (1958) with a smaller group of patients, and by Siegel (1973) in a study in New York City comparable in size to the British study of Manson and colleagues (1960). Recent evidence suggests, however, that V-Z virus (see Chapter 7) can very rarely cause congenital defects of a particular pattern. Cases with similar clinical features have been observed in several countries, and there is some laboratory evidence to support the occurrence of fetal V-Z infection. In addition, V-Z infection acquired late in pregnancy can cause severe disease in the newborn (Gershon, 1975).

These three prospective studies are in general agreement with respect to the incidence of congenital defects following maternal viral infections, but more detailed studies by Siegel and co-workers (1966) on the effect of these agents on fetal mortality and birth weight following such infections (Siegel and Fuerst, 1966) indicate that some of these viruses could also have an indirect adverse effect. Siegel et al. (1966) found an increase in the fetal death rate following rubella and mumps in pregnancy, but no such effect was noticeable after measles and chickenpox. The perinatal mortality was increased after rubella and also after hepatitis A virus (HAV) infection occurring late in pregnancy; in the latter case this appeared to be related to the severity of the maternal disease. Siegel and Fuerst (1966) found an increase in the frequency of prematurity* following rubella, measles, and hepatitis in pregnancy. In the case of rubella this appeared to be related to intrauterine growth retardation and presence of malformations resulting from early infection, but with hepatitis A and measles the outcome was probably related to early onset of labor induced by the severity of the maternal disease. This is probably an indication that the effects of various infectious agents on the fetus are mediated in different ways.

Mumps virus has been incriminated as a cause of congenital defects more often than

---

*The term "prematurity" used at that time would now more correctly be replaced by "low birth weight" or "small for gestational age."

Table 2–3. RUBELLA AND OTHER VIRAL INFECTIONS DURING PREGNANCY IN THE UNITED KINGDOM: NUMBER AND PROPORTION OF INFANTS WITH AND WITHOUT MALFORMATIONS IN CONTROL SERIES AND (6) VIRUS SERIES

Type of Case	All Infants					All Liveborn Infants				
	No. of Cases	Without Major Malformations		With Major Malformations		No. of Cases	Without Major Malformations		With Major Malformations	
		No.	%	No.	%		No.	%	No.	%
Control series	5611*	5431*	96.8	156*	2.8	5455*	5326*	97.6	128*	2.3
Rubella up to 12th week	192	160	83.4	30	15.6	183	154	84.2	29	15.8
Rubella 13th to 28th week	275	266	96.7	9	3.3	268	261	97.4	7	2.6
Chickenpox up to 12th week	73	70	95.9	1	1.4	70	69	98.6	1	1.4
Chickenpox 13th to 28th week	142	137	96.5	4	2.8	140	137	97.9	3	2.1
Measles up to 12th week	36	31	86.1	4	11.1	35	31	88.6	4	11.4
Measles 13th to 28th week	45	42	93.3	3	6.7	44	42	95.5	2	4.5
Mumps up to 12th week	115	112	97.4	2	1.7	113	111	98.2	2	1.8
Mumps 13th to 28th week	230	218	94.8	8	3.5	224	219	97.8	5	2.2
Poliomyelitis up to 12th week	8	5	62.5	1	12.5	6	5	83.3	1	16.7
Poliomyelitis 13th to 28th week	24	24	100.0	0	–	24	24	100.0	0	–
Influenza up to 12th week	41	41	100.0	0	–	41	41	100.0	0	–
Influenza 13th to 28th week	99	92	92.9	7	7.1	97	91	93.8	6	6.2

*In all series a few were not stated, so that the total number of cases does not agree with subtotals in all cases.
From Manson, M. M., et al.: Rubella and other virus infections during pregnancy. Rep. Publ. Hlth. Med. Subj. 101, 1960.

any virus except rubella (Rhodes, 1960), but proof is still lacking. Ylinen and Jarvinen (1953) in Finland found a high incidence of malformations in children whose mothers had parotitis in the first trimester (22 per cent), compared with 10 per cent when the illness had occurred in the second and third trimesters. The prospective study reported by Siegel and co-workers (1966) identified a higher rate of spontaneous abortion following mumps in pregnancy but found no evidence of fetal damage. The association between exposure to mumps in pregnancy and primary endocardial fibroblastosis in the offspring is not regarded as sufficiently strong, and the subject requires further study. Mumps virus has been isolated from a fetus spontaneously aborted at 10 weeks following clinical mumps in the mother early in pregnancy. This case report demonstrates that mumps virus can cross the placenta and cause fetal infection, but no other conclusions can be drawn (Kurtz et al., 1982).

The outcome of the cases complicated by maternal influenza detailed in the report of Manson and colleagues (1960) was unusual in that an excess number of deaths from a variety of unremarkable causes occurred in infants in the second year of life. The diagnosis of influenza was made on clinical grounds, and the cases concerned were associated with influenza between the thirteenth and twenty-eighth weeks of pregnancy. The role of maternal influenza as a cause of congenital defects is as controversial as that of mumps, but there are important differences in the pathogenesis of the two infections that must be taken into account. As already stated, there is no viremic phase in influenza, and so in theory the fetus is unlikely to be *infected* as a result of viral invasion. Fetal infection seems to be an important process that subsequently leads to fetal damage with other viruses such as rubella and CMV. This is not to say that a fetus cannot be damaged indirectly by maternal influenza, toxemia, hyperpyrexia, or other metabolic disturbances or by medication with salicylates and other antipyretic drugs. Another factor relevant to the possible relationship between maternal influenza and fetal damage is the lack of consistency in the reporting of any increase in congenital defects following pandemics and major epidemics of influenza in the past few decades, especially during the Asian influenza epidemic of 1957 and with the Hong Kong strains in the late 1960's.

There is no reliable evidence to suggest that HAV or the enteroviruses are contributory causes of congenital defects (Siegel, 1973), despite one report linking Coxsackie B infection in pregnancy with congenital heart disease (Brown and Evans, 1967).

Smallpox vaccine could undoubtedly cause fetal death and fetal damage, particularly after primary vaccination, but is of little consequence now that smallpox has been eradicated from the world. However, the association between smallpox vaccine and fetal infection justifies the recommendation that smallpox vaccine and other live vaccines be contraindicated in pregnancy. Live attenuated rubella vaccines administered inadvertently during pregnancy have been shown rarely to infect the fetus, and in one case, structural damage to the lens of the eye has been reported (Modlin et al., 1975). However, new facts regarding the teratogenicity of rubella vaccines have now come to light and are discussed in subsequent chapters on rubella and prevention (Chapters 3 and 15).

Bibliography

Abortion Act: An Act to amend and clarify the law relating to termination of pregnancy by registered medical practitioners. Elizabeth II. Her Majesty's Stationery Office, London, 1966, Chapter 87.

Alford, C. A., Neva, F. A., and Weller, T. H.: Virologic and serologic studies on human products of conception after maternal rubella. N. Engl. J. Med. *271*:1275–1281, 1964.

Bradford Hill, A., Doll, R., Galloway, T. M., and Hughes, J. P. W.: Virus disease in pregnancy and congenital defects. Br. J. Prev. Soc. Med. *12*:1–7, 1958.

Brown, G. C., and Evans, T. N.: Serologic evidence of coxsackievirus etiology of congenital heart disease. J.A.M.A. *199*:183–187, 1967.

Cooper, L. Z., Zirling, P. R., Ockerse, A. B., Fedun, B. A., Kiely, B., and Krugman, S.: Rubella: clinical manifestations and management. Am. J. Dis. Child. *118*:18–29, 1969.

Dudgeon, J. A.: Infective causes of human malformations. In Human malformations. Br. Med. Bull. *32*;77–85, 1976.

Dudgeon, J. A., Butler, N. R., and Plotkin, S. A.: Further serological studies on the rubella syndrome. Br. Med. J. *2*:155–160, 1964.

Gershon, A. A.: Varicella in mother and infant: problems old and new. In Krugman, S., and Gershon, A. A. (eds.): Infections of the Fetus and Newborn. Progress in Clinical and Biological Research, Vol. 3: New York, Alan R. Liss Inc., 1975.

Koplan, J. P., and Axnick, N. W.: Benefits, risks, and costs of viral vaccines. Prog. Med. Virol. *28*:180–191, 1982.

Kurtz, J. B., Tomlinson, A. H., and Pearson, J.: Mumps virus isolated from a fetus. Br. Med. J. *284*:471, 1982.

Manson, M. M., Logan, W. P. D., and Loy, R. M.: Rubella and other virus infections during pregnancy. Rep. Publ. Hlth. Med. Subj. No. 101, 1960.

Modlin, J. F., Brandling-Bennett, A. D., Witte, J. F., Campbell, C. C., and Myers, J. D.: A review of 5 years experience with rubella vaccine in the United States. Pediatrics 55:20–29, 1975.

Nahmias, A. J., Visintine, A. M., Reimer, C. B., Buono, I. D., Shore, S. L., and Starr, S. E.: Herpes simplex virus infection of the fetus and newborn. In Krugman, S., and Gershon, A. A. (eds.): Infections of the Fetus and Newborn. Progress in Clinical and Biological Research, Vol. 3. New York, Alan R. Liss Inc., 1975.

Rhodes, A. J.: Virus infections and congenital malformations. In Congenital Malformations: Papers and Discussions Presented at the 1st International Conference on Congenital Malformations, London. Philadelphia, J. B. Lippincott Company, 1960, pp. 106–116.

Siegel, M.: Congenital malformations following chickenpox, measles, mumps and hepatitis. J.A.M.A. 226:1521–1524, 1973.

Siegel, M., and Fuerst, H. T.: Low birth weight and maternal virus diseases: a prospective study of rubella, measles, mumps, chickenpox and hepatitis. J.A.M.A. 197:680–682, 1966.

Siegel, M., Fuerst, H. T., and Peress, N. G.: Comparative fetal mortality in maternal virus diseases. N. Engl. J. Med. 274:768–771, 1966.

Ylinen, O., and Jarvinen, P. A.: Parotitis in pregnancy. Acta Obstet. Gynecol. Scand. 32:121–132, 1953.

3

Rubella

HISTORICAL INTRODUCTION

The causal relationship between maternal rubella in pregnancy and congenital defects was first recognized by the late Sir Norman Gregg in 1941 following the extensive epidemic of rubella in Australia between 1939 and 1941. Although it is clear from the literature that similar defects had occurred before, the significance of cause and effect had not been appreciated. Data obtained from retrospective surveys recorded by Lancaster (1954) pointed to an increase in the births of deaf children at irregular intervals between the years 1893 and 1940 in England, Iceland, Australia, and New Zealand. Cases of infants who had congenital defects, including cataracts, deafness, and heart disease, and whose mothers had had rubella in early pregnancy had been reported from the Children's Research Foundation in Cincinnati between 1930 and 1936 by Beswick and co-workers (1949), but the significance of the association between the maternal illness and the defects had not been appreciated. It is also possible that some cases of cataracts encountered in earlier surveys of deaf children with retinitis pigmentosa had been caused by maternal rubella infection (Fraser, 1964).

The extent of the rubella epidemic in Australia from 1939 to 1941 and the subsequent birth of so many children with the same type of deformity in widely separated areas of the continent of Australia may well have been the factors that drew Gregg's attention to the causal relationship, but whatever the reason it must be acknowledged that it was because of Gregg's intuition and sense of inquiry that

the relationship was established. Similarly, it may have been the extent and severity of the rubella epidemics of the years 1962 to 1964, together with newly developed facilities for the investigation of the disease, that drew the attention of pediatricians and virologists of the present generation to the wider clinical impact of intrauterine rubella upon the fetus.

Gregg (1941) reported his observations to the Ophthalmological Society of Australia in a paper entitled "Congenital Cataract Following German Measles in the Mother." He recorded a series of 78 infants with congenital cataracts from different parts of Australia, 67 of whose mothers had had rubella early in their pregnancies, most frequently in the first or second month; in some cases the mother had not at the time realized that she was pregnant. The cataracts were usually bilateral; the infants were usually small and ill-nourished, with feeding difficulties, and many also had congenital heart disease. Microphthalmus was also common, and irregular areas of pigmentation were noticed in the retinas of several patients. Several other defects, such as buphthalmus and a transient corneal haze, were also recorded by Gregg. Twenty-six of the 35 infants were first-born children, three were second-born, and the remaining six were third- or later-born offspring.

This episode of a "clustering" of congenital cataracts in different parts of Australia and the association of defects with a history of rubella in pregnancy led Gregg to believe that these defects were not purely developmental but caused by some toxic or infective agent. He expressed his opinion in the following terms:

13

Table 3–1. **THE OCCURRENCE OF CONGENITAL DEFECTS IN CHILDREN FOLLOWING MATERNAL RUBELLA IN PREGNANCY IN NEW SOUTH WALES IN 1940***

Defect	No. of Cases	Defect	No. of Cases
Deaf-mutism	78	Eye and heart disease	4
Deaf-mutism and heart disease	15	Heart disease	4
		Deaf-mutism, eye and heart disease	6
Eye disease	4	No defects	5

*Details of 116 cases: 111 with defects, 5 apparently normal.

From Gregg, N. M., et al.: Occurrence of congenital defects in children following maternal rubella during pregnancy. Med. J. Aust. 2:122–126, 1945.

I believe that these figures, with the noticeably high incidence in the children of primiparae, afford confirmatory evidence of the close association between congenital cataract in the baby and maternal infection. For it was this young adult group, to which the primiparae belong, that was particularly affected by the epidemic of "German Measles."

Gregg made several other predictions that have since proved correct. In his first paper he wrote,

It is difficult to forecast the future of these unfortunate babies. We cannot at this stage be sure that there are not other defects present which are not evident now, but which may show up as development proceeds. The cardiac condition also tends to make the prognosis doubtful. One baby who had survived two operations some months ago suddenly died quite recently at the age of seven months. The possibility of the appearance of neurotropic manifestations at a later date will be kept in mind. The prognosis for vision depends on the presence or absence of nystagmus and, of course, on the condition of the retina and choroid.

In a subsequent analysis of the annual incidence of maternal rubella infection, Gregg and his associates (1945) found that 136 cases had been reported in New South Wales between 1923 and 1942, with a peak incidence of 116 cases in 1940. Of these 116 women, 111 gave birth to malformed children and five to apparently normal children. The defects are detailed in Table 3–1, and their relationship to the onset of maternal infection is displayed in Table 3–2. Gregg's data also showed that defects were not apparent in cases in which maternal infection had occurred after the sixteenth week of gestation (see Table 3–2).

The association between congenital deafness and maternal rubella was first recognized in 1943 by Swan and co-workers (1943) and independently at about the same time by Gregg (1944). Swan and his associates (1943; Swan et al., 1946) collected data on 101 cases of congenital malformations following rubella in early pregnancy and found that the malformations most frequently encountered were microcephaly (62 per cent), cardiac disease (52 per cent), deaf-mutism and deafness (48 per cent), cataract (10 per cent), and mental deficiency (5 per cent). The cases of deafness encountered by Gregg and colleagues (1945) in the New South Wales survey were similar to those reported by Swan et al. (1943) except that the children studied did not appear to be totally deaf. "Although they did not respond to the human voice, they could hear loud, high-pitched sounds such as a whistle, a bell, or hand-clapping." Similar cases were observed by Carruthers (1945), who considered the deafness to be of the nerve type and unrelated to defects of the external or middle ear. The first clue to the pathological cause of the lesion was found in one of Carruthers's patients, who died of congenital heart disease and in whom a marked failure of differentiation of the cells forming the organ of Corti was discovered.

Confirmation of the association between maternal rubella and congenital malformations soon came from other Australian sources (Carruthers, 1945; Patrick, 1948) and from many other parts of the world. In the United States many cases were reported; a detailed review of these can be found in a paper by Wesselhoeft (1947). In Great Britain cases were reported by Hope Simpson (1944), although a note of skepticism was expressed in an annotation in the Lancet ("Rubella and Congenital Malformations," 1944) that stated,

There have been plenty of examples in medical history of a clinical picture suddenly emerging out of jigsaw pieces at which generations of doctors have gazed unseeingly. Gregg, in South Australia [as reported; should have read New South Wales], may have provided another example by connecting a rubella-like illness in the mother with cataract and other congenital abnormalities in her child: but though the possibility remains, he cannot yet be said to have proved his case. . . .

The lay public have always held that congenital malformations have an extrinsic explanation—from being frightened by a dog to falling downstairs—and it will be strange if the influence of a mild illness in the first months of pregnancy, accompanied by a rash, has escaped attention.

Table 3–2. DETAILS OF 136 CASES OF CONGENITAL DEFECTS REPORTED FROM NEW SOUTH WALES, 1923–1942*

Congenital Defects	Time of Onset of Maternal Infection in Months During Pregnancy								Total
	First	Second	Third	Fourth	Fifth	Sixth	Seventh	Undetermined	
Deaf-mutism	1	30	31	15	—	—	—	8	85
Deaf-mutism and heart disease	1	8	6	2	—	—	—	—	17
Heart disease	1	1	2	1	—	—	—	—	5
Eye disease	1	3	2	—	—	—	—	—	6
Eye and heart disease	3	5	—	—	—	—	—	—	8
Deaf-mutism, eye disease, and heart disease	6	2	—	—	—	—	—	—	8
Deaf-mutism and eye disease	—	1	—	—	—	—	—	—	1
No apparent defects	1	—	1	1	2	—	1	—	6
Total	14	50	42	19	2	—	1	8	136

*Includes the 116 cases referred to in Table 3–1.
From Gregg, N. M., et al.: Occurrence of congenital defects in children following maternal rubella during pregnancy. Med. J. Aust. 2:122–126, 1945.

For 20 years following Gregg's discovery little progress was made either in the understanding of the pathogenesis of rubella, including the mechanisms of fetal damage, or in the development of a means of prevention, although some experiments carried out in human volunteers by Krugman and Ward (1954) yielded some useful though limited data. In 1962 rubella virus was isolated by cell culture techniques by two independent groups of investigators (Parkman et al., 1962; Weller and Neva, 1962). This discovery led inevitably to the development of new techniques for the diagnosis and prophylaxis of rubella and also for the detailed study of the effects of the virus upon the fetus. This latter result was of fundamental importance, and the newly developed procedure for detecting rubella virus and antibody was soon put to the test. In 1962, rubella appeared in epidemic form in Europe and later spread to the United States, where a major pandemic started in 1964, lasting into 1965. Many thousands of children were born during this period (1962 to 1965) with multiple handicaps as a result of intrauterine rubella.

The symptoms most commonly encountered in Australia in the 1940's had been cataracts, heart disease, and deafness, either singly or in combination. These were usually referred to as the "rubella syndrome." Following the extensive epidemics of 1962 to 1965 several "new" manifestations were encountered for which various names were used, such as the "expanded rubella syndrome" and "acute disseminated neonatal rubella." These terms did not contribute much to our understanding of the problem, and the term "congenital rubella" proposed by Dudgeon (1966) has now come to be generally accepted; it is, moreover, in keeping with the terminology used for other intrauterine infections, such as congenital syphilis, toxoplasmosis, cytomegalovirus, and varicella-zoster.

NATURAL HISTORY

The natural histories of postnatal and prenatal rubella must be considered together because the two are so closely related. *Postnatal rubella* is an acute, self-limiting infectious disease following which there is long-term immunity. Infection takes place via the respiratory route, and nasopharyngeal secretions are the principal source of infection.

Current information indicates that the causative virus consists of a single antigenic type, although there is some evidence from Kono (1969) that strains of virus isolated in Japan in the late 1960's were less virulent than strains isolated in other parts of the world; this finding has never been substantiated. Subclinical primary infection is more common in rubella than in measles, and reinfection, which is usually asymptomatic, occurs not infrequently. On the whole rubella is probably less infectious than measles, even when both clinical and subclinical infection rates are taken into account. The difference in the age-specific incidence rates for the two diseases is the best indication of this fact. Nevertheless, rubella can cause widespread disease in all susceptible age groups in communities where it is not generally endemic. An example was the epidemic of rubella in the Pribilof Islands in 1963, in which virtually all individuals born after the previous epidemic of 1941 were infected (Brody et al., 1965). The peak incidence of rubella infection is in childhood and early adolescence, but, again in contrast to measles, a significant proportion of the adult female population escapes infection in childhood and remains susceptible during the period of childbearing. In most countries rubella is a disease of late winter and spring, extending into the early summer months.

Prenatal rubella infection differs in several important respects from postnatally acquired infection. Instead of being a mild, self-limiting disease, intrauterine rubella is often associated with a severe disseminated infection and a chronic infective state that persists throughout fetal life and for many months after birth. The extent of fetal infection is reflected in the number of organs that may be affected. In some cases infection may be so severe as to be incompatible with life, and fetal death ensues; the dysfunction in those who survive depends on the organs involved and the extent of the damage to them. Not all the consequences of fetal infection are evident at birth; some of the late consequences, coming on several months or even years after birth, may be related indirectly to the chronic infective state that is such a prominent feature of intrauterine rubella. Another feature is the varied response of the fetus to infection. Disseminated infection does not always occur; a single organ may be involved, or the fetus may contract a subclinical infection or escape infection altogether.

Epidemiology

Since the introduction of vaccination against rubella in about 1970, the epidemiology of the disease has changed in many countries where active vaccination campaigns have been in progress. The present epidemiologic status of rubella must be considered against this background.

Postnatal Rubella Prior to Vaccination

Rubella has a worldwide distribution, but marked variation in the incidence of the disease is encountered from one country and one continent to another. As already stated, the incidence of rubella is difficult to estimate because of the frequency of subclinical infection and the resemblance between rubella and other viral exanthemata. Nevertheless, a broad view of the worldwide incidence of the disease can be gained from scrutiny of the distribution of reported cases of rubella and the incidence rates for age groups in countries where it is notifiable. A second and more reliable approach, that of seroepidemiology, uses the incidence of rubella antibody in different age groups of both sexes within a population to distinguish the proportion of susceptible individuals from the proportion of those who are immune. Both forms of epidemiological survey are essential in assessing the effect of vaccination.

Before vaccination was introduced in the United Kingdom in 1970, rubella was notifiable in only four large cities or county boroughs. Now a broader system of voluntary reporting has been introduced. In the early 1970's rubella was notifiable in only eight of the 31 countries making up the European Region of the World Health Organization (WHO, 1973). Following the worldwide pandemic of 1963 to 1965, rubella became notifiable throughout the United States, whereas previously it had been notifiable in only six states.

The worldwide epidemicity of rubella is more variable and less regular than that of measles. Three broad epidemic patterns of rubella exist. *In continental populations* in the developing countries of the Northern and Southern Hemispheres, epidemics tend to occur every 9 to 10 years, with scattered outbreaks in between and with major epidemics or pandemics at intervals of 30 to 40 years. The epidemicity of rubella in the United Kingdom and the United States (Witte et al., 1969) has not been dissimilar. A different periodicity, with epidemics occurring every four to five years, has been observed in Czechoslovakia and Poland (WHO, 1973).

In densely populated areas rubella epidemics probably occur yearly as the result of a continuous low infection rate. As the disease is generally mild, except in its effect on the fetus, infection may pass unnoticed. In contrast, *in isolated areas,* such as the Pribilof Islands in Alaska, introduction of rubella into a virgin population results in an extensive epidemic affecting the susceptible population of all age groups not previously exposed (Brody et al., 1965).

Worldwide data on the global incidence of rubella have been obtained from several serological surveys (Rawls et al., 1967; Cockburn, 1969). Because the tests employed when these studies were performed were variable and the antibody titer for distinguishing between susceptible and immune individuals was set at an arbitrary level of one in 40, only a general impression can be gauged from these data. Despite these reservations, there appeared to be a remarkably uniform distribution of rubella antibody in various age groups throughout the five continents. Among 17 to 22 year olds, antibody was found in approximately 80 per cent of the 12 of the 25 study groups and in over 70 per cent of the 20 participating countries. The proportion of pregnant women (age unspecified) with antibody (i.e., presumably immune) was 85 per cent or more in eight of the study groups. Unexpectedly low figures for the number of immune pregnant women (42 per cent) were found in two cities in Hawaii. Similarly, Sever and co-workers (1964) found that 18 per cent of 600 women aged 14 to 44 years had no detectable neutralizing antibody and that the incidence of susceptibility was higher in black (21 per cent) than in white women (14 per cent). Further studies by Sever et al. (1965) also revealed a higher rate of susceptibility to rubella in pregnant women in Hawaii (50 per cent). Nagayama and colleagues (1966) found that 35 per cent of pregnant women aged 18 to 40 years in Fukuoka in southern Japan were seronegative.

Serological data on the incidence of rubella antibody in populations in different parts of the world are shown in Tables 3–3 and 3–4. This is important information because the

Table 3–3a. EPIDEMIOLOGICAL DATA ON ANTIBODY STATUS IN NINE EUROPEAN COUNTRIES
(Percentage Frequency of Rubella Antibody According to Age)*

Age Group (Years)	Algeria	Czechoslovakia†	France†	Germany‡	Hungary†	Poland	Sweden	USSR	UK
1–4	NK	20	NK	28.0	43.0	44.0	0	20	7
5–9	60.0	25–63	51	52.8	50.0	71.7	65	65	40
10–14	80.0	64.8–86.6	62	69.7	58.0	84.7	72	72	40–60
15–19	99.7	86.6–92.1	81	83.4	74.0	92.9	90	90	71
20–30	89.5	92.1–96.5	87	89.6	85.5	95.9	96	95	80

*NK = not known.
†Data obtained by neutralization test during period from 1966 to 1967.
‡Data from Stuttgart area.
From World Health Organization: Prevention of Rubella. Report by a working group convened by the Regional Office for Europe of the World Health Organization, Budapest, June 12–16, 1972. Copenhagen, WHO, 1973.

Table 3–3b. SEROEPIDEMIOLOGICAL DATA ON RUBELLA ANTIBODY STATUS IN VARIOUS COUNTRIES IN AFRICA, ASIA, OCEANIA, AND THE AMERICAS
(Percentage Frequency of Rubella Antibody According to Age)*

Age Group (Years)	Africa			Asia		Japan		Oceania	
	Togo	Kampala	Lagos	Saigon	Singapore	Fukuoka	Ohstu	Melbourne	Papua, New Guinea
17–22*	64	—	—	—	76	—	31	77	—
23–29*	—	—	—	—	75	64	34	74	—
30–35*	—	—	—	—	(100)	68	38	83	89
Adult females†	—	85.5	85.4	92.9	—	—	—	—	—

Age Group (Years)	Americas					United States	
	Buenos Aires	Sao Paulo	Kingston, Jamaica	Ottawa	Ontario	Atlanta	11 Cities
17–22*	83	76	52	86	70	82	75
23–29*	87	77	67	88	80	88	79
30–35*	79	83	—	93	—	84	86

*Data obtained from WHO Collaborative Study, the age groupings of which are retained (Rawls et al., 1967; Cockburn, 1969).
†Ages are not specified but vary from 17 to 30 years.

Table 3–4. **INCIDENCE OF RUBELLA ANTIBODY IN VARIOUS GROUPS IN THE UNITED KINGDOM BEFORE AND AFTER THE INTRODUCTION OF RUBELLA VACCINATION IN 1970**

Groups	Average Age in Years	No. Tested	No. Seropositive	% Seropositive
	Period Prior to Vaccination, 1965–1970			
Nurses at Children's Hospital, London				
Prior to training	18	751	536	71.4
During training	23	178	144	81.9
London Obstetric Hospital				
Primiparae	24	263	228	86.7
Multiparae	28	308	260	84.4
University students*				
Female	18–21	300–500 annually		80.0
Blood donors*				80–82
Female	18–29	3000–4000 annually		82–90
Male	18–29			
	Post-Vaccination Era, 1976–1982			
Nurses at Children's Hospital, London				
1973–1976	18	604†	510	84.4
1977–1982	18	426†	403	94.6
University students*				
Female	18–21	–	–	94.0
Male		–	–	80–86
Blood donors*				
Female	18–21	–	–	94.97
Male		–	–	88–90

*Data from Clarke, M., et al.: Surveys of rubella antibodies in young adults and children. Lancet *1*:667–669, 1983. Sera were tested by hemagglutination inhibition until 1976, then by single radial hemolysis.
†Rate of vaccination increased from 33 per cent in 1973 to 1976 to 77 per cent in 1977 to 1982.

incidence of antibody, particularly in women of childbearing age, is a sound measure of the incidence of natural immunity. However, it should not be taken for granted that the incidence of rubella is uniform throughout the world, and health authorities need information on incidence to make decisions about the necessity of immunization. It could be argued that where 15 to 20 per cent of the adult female population remains susceptible there is probably a need for vaccination. When the level of suseptibility is 10 per cent the need for vaccination becomes debatable, and when the figure is 5 per cent the likelihood of congenital rubella's being a public health problem is probably low.

Postnatal Rubella Since the Introduction of Vaccination

As rubella is not generally notifiable in the United Kingdom, changes in incidence of the disease cannot be assessed by recording age-specific attack rates. The data shown in Table 3–4 give an indication of the trend in the rubella antibody status of the young adult population in the United Kingdom before and after the introduction of rubella vaccination. The groups included are not necessarily representative of the population of the whole country, but they come from a wide area and have been carefully studied by the same investigators over a period of years. There is discernible a downward trend in the percentage of seronegative females of childbearing age in the United Kingdom, and percentages are lower for females than for males of the same age. This pattern is evident both in the group of university students and among blood donors. It would be surprising if similar trends were not taking place in other countries where vaccination against rubella has been introduced.

Despite the continuing downward trend in the proportion of seronegative women in the United Kingdom, as reflected by the studies of Clarke and co-workers (1983), this pattern may not be applicable to all ethnic groups. Peckham and her colleagues (1983) have shown a marked difference in susceptibility to rubella among women of different ethnic groups attending a London teaching hospital. The percentage of these adult women attending the hospital who were seronegative (<15 IU/ml) for rubella was 9 per cent for whites, 10.3 per cent for blacks, 16.5 per cent for Indians and Pakistanis, and 25.8 for Chinese. Women born outside the United Kingdom were nearly twice as likely to be seronegative as those born in the United Kingdom.

In the United States, the reporting of rubella is widespread throughout the country, and the data shown in Table 3–5 reveal the changing pattern of reported rubella by age group. The most striking examples of this can be seen in the age-specific incidence rates for three major areas for three periods, 1966 to 1968 (before rubella vaccine licensure), 1975 to 1977 (in the middle of the vaccination program), and 1980 to 1981 (when the program was being fully implemented throughout the nation) (Orenstein et al., 1983). The overall incidence rate has decreased in the age groups 5 to 9, 10 to 14 and 15 to 19 years, but not at the same rate. The continuing downward trend in incidence rates has been observed in many parts of the United States, both among those under 5 years old and among 15 to 19 year olds (Bart et al., 1983). However, the present situation is by no means uniform, as persons of 15 years of age and older accounted for a much higher proportion of cases in 1982 (62 per cent) than in 1981 (37 per cent) (MMWR, 1983).

Even when allowance is made for variation in regional reporting of rubella, it would appear that at present a significant number of women of childbearing age are still susceptible to rubella.

Prenatal Rubella Prior to Vaccination

Congenital rubella defects have been reported from most countries of the world following Gregg's original report in 1941. These have been fully documented in reports from Sweden (Lundström, 1962), from the United Kingdom (Manson et al., 1960), from the United States (Rubella Symposium, 1965), and from many other parts of the world (International Conference on Rubella Immunization, 1969). As expected, there was a close correlation between the incidence of rubella in the countries concerned and the occurrence of rubella-type defects.

The fact that rubella is generally acquired later in life than measles means that a proportion of adolescent and young adult females remain susceptible during the vulnerable age of childbearing. As childbearing age varies so much from one part of the world to another, the difficulty in assessing the risk of fetal damage from congenital rubella is confounded. It has already been suggested that where the incidence of natural rubella infection is low the risk of congenital rubella defects being encountered is correspondingly high and *vice versa*. Factors other than age, such as sex and genetic and socioeconomic influences, may also have a bearing on the incidence of congenital rubella defects, but their impact is difficult to define precisely.

Table 3–5. **PER CENT DISTRIBUTION OF REPORTED RUBELLA CASES* AND INCIDENCE RATE†**
BY AGE GROUP, FOR ILLINOIS, MASSACHUSETTS, AND NEW YORK CITY,
1966–1968,‡ 1975–1977,‡ AND 1980–1981‡

Age Group (Years)	1966–1968			1975–1977			1980–1981		
	No.	% of Total	Incidence Rate	No.	% of Total	Incidence Rate	No.	% of Total	Incidence Rate
<5	1294	21.6	63.3	160	9.8	9.8	81	30.0	4.9
5–9	2304	38.5	101.3	233	14.2	11.6	65	24.0	3.9
10–14	1020	17.0	44.0	229	13.9	11.2	45	16.6	2.4
15–19	759	12.7	35.7	634	38.7	27.4	31	11.4	1.4
20+	610	10.2	3.7	384	23.4	2.3	49	18.1	0.3
Total	5987	100.0	24.3	1640	100.0	6.7	271	100.1	1.1

*Cases of unknown age excluded.
†Reported number of cases per 100,000 population.
‡Yearly averages.
From Orenstein, W. A., et al.: Symposium on Conquest of Agents That Endanger the Brain, Baltimore, October 28–29, 1982. In press, 1984.

Recognition of the types of defect associated with congenital rubella is also important. Typical cases were noted in a general hospital with a large pediatric department in Saigon, South Vietnam (Evans and Evans, 1966) and in antenatal clinics in Kampala, Uganda (Dudgeon, 1967) because the observers were on the lookout for them. Similar observations have been made from Zimbabwe, Rhodesia (Axton et al., 1979). However, in Japan, where the incidence of rubella antibody is similar to that in European countries and North America, very few children with congenital defects have been seen. The reason why congenital rubella appears to be less common in Japan than in other countries, including adjacent territories, is not clear. Lack of recognition and lack of reporting may be part of the matter but are not the whole answer (Best et al., 1974). Only 47 cases of congenital rubella were identified through a questionnaire sent out on a nationwide basis at the end of a five-year period when rubella had been prevalent in Japan. This number is considerably smaller than the number that would be reported in similar circumstances in the United Kingdom, which has only half the population of Japan. Although there are reported differences between the susceptibility rates of Japanese women in the southern provinces and those in the north, they do not provide a complete explanation for the low incidence of congenital rubella in Japan as a whole. In 1965 an extensive rubella epidemic occurred on the island of Okinawa, which has a predominantly Japanese population of just under 1 million. This resulted in the birth of some 342 rubella-affected infants (Hirayama, 1970). Kono and his associates (1969, 1971) suggested that this was due to the importation of virulent rubella strains from United States military bases, whereas Hirayama (1970) considered the main reason for the large number of congenital rubella–affected babies to be due to the fact that 40 per cent of the adult women of Okinawa were susceptible at the time.

Another extensive epidemic occurred in Japan in 1975 to 1977, and again the incidence of cogenital rubella appeared to be less frequent than that following epidemics in the United States and on Okinawa (Shishido et al., 1979).

An exceptionally high incidence of congenital rubella syndrome (CRS) was reported in children born in Ryuku after the extensive rubella epidemic there in 1964 and 1965, whereas the incidence of CRS in the nearby Amami Islands was low (Ueda et al., 1978). Retrospective serological studies suggested that the high rate of CRS in the Ryuku Islands was probably due to a low level of antibody in the population rather than to any difference in virulence between strains of rubella virus in Japan and surrounding areas.

The epidemic of rubella defects in Iceland following maternal rubella in 1963 and 1964 was noteworthy for the high incidence of severe hearing loss without accompanying defects such as cataracts or heart disease (Baldursson et al., 1972). No obvious explanation for this unusual manifestation of epidemic congenital rubella has been forthcoming. It cannot be explained by lack of recognition, as the children were carefully examined for cataracts and heart disease.

The extent to which these reported regional differences in the incidence of congenital rubella are real is by no means clear.

The epidemicity of congenital rubella parallels that of the natural disease. During the past 30 years, two major epidemic periods of rubella have left in their wake many children damaged by intrauterine rubella. The first period was from 1940 to 1943 when, following the Australian experience, congenital rubella defects were recognized all over the world. A similar episode, with an increased number of births of congenital rubella–affected children, occurred from 1962 to 1964 in Europe, particularly in the United Kingdom (Dudgeon, 1965) and Iceland (Baldursson et al., 1972); this increase was followed a year later by the catastrophic pandemic in the United States (Rubella Symposium, 1965). These periodic occurrences are probably a reflection of a gradual increase in the number of susceptible persons in the population, which facilitates the spread of virus through the community.

The association between epidemics of rubella and the subsequent birth of children with perceptive deafness has already been noted (Lancaster, 1954). Fisch (1969), in studying congenital deafness in 774 children in relation to epidemics of rubella in the United Kingdom, found that the incidence attributable to maternal rubella varied from 4.1 per cent to 6.5 per cent during a nonepidemic period (1962 to 1963) to 37 per cent to 40 per cent after an epidemic period (1964 to 1966). These figures were based on a history of clinical rubella in the mother and are probably underestimates, since the effect of subclinical maternal infection can be de-

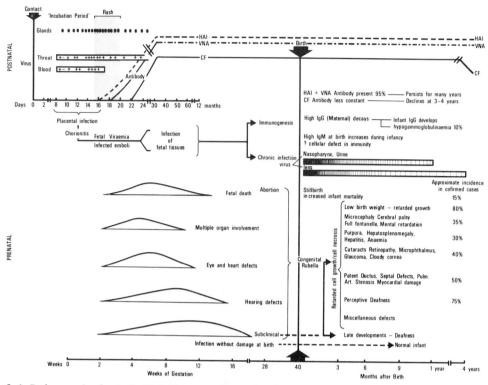

Figure 3–1. Pathogenesis of rubella. This illustrates the mode of spread of virus in postnatal rubella and the mode of spread to the placenta and fetus when rubella is contracted during pregnancy. The approximate incidence of defects in confirmed cases is shown to the right of the figure.

termined only by serological tests on the children. An even closer association in time between epidemic rubella in the population and congenital rubella deafness in children has been recorded by Anderson and co-workers (1970) in their observations on the relationship between the birth of children with congenital deafness in Sweden and preceding epidemics of rubella in the Swedish Armed Forces. Stuckless (in press), in an extensive review of the causation of deafness in children in the United States, estimated that between 5 and 6 per cent of deafness was related to congenital rubella and was even greater following an epidemic period.

Prenatal Rubella Since the Introduction of Vaccination

Although changes in the incidence of congenital rubella are becoming apparent as the result of vaccination programs in some countries, the conquest of congenital rubella has not yet been achieved. In the United States the incidence of CRS, as reported to the National Congenital Rubella Syndrome Registry (NCRSR) and the Birth Defects Monitoring Program (BDMP), showed a progres-

sive decline during the period from 1971 to 1978 (Centers for Disease Control, 1980), but cases are still occurring despite extensive vaccination coverage. An outbreak of congenital rubella, in which 31 infants with CRS were identified, was reported from Chicago in 1978; none of the mothers had been vaccinated (Lamprecht et al., 1982).

Congenital rubella continues to occur in the United Kingdom and is likely to do so until a greater proportion of susceptible individuals are protected by vaccination.

Pathogenesis

Details of the various stages in the pathogenesis of postnatal and prenatal rubella are shown in Figure 3–1.

Postnatal Rubella

Details concerning the mode of spread of virus throughout the body following primary infection were originally determined from experiments in human volunteers carried out by Krugman and his associates (Krugman et al., 1953; Krugman and Ward, 1954) and later by some of the same workers employing newly developed laboratory techniques for virus isolation and detection of rubella neutralizing antibody (Green et al., 1965).

The incubation period between contact and onset of the rash in rubella is usually 16 to 18 days but may vary from 14 to 21 days. Virus can usually be recovered from the nasopharynx as early as seven days before the onset of the rash—at the same time that lymphadenopathy usually becomes detectable—and for 10 to 14 days after the rash has disappeared. Although virus can be recovered from the nasopharynx for such a long time after the rash, the amount of virus present during this period is probably on the decline, and, in practical terms, the patient can be regarded as noninfectious a few days after the rash has disappeared. Virus can be recovered from the blood for up to seven days before the appearance of the rash, but thereafter it disappears rapidly from the blood stream. Maternal viremia is undoubtedly the important phase in the pathogenesis of fetal infection, as it is thus that virus passes from the maternal blood stream to the placenta and then to the fetus. It is probable that by the time of the appearance of the rash the placenta and possibly the fetus are already infected. The same pattern of virological events occurs in subclinical rubella infection.

Immunity in Postnatal Rubella. Circulating antibody appears within one or two days after the viremic phase and the onset of the rash; thereafter it increases rapidly (see Fig. 3–1). The original method of measuring antibody was by the virus neutralization (VN) test. However, valuable though this test is as one of the most reliable procedures for detecting antibody, it is not practicable for modern diagnostic or seroepidemiological surveys. Rubella antibody can now be measured by a series of well-defined *in vitro* techniques: the hemagglutination-inhibition (HI) test (Stewart et al., 1967), the immunofluorescence (IF) test, the single radial hemolysis (SRH) test, and the radioimmunoassay (RIA). These and other tests (Lennette and Schmidt, 1969), details of which are discussed later, probably all measure the same classes of antibody, namely, IgG, IgM, and IgA. The antibody detected by any of the methods is similar in time of appearance, but varies both in duration and in level according to the sensitivity of the test. For practical purposes, the HI test is still widely used for diagnostic work and evaluation of the response to vac-

cination, whereas the SRH technique is most suitable as a screening procedure.

Antibody measured by the HI test or other appropriate procedure can usually be detected by the second or third day after the rash appears, or even earlier. It reaches a peak about 21 to 28 days later and then gradually falls to a slightly lower plateau at which it persists for many years. Although there is considerable variation in the level of antibody from one individual to another, most individuals retain HI or VN antibody indefinitely once infected. Some observers (Leerhöy, 1968) have found that neutralizing antibody reaches a maximum titer several weeks after HI antibody, but this is not the general experience and may be a reflection of the sensitivity of the test procedures used.

Complement-fixing (CF) antibody develops more slowly than HI or VN and does not usually reach a peak titer for four to six weeks after the rash has appeared. It does not persist for as long as VN or HI antibody and has usually fallen to undetectable levels within five years of primary infection. Interpretation of the significance of CF antibody depends on the nature of the CF antigen employed in the test, as two antigens, the soluble and the cell-associated antigen, have been described (Schmidt and Lennette, 1969). Late development and rapid decline is a feature of CF antibody measured by the soluble antigen (Vesikari et al., 1971). The response of CF antibody detected by the glycine-extracted antigen more closely parallels that of HI and VN antibody but is usually somewhat later to appear. A probable explanation for the discrepancy between the results with the two antigens is that the CF test, unlike the HI test, does not measure IgM antibody, the appearance of which invariably precedes that of IgG antibody in primary infections. The CF test is now of less value in many situations as there are more sensitive and more practical methods for detection of IgM-specific rubella antibody, which is of great importance in the detection of recent primary infections.

Even if antibody is found to have fallen to very low levels, experience has shown that reinfection or vaccination will invariably result in a booster-type IgG antibody response. Complete loss of antibody and reversion to a susceptible state is very rare.

Primary rubella infection is associated with an initial response in IgM-specific antibody followed by an increase in IgG antibody, whereas in cases of reinfection the response is an increase in IgG antibody, characteristic of which is a rapid response of the booster type (Cooper, 1968; Horstmann et al., 1969). The earliest observations of these responses were made by means of the two mercaptoethanol (2 ME) procedure. Antibody of the IgM class is sensitive to 2 ME, whereas IgG antibody is not. More sensitive tests for detection of IgM antibody, such as the IF test and RIA, have now been developed; these have important practical implications for the diagnosis of recent primary infections and congenital rubella infection. The length of time that IgM is found to persist depends to a large extent on the sensitivity of the test employed to detect it.

It is important to be able to distinguish a recent primary infection, clinical or subclinical, from a reinfection because in the former there is a definite risk to the fetus, whereas in the latter the risk is remote.

Immunity to rubella is long-lasting, and in most persons it is lifelong. Second clinical attacks of rubella are not infrequently reported, but unless both the first and subsequent attacks are substantiated by virological tests little credence can be placed on a previous history of rubella. It is probable that immunity to rubella, like immunity to many other viral infections, is dependent on the presence of specific humoral immunity and cellular immune mechanisms that follow from the sensitizing effect of the primary infection. What is not known is whether antibody persists indefinitely after the initial infection or whether part of the viral genome persists in a noninfectious form to provide a continuing antigenic stimulus, thus maintaining immunity. It could be argued that long-term immunity to rubella in the absence of re-exposure, like immunity to many other diseases such as measles and poliomyelitis, depends upon the effect of the initial antigenic stimulus.

Reinfection in Postnatal Rubella. Although immunity to clinical disease is sound, immunity to reinfection is less durable. Reinfection undoubtedly occurs and is of special consequence in relation to the risk to the fetus. It is usually asymptomatic and can be demonstrated only by laboratory tests. The crucial problem is to determine whether viremia occurs, even for limited periods. This is of some concern, as cases of reinfection with symptomatic disease have been reported.

The rubella epidemic in the Pribilof Islands (Brody et al., 1965) clearly demonstrated the difference in the clinical attack rate for persons in the susceptible age group, 15 to 21 years old, and those over 21, who had been exposed in a previous epidemic and in whom clinical disease was strikingly absent. Virtually all individuals with asymptomatic infection had a fourfold or greater rise in neutralizing antibody. Parkman (1969) reported that 2 per cent of military recruits with rubella antibody (26 men) showed a booster antibody response during a rubella epidemic. Intense clinical surveillance at the time failed to reveal any signs of symptomatic disease.

Horstmann and her colleagues (1970) carried out a detailed clinical and virological study on military recruits exposed to a rubella epidemic in 1969. This involved a study of 190 military personnel (151 from Hawaii and 39 from the U.S. mainland), including groups of susceptible subjects and others known to be immune either as a result of recent rubella vaccination or naturally. The results, which are summarized in Table 3–6, show a clear-cut difference in the clinical attack rate between the susceptible (34.5 per cent) and the two immune groups (0 per cent). There is also a clear difference in the number of recruits from whom virus was isolated in the susceptible group (who had either clinical or subclinical disease) and the two immune groups. The serological responses of the susceptible and the immune groups were significantly different as well. One hundred per cent seroconversion was observed in the susceptible recruits, and there was an 80 per cent increase in antibody in the group vaccinated only a few months previously; however, only 3.4 per cent of the naturally immune subjects showed a booster response. It appeared from this study that the risk of reinfection was related to the level of antibody at the time of exposure; the lower the level of HI and CF antibody, the greater the risk of reinfection, and *vice versa.*

Laboratory studies using the 2 ME procedure for testing sera have shown that the antibody response is rapid and of the IgG type in cases of reinfection (Cooper, 1968; Horstmann et al., 1969). Tests more sensitive in distinguishing between IgM and IgG antibody have fully confirmed these early observations. It is against this background that reports of reinfection with symptomatic disease in naturally immune subjects, and reports, in some cases, of fetal damage, must be examined.

Horstmann and co-workers (1969) ob-

Table 3–6. DATA ON RUBELLA INFECTION AND REINFECTION OF SUSCEPTIBLE, VACCINATED, AND NATURALLY IMMUNE PERSONS EXPOSED IN AN EPIDEMIC

No. of Men Exposed	No. Susceptible		No. Vaccinated	No. Naturally Immune
190	26 (13.7%)		15	149
			(86.3%)	
No. with clinical rubella	9 (34.5%)		0	0
No. with subclinical rubella		17 (65.5%)	12 (80%)	5 (3.4%)
No. from whom virus isolated	6 (66.6%)	5 (29.3%)	1 (6.2%)	0
No. with fourfold rise in antibody*	9	17	12 (80%)	5 (3.4%)
	(100%)			

*Serological response measured by fourfold increase in hemagglutinin-inhibiting, complement-fixing, and/or precipitating antibodies.

Data from Horstmann, D. M., et al.: Rubella: reinfection of vaccinated and naturally immune persons exposed in an epidemic. N. Engl. J. Med. *283*:771–778, 1970.

served two young boys, aged 15 and 17, who were both exposed to rubella in an epidemic in an institution. At the height of the epidemic the HI titer in the 15 year old was 64 to 128 (reciprocal titers); it then rose to 2048. No IgM antibody was detected, and no symptoms were recorded. The 17 year old boy had an HI titer of 64; he developed clinical rubella with a rash and a booster response of antibody to a titer of 256. No virus was recovered from the throat washings of either patient. Wilkins and colleagues (1972) observed clinical reinfection in a 50 year old nurse participating in a rubella vaccine trial. She had demonstrable HI and VN antibody prior to the onset of symptoms of rubella complicated by arthritis. This finding suggested that viremia had occurred.

Details of nine other cases of reported reinfected are listed in Table 3–7. The patient (Case 1) observed by Strannegard and co-workers (1970) contracted rubella during an epidemic in Sweden in 1969 and developed a rash and lymphadenopathy. Because she was in the first trimester of pregnancy a termination was performed, and it was reported that the fetus was small for gestational age. Serum specimens had been collected 3 weeks before the onset of illness and 5 to 10 days after the onset of the rash. The serological details presented in Table 3–7 show that HI antibody but no VN antibody was present before exposure. Both HI and VN antibodies increased after infection and IgG and to a lesser extent IgM were detected in the respective serum fractions tested between 1 week and 24 weeks after onset of the rash. On the basis of the presence of IgG antibody in the pre-infection serum, the authors concluded that this was a case of rubella reinfec-

tion, occurring in an adult many years after a reputed attack of rubella as a child, but the absence of detectable VN antibody in this specimen and the detection of some IgM activity in the sera obtained 5 and 10 days after the rash point to the possibility of a primary infection. The interpretation must depend on the validity of the tests for HI and VN antibody.

Boué and colleagues (1971) observed three women who were exposed to rubella in early pregnancy (Cases 2–4). No symptoms developed; a significant rise in HI antibody was detected, but the sucrose density gradient test showed no increase in the IgM fraction. All three patients gave birth to normal children. Although no VN tests were carried out, it is reasonable to conclude that these three patients were reinfected but did not develop viremia; it can also be concluded that the fetuses were not infected, in view of the absence of IgM antibody in the infants' sera.

The case reported by Haukenes and Haram (1972) (Case 5) is of interest in that it deals with "full-blown" clinical rubella in a pregnant woman who four months previously had had an HI titer of 20 in two serum specimens. On the day the rash appeared the titer was still 20, but it rose to 640 two weeks later. Specific IgM but no CF antibody was detected. Serum analysis at first indicated that the HI activity was in the IgG fraction, but a subsequent reanalysis by Haukenes and co-workers (1973) revealed that the HI activity was probably due to the presence of lipoproteins and not to rubella antibody. The conclusion is that this was a case of primary infection, not one of reinfection.

The case reported by Northrop and colleagues (1972a and b) (Case 6) is somewhat

Table 3–7. **SUMMARY OF CASES OF RUBELLA REINFECTION REPORTED AFTER NATURAL RUBELLA**

Case Details and Investigators	Symptoms	Pre-exposure Rubella Antibody Levels in the Mother				Interval Between First Serum Tested and Specific Exposure to Reinfection	Post-exposure Rubella Antibody Levels in the Mother					Virus Isolation Studies on Fetus or Newborn	Rubella-Specific IgM on Cord Blood or Infant's Serum	Clinical Details on Fetus	Comments
		HI	VN	CF	IgM		HI	VN	CF	IgG	*Specific* IgM				
1. Pregnant woman Aged 35 years (Strannegard et al., 1970)	Rash Lymphadenopathy	80	<4	NT	NT	3 weeks	640	128	NT	±	± (trace)	NT	NS	Small for dates	Presumed reinfection or possible primary infection
2. Pregnant woman Aged 29 years (Boué et al., 1971)	Nil	40	<8	<8	—	3 months	280	NT	<8	+	—	NT	—	Normal, not infected	Reinfection
3. Pregnant woman Aged 24 years (Boué et al., 1971)	Nil	30	NT	NT	—	1 week after exposure	320	NT	NT	+	—	NT	—	Normal, not infected	Reinfection
4. Pregnant woman Aged 23 years (Boué et al., 1971)	Nil	20	NT	NT	—	1 week after exposure	320	NT	NT	+	—	NT	—	Normal, not infected	Reinfection
5. Pregnant woman (Haukenes and Haram, 1972)	"Full blown clinical rubella" with rash	20	NT	NT	NT	4 months previously and on day of exposure	640	NT	NT	+ (negative on re-test)	+	NT	NS	NS	Primary infection as a result of re-test
6. Pregnant woman (Northrup et al., 1972a and b)	Rash and arthritis	20	<10	NT	—	Second day of rash	320	<10	NS	+	—	+ on conceptus	NT	Therapeutic abortion	Presumed reinfection
7. Pregnant woman (Eilard and Strannegard, 1974)	Nil	640	<5	NT	NT	? 6 months, during second pregnancy	640	20	8	NS	—	—	+ cord blood	Multiple defects consistent with congenital rubella	Presumed reinfection ?Subclinical primary infection
8. Pregnant woman Aged 22 years (Forsgren et al., 1979)	Nil	20	<1	4	NS	1 year	160	20	512	NS	NS	+ at 1½ weeks	– at 1½ weeks + or 7 weeks	Normal, but infected	Reinfection ? Subclinical primary infection
9. Pregnant woman (Partridge et al., 1981)	Nil	400	40*	256	—	3 years	50	NT	4	+	—	+	—	Bilateral cataracts Retinopathy Microcephaly Died at 3½ years	Reinfection

HI = hemagglutinin-inhibiting antibody; CF = complement-fixing antibody; VN = virus neutralizing antibody; IgM = rubella specific IgM antibody; IgG = rubella IgG Antibody; NT = not tested; NS = not stated.
*Tested in another laboratory.

different. The patient developed clinical rubella in the seventh week of pregnancy and had an HI antibody titer of 20 on the second day of the rash; it rose to 320 two weeks later. Serum samples contained IgG but no IgM antibody (Northrop et al., 1972b). Following termination of the pregnancy rubella virus was recovered from the conceptus. This was presumed to be an instance of clinical reinfection with viremia leading to fetal infection, although, as Robbins (1972) pointed out, a titer of 20 on the second day of the rash in primary infections is not uncommon, whereas reinfection with symptomatic disease, as in this case, is rare. Whether this was a case of reinfection or primary infection hinges upon the tests for IgM antibody, which was clearly absent in both serum specimens. Reinfection seems to be the more likely explanation in this case. Similarly, the case reported by Eilard and Strannegard (1974) (Case 7), in which the fetus had evidence of multiple defects and IgM antibody was found in the cord blood, may also have been a case of subclinical primary maternal infection. HI antibody was present in the first serum but VN antibody was not detected, whereas it was found in the postinfection sample.

A further case, in which detailed virological investigations were performed, was reported by Forsgren and co-workers (1979) (Case 8). The patient, aged 22 years, gave birth to a boy who, although clinically normal, showed evidence of congenital rubella infection. Rubella antibody was detected in the mother's sera prior to and after the pregnancy, which was normal. Rising titers of HI and CF antibody were detected, and the hemolysin-in-gel test was also positive. No VN antibody was detected until six months after the birth of the child. Virological evidence of congenital rubella infection was obtained, but, surprisingly, the VN antibody test on the child was negative.

An unusual case of possible reinfection was reported by Partridge and co-workers (1981) (Case 9). The patient had had several serological tests for rubella antibody performed on three occasions prior to a pregnancy that was uneventful. Adequate levels of HI and CF antibody, and specific IgG were present in all three samples. She gave birth to a severely damaged infant from whom rubella virus was isolated. The child died at the age of three years, seven months. Two of the pre-exposure sera (taken 15 and 21 months prior to conception) were subsequently tested

for VN antibody, and both were positive at a titer of 1 in 40 by a sensitive test (Best et al., 1981). It can, therefore, only be concluded that rubella reinfection occurred, despite the presence of appreciable levels of HI, CF, and VN antibody. Chang (1974) has suggested that "while rubella re-infection is usually a benign condition, during pregnancy it often causes disseminated infection of the fetus or its products." The evidence referred to here and summarized in Table 3–7 would suggest that the reverse is the case and that reinfection may occur very rarely, for reasons that are not apparent. It is concluded that reinfection in pregnancy may occur in the naturally immune and in the vaccinated, but the risk to the fetus when this happens is very small indeed. In the opinion of Boué and co-workers (1971), the fetus is not likely to be at risk if serum fractionation studies show only rubella IgG antibody to be present. It is therefore reasonable to assume at present that if there is no evidence of rubella-specific IgM in cases of subclinical reinfection, the fetus is probably not at risk. Nevertheless, in view of the importance of the possibility of fetal damage following reinfection, great care must be taken in carrying out serological tests. In cases of doubt the VN test is most reliable, particularly since methods for pretreating sera for the HI antibody that require the removal of β-lipoprotein may remove specific antibody as well as the nonspecific inhibitors. This subject is dealt with in more detail in the section on laboratory diagnosis.

Prenatal Rubella

In contrast to postnatal rubella, which is a self-limiting disease, rubella contracted *in utero* frequently leads to a disseminated infection with visceral involvement and a chronic infective state, with persistence of virus throughout fetal life and after birth (Alford et al., 1964; Cooper and Krugman, 1967). The various possible sequences of events leading up to the birth of a child following primary maternal rubella are outlined in Figure 3–1. These data have been collated by numerous investigators who have carried out virological studies of the products of conception obtained by therapeutic abortion following exposure of the mother to rubella in pregnancy and of infants with congenital rubella in the early months of life (Rubella Symposium, 1965; International Symposium on Rubella Vaccines, 1969).

It now seems evident that fetal damage in

whatever form results from fetal infection, but although infection of the fetus following maternal infection in the vulnerable period of the first trimester and early second trimester is common, it does not necessarily follow that the fetus will be damaged (Dudgeon, 1969a). The fetus may escape infection or, having been infected, may be capable of reacting without suffering irreversible damage. The finding of small foci of infected cells in apparently normal tissues by means of immunofluorescence supports the latter possibility (Woods et al., 1966). The observations of fetal infection without overt disease in twin pregnancies provides further evidence (Dudgeon, 1965a; Forrester et al., 1966). In some cases identical twins exposed to intrauterine rubella have shown evidence of fetal infection without damage, and in others one twin has shown no evidence of infection while the other has been severely damaged.

The results of fetal infection after the first trimester of pregnancy have been studied in detail by means of improved serological techniques. Cradock-Watson and co-workers (1979) have shown a good degree of correlation between the IF technique and the RIA method for detecting rubella-specific IgM antibody. In a study of 304 infants whose mothers had had rubella at various stages after the first 12 weeks of pregnancy, it was found that the risk of fetal infection varied considerably at different stages of gestation (Cradock-Watson et al., 1980). Tests for rubella IgM antibody (IF and RIA) and for persistence of rubella IgG antibody (IF and RIA) revealed the following facts. IgM antibody was detected in 28 of 50 infants (56 per cent) following maternal rubella at 12 to 16 weeks of pregnancy, in 12 per cent at 24 to 28 weeks, in 19 per cent at 28 to 36 weeks, and in 58 per cent during the last month of pregnancy. Altogether IgM antibody was detected in 77 of 260 infants (29 per cent) whose mothers had rubella after the first trimester. The incidence of IgG antibody persistence was greater, as some infants had IgG antibody but no detectable IgM antibody. IgG was found to persist in 22 of 31 infants (71 per cent) after maternal rubella at 12 to 16 weeks; it fell to 28 per cent at 24 to 28 weeks and rose to 94 per cent during last month.

In all, 94 of 190 infants (49 per cent) showed persistence of IgG antibody following maternal rubella after the first trimester. Thus, the rate of fetal infection can be esti-mated at a figure between 29 and 49 per cent. In this study 302 of the 304 infants survived beyond the neonatal period (there was one stillbirth and one early neonatal death at 17 days; this infant was IgM-positive). Of the 302 surviving infants only five had obvious abnormalities, and only one of these, which was IgM-negative, had a rubella-type defect (pulmonary stenosis; this infant had no other stigmata of congenital rubella). These findings could be interpreted as related to changes in the permeability of the placenta at different stages in pregnancy.

These results have been confirmed by a study of the consequences of maternal rubella in over 1000 women exposed at successive stages of pregnancy (Miller et al., 1982). Forty per cent of the women exposed continued their pregnancies to term, and it was found that the incidence of fetal infection and fetal damage varied considerably. The congenital or fetal infection rate was 80 per cent following maternal rubella in the first 12 weeks of pregnancy; 67 per cent at 13 to 14 weeks; and 25 per cent at the end of the second trimester; this rate rose again to 60 per cent and then to 100 per cent in the latter stages of pregnancy. The incidence of fetal damage was very different. Nine of nine infants exposed in the first 11 weeks of gestation were found to have defects of the heart or deafness; at 11 to 12 weeks, two of four infants had signs of deafness, as did nine of 26 infants (35 per cent) exposed between 13 and 16 weeks. In infants whose mothers had had rubella after the sixteenth week of pregnancy, no signs of rubella defects were detectable at the mean age of the follow-up, which was 26 months. Surprisingly, none of the 11 infants whose mothers had asymptomatic rubella showed evidence of fetal infection or damage. The number of cases in this study is small, but the investigation reveals a higher incidence of defects in the first 11 to 12 weeks than has previously been reported. At the same time, it confirms earlier reports of differences between the fetal infection rate and the fetal damage rate and supports findings that there is little evidence of fetal damage following maternal rubella after the sixteenth week of pregnancy.

Placental-Fetal Infection. The first clue that the fetus might become infected as a result of maternal rubella came from Selzer (1963, 1964), who showed by histological studies on the products of conception that the placenta and fetus had been infected. Rubella virus was also isolated from an aborted fetus. Later, Kay and his colleagues (1964) recovered rubella virus from a fetus at the twenty-third week of gestation, 18 weeks after the maternal infection. In a detailed study carried out by Alford and co-workers (1964), virus was recovered from 47 per cent of the products of conception. Virus was recovered both from the placenta and from fetal tissues; moreover, in a few cases in which hysterectomy had been performed and an intact sac thereby obtained (thus reducing the risk of viral contamination from the placenta) virus was recovered from the placenta, amniotic fluid, and numerous fetal organs—brain, heart, skin, muscle, and heart blood. In this study of 51 patients, virus was recovered more readily from fetal tissues following maternal infection in the first eight weeks of pregnancy than in the second eight weeks, whereas placental infection could be demonstrated with the same frequency throughout the period of gestation from one to 14 weeks. Essentially similar results with isolation rates of between 50 and 60 per cent were obtained by other investigators by means of simultaneous inoculation of placental and fetal tissues directly into monolayer cell cultures (Horstmann et al., 1965; Monif et al., 1965; Heggie, 1967).

Rawls and co-workers (1968) achieved a higher rate of virus isolation (90 per cent) from both the placenta and fetal tissues by trypsinization of the tissues than by direct inoculation of monolayer cultures. Thompson and Tobin (1970) recovered virus from the products of conception in 29 of 32 cases (91 per cent) and from 15 of 17 fetuses when an intact sac was obtained. Virus was recovered from numerous fetal organs—the eye, brain, lung, liver, and kidney—and no difference was observed in the isolation rate from fetuses whose mothers had had serologically proven rubella in the first (four of five), second (16 of 18), or third four weeks (nine of 11) of pregnancy. The data obtained by Thompson and Tobin (1970) do not substantiate the view that the placenta acts as a barrier to fetal infection, as was originally indicated by Alford and colleagues (1964), but this difference could be due to the use of improved laboratory methods that have evolved in the intervening years. Thompson and Tobin's results are in conformity with the serological and other findings, already described, of Cradock-Watson and co-workers (1980) and Miller and co-workers (1982).

The observation of Banatvala (1969) that fetal tissues obtained between the sixteenth and twenty-sixth weeks of gestation support the growth of virus as well as those obtained during the tenth to twelfth weeks backs findings that the fetus may be infected at any stage in pregnancy, although the risk varies from early to late pregnancy. But this does not explain why the fetus is not necessarily damaged as a result of infection. The explanation probably lies in the possible mechanisms that cause fetal damage, a subject discussed later. Dudgeon (1969a) has concluded that the fetus, despite being infected, can "cure" itself of the infection. This view is in keeping with the frequent observation that not all mothers who had had clinical rubella in the first trimester have clinically affected children.

The Rubella–Infected Infant. The chronic infection contracted *in utero* persists into postnatal life. Congenital rubella–infected infants have been found to excrete virus from the nasopharynx and urine during the first four weeks of life (Alford et al., 1964). Virus can also be recovered from numerous organs of infants with congenital rubella who die in infancy. A high virus-isolation rate has been reported by Cooper and co-workers (1965) in 58 of 70 congenital rubella–infected infants with neonatal purpura. Details of the virus-excretion rate in infants with congenital rubella from the data of Cooper and Krugman (1967) are shown in Figure 3–2. Eighty-one per cent were found to be excreting virus at birth, 33 per cent at six months, and 11 per cent at one year of age.

Infectiousness of the Congenital Rubella–Infected Infant. Congenital rubella–infected infants are a source of contagion. A number of medical and nursing personnel have contracted rubella as a result of contact with virus-excreting rubella-infected infants (Cooper et al., 1965). Other reports have drawn attention to the high rate of infection among seronegative susceptible student nurses caring for infants born with rubella infection following maternal rubella in pregnancy (Schiff and Dine, 1965) and also after inapparent maternal infection (Avery et al., 1965). For practical purposes these infants are seldom contagious after they reach three months of age, although they may still be excreting virus. The reason for this noncontagiousness may be quantitative, inasmuch as the amount of virus being "shed" by congenitally infected infants at three months of age or after is small and is unlikely to be sufficient to result in transmission. Virus does not appear to persist in the nasopharynx and urine

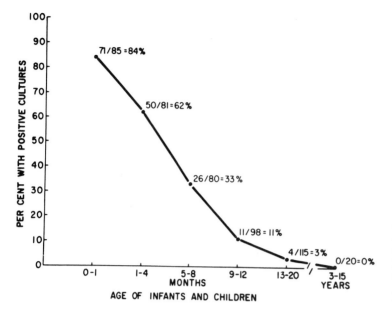

Figure 3–2. The incidence of virus excretion in congenital rubella by age. (From Cooper, L. Z., and Krugman, S.: Clinical manifestations of postnatal and congenital rubella. Arch. Ophthalmol. 77:434–439, 1967. Copyright 1967, American Medical Association.)

in older patients (aged five to 22 years) with congenital defects (Sever and Monif, 1965). On the other hand, virus has been found to persist in various organs, such as the lens, the inner ear, and the brain, for prolonged periods.

Immunogenesis in Prenatal Rubella. Another feature that distinguishes prenatal from postnatal rubella infection is the immunological response that results from intrauterine infection. At first sight it seems probable that some immunological mechanism, possibly a defect in cellular immune function or interferon production or both, is responsible for the chronic infective state, but proof of this is lacking (Marshall, 1971). Failure to establish a defect in cell-mediated immunity may be due to technical methods, as Fuccillo and co-workers (1974) have indicated.

In 1963, Plotkin and colleagues (1963) reported that children with rubella syndrome defects possess neutralizing antibody at an age when maternally transmitted antibody should have disappeared. This finding was soon confirmed by Weller and co-workers (1964) and later by Dudgeon and co-workers (1964) and Butler and co-workers (1965).

At the time it was generally assumed that an infection acquired *in utero*, or soon after birth, would render the infant immunologically tolerant to the microorganism and that the infant would be incapable of responding with antibody production to that organism. This theory was based on the concept of immunological tolerance put forward by Burnet and Fenner (1949) to explain the absence

of antibody formation in lymphocytic choriomeningitis (LCM) infection of mice. That this does not apply to the human situation now seems clear, although there are a few reported instances in which antibody has not been detected (Plotkin et al., 1966; Hardy et al., 1969a), and some cases have been encountered that were found to be seronegative although they appeared to be clinically typical of congenital rubella. The child described by Plotkin and co-workers (1966) was also found to have hypogammaglobulinemia, as well as multiple defects, and continued to excrete rubella virus for many months. Cooper and colleagues (1971) reported a higher rate of loss of rubella HI antibody in children with congenital rubella than have other observers. Fifty (18.5 per cent) in a group of 270 congenitally infected children had no detectable antibody by the age of five years. Despite these findings, Weller and co-workers (1964) believed that a retrospective diagnosis of congenital rubella could be made by serological tests for rubella antibody. This view is well substantiated by numerous previously mentioned reports in which such serological tests were carried out at an age when maternal antibody should have disappeared and before postnatal infection had been acquired (see the later discussion of surveillance).

Immunogenesis starts at about the sixteenth to the twentieth week of pregnancy. Alford and colleagues (1964) found that the titers of neutralizing antibody in fetal heart blood and amnionic fluid collected 12 to 16 weeks following termination of pregnancy were very much lower than those in the corresponding maternal blood specimens. Both fetal and maternal antibody were largely composed of 7S (IgG) antibody. In congenital rubella–infected newborns the antibody levels are usually similar to those of the mothers or even higher. The response of CF antibody is less constant. In some patients a rising titer has been demonstrated, in others a fall in titer has been detected, and in still others the levels remain constant throughout the first year of life (Hayes et al., 1967).

Immunoglobulin Levels. Intrauterine infection also produces changes in the principal serum immunoglobulins, IgG, IgM, and IgA. Alford (1965) and Bellanti and co-workers (1965) made the important observation that rubella antibody in congenital rubella–infected infants is contained in the IgM fraction. As IgM does not cross the normal placenta, it was assumed that this was evidence of fetal antibody production. Soothill and colleagues (1966) found that total serum IgM levels were raised in the cord blood and sera of infants with congenital rubella and remained elevated for several months. Rarely, very high levels have been observed (Hancock et al., 1968). Conflicting evidence has been produced concerning whether the IgM level is related to the extent of clinical damage. McCracken and co-workers (1969) found appreciably lower or normal IgM levels in children with mild clinical forms of congenital rubella, whereas Alford and colleagues (1967; 1968) found elevated levels in cases of subclinical infection. Congenital rubella–infected infants also have raised levels of IgG that usually persist without any incidence of the normal "physiological trough" at two to three months of age (Soothill et al., 1966; Marshall, 1971). A few cases of acquired hypogammaglobulinemia have been reported, but this is a most uncommon finding (Plotkin et al., 1966; Soothill et al., 1966; South and Good, 1966). Some congenital rubella–infected infants also have raised levels of IgA at birth, but these are not as constant as are raised levels in the IgM response.

Persistence of Antibody in Congenital Rubella. Initial studies indicated that rubella antibody persists in patients with congenital rubella for many years, if not indefinitely (Dudgeon et al., 1964; Sever and Monif, 1965). However, subsequent reports have cast doubt upon this view. Kenrick and co-workers (1968) found that six of the original

50 patients with congenital rubella from the Australian epidemic of 1940 to 1941 had no detectable HI antibody when examined at the age of 25 years. They also believed that these patients were not immune because they had had clinical rubella. Hardy and her colleagues (1969b) also found a four-fold or greater decline in antibody in 18 of 20 patients, and in 50 per cent no detectable HI antibody could be detected. Florman and co-workers (1970) found that a number of deaf children born to mothers who had had a rubella-like rash in pregnancy were seronegative and failed to develop an immune response following administration of HPV-77 rubella vaccine. These findings have to some extent been corroborated by Hosking and colleagues (1983) in a study of rubella-deaf individuals and those with familial deafness. Both groups of deaf persons, aged three to 28 years, and a control group of 12 nerve-deaf patients, and 17 adult hospital staff personnel (aged 19 to 43 years) were tested for rubella HI antibody, for lymphocyte responsiveness to rubella antigen, and for response to rubella vaccine (Cendevax). The eight rubella-deaf individuals all had detectable HI antibody and therefore did not develop any increase after vaccination, but none showed any *in vitro* lymphocyte responsiveness to rubella antigen. On the other hand, the non–rubella-deaf individuals and control subjects who had detectable rubella HI antibody showed a positive lymphocyte response, whereas those without antibody did not. Similarly, only those without HI antibody responded to an injection of rubella vaccine. Although the authors were not able to prove their hypothesis, they postulated that patients rendered deaf as a result of intrauterine rubella should fail to show a lymphocyte response to rubella antigen later in life and, if the antibody test and lymphocyte response were both negative, should fail to respond with antibody after vaccination. In contrast, non–rubella-deaf patients and normal individuals should respond.

These findings are in agreement with those of Buimovici–Klein and colleagues (1979), who demonstrated an impaired cell-mediated response in congenital rubella patients that correlated with gestational age at the time of infection. Surprisingly, none of the eight rubella-deaf subjects studied by Hosking and co-workers (1983) showed a loss of HI antibody. Considering their age (seven to 24 years), this antibody persistence is in contrast to the findings of Hardy and colleagues

(1969b) and Cooper and colleagues (1971). In a detailed study of 91 patients with multiple congenital defects, Marshall (1971) found that only one child was without detectable antibody. Little difference in titer was detected between those with multiple defects and those with single defects. There was no apparent decline of antibody with age, as can be seen from Figure 3–3. However, some loss of antibody was observed in a group of children who had acquired subclinical intrauterine rubella infection (Marshall, 1971).

Cell-Mediated Immune Response. A fully functional cell-mediated immune mechanism is necessary for recovery from viral infections. The fact that rubella virus can persist in the presence of a virtually normal response points to a possible defect in cellular immunity. Several workers have demonstrated a failure of delayed-type hypersensitivity to dinitrofluorobenzene (Cooper, 1968; White et al., 1968). Similar findings have also been reported with a Candida antigen. Attempts to measure cell-mediated immunity by observing the response of peripheral lymphocytes to mitogenic stimulation with phytohemagglutinin (PHA) have led to a number of contradictory results. Olson and co-workers (1967; 1968) found that congenital rubella–infected newborns failed to respond to PHA, whereas older infants did. Simons and Fitzgerald (1968) could not confirm this nonresponsiveness, although they showed that it was less marked in younger infants than in older patients. White and colleagues (1968) also found diminished lymphocyte responsiveness to other antigens, such as diphtheria and tetanus toxoids, and to vaccinia virus. Marshall (1971), in a study of 10 infants with congenital rubella, found no difference in PHA response between the infants and adults controls. Four of six patients younger than eight weeks of age, who were at the time shedding virus, showed a response to PHA stimulation. The patients also showed a response to diphtheria and tetanus antigens following immunization, but a surprising finding was the increase in the spontaneous reactivity of lymphocytes in the younger patients. Whatever the reason for this finding and for discrepancies in results so far reported (some of which may be due to the techniques employed), there is no clear evidence yet of a defect in cellular immunity, although on clinical and histological grounds some such defect might be expected. Further work, in particular the measurement of lymphocyte transformation with an inactivated rubella antigen, is needed to test this hypothesis.

Interferon Production. The role of interferon in limiting congenital rubella infection is not well understood. Mims (1968) has postulated that persistence of infection is due to poor interferon production, but this is difficult to prove. Desmyter and co-workers (1967) failed to demonstrate interferon in the serum or urine of young infants with congenital rubella, although these subjects were found capable of a normal interferon production to measles vaccine later in childhood. Marshall (1971) also failed to detect interferon in the serum or urine of five infants. Rawls and colleagues (1968) were unable to detect interferon in chronically infected fetal cell cultures and postulated that infection of fetal cells at an early stage in embryonic life might lead to rubella-specific tolerance to interferon. This possibility cannot be confirmed at present, but the fact that rubella virus is a poor interferon inducer, rather than the age of the cells, may be responsible for lack of interferon production. Human fetal leukocytes from a 16-week fetus are undoubtedly capable of producing interferon in response to other viruses, such as Sendai virus. Cantell and co-workers (1968) and Banatvala and co-workers (1973) have shown that rubella virus can induce interferon in fetal cells of 10 to 22 weeks' gestation but, generally, the levels were lower than those seen with Sendai virus. Banatvala et al. (1973) found marked variation among both high-passage and low-passage rubella virus strains in their capacity to induce interferon. They also observed that higher levels of interferon were detectable in placental cultures than in cultures prepared from lung, spleen, or blood. A number of Japanese rubella vaccine strains, reputed to be less teratogenic than most rubella virus strains, induced the highest levels of interferon in placental cultures, whereas little difference was detected between the Japanese and other strains in lung or blood cultures.

Pathology of Congenital Rubella

Detailed descriptions of the pathological aspects of congenital rubella can be found in papers and review articles by Töndury (1962), Töndury and Smith (1966), Driscoll (1969), and Esterly and Oppenheimer (1973). The wide variety of gross anomalies, such as

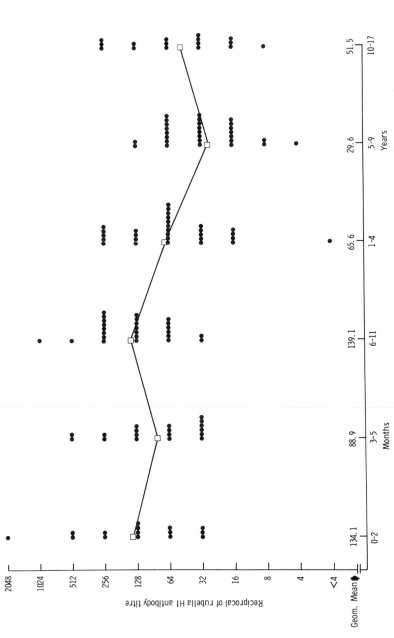

Figure 3–3. The persistence of antibody in single congenital rubella. The circles represent tests on single patients and not sequential studies on the same patients. The geometric mean antibody titer is shown in a continuous line joining open squares. Only one child in the series of 132 showed a loss of antibody. (Courtesy of Dr. W. C. Marshall, The Hospital for Sick Children, Great Ormond Street, London.)

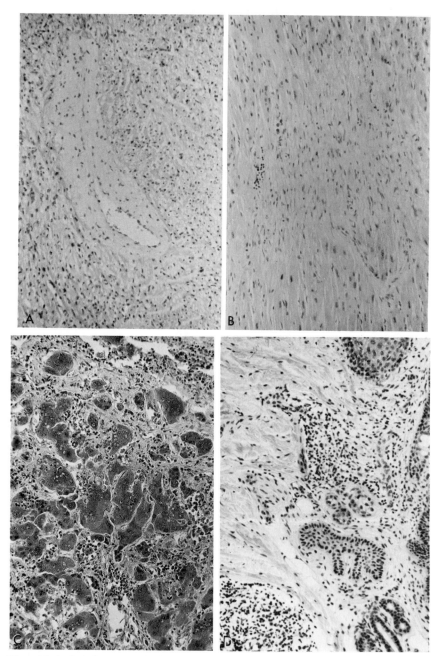

Figure 3–4. Histopathological changes caused by congenital rubella. (By permission of the Board of Governors, The Hospital for Sick Children, Great Ormond Street, London.) A, Intimal thickening of a blood vessel in a fatal case of congenital rubella. ×100. B, Myocardial necrosis. ×100. (By permission of the Board of Governors, The Hospital for Sick Children, Great Ormond Street, London.) C, Liver biopsy specimen showing giant cell hepatitis. ×100. (Courtesy of Professor Harold Stern, St. George's Hospital, London.) D, Skin biopsy specimen from the chronic rash of an infant with congenital rubella, showing round cell infiltration. ×100. (By permission of the Board of Governors, The Hospital for Sick Children, Great Ormond Street, London.)

those affecting the cardiovascular and central nervous systems, are described in the relevant clinical sections of this chapter; this section is primarily concerned with the histopathological manifestations of the lesions, examples of which are shown in Figure 3–4.

The Placenta and Chorion. No consistent, characteristic gross lesions have been found in the placenta, although small placental size has been described in a few cases. In many placentae from late terminations shrunken and fibriotic villi were found. Driscoll (1969) found evidence of deciduitis with inclusion bodies in both degenerating and intact decidual cells. Necrosis of endothelial cells in villous capillaries was a frequent finding, as was necrosis of the chorionic epithelium and endothelium.

The Cardiovascular System. The most commonly encountered cardiovascular lesions are persistent ductus arteriosus and stenosis of the pulmonary artery and its branches. Arterial intimal proliferation is exceedingly common. It was first described by Campbell (1965) and was found to be common in fatal cases of congenital rubella following the 1964 to 1965 pandemic. The degree of intimal proliferation can be so extensive as to be occlusive (Esterly and Oppenheimer, 1973), whereas the internal elastic lamina and media are usually unaffected. A unique feature of congenital rubella is that it tends to affect the major arteries, the pulmonary circulation, and the aorta, whereas the smaller arteries in both pulmonary and systemic circulation tend to be spared.

Histological study of the persistent ductus arteriosus in congenital rubella reveals that this is probably due to an arrest in the development of the ductus. The internal elastic lamina is found under a very thin intima, which consists of endothelium and an extremely thin subendothelial layer. Fine elastic fibers are found in the media, but the number of smooth muscle cells appears to be reduced. These changes are consistent with an arrest in the development of the vessel rather than with formation of a grossly abnormal structure (Gittenberger-de-Groot et al., 1980). Hypoplasia of the abdominal aorta has been reported in an adult female, aged 23 years, with stigmata of congenital rubella. Whether the hypoplastic vessel with irregular elastic plaques and no inflammatory changes seen in this woman resulted from intrauterine rubella is not clear (Limbacter et al., 1979).

Focal myocardial necrosis and scarring is not an infrequent finding and, as in other organs affected in congenital rubella, there is usually a surprising lack of any inflammatory reaction (see Fig. 3–4).

Hypoplasia of vessels and mineralization have also been described. Many observers feel that obliterative angiitis may well be one of the most pathological lesions in congenital rubella (see Fig. 3–4), although there are undoubtedly other processes that contribute to the causation of defects in this disease.

The Ocular System. The main ocular lesions are cataracts, retinopathy, and microphthalmus. Originally recognized by Gregg, cataracts are of the utmost importance because of their frequency and disabling consequences. Many of the histopathological lesions found in the lens are also pathognomonic of congenital rubella (Wolff, 1973). The primary and secondary lens fibers are formed during the eighth week of gestation, at a period when the maximum blood supply to the lens is being developed. These fibers may be directly damaged by the cytopathic effect of rubella virus, which delays their development; the virus may also remain latent, able to cause further damage at a later date. Retention of the nuclei in the lens fibers is characteristic of rubella cataracts, and areas of central necrosis with pyknotic nuclei in areas of degeneration are commonly found.

Similarly, infection between the seventh and eighth week of gestation may produce delay in development of and pathological lesions in the iris and ciliary body. Atrophy of the iris stoma, hypoplasia, or absence of the dilator muscles of the iris, with vacuolization and focal necrosis of the pigment epithelium of the iris and ciliary body, may be encountered. Failure of cleavage of the angle of the anterior chamber is also a fairly constant finding (Wolff, 1973).

Zimmerman and Font (1966) described a nongranulomatous uveitis with diffuse and focal infiltration of the anterior uvea by lymphocytes and plasma cells. They regarded these changes as pathognomonic of congenital rubella. Thus, these pathological lesions together represent the end result of the cytotoxic action of the virus. Retarded growth occurs early in intrauterine life, and secondary focal infiltration of cells, characteristic of an inflammatory response, may develop later, even after birth. Microphthalmus is another common feature of congenital rubella and yet another manifestation of retarded growth.

One of the most characteristic features of congenital rubella is the presence of a pigmentary retinopathy that is often referred to as rubella retinitis. The lesions, which consist of "pepper and salt" areas, result from foci of degeneration and from an absence or irregular distribution of the retinal pigment epithelium. They are different from the lesions of inflammatory chorioretinitis seen in congenital toxoplasmosis and cytomegalic inclusion disease.

Choroidal neovascularization, with subsequent hemorrhage and disciform scarring accompanied by visual loss, has been encountered in a number of cases of congenital rubella with retinopathy (Deutman and Grizzard, 1978; Frank and Purnell, 1978). The neovascularization and hemorrhages appear to be limited to the subpigment epithelial space and develop as a late manifestation of intrauterine rubella in late childhood and adolescence. Unlike rubella retinopathy, which seldom affects visual acuity, disciform degeneration has a serious effect on vision (see Fig. 3–11).

The Auditory System. No major anatomical defects have been found in the temporal bones, but localized lesions have been found in the inner ear. These are mainly confined to the stria vascularis, Reissner's membrane, and the tectorial membrane. Necrosis of the epithelium of the cochlea with damage resulting from small hemorrhages and inflammatory cells in the stria vascularis is a common finding. The main histopathological changes observed by Friedmann (1974) consisted of inflammation and necrosis, with adhesions between Reissner's membrane and the tectorial membrane. The latter may be found retracted away from the organ of Corti and covered by inflammatory cells. In some cases studied by Friedmann and Wright (1966) the morphological differentiation of the organ of Corti was as advanced as could be expected, but the degeneration and inflammatory changes were consistent with damage occurring after organogenesis (see Fig. 3–5). Such changes would undoubtedly lead to profound deafness in the child, but as the inflammation is an ongoing process, it could also explain the late onset of deafness in childhood.

The other form of deafness encountered in congenital rubella is probably related to a central lesion in the brain, resulting in a form of central auditory imperception.

The Liver. The chronic infective state so characteristic of congenital rubella may result in liver damage, including hepatomegaly and focal necrosis of parenchymal cells with bile stasis and an infiltration of inflammatory cells. This is often associated with the presence of syncytial giant cells indistinguishable from giant cell hepatitis of unknown etiology (see Fig. 3–4).

The Reticuloendothelial System. Splenomegaly and, much less commonly, a small, shrunken spleen may be seen. The thymus is usually small, and both organs may show lymphopenia microscopically. In the lymph nodes well-developed germinal centers and plasma cell production may be found earlier than one would expect (Singer et al., 1969), and this finding corresponds with the elevated levels of IgM. In older infants, however, germinal centers may be absent (Singer et al., 1969), and thymic dysplasia may be seen (Thorburn and Miller, 1967; Berry and Thompson, 1968; Garcia et al., 1974).

The bone marrow is usually normal or hyperplastic, but often there is a paucity of megakaryocytes, which may be associated with thrombocytopenic purpura, particularly in the neonatal period (Plotkin et al., 1965a). Phagocytosis of erythrocytes and other cells by macrophages in the bone marrow is not uncommon (Zinkham et al., 1967).

The Lung. An interstitial pneumonitis may occur in congenital rubella. The main histopathological findings are a chronic interstitial infiltration and mononuclear cells and lymphocytes similar to those encountered in other viral infections of the lung. Phelan and Campbell (1969) have described the pathological features, which include an early florid stage, with extensive inflammatory infiltration and hyaline membrane filtration, followed by a varying degree of interstitial fibrosis and scarring. Cases of desquamative interstitial pneumonitis associated with circulating IgM antigen-antibody complexes have been described (Boner et al., 1983). This supports the hypothesis that part of the pathogenesis of late-onset disease in congenital rubella may involve antigen-antibody complexes containing rubella virus antigen.

The Central Nervous System. The main clinical manifestations involving the central nervous system are microcephaly and an acute meningoencephalitis. Microscopically, the most common finding is focal meningoencephalitis with chronic inflammatory infiltration of the meninges. Occasional infiltration around the small vessels may also be seen (Rorke and Spiro, 1967), but this is less extensive than in congenital toxoplasmosis and cytomegalovirus infection. In contrast, rubella encephalitis in the adult, although rarely fatal, tends to result in more extensive and widespread necrosis of the cortex and basal ganglia, with diffuse macroglial and microglial reactions. A rare form of chronic progressive panencephalitis has also been described (Townsend et al., 1975; Weil et al., 1975). A mild degree of atrophy of cerebral

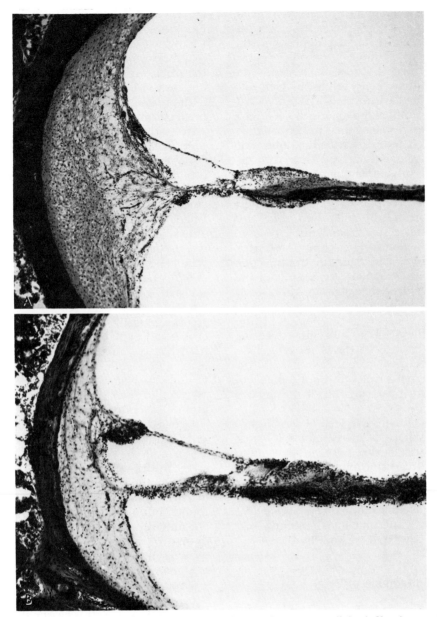

Figure 3–5. The most notable feature in the infantile cochlea is inflammatory cellular infiltration on the tympanic surface of the basilar membrane and the congested spiral ligament. Reissner's membrane is adherent to the atrophic vascular stria. ×50. B, Apical coil of right infantile cochlea. The most notable feature is a globular mass of granulation tissue in the angle between the atrophic vascular stria and the adherent Reissner's membrane. There is also marked cellular infiltration of the spiral ligament and of the basilar membrane. The tectorial membrane is deformed and is adherent to Reissner's membrane. ×60. (From Friedmann, I.: The Pathology of the Ear. Oxford, Blackwell Scientific Publications, 1974, pp. 418–419.)

gyri was noted in one case, with shrinking of the cerebellum, lens, and medulla. Slight thickening of the leptomeninges was also found. Microscopic sections revealed diffuse destruction and astrocytosis within the white matter, with perivascular collections of lymphocytes and amorphous, dark-staining deposits within the walls of small blood vessels.

Electron microscopic examination of the lesions confirmed the presence of numerous plasma cells. Reactive astrocytes in the affected areas were characterized by abundant cytoplasm, and nuclear bodies were frequent in such cells when they were observed under the electron microscope (Townsend et al., 1976). The most prominent pathological finding in the brain of a case studied in detail by Townsend and co-workers (1976) was numerous amorphous vascular deposits in the white matter in addition to the other lesions already described. The vascular lesions were more diffuse than those seen in children with congenital rubella who died without neurological deterioration. The amorphous deposits in the vessel walls, their ultrastructure, and the raised levels of rubella antibody in serum and spinal fluid, together with increased levels of gamma globulin in the cerebrospinal fluid, suggested that these deposits were due to precipitated globulins. These findings, along with the elevation of gamma globulin in the cerebrospinal fluid, pointed to local production of IgG within the central nervous system. Circulating immune complexes containing rubella-specific antigen and antibody have been described in two cases of progressive panencephalitis (Coyle and Wolinsky, 1981). The general histological picture resembled that seen in subacute sclerosing panencephalitis associated with measles virus.

The Bones. Involvement of bones, particularly of the metaphyses of the distal end of the femur and proximal end of the tibia, is common.

Histological lesions are seen at the lines of ossification. There is increased osteoblastic and osteoclastic activity, poor mineralization of osteoid, and distortion of the columnar orientation of newly formed bone spicules.

The Teeth. Necrosis of the epithelial cells forming the dental lamina and absence of the analage of permanent dentition have been described (Töndury and Smith, 1966).

Possible Mechanisms of Fetal Damage

Symptoms in viral diseases are usually ascribed to tissue damage resulting from cell destruction caused by viral replication. Cell necrosis is the predominant feature in infections such as yellow fever, smallpox, herpes simplex, and influenza, but cell destruction with cytolytic changes cannot be held to explain all of the clinical manifestations seen in every viral infection. It is probable that immunopathological processes are responsible for the exanthemata in rubella and measles and also for the perivenous demyelination in the postinfectious encephalitides. Some other viruses produce their effect by dysfunction without much evidence of cell damage; still others do so by a slow progressive degeneration, with persistence of the infectious agent, or by tumor destruction and cell dysfunction, for which several alternative mechanisms may be responsible. Possible mechanisms of the effects caused by congenital rubella are outlined in Figure 3–6 and Table 3–8.

Depression of Mitotic Activity. Human fetal cultures infected *in vitro* with rubella virus undergo a reduced rate of division and eventually cease to proliferate (Plotkin et al., 1965b). Similarly, cell cultures from infected infants show a reduced rate of growth. This reduced growth rate could be the result of chromosomal damage, as suggested by Chang and co-workers (1966), but Plotkin and Vaheri (1967) put forward the alternative hypothesis that it could be due to a soluble mitotic-inhibitory factor that they had demonstrated in human fibroblast cultures infected with rubella virus. This finding has not, however, been confirmed (Marshall, 1971). Clinically, a general depression of mitosis could explain the low birth weight that is such a constant feature in congenital rubella, and it would also be in accord with the findings of Naeye and Blanc (1965), in that many organs in congenital rubella–infected infants have a reduced number of cells.

Cytolytic Changes. Cell necrosis is seldom very marked in congenital rubella, but focal lesions may be seen in isolated organs such as the heart muscle, the liver, the organ of Corti, and, to a lesser extent, the brain. Signs of an inflammatory response are seldom found, but occasionally scar tissue may be encountered—for example, in the myocardium—indicating that the fetus is capable of overcoming an infection (Woods et al., 1966; Dudgeon, 1969a).

Vascular Damage. The vascular changes encountered in congenital rubella are of prime importance. It is reasonable to suggest that obliterative angiopathy of the small blood vessels in the placenta and the fetus occurring at a critical stage of fetal growth could result in damage to fetal organs (Kistler, 1973).

Virus Persistence. Not all the changes seen in congenital rubella are caused at the time of fetal infection; some may result from damage at a later date. Persistence of rubella virus in various organs such as the inner ear, the lens (Reid et al., 1966; Menser et al., 1967b), and the brain could be the cause of some types of late-onset disease. The loss or deterioration of hearing encountered in some children later in life could be the result of reactivation of persistent virus in the inner

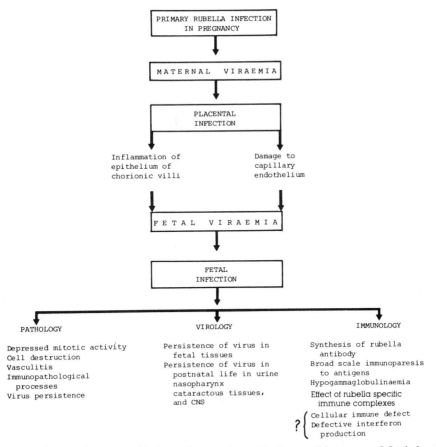

Figure 3–6. The pathogenesis of congenital rubella, together with the possible causes of fetal damage and the response of the fetus to infection. (Adapted from Marshall, W. C.: Immunological studies of intrauterine rubella. Ph.D. thesis. University of London, 1971.)

Table 3–8. **MECHANISMS OF FETAL DAMAGE IN CONGENITAL RUBELLA**

Pathological Process	Effect on Fetus
Placenta	
Deciduitis sclerosing angiopathy, villous inflammation	Diminished blood supply, intrauterine growth retardation
Fetus	
Reduced mitotic activity, chromosomal breaks	Intrauterine growth retardation, malformations, diminished number of cells per organ
Cytolytic changes	Damage to myocardium, inner ear, liver, etc.
Vasculitis, endothelial necrosis of blood vessels	Vascular anomalies
Persistence of virus	Meningoencephalitis, ? late onset of deafness and progressive panencephalitis, ? poor results of cataract surgery
Immunopathological	Late-onset disease: lung and skin lesions

ear. Also, the reactivation of persistent virus may cause cataracts to develop some time after birth and may explain the progressive panencephalitis encountered in late childhood.

Immunopathological Reactions. Not all of the symptoms of congenital rubella can be explained by the mechanisms so far discussed, and it seems reasonable, for example, in cases of late-onset disease and lesions of the skin and liver, to look to an immunopathological cause. It may be that the chronic rubelliform rash occasionally seen as such a manifestation can be explained on the basis of an antigen-antibody reaction. Marshall and colleagues (1975) have reported the isolation of rubella virus from a skin biopsy specimen of one such patient. The histopathological lesions are essentially similar to those observed in the exanthemata of infections such as measles, which are almost certainly due to delayed-type hypersensitivity (see Fig. 3–4D). The hypothesis that some forms of late-onset disease are related to circulating immune complexes of antigen and antibody is substantiated by their detection in two reported cases of desquamative interstitial pneumonitis (Boner et al., 1983).

Reports from Tardieu and co-workers (1980) and Coyle and co-workers (1982) underline the increasing recognition of the importance of rubella-specific immune complexes in the pathogenesis of late-onset clinical problems in congenital rubella. The patients investigated by Tardieu et al. (1980), none of whom had been particularly ill at birth, suffered a sudden onset of serious illness in the first year of life. The older patients investigated by Coyle et al. (1982) presented a different picture, with a gradual onset of a variety of symptoms of no great severity. In both groups, however, rubella-specific immune complexes were clearly associated with the late onset of symptoms.

The Consequences of Fetal Infection

The possible consequences of a primary maternal rubella infection on the fetus are summarized in Figure 3–7. Infection of the fetus may lead to an increased risk of spontaneous abortion, stillbirth, and death in the perinatal period and in infancy. Fetal infection may lead to congenital malformations, with structural damage to vital organs such as the eye, heart, and ear; to congenital disease in infancy, with damage to the liver and hemopoietic systems; or to late-onset disease in infancy, with rubelliform rashes, generalized lung disease, and, rarely, hypogammaglobulinemia. Equally important is the fact that an infected infant may appear "normal" and undamaged at birth and remain so, but others may manifest evidence of damage, particularly loss of hearing, in later infancy or early childhood (Peckham et al., 1979).

Finally, the fetus, in spite of exposure to maternal infection in the early weeks of pregnancy, may not become infected and will remain normal. On the other hand, an infant who has been infected and shows laboratory evidence of this, but is clinically normal at birth, is at risk of developing a defect later in life.

Maternal Rubella and the Risk to the Fetus

Two factors predominate in determining the risk to the fetus: the immune status of the mother and the gestational age at which rubella infection occurs.

Effect of Maternal Immune Status. The main risk to the fetus is related to primary rubella infection contracted in pregnancy. As already stated, the risk from reinfection is very remote, and even in authentic cases of laboratory-proven reinfection (see Table 3–7)

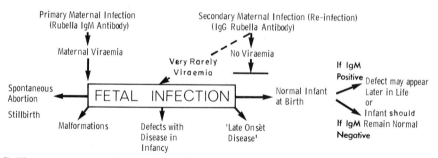

Figure 3–7. The consequences of intrauterine rubella, including the spectrum of fetal damage that may ensue.

it is difficult to understand how viremia can occur in the presence of circulating antibody.

The evidence that primary maternal rubella constitutes the main risk stems from repeated observations, starting with those of Gregg in 1941 and confirmed during the rubella pandemic of 1963 to 1965, that clinically diagnosed rubella contracted early in pregnancy frequently resulted in defects of a particular type in the offspring. Surveillance of congenital rubella defects has also confirmed that the risk to the fetus is as great after subclinical rubella as after clinical disease. In the United Kingdom program for congenital rubella surveillance only 45 per cent of mothers with a child with congenital rubella gave a history of a rash in pregnancy. Twenty five per cent of mothers were unaware of any illness throughout their pregnancies (Dudgeon et al., 1973; Sheppard et al., 1977).

The Effect of Gestational Age on the Fetus. The gestational age at which maternal infection occurs is crucial in determining the outcome with respect to fetal death, infant mortality, and the incidence of malformations and defects. Whatever the outcome may be, death or defect, it is almost certainly the direct consequence of fetal infection.

Prenatal and Infant Deaths. It is not altogether surprising, given its pathogenesis, that rubella in pregnancy leads to an increase in prenatal and infant deaths. This was established in the study on "rubella and other virus infections during pregnancy" carried out in the United Kingdom between 1950 and 1952 (Manson et al., 1960) (hereafter referred to as the U.K. study). Similar findings were observed by Lundström (1962) in Sweden during a similar period, 1950 to 1951 (hereafter referred to as the Swedish study).

The findings relating to the outcome of pregnancies complicated by rubella in the U.K. study are summarized in Table 3–9. The figures for the "expected" outcome were calculated from the accumulated experience of all control cases (5717) selected before the subjects in the various virus groups (rubella, measles, chickenpox, mumps, poliomyelitis, and influenza) were identified. "The calculations were made in such a way that the proportions chosen at each stage of pregnancy were the same as in the respective virus group, that is, the controls were standardized for the period of risk." A broad comparison between the nationally observed rates and the control series for 1950 through 1952 showed that the control group was

representative of the United Kingdom as a whole in terms of stillbirths, live births, and infant mortality and thus was suitable for comparison with the virus-infected group.

In all respects the outcome of the pregnancy was less favorable following maternal rubella up to the twelfth week than in successive stages of pregnancy. An analysis of the records for rubella between the thirteenth and sixteenth weeks of pregnancy did not reveal any increase in spontaneous abortion, stillbirths, or infant deaths in the first two years of life. Thus, gestational age was established as a crucial factor in determining these particular adverse effects on the fetus.

In the Swedish study four groups were studied. The *rubella (R) group* of 1146 pregnant women who contracted clinical rubella, the *nonimmune* exposed *group* (NE) of 951 women who had no clinical illness and had no knowledge of a previous attack of rubella, the *immune* exposed *group* (IE) of 398 women who were considered to be immune, and the *control group* of 2580 pregnant women who had no known contact with rubella during their current pregnancy. There appeared to be no increased incidence in spontaneous abortions in women with rubella in the first 4 months of pregnancy (54 of 726 [7 per cent] compared with 24 of 486 "nonimmune" women [5 per cent] and 15 of 194 "immune" women [8 per cent]). On the other hand, a difference was noted in the incidence of late abortions (sixth month or later): the rate was 3.2 per cent in the rubella group and 0.6 per cent and 1.1 per cent in the "nonimmune" and "immune" groups, respectively, compared with 0.8 per cent among the control subjects (Lundström, 1962). This difference was significant. However, as many women contracting rubella in the early part of the study (i.e., before July 1, 1951) were not treated as study subjects, there was no reliable estimate of early abortions. Later it was found that the incidence of abortions referable to rubella in the first four months of pregnancy was 15.6 per cent, compared with the overall incidence of 10 per cent in Sweden for that period (Lundström, 1962).

The stillbirth and infant mortality rates in the Swedish study were lower than those in the U.K. study, but this may reflect a national disparity since the control and national rates for the United Kingdom were higher than those for Sweden. Lundström (1962) recorded 13 stillbirths out of 459 births (2.8 per cent) following first-trimester rubella, compared with 14 stillbirths out of 701 births

Table 3–9. OUTCOME TO INFANT IN PREGNANCY COMPLICATED BY RUBELLA ACCORDING TO THE STAGE IN PREGNANCY COMPARED WITH THE EXPECTED OUTCOME CALCULATED FROM THE EXPERIENCE OF STANDARDIZED CONTROL GROUPS

Rubella Stage of Pregnancy	No. of Cases	Observed/ Expected	Abortion		Stillbirths		Born Alive but Dead at 2 Years		Alive at 2 Years	
			No.	%	No.	%	No.	%	No.	%
Up to Week 12	202	Observed	10.0	5.0	9.0	4.5	14.0	6.9	169.0	83.6
Standardized controls		Expected	4.9	2.4	4.8	2.4	4.9	2.4	187.4	92.8
13–28th week	276	Observed	1.0	0.4	7.0	2.5	9.0	3.3	259.0	93.8
Standardized controls		Expected	2.0	0.7	7.6	2.8	7.3	2.6	259.1	93.9
29th week or later	96	Observed	—	—	4.0	4.2	1.0	1.0	91.0	94.8
Standardized controls		Expected	—	—	2.1	2.2	2.3	2.4	91.6	95.4
All rubella cases	578	Observed	11.0	1.9	20.0	3.5	24.0	4.2	523.0	90.4
Standardized controls		Expected	6.9	1.2	14.6	2.5	14.6	2.5	541.9	93.8

Data from Tables 5 and G in Manson, M. M., et al.: Rubella and other virus infections during pregnancy. Rep. Pub. Hlth. Med. Sub. No. 110, 1960.

(2.0 per cent) in the control series. Figures for infant deaths were 18 of 446 (4.0 per cent) for the rubella cases and 9 out of 687 for the controls (1.3 per cent). The differences in the rates of stillbirths and infant deaths in the rubella and control groups were significant in both the U.K. and the Swedish studies and are in general accord with other reports on spontaneous abortions, stillbirths, and infant deaths following maternal rubella reported between 1946 and 1960 (summarized by Lundström [1962], tables 6 and 11). The incidence of spontaneous abortions following maternal rubella reported in thirteen prospective studies varied from zero to 36 per cent in one study reported by Siegel and Greenberg (1960), (see Lundström 1962, Table 6).

Incidence of Defects in Relation to Gestational Age. The original observations of Gregg (1941, 1944) and, more especially, of Swan (1949), which were the result of retrospective surveys, overemphasized the incidence of congenital defects following maternal rubella. Initial estimates by Swan (1949) put the incidence of congenital malformations following maternal rubella in the first trimester as high as 80 to 90 per cent. Subsequent prospective studies have revealed a considerably lower figure. Details of five such studies are summarized in Table 3–10.

Several points should be noted in interpreting the figures shown in this table. First, the recording of the incidence of congenital malformations and defects was based on a clinical diagnosis of rubella in pregnancy, as no laboratory tests for confirmation of the diagnosis could be made at the time. Secondly, several of these studies were undertaken between 1950 and 1957, when rubella was epidemic but before the full impact of congenital rubella, as revealed by the rubella pandemic of 1963 to 1965, was appreciated. The defects recorded were mainly those of the rubella syndrome—cataracts, perceptive deafness, and heart disease—seen singly or in combination, but both the U.K. and the Swedish studies did include a number of defects not normally associated with congenital rubella (e.g., pyloric stenosis, atresia of the esophagus and duodenum, and imperforate anus). Thirdly, the studies carried out in the United Kingdom and Sweden included matched controls for comparison. In the U.K. study there were 578 cases of rubella in pregnancy observed and 547 live infants were born to those mothers [the data in Table 3–10 refer to 543 of these 547 liveborn infants (in 4, the date of onset of rubella was not stated), as in Table L of the U.K. study newborns delivered up to the date week of pregnancy (11) and stillbirths (20) have been excluded and in a further four the onset of rubella was not stated]. Of these 543 documented liveborn infants with rubella, there were 24 (13.3 per cent) with major malformations born in the first trimester (non-rubella defects having been excluded). By comparison 2.3 per cent of 128 control subjects had major malformations. In the Swedish study there were 46 cases of rubella syndrome defects among 463 infants born to women who had had rubella in the first trimester (10 per cent), compared with 5 such cases out of 712 control subjects (0.7 per cent).

In looking at the incidence of defects in the fourth and subsequent months, as recorded in Table 3–10 and in the original reports, it is necessary to distinguish at what week of pregnancy maternal rubella occurred (not recorded by Lundström [1962]) and the age at which the assessment of defects was carried out. In the U.K. study, initial assessment was made as soon after birth as possible, but continuing evaluations were performed in some areas up to the second year of life; in the Swedish study, assessment took place between one and three years of age. In both studies, additional assessments for deafness were carried out, revealing an increased incidence with age; cases of deafness were also identified as having occurred following maternal rubella after the twelfth week of pregnancy. In a follow-up by Jackson and Fisch (1958) of 57 children in the original U.K. study, additional cases of congenital perceptive deafness were identified in 14 of 57 children (24.5 per cent, compared with 6.0 per cent in the original assessment), eight of which had resulted from maternal rubella between the twelfth and fourteenth weeks. No cases of deafness were detected among children whose mothers had had rubella after the fourteenth week, and no other major defects were encountered that had not been recognized in the original assessment. A further study of 156 of the original 547 liveborn children throughout England, Wales, and Scotland identified additional cases of perceptive deafness, of which three had followed rubella between the thirteenth and sixteenth weeks of pregnancy (Manson et al., 1960).

In a later follow-up study of 46 children

Table 3–10. INCIDENCE OF CONGENITAL RUBELLA DEFECTS FOLLOWING RUBELLA IN PREGNANCY

Study Country and Year of Occurrence	Gestational Age When Maternal Rubella Occurred (No. of Cases of Rubella Syndrome Defects per No. of Women Exposed at Specified Time in Pregnancy [%])				
	1st Month	2nd Month	3rd Month	4th Month	5th Month and Later
Lundström (1962) Sweden, 1951	13/113 (11.5)	18/150 (12.0)	15/186 (8.1)	3/204 (1.5)	2/468 (0.4)
Manson et al. (1960)* United Kingdom, 1952	6/45 (13.3)	10/61 (16.3)	8/77 (10.3)	2/72 (2.7)	0/288 (–)
Liggins and Philips (1963) New Zealand, 1959	2/2 (100)	6/12 (50.0)	2/15 (13.3)	2/16 (12.5)	0/44 (–)
Pitt and Keir (1965) Australia, 1950–1955	3/5 (60.0)	4/12 (33.3)	11/32 (34.4)	2/35 (5.7)	0/19 (–)
Siegel et al. (1971) United States, 1957–1963 United States, 1964	0/4 (–) 2/7 (28.6)	9/11 (81.8) 18/26 (69.2)	6/34 (17.6) 25/50 (50.0)	7/49 (14.3) 11/62 (17.7)	4/31 (12.9) 4/33 (12.1)
Total	26/176 (14.8)	65/272 (23.9)	67/394 (17.0)	27/438 (6.1)	10/883 (1.1)

*Non–rubella-type defects have been excluded from this series.

only one case among the 46 children whose mothers had had rubella in the second trimester.

More accurate information on the correlation of gestational age with the time of maternal rubella and the type of rubella defect is revealed in a study by Ueda and colleagues (1979). They carried out a study on 55 children with congenital rubella, 40 in Japan and 15 in Seattle, Washington. The gestational age was calculated as the number of days from the last menstrual period (LMP) until the onset of the rash in the mother. The number of defects in the series, together with the stage in gestation, measured in days, at which the rash occurred, is shown in Table 3–11. The wide scatter in time at which the defects occurred is evident. Many of the children suffered from combined defects, such as cataracts, heart disease, and deafness. Retinopathy was present in almost all patients with congenital rubella.

Data based on a clinical and virological study of confirmed rubella at successive stages in pregnancy have been reported by Miller and her colleagues (1982). Over 1000 women with confirmed rubella infection at different stages of pregnancy were followed up prospectively. Of the 960 women for whom the outcome of pregnancy was known, 523 (54 per cent) had therapeutic abortions and a further 36 (4 per cent) had spontaneous abortions. A total of 273 children, of which 102 were seropositive and were presumed to have been infected *in utero,* were followed up after birth. Of the 102 infected infants, it was found that the number of infants exposed at 11 weeks' gestation or before who had defects was 100 per cent (nine of nine); at 11 to 12 weeks it was 50 per cent (two of four); at 13 to 14 weeks it was 17 per cent (two of 12); and at 15 to 16 weeks it was 50 per cent (seven of 14). No defects were identified thereafter. The number of defects encountered was higher than in previous studies, but it must be emphasized that the outcome to the fetus in a large number of cases could not be determined because so many pregnancies were terminated.

Similar findings have been observed in Sweden and Denmark. Grillner and co-workers (1983), in a retrospective study, observed three cases of deafness among 65 children aged four to seven years who had been exposed to rubella during gestation. Sixty-two children had normal hearing, but one case of deafness followed maternal rubella at 12 weeks and two cases followed it at 14 weeks. In a further prospective study of 118 cases of rubella in pregnancy, one defect was encountered following maternal rubella at 15 to 16 weeks, and one defect was found among 12 children infected following the disease at the seventeenth week of gestation. In Denmark, the effect of maternal rubella on 209 infants exposed after the twelfth week of gestation was studied by Kejtorp and Mansa (1980). Rubella was confirmed serologically, and the infants' sera were studied for IgM rubella antibodies. Rubella defects, of which hearing impairment was the most commonly encountered, were observed in 30 to 40 per cent of all children infected during the first 14 weeks of gestation. Thereafter, the figure fell to one in 10 for the fifteenth and sixteenth weeks and to zero thereafter.

Preconceptional and Early and Late Pregnancy Infections. A few cases of preconceptional rubella followed by the birth of an infant with a rubella-like defect have been reported. Gregg (1941) referred to one such case as having occurred as a result of rubella three months before conception. Wesselhoeft (1947) also described abnormalities of the rubella syndrome following rubella at this stage. Lundström (1962) observed that in 22 cases rubella was reported to have occurred within one month prior to the LMP. Two children with the rubella syndrome were identified, suggesting that this is an "at-risk" period. However, as Lundström (1962) noted, it was probable that the two cases in question were actually referable to the RI (Lundström classified the cases thus: RI = rubella in first month, RII = rubella in second month, RIII = rubella in third month, and RIV = rubella in fourth month). Seven women had had rubella 34 days to four months prior to the LMP. They gave birth to normal children, but two of these had birth weights of less than 2500 grams. Sever and his colleagues (1969) encountered seven patients in whom rubella had occurred zero to 28 days before conception. The result was one case of congenital rubella (infection 21 days before conception), one abortion, one stillbirth, one child with multiple defects in infancy, and three normal children. They also observed 58 patients in whom rubella had occurred in the second trimester (13 to 26 weeks after conception), in addition to 42 in whom it had occurred during the first trimester. Nine of the 58 women with second-trimester infections had elevated total IgM levels, and six cases of congenital rubella and

Table 3–11. **CONGENITAL RUBELLA SYNDROME: CORRELATION OF GESTATIONAL AGE AT TIME OF MATERNAL RUBELLA WITH TYPE OF DEFECT***

			Heart Disease						
Study Group	Total	Cataract		PDA	PS-PAS	VSD	Murmur	Deafness	Retinopathy	No Major Defects
Ryuku Islands and Kyushu, Japan	40	8	7					32	35	7
Seattle, Washington	15	5	11					14	13	1
Total	55	13	18					46	35	8
Gestational age in days between LMP and onset of rash	—	26–57		25–62	36–71	31–93	16–47	16–131	16–131	5–182

No. of Patients

*PDA = persistent ductus arteriosus; PS = pulmonary stenosis; PAS = pulmonary artery stenosis; VSD = ventricular septal defect; LMP = last menstrual period.

Data from Ueda, K., et al.: Congenital rubella syndrome: correlation of gestational age at time of maternal rubella with type of defect. J. Pediatr. 94:763–765, 1979.

four suspected cases were reported in the offspring. Among the six infants born after maternal rubella between the fifteenth and twenty-second weeks, there was one case of microcephaly, deafness, and failure to thrive; two cases of peripheral pulmonary stenosis; and three cases of deafness, one of which also had an inguinal hernia, heptospleno-megaly, and purpura. The four suspected cases showed less obvious signs of congenital rubella; one child had microcephaly with suspected mental retardation, one was deaf, and the other two were suspected to be mentally retarded. Overall, the risk must be considered low and is difficult to quantify.

Hardy and her colleagues (1969a) have also reported on the possible adverse outcome following maternal rubella after the first trimester of pregnancy. They observed 24 women who contracted rubella, confirmed by laboratory tests, between the fourteenth and twenty-first weeks of pregnancy. Twenty-two were delivered of liveborn infants, a therapeutic abortion was performed in one case, and one woman gave birth to a macerated stillborn infant. Seven of the 22 liveborn infants who had been followed up for up to two years remained normal. One had an elevated total IgM at birth, but all had lost detectable rubella antibody by six months of age. Fifteen of the remaining liveborn children were suspected of being abnormal during infancy. Six of these had elevated IgM serum levels, and 10 had detectable antibody after six months of age, from which it can be assumed that they had been infected *in utero.* Most of the infants, both normal and affected, were of normal birth weight for gestational age, and the affected infants did not exhibit any severe problems during the neonatal period. Twelve children were found to

have normal communication skills, but six had a significant decrease in auditory sensitivity, and two had suspected hearing loss and delayed language development. Four children were found to have cardiac murmurs, and two of these probably had peripheral pulmonary stenosis.

As far as rubella infections later in pregnancy are concerned, the weight of the present evidence suggests that the risk of fetal damage, as opposed to fetal infection, is low after the sixteenth week. Thus the cases of defects following maternal rubella in the fifth month or later recorded in Table 3–10 should be viewed with caution. The two cases seen in the Swedish study, one heart defect and one case of deafness, could have been expected in the normal population. The same applies to the three cases recorded by Siegal and co-workers (1971). One heart defect and two cases of deafness could have resulted from causes other than rubella.

The Incidence of Specific Malformations and Defects. The incidence of specific malformations and defects affecting different organs was reported by Cooper and his colleagues (1969) following the rubella pandemic of 1964 to 1965 in the United States. Details on 376 congenital rubella–infected children at Bellevue Hospital, New York City, are shown in Table 3–12, together with the clinical manifestations and the stage of pregnancy when maternal rubella occurred. The incidence of most defects was higher when rubella occurred in the first two months of pregnancy than when it occurred in the third and fourth months, except for deafness, which occurred consistently in children exposed throughout the first four months of gestation. It is expected, however, that if the cases attributable to infection during the

Table 3–12. **CLINICAL MANIFESTATIONS OF CONGENITAL RUBELLA CORRELATED WITH TIME OF MATERNAL INFECTION***

Defect	Month of Pregnancy					No Clinical Rubella	Insufficient Information
	First	Second	Third	Fourth	>Fourth		
Neonatal purpura	14 (23%)	43 (41%)	7 (9%)	2 (5%)	0	12 (24%)	7
Heart disease	34 (57%)	62 (58%)	17 (21%)	2 (5%)	1 (6%)	29 (58%)	7
Cataract or glaucoma	30 (50%)	31 (29%)	6 (7%)	0 (—)	0	28 (56%)	2
Deafness	50 (83%)	76 (72%)	55 (67%)	21 (49%)	0	30 (78%)	11
Neurological deficit	34 (57%)	63 (59%)	20 (24%)	11 (26%)	0	33 (66%)	8
Total children	60	106	82	43	16	50	19

*Data on 376 cases of congenital rubella, showing total number of cases per month of pregnancy with percentages in parentheses.

From Cooper, L. Z., et al.: Rubella: clinical manifestations and management. Am. J. Dis. Child. *118*:18–29, 1969.

fourth month were broken down according to the week of pregnancy in which maternal rubella occurred, it would be found that the infections causing deafness and neurological deficit had occurred in the early part of the month, that is to say, between the thirteenth and sixteenth weeks.

Consequences of Maternal Rubella: A Synthesis

In all of the prospective studies that have been reported, the following points have emerged:

1. The risk to the fetus is greater following maternal rubella in the first eight weeks of pregnancy than in the second.

2. Although the first trimester has traditionally been regarded as the most "at risk" period, there is no clear cutoff point at the twelfth week of gestation. Malformations of the heart and eye are uncommon after this period, but they do occur. However, it is important in such cases to record the stage of gestation as precisely as possible in days or weeks between the onset of the LMP and the onset of the rash in the mother.

Hearing defects undoubtedly occur following rubella in the fourth month of gestation, but few appear to occur after the sixteenth week. The rare cases of deafness reported at the seventeenth (Grillner et al., 1983) and eighteenth (Ueda et al., 1979) weeks of gestation must be regarded as exceptions. For practical purposes, the first 16 weeks of pregnancy must be regarded as the period of greatest risk.

3. Nevertheless, the effect of rubella after this period needs careful scrutiny in view of the findings by Cradock-Watson and co-workers (1980) and Miller and co-workers (1982) on the incidence of fetal infection after the first trimester. Careful follow-up of such cases is essential in order to determine whether fetal infection after the sixteenth to twentieth weeks does lead to damage that may become apparent only later in life. This is particularly important in view of the reports by Hardy and her colleagues (1969a) and Lundström and co-workers (1974). The reports by Sever and co-workers (1969) and Hardy and co-workers (1969a) are at variance with the views of other investigators, particularly those of Cradock-Watson and colleagues (1980) and Miller and colleagues (1982). Nevertheless, in view of the fact that

fetal infection can occur beyond the second trimester, these reports merit careful study. That most of the children studied by Hardy and her colleagues were apparently normal at birth but developed disabilities in hearing, speech, and motor development later in life could be explained as the result of a continuing infection contracted *in utero* and causing damage after birth. This is consistent with observations of the late onset of deafness in children with congenital rubella and of the deterioration in hearing in some of those children. A long-term follow-up by Lundström et al. (1974) on the effects of maternal rubella on recruits for the Swedish Army revealed a number of hearing defects sufficiently severe to prevent acceptance for military service in those recruits whose mothers had had rubella in the fourth and fifth months of pregnancy. These findings are at variance with those of other reported surveys. All reports concerning the effect of maternal rubella after the first trimester of pregnancy indicate that children born after such pregnancies should be closely observed to assess their developmental progress. Despite the paucity of documented evidence on the incidence of defects from maternal rubella contracted beyond the twentieth week of pregnancy (and because in many studies the incidence of defects has been related to the month of gestation rather than to the week), it can only be concluded from the data shown in Tables 3–10 and 3–11 that the risk beyond the twentieth week is small and cannot as yet be quantified.

CLINICAL ASPECTS

The original descriptions of congenital defects associated with maternal rubella made by Gregg and others in the 1940's mainly concerned those involving the eye, the heart, and, later, the auditory system. The triad of symptoms—cataracts, heart disease, and deafness—came to be known as the rubella syndrome. Both Gregg (1941, 1944) and Lundström (1962) also referred to other manifestations: that the affected infants were often ill-nourished and that they were small at birth for their gestational age and subsequently underweight for their age. Microcephaly was often present. The present concept of the rubella syndrome is different. The spectrum of clinical manifestations is wider and more varied. New defects and other evidence of fetal infection have been identified, all of which are included under the broad term "congenital rubella" or congenital rubella syndrome (CRS).

A list of the clinical manifestations encountered in congenital rubella is shown in Table

Table 3–13a. CLINICAL ASPECTS OF CONGENITAL RUBELLA

General
Intrauterine growth retardation; spontaneous abortion; stillbirth; small for gestational age; failure to thrive; increase in neonatal and infant mortality; slow development in infancy and early childhood

Ocular
Cataracts; pigmentary retinopathy; microphthalmus; glaucoma; cloudy cornea; macular degeneration of the retina; iris hypoplasia; strabismus

Cardiovascular Lesions
Persistent ductus arteriosus (PDA); PDA and pulmonary arterial lesions; pulmonary arterial lesions: (1) hypoplasia of artery, (2) supravalvular stenosis, (3) valvular stenosis, (4) peripheral branch stenosis; renal artery stenosis; ? cerebrovascular stenosis; aortic stenosis; ventricular septal defects and tetralogy of Fallot; myocardial damage; neonatal myocarditis

Auditory
Sensorineural deafness; central auditory imperception; deafness with speech defects, with or without mental retardation; ? delayed speech with normal hearing and intelligence

Central Nervous System
Microcephaly; full anterior fontanelle; meningoencephalitis; mental retardation; lethargy; hypotonia; irritability; unreactive, hypotonic infant; late onset of irritability and hypotonia; late onset of convulsions and "meningitis"; progressive panencephalitis; autism

Visceral
Hepatosplenomegaly; hepatitis and jaundice

Hematological
Neonatal thrombocytopenic purpura; anemia; hemolytic anemia

Osseous
Osteopathy; lack of calcification of osteoid

Pulmonary
Interstitial pneumonitis

Immunological
Chronic rubelliform rash; thymic hypoplasia; dysgammaglobulinemia; circulating immune complexes

Miscellaneous
Adenopathy; thymic hypoplasia; hypogammaglobulinemia; recurrent or persistent infections; chronic diarrhea; growth hormone deficiency; diabetes mellitus; dermatoglyphic abnormalities; hypothyroidism

3–13a and in Tables 3–14 and 3–15. These lists attempt to identify those malformations and defects that are commonly associated with congenital rubella, either singly or in combination, and that are presumed to be the result of intrauterine rubella infection. It does not follow that all defects associated with proven cases of congenital rubella such as inguinal hernia, cryptorchidism, and meningomyelocele are causally related in intrauterine rubella infection. Some of these are listed in Table 3–13b. Many such defects were identified by Lundström (1962) in the Swedish survey, but only meningomyelocele and cryptorchidism following first-trimester rubella appeared to be on the borderline of significance when compared with defects arising in cases of rubella in the second and third trimesters and in the control cases. If account is taken of the pathology and pathogenesis of congenital rubella, there is reason to accept that such defects could be causally related but they do not occur with the consistency that would be expected. The prevalence of many of these defects in the population is such that one might expect them to occur in individuals with congenital rubella as additional and unassociated defects.

Cooper (1975) has placed the various clinical manifestations of congenital rubella into three main groups: transient, permanent, and developmental. This grouping is useful for purposes of prognosis and management. Included in the first category (transient) are the defects present in the newborn period and early infancy, such as low birth weight, purpura, thrombocytopenia, hepatitis, large anterior fontanelle, and some cases of me-

Table 3–13b. DEFECTS REPORTED IN THE RUBELLA SYNDROME BUT NOT PROVEN TO BE CAUSALLY RELATED*

Anencephaly	Tracheobronchial atresia
Hydrocephaly, seizures,	or fistula
ptosis of the eyelid	Pyloric stenosis
Meningomyelocele**	Umbilical hernia
Retrolental fibroplasia	Myxedema
Hypospadias	Renal and adrenal
Cryptorchidism**	anomalies
Harelip and cleft palate	Syndactyly, polydactyly
Situs inversus	Talipes
Inguinal hernia	Mongolism
Intestinal atresia	Intussusception

*Some of the defects referred to in the reports by Manson and co-workers (1960) and by Lundström (1962).

**The only two defects considered by Lundström (1962) to be of borderline significance.

ningoencephalitis. Also included are some of the manifestations of the late-onset disease, such as pneumonitis and lymphadenopathy. The permanent sequelae, which include the major malformations such as cataract, heart disease, hearing loss, and microcephaly, are the most serious, but progress in medical and surgical treatment means that much can now be done to alleviate their effects. The developmental problems are frequently not recognizable at birth but become apparent during the early years of life. Deafness is such an example; hearing loss may not become apparent until the child is four to five years of age, or a hearing loss already present may worsen. Other disorders in this category are mental retardation and behavioral disorders; arterial stenosis, such as pulmonary artery stenosis; diabetes mellitus and thyroid disorders; immune complex disease; thymic hypoplasia and dysgammaglobulinemia; and, finally, progressive panencephalitis. The occurrence of these developmental problems necessitates careful and repeated evaluation of children with congenital rubella.

The spectrum of disease in congenital rubella is illustrated in Figures 3–8 through 3–14.

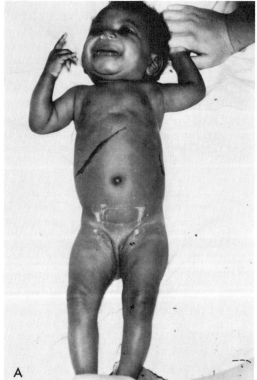

Figure 3–8. A, An infant with a severe case of congenital rubella with neonatal jaundice, hepatosplenomegaly, failure to thrive, and marked lymphadenopathy. The child later became severely deaf in both ears. She was born after 38 weeks' gestation and weighed 4 lb 2 oz; her case was diagnosed by virus isolation and persistence of rubella antibody. There was no history of maternal rubella. B, The same child as in A, with bilateral cataracts first observed at six weeks of life. (By permission of the Board of Governors, The Hospital for Sick Children, Great Ormond Street, London.)

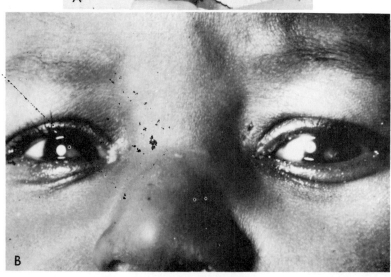

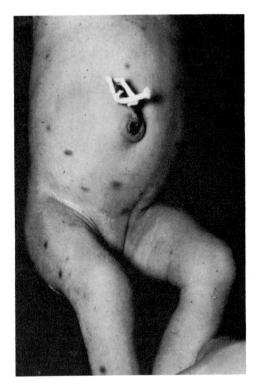

Figure 3–9. Two day old infant with severe neonatal purpura, enlarged anterior fontanelle, bilateral corneal edema with increased ocular tension, osteopathy, and persistent ductus arteriosus. Platelets fell to 17,000/cu mm. She weighed 3 lb at birth. There was a history of maternal rubella at eight weeks' gestation. The infant died at six weeks of age from heart failure and severe hepatic involvement due to hepatitis. The infant's case was diagnosed by virus isolation and persistence of rubella antibody. (See the color frontispiece illustration.) (By permission of the Board of Governors, The Hospital for Sick Children, Great Ormond Street, London.)

Figure 3–10. Pigmentary retinopathy. (See the color frontispiece illustration.) (By permission of the Board of Governors, The Hospital for Sick Children, Great Ormond Street, London.)

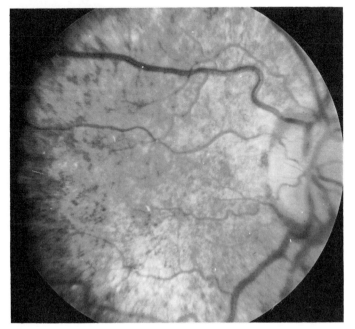

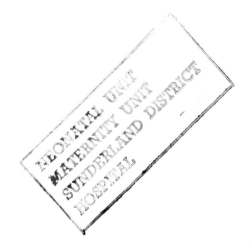

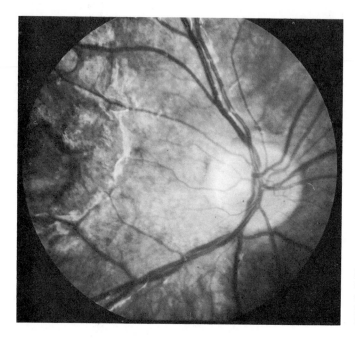

Figure 3–11. Disciform degeneration of the macula. (By permission of Mr. David Taylor and the Board of Governors, The Hospital for Sick Children, Great Ormond Street, London.)

Figure 3–12. Chronic rubelliform rash. (See Fig. 3–4D for histopathological changes in a skin biopsy specimen.) (By permission of the Board of Governors, The Hospital for Sick Children, Great Ormond Street, London.)

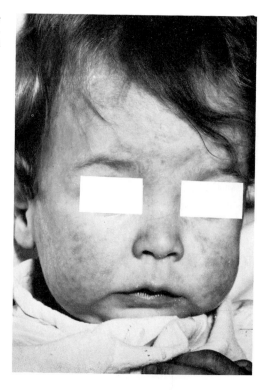

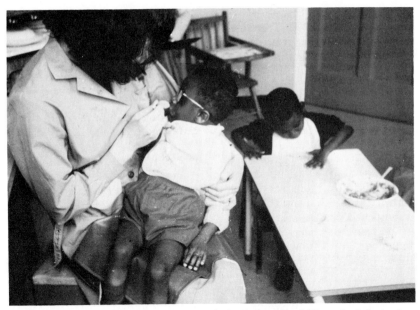

Figure 3–13. Two severely damaged children with congenital rubella. The child on the left also has severe cerebral palsy. (Courtesy of Professor K. S. Holt, The Hospital for Sick Children, Great Ormond Street, London.)

Fetal and Infant Mortality

An increase in fetal mortality has been reported by several investigators (Manson et al., 1960; Siegel et al., 1966). Premature delivery and stillbirths are not important features of congenital rubella, but intrauterine growth retardation is extremely common. In a prospective study of the effect of maternal viral infections on birth weight, Siegel and Fuerst (1966) found that the majority of

rubella-infected infants were born after the thirty-sixth week of gestation but that there was a high incidence of low birth weight (less than 5 lb, 8 oz, or 2500 gm). For infants congenitally infected with measles and hepatitis (presumed to be HAV), delivery usually occurred before the last month of gestation.

A low birth weight for normal gestational age (small for gestational age), due to intrauterine growth retardation, was found to be the most prominent and constant character-

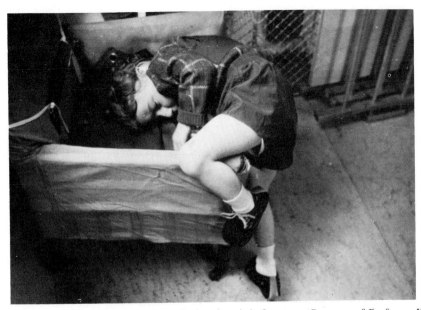

Figure 3–14. A deaf, partially sighted child who displayed autistic features. (Courtesy of Professor K. S. Holt, The Hospital for Sick Children, Great Ormond Street, London.)

istic of congenital rubella–infected infants born during the pandemic of 1962 to 1964. Cooper and co-workers (1965) found that as many as 60 per cent of affected infants fell below the tenth percentile, and 90 per cent fell below the fiftieth percentile. Intrauterine growth retardation and subsequent retardation in postnatal growth is seldom the sole manifestation of congenital rubella. Lejarraga and Peckham (1974) have shown that the mean birth weights of children exposed to maternal rubella without acquiring defects do not differ significantly from the fiftieth percentile or from one another but that those of infected infants with defects are significantly lower. Similarly, the head circumference was smaller in children with defects, even when pigmentary retinopathy was the sole defect.

The mortality rate of infants with congenital rubella is high, particularly when the infection is associated with a low birth weight and multiple defects. The mortality rate in the 58 infants with neonatal purpura and other defects studied by Cooper and co-workers (1965) was 20 per cent.

Congenital Malformations

The main malformations resulting from damage during the period of organogenesis are found in the eye (cataracts and retinopathy), the heart (persistent ductus arteriosus and pulmonary stenosis), and the ear (sensorineural perceptive deafness). Apart from deafness and, to a lesser extent, retinopathy, these usually occur in combination with other defects. They are described in greater detail in the sections on the various organ systems involved.

Ocular Defects

The main ocular defects encountered in congenital rubella are listed in Table 3–13a.

Cataracts. Cataracts, which are among the most common defects in congenital rubella, may be unilateral or bilateral (see Fig. 3–8). Two main types of cataract were described by Gregg (1941) and others (Roy et al., 1966). One type consists of a central, densely white, pearly lesion and a small clear zone between the lesion and the border of the iris. In the second type the density is more uniform throughout, with less contrast between the central and intermediate zones. Rubella cat-

aracts, which are usually subtotal, are generally present at birth, but they may not become evident until several weeks after birth. In a series investigated by Murphy and colleagues (1967), cataracts were first noted in 11 infants in the first four weeks of life, in 10 between four and 12 weeks, and in two others between three and nine months. Retinopathy and microphthalmus were associated with cataract formation in several cases, particularly unilateral cataract formation.

Pigmentary Retinopathy. This is a common abnormality and of great diagnostic significance. Retinopathy is more often unilateral than bilateral and may be the only defect present. Roy and co-workers (1966) described 17 cases.

Retinopathy (see Fig. 3–10 and the frontispiece, Fig. C) results from lack of pigment formation and is a nonprogressive condition. The pigmentary areas vary in size and form, from fine "pepper and salt" areas to larger ones, sometimes scattered throughout the retina and sometimes confined to the peripheral zones. Retinopathy is difficult to detect in the presence of cataracts. It rarely, if ever, affects visual acuity.

Disciform Degeneration of the Retina. Patients with pigmentary retinopathy may subsequently develop loss of vision due to subretinal neovascularization and disciform scarring of the macula, although the exact association between the two conditions is unclear. Although progressive changes in the fundus have been noted in children with pigmentary retinopathy (Collis and Cohen, 1976), it has usually been regarded as a benign disease. Frank and Purnell (1978) reported two patients, aged 17 years and 11½ years, both of whom presented with sudden loss of vision. The mothers of both patients had had a febrile illness with a rash in the first trimester of pregnancy. The 17 year old patient had no detectable abnormalities at birth. At the age of 17 years the patient complained of decreasing vision in the right eye. Visual acuity was found to have decreased in that eye to 6/60 from 6/6 two years previously. Pigmentary clumping in the macula was noted, together with a subretinal neovascular membrane surrounded by a hemorrhage. Nine months after her initial visit, a disciform scar had formed. The left eye was normal. The 11½ year old girl complained of loss of vision in the left eye for three weeks. Retinitis and deafness had been noted in the first year of life. Two years prior to the sudden loss of vision, visual acuity had been recorded as 6/6 (RE) and 6/75 (LE). Later it was reduced to 0/21 (LE). Diffuse pigmentary clumping of the retina in both eyes was noted, and in the left eye a subretinal neovascular membrane with surrounding hemorrhage was detected. Over a period of weeks, visual acuity in the affected left eye decreased to 0/60. Deutman and Grizzard (1978) described three similar cases in children aged 7 to 14 years, all of whom had congenital perceptive deafness. Loss of vision was sudden in two cases but less obvious in the third patient. The retinal changes were similar to those described by Frank and Purnell. The retinal lesions illustrated in Figure 3–11 were observed in a 10 year old boy who had had surgery for a cataract in his microphthalmic left eye when he was three years old. The visual acuity in the right eye was never below 3/10. The acuity in the right eye was 6/5 unaided, despite a moderate pigmentary stippling of the macula. When he was nine years old he complained of a sudden loss of vision in the right eye. The cause was a disciform degeneration of the macula (Taylor, 1983).

Microphthalmus. This is often found in association with congenital cataract. Gregg (1944) found that 60 per cent of patients with unilateral cataracts had microphthalmus. If it is present in both eyes, it may be difficult to recognize for lack of a normal eye for comparison. Wolff (1973), in a study of 328 cases of congenital rubella, found microphthalmus in 30 eyes. It was frequently bilateral and in 24 cases was associated with cataract and retinopathy.

Glaucoma. This is much less common than cataracts but is of great importance because of the imminent danger to sight that it presents unless surgical treatment is instituted. Of the 58 cases of congenital rubella in the newborn reported by Cooper and colleagues (1965), 3 per cent had glaucoma. Weiss and co-workers (1966) described eight cases, in six of which glaucoma was bilateral. Seven of the children had other rubella defects. Glaucoma normally occurs in the neonatal period, but one infant reported by Weiss et al. (1966) first manifested the disease at eight months of age. Differential diagnosis between glaucoma and a corneal haze should be made under anesthesia, when corneal edema will be detected as a result of the raised intraocular pressure. The edematous, enlarged corneas with deep anterior chambers may be difficult to recognize in infants with microphthalmus, in whom the anterior chamber is shallower than normal.

Strabismus. In the study by Wolff (1973) already referred to, strabismus was encountered in 58 of 328 cases. In many of these, both esotropic and exotropic, strabismus was associated with other ocular defects. Lundström (1962) also encountered a slightly higher incidence of strabismus following rubella in the first trimester, and it was associated with other ocular defects.

Nystagmus. Gregg (1941) encountered nystagmus in many of the patients referred to him, usually in association with cataracts. Of the subjects studied by Wolff (1973), 42 children had nystagmus and 24 had cataracts. In others, psychomotor retardation, glaucoma, strabismus, or retinopathy was present.

Transient Corneal Haze. This is a comparatively rare feature that usually resolves spontaneously. It is not associated with raised intraocular pressure and does not require treatment.

Defects in the Iris. The pupil in the congenital rubella–infected patient may respond sluggishly to light, and the iris may appear atrophic. Iris hypoplasia is frequently associated with cataract and microphthalmus.

Cardiovascular Disease

Defects of the Great Vessels. Most forms of cardiac disease seen in congenital rubella are of the acyanotic type, and they are generally less complex than other forms of congenital heart disease. The cardiac lesions in 96 children studied by Kiely and colleagues (1975) consisted of 66 cases of persistent ductus arteriosus (PDA), this being the only cardiac lesion in 19 cases; 47 cases of pulmonary artery stenosis (PAS) involving the main artery and its branches, PAS being the sole cardiac lesion in seven children; and 37 cases of pulmonary valvular stenosis, usually in association with PDA and PAS. Other lesions, such as aortic and renal artery stenosis, were encountered with septal defects, and tetralogy of Fallot was also observed.

A high incidence of pulmonary arterial lesions was also noted by Hastreiter and co-workers (1967). In 34 of 37 patients the cardiovascular lesions were limited to the great vessels and ductus arteriosus. Twenty-six patients had pulmonary arterial lesions and associated PDA, six had isolated pulmonary lesions, and three had complex and multiple cardiovascular lesions. Pulmonary artery involvement with or without associated PDA has also been recorded by Franch and Gay (1963), Liggins and Phillips (1963), Korones and colleagues (1965), and Sperling and Verska (1966). This high frequency of pulmonary arterial involvement was not observed, however, in a combined clinical and virological study of cases of congenital heart disease (CHD) at the Hospital for Sick Children, Great Ormond Street, London (Starkova and Ebrahim, 1972). During a three-year study of 580 cases of CHD, 60 cases of PDA were diagnosed, but only 12 were considered likely to be attributable to maternal rubella. All 12 cases had low birth weights and were associated with other rubella defects. In eight of the 12 patients, PDA was the sole cardiac defect; four of these patients also had pulmonary stenosis (two with valvular and two with peripheral pulmonary stenosis). In the remaining 48 patients with PDA, in whom it was the only cardiac defect, none of the other defects were of the type encountered in congenital rubella, and the birth weights were not abnormally low.

Other peripheral arterial lesions, such as renal artery stenosis, have been reported in three cases of congenital rubella with other associated defects by Menser and co-workers (1966, 1967c). Renal artery stenosis associated with hypertension has been observed by Esterly and Oppenheimer (1973) in a series of 13 cases of congenital rubella. The cerebral vasculature has so far received little attention from investigators, but it is conceivable that stenotic lesions are present in cerebral vessels and play a role in the focal neurological features that are sometimes observed.

Neonatal Myocarditis. Damage as the result of necrosis to myocardial muscle fibers may lead to severe illness in the newborn period. Four infants with such damage, each with an associated PDA, were observed by Korones and colleagues (1965); two of these children died. The clinical course in the four infants was characterized by left-sided cardiac failure during the first few days of life. In the two infants who survived, there was no evidence of myocardial injury until the second and third weeks of life. Another 10 cases in infants with electrocardiographic (ECG) changes pointing to myocardial damage due to ischemia have been reported by Ainger and co-workers (1966). Seven of these infants died. The three who survived had ECG changes compatible with myocardial infarc-

tion as it is seen in adults. Three additional infants were found to have evidence of healed infarction at birth, a fact suggesting that myocardial damage had occurred *in utero*. This type of lesion may explain some of the sudden cases of cardiac arrest or cardiac failure without evidence of structural abnormalities that are encountered in infants with congenital rubella.

Hearing and Speech Defects

Perceptive or Sensorineural Deafness. Perceptive or sensorineural deafness is the most common manifestation of congenital rubella, and it is also one of the few defects that occurs alone. The hearing loss is frequently bilateral and of equal severity in both ears, but in some cases the loss in one affected ear may be slight or moderate. Unilateral deafness also occurs, and such cases are of special importance because they may go undetected, as a result of which the child's speech development may be affected.

The importance of continual reassessment of children known or thought to have been exposed prenatally to rubella is borne out by the increased incidence of deafness in children reported to be normal at birth. Several long-term follow-up investigations of children suspected to be suffering from deafness as a result of intrauterine rubella have shown that the incidence of perceptive or sensorineural deafness may increase from around 6 per cent in the first two years of life to approximately 20 per cent or greater later in childhood (Jackson and Fisch, 1958; Manson et al., 1960; Barr and Lundström, 1961; Sheridan, 1964; Butler et al., 1965). This was particularly evident in a study reported by Peckham (1972) of a group of 84 children who had been exposed to intrauterine rubella. When first assessed for signs of hearing loss at one to four years of age, 23 per cent were found to be deaf; when reassessed six to eight years later, another nine of the 49 children with rubella antibody (seropositive) were found to be deaf. No other rubella-type defects were encountered, and no further defects were found in any of the children without rubella antibody (seronegative).

Clinical and serological studies for rubella antibodies in 139 children with severe hearing loss at a center for hearing and speech defects in London revealed a high incidence of rubella antibody (54 per cent) in children aged six months to six years, both in the children who had a history of maternal rubella or contact during gestation and in those who had no such history. The incidence of rubella antibody in these children was considerably higher than that in a randomly selected control group (7 per cent) made up of children attending hospital outpatient clinics. These data reported by Gumpel and co-workers (1971) indicate that intrauterine rubella may have been responsible for approximately 25 per cent of cases of congenital perceptive or sensorineural deafness diagnosed as deafness of unknown etiology. The frequency with which sensorineural deafness may result from maternal rubella has been well established in a study by Peckham and her colleagues (1979) on a group of children referred to a hearing and speech center in London. Over a four-year period 568 children aged six months to four years were examined clinically and by serological tests. Of the 349 children with sensorineural deafness, 83 (23.8 per cent) had rubella antibody, whereas only 19 (8.7 per cent) of the remaining 219 children in whom sensorineural deafness had been excluded had antibody. The usefulness of serological tests in identifying cases of congenital rubella deafness was confirmed. A striking difference was found between the seropositive and seronegative deaf children. The former had far fewer associated defects and histories of adverse perinatal events, as well as fewer family histories of deafness.

Severe deafness was a prominent feature following a rubella epidemic in Iceland in 1963 to 1964 (Baldursson et al., 1972). Thirty-seven children with rubella syndrome were detected; none had cardiac or ocular defects, but all had varying degrees of hearing loss. Many of the children had behavioral disorders but normal intelligence. Deafness was also a prominent feature of the rubella epidemic in Trinidad in the West Indies between 1960 and 1962 (Karmody, 1968). Serological tests for rubella antibody performed on many of the children with deafness of unknown etiology indicated that maternal rubella in subclinical form was probably responsible for a high proportion of such cases.

Other Forms of Hearing Disorder. Although sensorineural deafness is the most common of all rubella defects, defective hearing does not always result from damage to the organ of Corti. Some children suffer from a form of central auditory imperception that is probably cerebral in origin, a condition in which, although they can hear certain sounds, they cannot compehend them. In such cases there is often a high incidence of speech disorders because the child cannot comprehend the spoken word. Precise evaluation of the factors responsible in these cases is extremely difficult, and it is possible that the lesion lies at cortical level. Ames and co-workers (1970) found that central auditory imperception was probably the cause for the failure of 30 of 118 children to respond to sound.

Speech defects and delayed onset of normal speech without evidence of hearing loss have been reported, but these do not appear to be important features of congenital rubella except when associated with other defects. Nevertheless, bearing in mind that the central nervous system may be severely involved in congenital rubella (Desmond et al., 1967), one must consider the possibility that speech defects may occur as part of the clinical spectrum resulting from an encephalitic process.

Central Nervous System Disease

Involvement of the central nervous system in congenital rubella is more common than it was originally thought to be, but it is usually found in association with other defects. Approximately 25 per cent of infants show signs of central nervous system involvement in the first few weeks or more of life. This is usually manifested by a full anterior fontanelle, irritability, and a raised level of protein in the spinal fluid. As the affected infant grows, other signs of microcephaly and mental retardation become evident. Desmond and her colleagues (1967) found some form of neurological disease to be present in 81 of 100 patients examined between birth and the second year of life. They described three main patterns of central nervous system disease. The first was characterized by lethargy, hypotonia, and a full anterior fontanelle at birth, followed later by irritability, disturbed sleep, intermittent head retraction, and arching of the back; more than half of 51 infants in this group showed a marked delay in motor development. A second pattern was seen in 11 patients who presented as small, unreactive, hypotonic infants who failed to gain weight and had delayed motor development. Symptoms of irritability similar to those of the first group tended to develop later in infancy, but subsequent improvement occurred. A third group of seven patients presented with a sudden onset of acute meningitis and convulsions. In two of these seven patients symptoms developed suddenly at three months of age; both had hepatitis and a raised protein level in the cerebrospinal fluid. The majority of these children had other manifestations of congenital rubella, including low birth weight and congenital defects.

Forty-four of the 64 surviving children had abnormal neurological findings at the age of 18 months, of which tone disturbances and head retraction with arching of the back were the most frequent.

Cooper (1968) reported similar findings. One hundred nine of 309 children with congenital rubella had some signs of psychomotor retardation, ranging from mild developmental delay to severe quadriparesis.

Autism. Behavioral disturbance is not uncommon in congenital rubella. A child with congenital rubella may be erratic, restless, disoriented, and unresponsive. In a study of 244 congenital rubella–infected children, Chess (1971) found 18 children with autistic features; 10 were diagnosed as autistic, and the remaining eight children showed some features of autism.

Behavioral Disorders. These have been well studied in a longitudinal observation by Chess and co-workers (1971; Chess, 1974). Of a group of 224 children initially studied at the age of four to five years, 210 were re-evaluated four years later. Half of the children had no apparent psychiatric disorders, but the remainder showed signs and symptoms of either mental retardation (26 per cent), reactive behavior disorder (18 per cent), cerebral dysfunction (12 per cent), autism (6 per cent), or neurotic behavior (3 per cent). Chess (1974) reviewed the degree of mental retardation in 54 children with congenital rubella at the age of eight to nine years. She found that 12 were in the borderline mild-moderate category and 36 had severe or profound retardation. In six children the degree of mental retardation could not be specified.

Intrauterine infections such as rubella are doubtless responsible for only a fraction of these disorders, but the observation that one virus can probably lead to disorders such as autism is an important one that merits further detailed virological investigation.

Chronic Encephalitis. Virological investigations showed that virus could be recovered from the cerebrospinal fluid or other sources in a high proportion of cases—from 50 per cent of those with mild involvement to 73 per cent with severe involvement. Rubella virus was isolated from the spinal fluid of several "normal" infants without obvious central nervous system disease, but those in whom virus persisted later had impairment of vision and hearing. Virus was also isolated from five of eight infants at 18 months of age whose sole defect was impaired hearing. The virus persisted in the cerebrospinal fluid throughout the first year of life in many cases and to 18 months of age in one patient. In many cases elevated cerebrospinal fluid protein was associated with pleocytosis (Desmond et al., 1967).

These findings were in conformity with an earlier report by Monif and Sever (1966) that rubella virus leads to a chronic infection of the central nervous system. Virus was isolated from the spinal fluid or brain of 17 infants who ages ranged from seven to 132 days.

Chronic Progressive Panencephalitis. A more progressive disorder of the central nervous system may also occur as a rare complication. Townsend and colleagues (1975) described three children with a presumptive diagnosis of congenital rubella in whom a progressive disease of the central nervous system developed during the second decade of life. This was characterized by ataxia spasticity, intellectual deterioration, and seizures. Rubella antibody was detected in both the serum and spinal fluid. In a similar case in a 12 year old boy with progressive dementia, ataxia, and myoclonic seizures, widespread brain involvement was suggested by the electroencephalographic recordings and by the histopathological examination at autopsy. Rubella virus was recovered from the brain by the cocultivation technique (Weil et al., 1975).

Progressive panencephalitis does not appear to be an effect only of intrauterine rubella infection, as a case has been reported in a 19 year old man who had developed clinical rubella at the age of seven (Wolinsky et al., 1976). The patient was referred for evaluation of dementia and had no stigmata of congenital rubella. The clinical and virological findings were in keeping with progressive panencephalitis associated with postnatally acquired rubella; they were similar in some respects to those of subacute sclerosing panencephalitis associated with chronic measles virus infection.

Miscellaneous Clinical Manifestations

Many of the other manifestations listed in Table 3–13a are found in different organ systems but tend to occur in combination either in the early newborn period or as a form of late-onset disease later in infancy.

Congenital Disease in Infancy. Some of the defects commonly encountered in the newborn period are listed in Table 3–14. Purpura associated with thrombocytopenia is a common manifestation of congenital rubella at this age. Cooper (1968) encountered 85 such cases in a total of 350 infants with congenital rubella. The lesions range in diameter from 2 to 10 mm. They may appear as scattered petechiae, often on the face and upper part of the trunk, or they may present as a diffuse macular rash covering the entire body. Purpura may be present at birth but more often appears within 48 hours after birth and resolves without specific therapy within three to four weeks.

Very rarely, a generalized rubelliform rash is seen in the newborn. The presence of this rash suggests that the fetus had prenatal rubella with a rash similar to that of the typical postnatal disease (see Fig. 3–12).

Hepatosplenomegaly. Enlargement of both liver and spleen is another common feature of the disseminated disease. These organs are usually found to be firm and to extend well below the costal margin.

Hepatosplenomegaly may occur in association with jaundice, which usually appears within 24 hours of birth. Hepatitis may occur without jaundice, with raised transaminase levels persisting for several weeks.

Enlargement of the liver alone may occur in patients with congestive heart failure.

Table 3–14. **CONGENITAL DISEASE IN INFANCY***

Intrauterine growth retardation with delayed somatic growth
Thrombocytopenia, purpura, anemia
Hepatosplenomegaly, jaundice, neonatal giant cell hepatitis
Myocarditis
Osteopathy
Lymphadenopathy
Thymic hypoplasia

*These disorders may be associated with the well-recognized congenital malformations of the heart, ear, and eye.

Osteopathy. Abnormal changes in the long bones of the upper and lower extremities and in the skull have been described by Rudolph and co-workers (1965) and Singleton and co-workers (1966). The most striking change in the long bones is an alteration in the trabecular pattern in the metaphyses, which is especially pronounced in the distal femoral and proximal tibial metaphyses. Areas of translucency are found in a longitudinal axis, as are irregularity and poor mineralization of the growth plate. The skull may be enlarged, and there may be a large anterior fontanelle.

Hematological Changes. Thrombocytopenia is the most common abnormality (Cooper et al., 1965; Horstmann et al., 1965; Rausen et al., 1967). Platelet counts vary from 10,000 to 100,000/cu mm, and in the series reported by Cooper and co-workers (1965) 85 per cent had counts below 90,000/cu mm. Thrombocytopenia is not affected by corticosteroid therapy, rarely leads to severe hemorrhage, and usually resolves spontaneously.

The hemoglobin concentration is usually normal at birth, although infected infants may have an increase in the number of normoblasts and reticulocytes. Anemia often becomes evident later in the neonatal period, with signs of a decline in hemoglobin concentration and of a reticulocyte response. A paucity of megakaryocytes has been noted in the bone marrow of infected infants. In most cases the abnormal hematological findings return to normal without treatment; the fact that several of the patients with anemia have died is probably related to the presence of multiple defects rather than a direct result of damage to the blood-forming organs (Cooper et al., 1965; Horstmann et al., 1965) or of damage caused by the blood-forming organs.

A case of congenital rubella with a Coombs-positive hemolytic anemia and hypoplastic bone marrow has also been observed in a seven month old infant (Miyazaki et al., 1979). The infant died at the age of nine months from congestive heart failure secondary to anemia with hypoplasia of all elements of the bone marrow, megakaryocytes, erythrocytes, and granulocytes.

Late-Onset Disease

From three to four months of age until the end of the first year of life the features characteristic of the newborn period, such as purpura and hepatosplenomegaly, recede, whereas others, such as central nervous system disorders and psychomotor retardation, become more apparent. Examples of these are shown in Figures 3–10 and 3–12 through 3–14.

Other clinical manifestations arise that are somewhat different and have been termed "late-onset disease" (Marshall, 1973). Some of these are listed in Table 3–15. They are not particularly common, but they can lead to severe disease. More important, however, is the light that these manifestations shed on the pathogenesis of congenital rubella. They may result from a persistent infection or an immunopathological process or both. A chronic rubelliform rash may occur at about three to four months of age. It is usually generalized, but it is unlike the rash in postnatal rubella in that it persists for many weeks. The rash has some of the features of that seen in histiocytosis. Biopsy of the skin lesions has revealed focal aggregations of small round cells in the dermis (see Fig. 3–4D). Rubella virus has been isolated from one such case (Marshall et al., 1975).

A more important manifestation is generalized lung disease. The main clinical features are cough, tachypnea, and cyanosis. The onset may be sudden but is usually gradual. Mortality is high, but the response to treatment with adrenocorticotropic hormone or corticosteroids is often dramatic (Marshall, 1973). These cases have all the features of an interstitial pneumonitis (Singer et al., 1967; Thorburn and Miller, 1967; Phelan and Campbell, 1969). The age of onset, the histopathological picture, and the response

to steroids suggest that the pneumonitis may be due to an immunopathological process.

These infants may show characteristic signs of failure to thrive, difficulties in feeding, slowness to gain weight, and persistent diarrhea. These symptoms are often recurrent and may be associated with an increased susceptibility to infection, particularly of the lung. Pulmonary infection complicated by *Pneumocystis carinii* carries an unusually high mortality (Lingeman et al., 1967; Phelan and Campbell, 1969; Marshall, 1973).

Two cases of desquamative interstitial pneumonia have been reported by Boner and co-workers (1983). The two infants, aged three months and five weeks, respectively, had pneumonitis, and histological investigation showed desquamative pneumonitis. Both had IgG deficiency and increased levels of circulating IgM antigen-antibody complexes. The younger infant, who had the more marked pulmonary interstitial pneumonitis, eventually died.

Several cases of hypogammaglobulinemia were described following the worldwide prevalence of congenital rubella in the 1960's (Soothill et al., 1966). In contrast to the normal finding in congenital rubella of high levels of IgG in the early months of life, several patients were found to have IgG deficiencies of sufficient degree to lead to antibody deficiency syndrome. All six subjects exhibited other manifestations of congenital rubella, but no further cases have been reported in recent years.

The importance of late onset of hearing loss or deterioration in hearing has been mentioned in a previous section. Late-onset speech defects may also develop, but it is extremely difficult to determine whether a delay in speech or some of the complicated language disorders in children that are unassociated with defective hearing are attributable to intrauterine rubella infection.

Table 3–15. **LATE-ONSET DISEASE IN INFANCY AND CHILDHOOD***

In Infancy	In Childhood
Chronic rubelliform rash	Sensorineural deafness
Interstitial pneumonitis	Central auditory
Recurrent pulmonary	imperception
infection	Diabetes mellitus
Chronic diarrhea	Thyroid dysfunction
Hypogammaglobulinemia	Hypothyroidism
Immune complex disease	Thyrotoxicosis
	Thyroiditis
	Growth hormone
	deficiency
	Immune complex disease
	Progressive
	panencephalitis

*These disorders may be associated with the well-recognized congenital malformations of the heart, eye, and ear.

Other Manifestations

Thymic Hypoplasia. Several cases of congenital rubella with thymic hypoplasia have been described (Berry and Thompson, 1968; Garcia et al., 1974). Vascular lesions similar to those found in other organs in congenital rubella are usually present in the thymus, and there is a paucity of lymphocytes, macrophages, and lymph follicles. All of the patients so far described have died.

Abnormal Dermatoglyphics. Some investigators have found a number of children with congenital rubella to have an increased number of whorls in their finger patterning. Purvis-Smith and Menser (1968) found that 28 per cent of rubella-infected infants had an increased number of whorls compared with that of the general population (7 per cent); and Gumpel (1972) observed a higher incidence among both Caucasian infants (38 per cent) and black children from the West Indies (36 per cent) with congenital rubella than among normal children (7 per cent). The mothers also had similar configurations. The significance of these findings is not understood.

Nagono and co-workers (1978) observed abnormal fingertip whorl patterns, fingertip loop patterns, and interdigital space patterns in children with congenital heart disease due to rubella. Ross (1979) found a statistically significant difference in the fingertip ridge pattern in the offspring of women exposed to rubella in pregnancy compared with a control group of children. It was found that the pattern profile differed in the two congenital rubella groups (10 children whose mothers were given gamma globulin following exposure and 29 whose mothers had not received globulin) and that both of these differed from the controls. A significant increase in whorls was found in the children whose mothers had not had globulin, as was an increase in ulnar loops in those to whose mothers globulin had been administered. This study was carried out as part of the Rubella Birth Defect Monitoring Project of New York University Medical Center.

Endocrine Disorders

Diabetes Mellitus. A case of congenital rubella with diabetes mellitus was described by Forrest and colleagues (1969). Later (1971) they described a high incidence of this combination in adult patients; one such patient had typical rubella pigmentary retinopathy. In three of these patients the onset was in childhood. Four cases in children were reported by Plotkin and Kaye (1970), and others were observed by Johnson and Tudor (1970). Menser and Reye (1974) believe that congenital rubella can cause diabetes in persons who are not genetically predisposed and that this may be due to a decrease in the number of functioning cells in the islets of Langerhans. This situation could be the result of a primary viral invasion or, more probably, a persistent viral infection. Support for the relationship comes from virological

studies by Cooper and co-workers (1965) and the discovery of histopathological lesions in the pancreatic arteries by Rorke and Spiro (1967). Bunnell and Monif (1972) reported extensive lymphocytic infiltration of the pancreas of a three month old child with congenital rubella who had died of respiratory insufficiency. It is possible that an immunopathological process similar to that put forward as the mechanism responsible for the lesions encountered in late-onset disease could lead to damage to the pancreas.

A further study on the incidence of diabetes mellitus following congenital rubella has been reported by Menser and colleagues (1978). Forty-five patients were re-examined. They were part of a group of 50 young adults, re-examined in 1967 (Menser et al., 1967c), who had been among the patients in Gregg's original series. Nine of these 45 patients (20 per cent) aged 24 to 29 years had symptoms of diabetes mellitus. All were suffering from deafness, and four had other defects (two cases of cataracts and two of retinopathy), but they were not a severely handicapped group. Only one was insulin-dependent. The authors also encountered eight cases of diabetes in a group of 318 patients with congenital rubella (including 15 adults). Their ages ranged from 18 months to 38 years. They were a much more severely handicapped group, and all eight were insulin-dependent. One patient also had had an episode of thyrotoxicosis. Menser and her colleagues (1978) refer to 24 additional cases of diabetes in congenital rubella patients in Australia, New Zealand, Sweden, the United States, and England. No cases of diabetes mellitus had been encountered in the United Kingdom between 1970 and 1977 under the National Congenital Rubella Surveillance Programme (Dudgeon et al., 1973; Sheppard et al., 1977), but two cases have since been reported in a further review of 482 cases in the U.K. Surveillance Programme (Smithells et al., 1978). The differences between the Australian and U.K. series are striking in this respect for which no obvious explanation is as yet forthcoming, although the differences in the incidence of the HL-A antigens (*vide infra*) may play a contributory role.

Cooper (1975) identified five cases of diabetes in a follow-up of 300 survivors of the 1964 rubella pandemic. He estimated the likelihood of diabetes in children with congenital rubella to be at least four times greater than that in the general population of children in New York under the age of 15 years. Previously, Cooper (1975) had isolated rubella virus from pancreatic specimens obtained at therapeutic abortion or autopsy.

Thyroid Disorders. Thyroid dysfunction has also been reported in association with clinical rubella. Two patients with thyrotoxicosis have been reported by Menser and co-workers (1978) and by Ziring and co-workers (1975). In addition, cases of thyroiditis have been observed by Comas and Bentances (1976), Nieburg and Gardner (1976), and Ziring and colleagues (1977). Hypothyroidism has been observed in several instances (Ziring et al., 1975; Hanid, 1976). A case of childhood myxoedema has been reported by Auruskin and co-workers (1982). Signs of myxoedema developed in a six year old female who was born with multiple congenital rubella defects. The features of hypothyroidism—except mental retardation, symptoms of which she had in the first year of life—were corrected by gradually increasing the amount of thyroid hormone administered. No other endocrine disorders, diabetes, or growth hormone deficiency were detected in this patient. Hypothyroidism has also been observed as a feature of congenital rubella (Cooper, 1975).

Growth Hormone Deficiency. Many patients with congenital rubella remain smaller than normal in infancy, but they subsequently grow at a normal rate (Michaels and Kenny, 1969). It has been suggested that the spurt in growth is related to the time of termination of the viral infection. Marshall (1973) reported that of 70 patients aged three to 19 years 40 per cent were below the tenth percentile and that this finding was more marked in those with multiple defects. Two cases of retarded growth were the result of growth hormone deficiency; both children have responded to treatment with human growth hormone (Preece et al., 1977).

Histocompatibility (HL-A) Antigens. It is well known that the incidence of some diseases varies among different ethnic groups. It is also recognized that there are marked differences among HL-A antigens in certain ethnic groups. Studies by Honeyman and Menser (1974) have shown that the frequency of HL-A antigens 1 and 8 appears to influence the incidence of rubella, among other diseases, and may be related to the incidence of rubella defects, among others. Related to this finding is the observation that the incidence of HL-A antigen 1 is very much lower in the Japanese population, where the incidence of congenital rubella is remarkably lower than in Caucasian populations. Although this low incidence may be due to the possibility that Japanese rubella virus strains are less teratogenic, it is also possible that there are genetic factors that determine susceptibility. Menser and co-workers (1974) have shown that congenital rubella–infected subjects, especially those with diabetes, have an increased frequency of HL-AB8, but not HL-ABW15, regardless of whether diabetes is insulin-dependent. Tissue typing in a case of congenital rubella and myxoedema (Auruskin et al., 1982) demonstrated HL-ABW6 antigens unlike those encountered in diabetes.

Immune Complexes in Late-Onset Disease

The presence of rubella-specific immune complexes has already been referred to in cases of interstitial pneumonia and progressive panencephalitis. It is probable that they play a more important role in the pathogenesis of late-onset disease than was hitherto thought to be the case. Several instances of an association between immune complexes and late onset of clinical problems affecting several organ systems have been reported by Coyle and co-workers (1982). Twenty-one of 63 congenital rubella–infected subjects, aged five months to 28 years, had circulating immune complex activity, and 21 of 31 congenital rubella patients had rubella-specific immune complex activity. The same was demonstrated in 39 of 65 subjects vaccinated against rubella but not in subjects either susceptible to or naturally immune to rubella. The 63 patients aged 5 months to 28 years included 19 patients with deafness with or without retardation, 22 patients with deafness and cataracts with or without retardation, and 22 patients with deafness, cataracts, heart disease, and retardation. Thus, this was a severely handicapped group.

Although there was no apparent change in the static stigmata of congenital rubella (i.e., cataracts or deafness), it was found that 10 of the 63 patients had recently developed a variety of new manifestations. These included proteinuria (three cases), abnormal liver function tests (two cases), abnormal glucose test and persistent antirubella IgM (one case), thyroiditis with reduced thyroid function (one case), generalized seizure disorder (one case), purpura (one case), and glaucoma (one case). All 10 of these patients had rubella-specific immune complexes, whereas these could be demonstrated in only 11 of the remaining 53 patients. The difference was highly significant (P < 0.001 by the Fisher exact test).

The relationship between immune complexes in vaccinated subjects is discussed in a later section.

The role of circulating immune complexes has been studied in detail in eight infants by Tardieu and colleagues (1980). Eight boys with congenital rubella were studied. Four had minimal or no symptoms at birth, and four had symptoms of cardiac disease with cataract, hepatosplenomegaly, or purpura. None of the patients was seriously ill during the first few months of life. At three to six months growth failure became evident. Neurological symptoms developed in two patients, but developmental milestones were normal in the remaining six. After a latent period between the ages of three and six months, all patients presented with an acute onset of severe clinical symptoms. These included interstitial pneumonia, diarrhea, skin rash, hepatosplenomegaly, rapid neurological deterioration, and purpura. Four developed an abnormal susceptibility to bacterial infections and two developed *P. carinii* infection. Six of the eight patients died. Low levels of rubella antibody were detected in the early months of life and during the acute phase of the severe clinical disease. The rubella HI titer increased after the acute phase of illness in five patients but remained low until the time of death in three patients. IgM antibodies were detected in six subjects. Immune complexes and rubella-specific immune complexes were detected in four patients in the acute phase of the illness. A disequilibrium of T- and B-lymphocytes was detected initially but was followed by a progressive correction of T- and B-lymphocyte percentages concomitant with the rise of serum IgM levels.

The Long-Term Effects of Intrauterine Rubella

The long-term effects of maternal rubella infection depend, to a great extent, on the age at which the initial assessment is made and on the progress that is made in medical and surgical treatment of the congenitally affected infant. Major improvements in cardiac and cataract surgery can do much to relieve these disabilities, as can the development of improved hearing aids for the deaf child. Gregg (1941) first drew attention to the fact that other abnormalities, not detectable at birth or soon thereafter, might appear as development proceeded. On the basis of a follow-up study of 50 of the original patients from the New South Wales epidemic of 1940 and 1941, however, Menser and colleagues (1967a, 1969) suggested that the prognosis is not as bad as might be expected. Subsequent studies have not supported this somewhat optimistic view except in cases where minimal damage has been caused or a single organ affected. The detailed studies by Cooper (1968, 1975) have clearly shown that many congenital rubella–infected children are severely handicapped. This finding is confirmed by a study of hospital-referred cases reported by Gumpel (1972). Eighty-five children were re-examined between three and 19 years of age. Only nine were able to attend normal school, and these were children with unilateral deafness or cataracts or a combination of these with a heart defect that was correctable by surgery. The remainder were at special schools for deaf and severely subnormal persons. Profound deafness combined with cataracts and brain damage made the prognosis extremely poor.

Incidence of Single and Multiple Defects

Every investigation of groups of patients with congenital rubella has revealed a high incidence of multiple defects, with sensorineural deafness and pigmentary retinopathy standing out as the most commonly encountered solitary defects. The incidence of 75 per cent for perceptive or sensorineural deafness mentioned in Figure 3–1 is remarkably similar to that of 76 per cent reported in the study of congenital rubella in 41 schoolchildren and adolescents done by Forrest and Menser (1970). With a few exceptions, such as 15 cases of congenital heart disease in the 41 children (37 per cent), their figures are similar to those presented in Table 3–16, which shows the incidence of rubella-type defects in three series of cases. The first was a retrospective series of 287 cases referred to or seen at the Hospital for Sick Children, Great Ormond Street, London; the second,

Table 3–16. **INCIDENCE OF RUBELLA-TYPE DEFECTS IN CASES OF CONGENITAL RUBELLA**

	Retrospective Figures Summarized by Dudgeon, U.K., 1963–1970	Cooper, U.S., 1967	National Congenital Rubella Surveillance Programme, U.K., 1971–1975
Number of cases	287	271	367
Low birth weight	75%	NS*	35% (10th percentile)
Cardiac defects	55%	52%	26%
Ocular lesions	50%	40%	18%
Cataracts			
Cloudy cornea			
Hearing defects	50%	52%	67%
Central nervous system defects	25%	40%	29%
Microcephaly			
Mental retardation			
Neonatal purpura, hepatosplenomegaly	30%	31%	31%
Deaths	15%	13%	6%

*NS = not stated.

a series of similar size studied personally by Cooper in the United States (Cooper, 1968); and the third, 367 suspected or confirmed cases reported to the National Rubella Surveillance Programme in the United Kingdom. The nature of rubella-type defects reported to the Surveillance Programme between 1975 and 1981 has not materially changed since the original reports by Dudgeon and colleagues (1973) and Sheppard and colleagues (1977). There are a number of differences in the incidence of these defects, the reasons for which are not immediately apparent. For example, in the early studies in the United Kingdom in 1962 and 1963, comparatively few cases of neonatal purpura were reported; now the incidence appears to be similar to that in the United States. Again in the United Kingdom, stenosis of the pulmonary artery was encountered less commonly as a cardiac defect than in the United States, despite the fact that in nearly all cases a definitive diagnosis is now made by catheterization and not only on clinical grounds.

More important to the overall incidence of multiple defects, however, whether it be 88 per cent (Forrest and Menser, 1970) or 79 per cent (Dudgeon, 1967), is the combination of defects which occur in these children.

The age at which defects most frequently present is shown in Table 3–17. The factors that most closely affect the child's ability to adjust are, first, the type of lesion (i.e., whether it is permanent or temporary); second, the organ involved; and third, the extent of the lesion (i.e., whether it is unilateral or bilateral). For example, a child with a cataract or deafness and a heart defect has a major advantage over a child with bilateral cataracts, bilateral deafness, cardiac disease, and mental retardation. This was well borne out in the study by Gumpel (1972) of congenital rubella in 85 patients at the Hospital for Sick Children, London, some of whom are included in the 287 cases referred to in Table 3–16.

The frequency of multiple defects became increasingly apparent after the 1964 pandemic, but this can be explained only partly by better investigational procedures. The crux of the matter lies in the propensity of rubella virus to damage the host by a variety of means. Multiple defects should be expected, not regarded as exceptional, and they should also act as a spur to preventive measures.

The Management of Congenital Rubella

The first and most important step in the management of congenital rubella is to establish a precise diagnosis by means of laboratory tests (see later discussion of laboratory tests and Chapter 14). These should be performed as early as possible if congenital rubella is suspected on clinical grounds, so that the management of the case, both short- and long-term, can be arranged. An accurate diagnosis is also important so that the parents can be reassured of the unlikelihood that such an event will occur in a future pregnancy. Continual assessment should be arranged and the parents advised of the im-

Table 3–17. **SOME COMMON ASSOCIATED DEFECTS ENCOUNTERED ACCORDING TO AGE***

In the Newborn	In Infancy	In Childhood
LBW CAT CHD		
LBW CHD TCP HS Jaundice		
CAT CHD		
LBW CAT CHD TCP HS Jaundice		
	LBW FTT CAT Retinopathy CHD MR ? Deaf	
	FTT Retinopathy CHD MR Deaf	
	FTT CAT CHD CP Deaf	
		Deaf MR Microcephaly
		Delayed development Deaf
		Deaf and/or retinopathy
	Deafness Retinopathy	Deafness

*LBW = low birth weight (synonymous with "small for dates" and "small for gestational age"); HS = hepatosplenomegaly; CAT = cataract; FTT = failure to thrive; CP = cerebral palsy; MR = mental retardation; CHD = congenital heart disease; TCP = thrombocytopenia.

portance of this, particularly in regard to the risk of late-onset defects such as deafness. The "normal" infant born to a mother who experienced a rubelliform rash in pregnancy is of particular importance. Follow-up should continue for at least five to seven years. The steps to be taken in the management of the child depend to a large extent on the age when symptoms first appear.

In the Newborn Period. Recognition and prompt treatment of heart failure are essential. Expert cardiological advice should be sought concerning the most appropriate time for the surgical correction of a cardiac lesion such as persistent ductus arteriosus or pulmonary stenosis. This will depend not only on the age of the child but also on the presence and severity of associated defects. In most cases surgery should be carried out in the first year of life or soon thereafter.

It may be necessary to correct anemia and thrombocytopenia by transfusion, but these two abnormalities are usually resolved without specific treatment. Corticosteroids are of no value in the treatment of thrombocytopenia.

All infants with congenital rubella are potentially infectious during the first six months of life (see Fig. 3–2), but for practical purposes it is unnecessary to keep hospitalized patients on infectious precautions after three to four months of age. It is important that female hospital personnel, doctors, nurses, and other staff attending these children have their rubella immune status determined on appointment to the hospital staff and that, if necessary, they be immunized with rubella vaccine. Precautions should also be taken to prevent female visitors who are pregnant or who might become pregnant from coming

into contact with the congenital rubella–infected infant during the period of contagiousness.

Detection of cataracts in babies with CRS is of the utmost importance, since the severe visual handicap that may result if inappropriate steps are taken is largely preventable by early and vigorous treatment. Detection is best carried out with the ophthalmoscope set so that objects at about 1 ft to 18 in are in focus to the observer, and the eye is inspected through the ophthalmoscope aperture with the instrument held 1 ft to 18 in from the eye. Normally there is a bright red reflection from the pupil; its absence may indicate an opacity in the refractive media, the most common cause of which is congenital cataract.

Bilateral cataracts, if sufficiently severe, require early surgery and optical correction with contact lenses starting as soon as possible. Unilateral cataracts also require vigorous treatment since the other eye may be affected by retinal degeneration later in life. This so-called disciform degeneration is not necessarily directly related to the pigmentary retinopathy commonly seen in congenital rubella, which is of little functional significance, but may be a late development that destroys central vision. Because of this surgery is warranted in cases of unilateral cataract.

Because of a severe inflammatory reaction following the aspiration method of cataract surgery, Scheie and colleagues (1967) recommended that surgery should not be undertaken in patients with congenital rubella until the age of 18 months. However, with the widespread use of steroids and improved surgical techniques to remove the lens completely, this delay is no longer warranted;

surgery should be undertaken as early as possible and contact lenses fitted shortly afterward (Taylor, 1982a and b).

Expert auditory assessment should be undertaken as early in life as possible and continued even when hearing appears to be normal. Careful checks should be made at approximately one year of age, at about two to three years, and again at school entry at four to five years. Hearing aids should be fitted as soon as this is practicable.

Later in Infancy and Childhood. The onset of generalized lung disease due to interstitial pneumonitis may be insidious, and treatment with corticosteroids is recommended. Nutritional requirements may require adjustment in cases of chronic and prolonged diarrhea. The rare cases of retarded growth owing to growth hormone deficiency or hypothyroidism require appropriate replacement therapy.

One of the most important aspects of the management of congenital rubella is to ensure an overall and regular developmental assessment. It is advisable that one physician be responsible for the coordination of a child's treatment. A child with cataracts and heart disease should have as complete an assessment as one with perceptive deafness, and *vice versa*. Children with cerebral palsy and muscular abnormalities require intensive and prolonged physiotherapy. As the child grows older, consideration must be given to the form of education best suited to his or her physical and mental condition. Every effort should be made to place the child in a normal school and to advise and encourage the parents. But again, continued reassessment is essential, particularly for the child with partial hearing loss, since deterioration may go undetected. Children in special schools for the deaf and handicapped should also be assessed at intervals because of the possibility that an original examination may have been incorrect.

Attempts to limit virus excretion by treatment with antiviral drugs such as amantadine have been largely unsuccessful (Plotkin et al., 1966).

LABORATORY ASPECTS

Properties of the Virus

Rubella virus was originally grouped with the unclassified RNA viruses. Holmes and Warburton (1967) and Holmes (1969) have suggested that because the virus has some morphological and biological properties in common with the arboviruses, such as the possession of a hemagglutinating antibody, it should be classified as an arbovirus. There is no indication, however, that an arthropod vector plays any role in the transmission of rubella. Andrews and co-workers (1978) have preferred that the rubella virus be classified as rubivirus, a member of the Togaviridae.

Morphology. Electron microscopy of both ultrathin and negatively stained preparations has revealed virions between 50 and 70 nm in diameter surrounded by an outer envelope 8 nm in thickness. Negatively stained preparations show that the virus is pleomorphic without obvious symmetry (Best et al., 1967). Kistler and colleagues (1967) found changes in the mucus-secreting cells of human embryonic nasal and tracheal organ cultures, and virus particles were seen at the cell surface, particularly between the microvilli. Some of the secretory cells contained large osmophilic inclusion bodies with distorted cell organelles and myelin whorls.

Chemical Composition. Infectious single-stranded RNA virus with a molecular weight of 3×10^6 daltons has been obtained from virions of infected cells (Hovi and Vaheri, 1970).

Physiochemical Properties. The virus is reasonably stable at 4° C in virus maintenance or transport medium for periods of up to one week. Initial studies on the buoyant density of the infectious virus particle revealed low figures of 1.085 to 1.120 gm/ml, depending on the techniques employed. Other studies revealed figures of 1.16 to 1.21 gm/ml (Magnusson and Skaaret, 1967; McCombs and Rawls, 1968).

The virus is sensitive to lipid solvents, ether, chloroform, and changes in pH. The optimal pH is 6 or 7; rubella virus is labile at pH 5 and rapidly inactivated at pH 3.

Hemagglutination. The virus causes agglutination of one or two day old chick red blood cells (Stewart et al., 1967). Hemagglutination is maximal at 4° C and less marked at room temperature (25° C). Erythrocytes of other species are also agglutinated by rubella virus, as are pigeon, goose, sheep, and tanned human cells. Enhancement of the hemagglutinating antigen (HA) can be achieved by treatment of virus-infected cultures with polysorbate 80 (Tween 80) (Furukawa et al., 1967; Halonen et al., 1967).

Antigenic Properties. Rubella virus consists of a single antigenic strain. In this respect it resembles measles virus and does not show any evidence of possessing serological subtypes or of undergoing the antigenic variation that is such a common feature of influenza and other respiratory viruses. Minor antigenic differences have been described by Fogel and Plotkin (1967) from kinetic neutralization and adsorption studies, but Banatvala and Best (1969), in a comparison of eight different attenuated or laboratory-adapted and recently isolated strains, could find no differences by HI tests.

Another method of detecting antigenic differences is by observing the morphology of plaques (Fogel and Plotkin, 1967; Lawrence and Gould, 1969). Differences in plaque size were observed by Lawrence and Gould (1969) among several virus strains, but they were not apparently related to the passage level or to the degree of attenuation. However, Doss (1972) found that differences in plaque size could be detected between some wild strains and vaccine strain, provided that the technique for measuring plaque size was carefully controlled.

Despite the lack of evidence of antigenic variation, the possibility that strains may vary in virulence cannot be dismissed. The extensive epidemics that occurred in the 1940's and 1960's may be explained on the basis of a highly susceptible population, a change in virulence in the virus, or both. It seems doubtful that the severity of the disease seen in patients with congenital rubella from 1962 onward can be explained entirely by better methods of clinical investigation. It has been reported from Japan that the incidence of congenital defects is very low, although the incidence of women of childbearing age susceptible to rubella is not dissimilar to that in countries in Europe and North America. Kono (1969) has postulated that this difference could be due to the fact that the indigenous Japanese strains are less teratogenic than virus strains isolated in Taiwan and in the United States. He produced some evidence in laboratory animals to support this hypothesis, but other workers have failed to substantiate his findings. Nevertheless, the possibility that strains of rubella virus may vary in virulence or undergo antigenic variation cannot be dismissed.

Rubella Antigens. Rubella virus consists of an HA antigen, complement-fixing (CF) antigens, and precipitating antigens.

The HA antigen is known to be located at the cell surface because hemadsorption has been observed in infected cell cultures (Lennette and Schmidt, 1969) and because virus particles have been observed at the cell surface by electron microscopy (Holmes and Warburton, 1967; Lennette and Schmidt, 1969).

Two *CF antigens* have been described: a large-particle antigen extracted from concentrated fluid-phase antigens and a smaller-particle antigen extracted from the cellular phase of infected cell cultures with alkaline-buffered saline. The two antigens can be separated by Sephadex-gel filtration (Schmidt and Lennette, 1969). The smaller-particle or soluble antigen has a lower buoyant density than the larger particle and is not associated with infectious or hemagglutinating activity, as is the larger particle. Schmidt and Lennette (1969) have shown that both antigens have a similar protein composition and that the small particle may be a subunit of the virus coat rather than an internal component.

Two *precipitating antigens* have been described by Le Bouvier (1969); they have been termed theta and iota antigens. The theta antigen also appears to be a surface antigen and may be a subunit of the HA antigen. Precipitins to it develop and persist in a manner similar to that of HI antibody, whereas anti-iota precipitin behaves more like the response to CF antibody: it appears more slowly and falls more rapidly. Some congenital rubella–infected infants continue to produce anti-iota precipitin for up to two years after the usual period of virus excretion. This indicates that virus synthesis is continuing.

Cultivation of Rubella Virus. The virus was first isolated in primary human cultures (Weller and Neva, 1962) and primary African green monkey kidney (AGMK) cultures (Parkman et al., 1962). Initially, evidence of virus replication was difficult to establish because the cytopathic effects in human amnion cultures were slow to develop and because in monkey kidney cultures replication could be detected only indirectly by the interference technique, that is, challenge inoculation of infected cultures with another virus capable of causing a cytopathic effect. As experience in handling rubella virus grew, it was realized that the virus can be cultivated in a wide range of cells, many of which are suitable for diagnostic purposes or for antigen or vaccine production. Details are discussed in Chapter 14 (Table 14–4 and Figs. 14–3 and 14–4).

Laboratory Diagnosis

A precise diagnosis of rubella can be made only by means of laboratory tests. There are several situations in which such tests, carried out at the appropriate time, can be of value. They can be used for epidemiological surveys to detect the incidence of susceptible persons in a population, in the determination of the immune status of a woman who acquires or is exposed to rubella in pregnancy, and in the general management of rubella in pregnant women. They are also of great value in the diagnosis of congenital rubella and in determining the effectiveness of rubella vaccines.

The laboratory procedures available for the diagnosis of intrauterine viral infections are described in detail in Chapter 14, but they are summarized here for the sake of convenience. The methods used for the collection of material and the main procedures for diagnosis—namely, (1) virus isolation, (2) serological tests for rubella antibody, and (3) tests for IgM- and IgG-specific antibodies—are detailed here.

At the time the first edition of this book was published in 1978, laboratory procedures for the diagnosis of virus diseases in general were undergoing a major transformation. Traditional tests based on isolation of the causative agent, together with tests that distinguished a rise in antibody between acute and convalescent sera, were being replaced by alternative techniques that were more sensitive and more reliable, and yielded results more quickly. This trend has continued, and there is now a wide range of laboratory procedures that can provide vital information both quickly and with precision. In order to derive the maximum benefit from the tests available and achieve a correct diagnosis in individual circumstances, it is incumbent on both clinicians and virologists to appreciate their complementary roles.

Two main situations now exist in which laboratory tests can play a significant part in the control of rubella and in the management of rubella in pregnancy and its consequences. Ultimately these circumstances should not arise, because when rubella immunization is properly utilized the ill-effects of rubella in pregnancy should no longer exist. Until that stage has been reached, however, much can be done to reduce the risk of congenital rubella infection and its consequences.

First, screening tests to detect an individual's rubella immune status play a vital part in the detection of those women who are susceptible and need protection by immunization. Secondly, a precise diagnosis of rubella following an illness or contact with rubella in pregnancy can now be made in most circumstances, so that appropriate advice can be given or action taken by a patient's physician. In these circumstances several general points should be borne in mind:

1. Virologists have available highly sensitive tests for detecting rubella antibody and rubella-specific IgM antibody. The choice of the test to be employed and its interpretation are matters for the virologist, but he or she must be guided by detailed information that the clinician should supply.

2. The emphasis in the laboratory diagnosis of rubella has moved away from virus isolation procedures (valuable though they are in special circumstances) to serological tests. The time of collection of serum specimens in relation to the onset of disease or date of contact with it is vital to the selection of the appropriate test as well as to the interpretation of the results.

3. The diagnosis of rubella must be based on a full understanding of the pathogenesis of the disease, the length of the incubation period, and the time of appearance of rubella antibodies and of IgM-specific antibody. The pathogenesis is depicted in Figure 3–1. The incubation period is usually 16 to 18 days, with a range of 14 to 21 days. Rubella antibodies appear soon thereafter, but the antibody response varies considerably from one individual to another as well as with the test employed. Some individuals have detectable HI antibody within 24 hours of the onset of the rash, or even earlier. In most cases HI antibody appears within five to seven days of the rash and increases rapidly thereafter, reaching a peak at 21 to 28 days after the rash appears. Antibody titers may decline up to 10-fold over the next five years, but again marked individual variation is encountered.

It is generally inadvisable to attempt to distinguish between a recent infection and one in the remote past on the basis of the antibody level in a single sample of serum, whether the level is expressed as the HI titer or in international units. In many individuals a high level of antibody may be suggestive of a recent infection, but this is not always the case. Similarly, a comparatively low titer (15 to 100 IU/ml) may indicate a past infection or the start of a rising titer. Unless two samples of sera, collected at appropriate times in relation to the incubation period, can be compared using the same test, it may be difficult to distinguish between a recent and a past infection without recourse to IgM estimates.

4. The selection of tests for rubella antibody detection and in particular for IgM-specific antibody must depend upon the experience and workload of individual laboratories.

Diagnosis of Postnatal Rubella

The laboratory tests outlined in Table 3–18 have a special relevance for the diagnosis of clinical illnesses suspected to be caused by rubella and for determining the immune status of women exposed to rubella in pregnancy. Equally important is the application of these refined techniques for the estimation of a woman's rubella immune status. Virus isolation tests have been included in the table, although they are of less practical value nowadays in view of the development of improved serological techniques.

The three situations following a clinical illness diagnosed as rubella that are outlined in Table 3–18 are the ones most commonly encountered. Provided the tests are correctly carried out with the necessary controls, it should be possible to make a definitive diagnosis if sera, especially repeat specimens, are collected at the appropriate times.

In cases of contact with rubella or suspected rubella it is important to allow sufficient time between the collection of specimens, bearing in mind the length of the incubation period and the fact that subclinical infection is common in rubella. If clinical disease develops in the exposed individual, tests can be carried out in the way described in Table 3–18 for an individual with illness and rash. If no disease develops within 14 to 21 days after contact, further tests should be performed to determine whether seroconversion has occurred. In both situations, clinical illness and contact with rubella, difficulties may be encountered in the interpretation of the significance of low levels of antibody in single serum specimens. These difficulties may be obviated by testing a further specimen for an increase in antibody or by testing for specific IgM. The presence of IgM antibody is strongly suggestive of a recent infection, whereas IgG suggests an infection in the past or, if associated with a rising titer, reinfection. IgM-specific antibody appears early in the disease and usually reaches a peak three to six weeks after onset of the rash. It may persist for several months after infection in some individuals (Al-Nakib et al., 1975). Tests for IgM antibody are now much easier to perform and yield valuable data as to the probability of a recent infection having occurred. There is now less reluctance on the part of clinicians to ask for such tests, and many laboratories are in a position to offer them (Cradock-Watson et al., 1979, 1980).

The screening tests based on radial hemolysis (RH) and HI tests, which compare test sera with control sera of known potency, are invaluable in determining an individual's immune status. In the majority of cases, the results are clear-cut, either "immune" or "susceptible." Few sera are found to have borderline levels of antibody. When these are encountered it is advisable to regard the individual as susceptible.

As a result of these tests a number of individuals will be identified who are susceptible and who therefore require vaccination against rubella at an appropriate time. In addition, cases of recent infection in pregnant women may be identified. The management of such cases depends on the risk of fetal damage and the gestational age at which infection has occurred. Clinicians need this information to make their judgments on the action to be taken.

Diagnosis of Prenatal or Congenital Rubella

The laboratory tests described in Chapter 14 and briefly summarized in the preceding paragraphs are equally valuable in the diagnosis of congenital rubella (see Table 3–19). They also have an important role to play in the surveillance of rubella vaccine immunization programs. The tests to be employed depend to a great extent on the age of the child.

In the Newborn Period. A retrospective diagnosis of intrauterine infection can be made either by isolation of the virus from the urine or nasopharynx, by the demonstration of IgM-specific antibody, or by both methods. The studies of Cradock-Watson and his colleagues (1979, 1980) have demonstrated the value and practicability of serological tests for rubella IgM antibody in infants with congenital rubella. The ability to recover virus from the congenitally infected child depends on his or her age and also on technical considerations. Virus isolation and

Table 3-18. LABORATORY DIAGNOSIS OF POSTNATAL RUBELLA*

Clinical Situation	Laboratory Test and Result	Interpretation	Action Required	Interpretation
1. Illness with rash in past 7 days	a. HI test < 15 IU	Susceptible	Repeat in 7–10 days	i. Rising titer indicates recent infection† ii. No change: not rubella
	b. HI test 15–100 IU	? Immune	Repeat in 7–10 days + IgM	i. No change and IgM negative indicates past infection ii. Rising titer and IgM positive indicates recent infection† iii. Rising titer and IgM negative indicates reinfection
	c. HI test 100–200 IU	? Recent infection ? Immune	Repeat in 7–10 days + IgM	i. Rising titer and IgM positive indicates recent infection† ii. No change and IgM positive indicates recent infection† iii. No change and IgM negative indicates past infection
	Virus isolation test with virus isolated from subject	Proof of infection, but usually impracticable because of time factor		
2. After contact with rubella within 7 days	a. HI test < 15 IU	Susceptible	Repeat in 14–21 days	i. No change: not infected or not rubella ii. Rising titer indicates recent infection†
	b. HI test > 15 IU	Immune	No action	
3. After contact within 14 days	a. HI test < 15 IU	Susceptible	Repeat as in 1a and + IgM	
	b. HI test > 15–100 IU	? Immune ? Recent infection	Repeat in 7 days + IgM	i. No change and IgM negative indicates past infection ii. Rising titer and IgM positive indicates recent infection† iii. No change and IgM positive indicates recent infection†
4. Screening tests for immune status	a. HI test > 15 IU		Rubella antibody detected: immune, no action unless recently exposed to rubella	
	b. HI test < 15 IU		Rubella antibody not detected: susceptible, *vaccinate*§	
	c. HI test = 8 IU/ml		Antibody detected in low titer: regard as susceptible, offer vaccine§	
	d. SRH‡ zone ≥ 15 IU		Antibody detected: probably immune unless recently exposed‡	
	e. SRH no zone		Antibody not detected: susceptible, *vaccinate*§	
	f. SRH zone < 15 IU		Antibody probably present in low titer: Regard as susceptible, *vaccinate*§	

*HI = hemagglutination-inhibition test; IU = international units/ml; SRH = single radial hemolysis (sometimes referred to as RH or radial hemolysis).

†Recent infection implies fetus at risk if subject is pregnant.

‡The routine test will not distinguish between a recent or past infection. Inquire if patient is pregnant and proceed as in 1b above.

§Vaccinate unless there are contraindications.

Table 3–19. **LABORATORY DIAGNOSIS OF PRENATAL AND CONGENITAL RUBELLA**

Test	Result	Interpretation
A. *In the newborn period*		
Virus isolation	Positive from urine, nasopharynx, lens, tissue etc.	Proof of diagnosis
	Negative	Does not exclude congenital rubella, therefore carry out serological test in parallel
Serology		
Cord blood for HI* and IgM	IgM positive	Evidence of congenital rubella
	IgM negative	Does not exclude congenital rubella, perform HI tests
HI on infant and mother	HI positive on both	Repeat at 4–6 months to detect persistence of HI in infant serum
B. *In infancy and early childhood*		
HI test on infant and mother	HI positive on both	Strongly suggestive of congenital rubella if antibody persists in infant; of greater significance if child under 4 years of age
	HI negative in infant or child	Congenital rubella not confirmed

*HI test for rubella IgG antibody or by another test deemed to be appropriate, e.g., RIA (see Chapter 14).

the test for IgM-specific antibody are of maximal value as diagnostic procedures in the first few weeks of life. The demonstration of a raised total IgM is of some value as a screening test, but this occurs in only approximately 50 per cent of confirmed cases of congenital rubella. Serological tests for HI antibody at this age are of little value because no distinction can be made between maternal and fetal IgG antibody. The tests should, therefore, be repeated at six to eight months of age.

Later in Infancy and Childhood. Since rubella antibody persists for prolonged periods in the congenitally infected infant, serological tests for HI antibody are particularly useful when carried out after six months of age (when maternally transmitted antibody will have largely disappeared) and before the fourth year of life, when antibody may be acquired as a result of natural exposure.

The use of these tests is discussed in further detail under Congenital Rubella and Vaccine Surveillance.

PREVENTION

General Considerations

The basic principles that govern the prevention of viral infections in the fetus and newborn are described in Chapter 15, but for the sake of convenience they are included here in summary form.

The occurrence of congenital rubella defects as a direct consequence of maternal rubella constitutes a *prima facie* case of a need for prevention. Before the introduction of rubella vaccination in the United Kingdom the total number of reported cases of congenital rubella defects was approximately 250 per annum (Dudgeon, 1972), but this figure was almost certainly an underestimate as it did not take into account the frequency of deafness due to rubella. The experience of the 1964 to 1965 pandemic highlighted the frequency of multiple defects and multiple handicaps and the suffering of the affected children and their families (Cooper et al., 1969). In purely financial terms, the cost of the medical, social, and educational services required by the pandemic exceeded $1 billion.

Theoretically, congenital rubella can be prevented by immunization, either passive or active, as with any other infectious disease, but there is an important difference in the approach to prevention of congenital rubella defects by immunization. The normal method of protecting an individual against an infectious disease such as diphtheria or measles is by active immunization prior to exposure. In the case of rubella it is different. The object is to protect the fetus indirectly by affording protection before a pregnancy is started, by immunization either in childhood or close to the age of childbearing. As many women of childbearing age are not immune to rubella, vaccination helps to bridge the gap left by nature by reducing the number of susceptible females who may contract the disease in pregnancy. The principle is not dissimilar to the indirect method of prevention of neonatal tetanus achieved by active immunization of the mother.

Passive Immunization

Much has been written during the past 25 years about the value, or lack of value, of passive immunization with immunoglobulin (IG). Since the matter is discussed in detail in Chapter 15, it is sufficient to say here that, whereas it is agreed that the use of IG for passive immunization *as a routine procedure* in rubella prevention is totally impracticable on several grounds, a case can be made for its use in special circumstances, such as those of a pregnant woman exposed to rubella who is anxious for the pregnancy to continue to term. This should in no way reduce emphasis on the need for active immunization at an earlier date to keep such an event from occurring. Details of IG dosage and of the essential laboratory tests to be carried out in association with its administration are also discussed in Chapter 15.

The important point to remember about passive immunization procedures in general is that they can be used either to prevent a disease or to modify its effect. This distinction is important. In the case of rubella complete suppression of infection is the objective, whereas with infectious hepatitis (virus A) or measles (before a measles vaccine became available) modification or suppression of symptoms was acceptable. As it is well known that subclinical rubella can cause fetal damage, it is essential to monitor the effect of administration of IG in cases of rubella in pregnant women by using serological tests to determine whether infection has occurred.

Active Immunization

Active immunization is the most effective form of prevention. Its advantage is that, given a satisfactory vaccine, the immunity that results is of long duration; in many circumstances, it could last as long as immunity produced by natural infection.

Active immunization can be achieved either by means of a killed inactivated product that is given in a series of injections spaced at intervals of several weeks and that

usually requires a booster inoculation, or by means of a live attenuated vaccine.

Requirements for a Rubella Vaccine. A number of basic criteria are required for a rubella vaccine, especially for a live attenuated product. There should be (1) an absence of undesirable reactions or side-effects, (2) no evidence of transmissibility to susceptible contacts, (3) no adverse effects on the fetus, (4) a satisfactory immune response that is long-lasting, and (5) a safe virus strain and cell substrate acceptable for vaccine production.

Killed Inactivated Rubella Vaccines. In theory, an inactivated rubella vaccine might offer certain advantages over a live attenuated vaccine because in the latter, although the virulence of the virus is modified, the risk always remains that the modified attenuated strain might still be teratogenic.

Attempts to produce such a killed rubella vaccine have been disappointing. Sever and co-workers (1963) and Frankel (1964) reported that formaldehyde-treated preparations induced antibody responses in susceptible persons, but Buynak and colleagues (1968) found that a purified and concentrated preparation failed to do so. There was also some doubt concerning whether the antibody responses that did occur resulted from small quantities of residual live virus in the vaccine. Beck (1969) reported that rubella virus could be readily inactivated by formaldehyde, ultraviolet irradiation, ether, and beta-propiolactone, but the preparations were not antigenic. By the time of this report, considerable progress had been made in the development of attenuated rubella vaccine strains, and the development of inactivated products had been abandoned on grounds of lack of antigenic potency. A further theoretical risk was that patients inoculated with an inactivated preparation might become sensitized and develop reactions similar to those observed following the use of killed measles vaccine.

Live Attenuated Rubella Vaccines. Experimental studies by Parkman and co-workers (1966) showed that rubella virus strains repeatedly subcultured in AGMK cultures became attenuated. The seventy-seventh passage virus (HPV-77) was shown to be of reduced virulence for monkeys in that it produced a nontransmissible inapparent infection with antibody conversion in all of the animals.

Meyer and his colleagues (1966, 1967) carried out clinical trials with the HPV-77 strain by subcutaneous inoculation of 51 susceptible children; 49 seronegative children were left unvaccinated as contact controls. None of the children manifested symptoms, all showed seroconversion, and pharyngeal excretion of the vaccine virus was detected intermittently in 75 per cent between the seventh and twenty-first days after inoculation. All unvaccinated contacts remained well, none excreted virus, and none showed evidence of seroconversion.

This trial raised a number of important issues regarding the development and use of attenuated rubella vaccines. Virus excretion from the nasopharynx following subcutaneous inoculation indicated that viremia had probably occurred. The excreted virus, although shown to be present in low titer, might lead to infection of a susceptible contact and, if administered to a susceptible pregnant woman, could cause damage to the fetus. At this time manufacturers and others responsible for vaccine development were becoming increasingly apprehensive about the problem of safety of vaccines prepared from monkey kidney cultures because of the risk of latent simian agents.

In view of the wide range of cell cultures in which rubella virus can be cultivated, the selection of an alternative type of cell substrate did not present an insurmountable problem, but the question of transmissibility and viremia did pose special problems because of the potential risk of transmission to a susceptible pregnant woman and subsequent fetal damage.

By 1969 a number of alternative rubella vaccines had been developed, and clinical trials were initiated in human volunteers to answer some of the questions raised by the earlier experimental studies. Details about some of these vaccines, together with information about the virus strain, seed virus, and cell substrate, are shown in Table 3–20. Details of the clinical trials, most of which were carried out with a limited number of vaccines,

have been fully reported at two international conferences. The first was held in London in 1968 (International Symposium on Rubella Vaccines, 1969) and the second at Bethesda, Maryland, in 1969 (International Conference on Rubella Immunization, 1969) (Dudgeon, 1969b).

The trials, involving immunization of many thousands of susceptible persons in many different countries and detailed clinical and virological investigations, established a number of facts relative to licensure of rubella vaccines for routine use.

1. In general, the vaccines did not cause any severe or untoward side-effects, except for joint reactions that appeared to be age- and sex-related in that they were encountered more often in adult females than in children or adult males. One vaccine prepared in dog kidney cell cultures (HPV-77DK12) caused more severe joint reactions than did other vaccines and was withdrawn by the manufacturer after licensure.

2. The vaccines tested were all immunogenic, producing satisfactory antibody levels and seroconversion in 85 to 98 per cent (in most cases closer to the latter figure) of the vaccinated subjects. Most investigators found that the antibody levels were approximately fourfold lower than those seen after natural infection.

3. No definite evidence of virus transmission from vaccinees to susceptible contacts was found, despite exhaustive studies and the fact that many thousands of doses had been administered. No evidence of transmission of infection was found in newborn infants whose mothers had been vaccinated in the postpartum period, even among those who were breast-fed. Four episodes of potential transmission from a vaccinee to a contact were reported as the result of serological tests, but at the time it was not possible to determine whether these were natural or vaccine-induced infections (Dudgeon et al., 1969; Lipman, 1969; Lefkowitz et al., 1970;

Table 3–20. **LIVE ATTENUATED RUBELLA VACCINES CURRENTLY LICENSED**

Vaccine Strain (Trade Name)	Cell Substrate for Preparation of Vaccine	No. of Passages Used for Seed Virus
Cendehill vaccine (Cendevax)	Primary rabbit kidney cell cultures	51st passage
Duck embryo HPV-77 DE5* (Meruvax)	Duck embryo cell cultures	HPV × 77 DE × 5
RA27/3 (Almevax)	Human diploid fibroblasts, W1-38 strain	27 passages in diploid cells
RA27/3 (Meruvax II)	Human diploid fibroblast cultures	27 passages in diploid cells

*HPV DE5 = high passage virus duct embryo fifth passage.

Schiff et al., 1970). These facts are all well documented in the reports of the international symposia already referred to (International Symposium on Rubella Vaccines, 1969; International Conference on Rubella Immunization, 1969). Because of their safety, relative lack of severe reactions, immune responsiveness, and lack of evidence of transmissibility, the vaccines listed in Table 3–20 were licensed in 1969 and 1970 for the routine prevention of rubella (Dudgeon, 1969b). The key questions of duration of immunity and possible adverse effect on the fetus remained for the time unanswered.

Vaccination Policy

The object of vaccination against rubella is to prevent congenital rubella infection and, therefore, rubella defects. The first discussions on future policy for rubella vaccination took place at the International Conference on Rubella Immunization in 1969. From this emerged two broad vaccination strategies, usually referred to as the United States (U.S.) and the United Kingdom (U.K.) strategies. Both have been maintained over the past decade and have remained substantially the same, although both have been amended and extended in their tactical application (Dudgeon, 1979; Hinman et al., 1979).

The U.S. approach was at first directed toward mass vaccination of prepubertal children of both sexes, with subsequent vaccination of children of both sexes from the age of one year onward (Centers For Disease Control [CDC], 1970; "ACIP Recommendations," 1972). This strategy was intended to break the chain of transmission among young children and thereby to reduce the risk of infection among adult women. It also presumed that vaccine-induced immunity would be lifelong and would provide protection for girls throughout their subsequent childbearing years. At this stage it was recommended that if combined vaccines, such as measles-mumps-rubella (MMR), were used, vaccination should not be performed before children reached the age of 15 months.

The U.K. strategy was, and is, different. It involved selective immunization of girls just before they entered the childbearing period by offering vaccination at 11 to 14 years of age. This approach was based on the presumption that vaccine-induced immunity might not be lifelong, and at the time the vaccination program was introduced in the United Kingdom in 1970 there was no way to be sure. It was presumed that vaccination close to the age of childbearing might be more likely than vaccination in early childhood to confer immunity throughout this vulnerable period. Furthermore, by restricting vaccination to females, natural infections would continue to occur in unvaccinated males, providing a booster effect by re-exposure to wild virus. Thus the two main vaccination programs concentrated initially either on mass vaccination of children or on selective immunization of older girls. Both strategies have since been considerably modified to include older at-risk groups, but without changing their main targets.

In the United States in 1969 and 1970 rubella vaccination was recommended for children of both sexes from one year of age to puberty. The emphasis was on the need to immunize children in kindergarten and elementary school. A cautious approach was taken to vaccinating postpubertal females because of the risk to the fetus if the vaccinee was pregnant. Therefore, routine immunization was not recommended unless the possibility of pregnancy could be excluded (Centers for Disease Control, 1970). In 1971 it was considered desirable to extend the vaccination program to include adolescent girls and adult females, subject to serologic testing and the subjects' avoidance of pregnancy (Centers for Disease Control, 1971). Between 1976 and 1978 a further expansion was recommended to include susceptible postpubertal females (subject always to contraindications), adolescent females, and males in population groups such as training colleges, military bases, and so forth. Serological testing was to be extended, where practical, to include testing of nonpregnant adult females, premarital testing, and antenatal and antepartum testing (Centers for Disease Control, 1980). In 1981 the Advisory Committee on Immunization Procedures (ACIP) endorsed the earlier recommendations and went somewhat further. Having taken into account the accumulated evidence resulting from the inadvertent administration of rubella vaccines to pregnant women, the ACIP concluded that there was little or no evidence of a teratogenic effect from the two vaccines currently licensed in the United States ("Recommendations of the Immunization Practices Advisory Committee (ACIP)" 1981). It stated, therefore, that "rubella vaccination should not be a reason to *routinely* recommend interruption of pregnancy. . . . The ACIP believes that the risk of vaccine associated malformations is so small as to be negligible" (italics added for emphasis).

As a result of this change in attitude, which is discussed further in a later section, less emphasis was placed on serological testing and more on questioning postpubertal females about whether they were pregnant or likely to be and on instructing them about the need to avoid pregnancy for three months after vaccination. Further emphasis was placed on the need to extend vaccination to at-risk adult groups, both female and male, and to provide proof wherever possible of rubella immunity by serological tests. Premarital screening was recommended, as was prenatal screening followed by postnatal vaccination where appropriate.

In the United Kingdom, the initial program instituted in 1970 recommended vaccination of girls between the ages of 11 and 14 years. In 1972 vaccination of women of childbearing age was made available on request for those shown by serological testing to be susceptible. In 1974 an intensive effort to vaccinate more girls aged 11 to 14 was made, and in 1976 a routine serological test for rubella antibody was made available to women attending family planning clinics. Postpartum vaccination was strongly recommended. In 1981 the initial age of vaccination for girls was reduced from 11 to 10 years.

Until 1981, these were the two main alternative vaccination policies used in different countries, but it must be emphasized that in some countries vaccination was strongly recommended whereas in others vaccine was made available without any clear-cut recommendations.

At that time, public health authorities in the United States were moving toward a progressive campaign to eliminate diseases such as measles and rubella by the use of combined vaccines together with an element of compulsion. The "compulsion" involved requiring a certificate of vaccination against six common communicable diseases, including rubella, prior to school entry. The U.S. program has already resulted in a noticeable decline in naturally acquired rubella, as well as in the reported incidence of congenital rubella. This effect, which was predictable, has been more noticeable than in the United Kingdom. A number of individuals and health authorities there have suggested that implementation of a program like the U.S. program would be more likely to solve the problem of the control of congenital rubella.

However, major changes in immunization policies should be undertaken only for good reason, and failure to implement a sound policy is not a good reason to give that policy up. Furthermore, it is difficult to underestimate the effect of the combined MMR vaccine in the United States in controlling both measles and rubella. As was pointed out at a conference in 1982 on "The Conquest of Agents That Endanger the Brain" (Dudgeon, 1983), the acceptance rate of measles vaccine in the United Kingdom is so low, around 50 per cent of those eligible, that a change to the U.S. scheme might be counterproductive. In the meantime, a third program was started in Sweden in January 1982 (Taranger, 1982). A comparison of the three schemes is shown in Table 3–21.

Information Gained Since 1969

An immense amount of information has been acquired since rubella vaccines were licensed in 1969 and 1970. This information is here considered as it relates to the requirements for a rubella vaccine set out earlier.

1. Vaccination reactions

The only reactions of any consequence experienced by the vaccinees have been arthritis and arthralgia. These were much more severe following use of the HPV-77 dog kidney vaccine than with other rubella vaccines, as a result of which HPV-77 dog kidney vaccine was withdrawn from the market. In a comparative trial of several rubella vaccines it was found that joint symptoms occurred frequently in adult females, in 23 per cent to 42 per cent of cases, depending on the vaccine used (Best et al., 1974). In general, these joint symptoms are seldom sufficiently serious to prevent an affected individual from normal activities unless frank arthritis occurs.

2. Transmissibility

No conclusive evidence of transmission from vaccinee to susceptible contacts has been recorded despite extensive use of vaccines, many millions of doses of which have now been administered. In the few reported cases already referred to, contact with wild virus could not be ruled out. Although rubella vaccine strains can be recovered from the nasopharynx, the amount of vaccine excreted appears to be in low titer and insuffi-

Table 3–21. **VACCINATION PROGRAMS AGAINST RUBELLA**
A Comparison of Three Different Programs to Prevent Congenital Rubella*

Country	Objective	Vaccine Schedule	Target Groups for Vaccination
United Kingdom Australia, Israel Some European countries Canada (some provinces)*	Selective immunization Protection of the individual	Monovalent rubella vaccine Single dose, 0.5 ml	1. Girls aged 10–14 years 2. Susceptible adult females 3. Postpartum vaccination following antenatal screening 4. Health care personnel, nurses (including males), doctors, hospital staff, teachers, play-group leaders, therapists, etc.
United States and North America	Eradication of rubella Break in transmission of virus Direct protection of those at risk	Mainly MMR† for children Monovalent for adults Single dose, 0.5 ml	1. All children over 12 months to puberty (at 15 months if MMR is used) 2. Adolescent and adult females (serological tests if practical) 3. Educational, health, and military groups 4. Premarital and prenatal screening for adult females
Sweden	Eradication of rubella, measles, and mumps in 10 years	MMR Two doses, 0.5 ml	1. All children at 18 months and 12 years (voluntary)

*Some Canadian provinces changed to U.S. Vaccination Program in 1983–1984.
†MMR = Measles, mumps, and rubella trivalent vaccine.

cient to be communicable. For practical purposes, rubella vaccine infections can be regarded as noncommunicable. Indeed, all vaccination programs currently in use are based on the acceptance of this fact. No restrictions need be imposed on vaccinated children who will inevitably come into contact with their mothers at home.

3. Adverse effect on the fetus: teratogenicity

The problems of teratogenicity and duration of immunity were the two most important factors under consideration at the time of vaccine licensure.

Administration of rubella vaccine is contraindicated at any stage in pregnancy (see Chapter 15) because there is no method to determine whether the process of attenuation is accompanied by a lack of teratogenicity. Until the development of such a test, which seems unlikely in view of the difficulty of adapting rubella viruses to an animal model system, it should be assumed that all vaccine strains could be teratogenic. Inadvertent administration of vaccine to pregnant women is bound to occur, since it may be given to a woman who does not know that she is pregnant at the time. The risk can be reduced by pretesting all adult women of childbearing age for rubella antibody. Only those suscep-

tible need be given vaccine and then only when precautions against pregnancy are observed. The logistical difficulties of performing screening tests for rubella antibody are considerable. This has been apparent in the evolution of rubella vaccination programs in the United States and the United Kingdom. If it is practical, serological testing should be incorporated into vaccination programs for adult females.

Reports of inadvertent rubella vaccination in women shortly before or after conception have been reported from the Centers for Disease Control (CDC), Atlanta, Georgia (1976). The details are summarized in Tables 3–22 and 3–23. For the 353 pregnancies listed, the immune status of the mothers was known in only 85 cases, and of the 71 susceptibles, 38 gave birth to liveborn infants, none with evidence of congenital rubella. It can be seen from Tables 3–22 and 3–23 that rubella vaccine virus can infect the placenta, cross the placenta, and produce fetal infection. In such cases, it must be assumed that the fetus might be damaged. Of a series of 19 pregnancies complicated by rubella vaccination that were studied by Fleet and co-workers, (1974), 10 went to term, eight were terminated, and one aborted spontaneously. The 10 liveborn infants were normal at birth and have so far shown no sign of infection. Virus was recovered from the eye of one of the

Table 3–22. **OUTCOME OF PREGNANCIES IN WOMEN RECEIVING RUBELLA VACCINE SHORTLY BEFORE OR AFTER CONCEPTION (Accumulated Data Through 1976)**

| Prevaccination Immunity Status | No. of Cases | Outcome of Pregnancy | | | |
| | | Abortion | | Delivery of Live Infant | Unknown |
		Therapeutic	*Spontaneous*		
Susceptible	71	29	3	38	1
Immune	14	1	0	13	0
Unknown	268	124	14	122	8
Total	353	154	17	173	9

From Centers for Disease Control: Rubella Surveillance, July 1973–December 1975; p. 11. Issued August 1976.

aborted cases; the other eye showed histological changes in the lens fibers.

Additional studies by Modlin and co-workers (1976) showed that 21 per cent of women known to be susceptible who elected to have a therapeutic abortion following rubella vaccination had rubella-virus culture-positive abortion specimens. Virus was isolated from tissues in nine cases, including the fetal eye in two cases, the fetal kidney in one, and the placenta or undifferentiated products of conception in the remainder. Six of the nine virus-positive specimens came from susceptible women. In contrast, it was found that none of the 172 pregnancies that went to term resulted in an abnormal birth, including those of 38 women known to be susceptible. This figure of 21 per cent culture-positive material noted by Modlin et al. (1975) is similar to that of 25 per cent reported by Vaheri and colleagues (1972), in whose study virus was isolated from the fetal kidney in one of 24 fetal specimens. The accumulated evidence by 1976, six years after vaccine licensure, indicated that vaccine virus can cross the placenta and infect the fetus but

that the risk of fetal infection and of fetal damage is difficult to estimate. A distinction must be made between placental infection and fetal infection, and unless care is taken to culture placental and fetal tissues separately a false impression of the risk can be gained.

Recent evidence from the United States, however, casts a new light on the teratogenicity of rubella vaccines currently in use. Since 1969 the CDC has maintained a registry of all women who received HPV-77 or Cendehill vaccine within three months prior to conception and in the first trimester of pregnancy. An analysis of the first 88 pregnant women, known to be susceptible, who had been vaccinated and carried their pregnancies to term revealed no evidence of abnormalities at birth. Two cases of fetal infection were identified (Preblud et al., 1980). The registry also includes data on 164 women whose immune status was unknown at the time of vaccination and who carried their pregnancies to term. No abnormalities were noted at birth, but three infants were born with positive IgM titers (Preblud et al., 1980).

Table 3–23. **CHARACTERISTICS OF PATIENTS WITH RUBELLA VACCINE–LIKE VIRUS ISOLATED FROM THERAPEUTIC ABORTION SPECIMENS**

Prevaccination Immunity Status	Gestation at Abortion (Weeks)	Interval Between Vaccination and Abortion (Weeks)	Tissues Positive for Rubella Virus
Susceptible	6	4	Undifferentiated products of conception
Susceptible	8	5	Decidua
Susceptible	14	5	Placenta
Susceptible	13	20	Fetal eye
Susceptible	13	6	Products of conception, fetal bone marrow
Susceptible	7	9	Products of conception
Unknown	14	16	Placenta, fetal eye
Unknown	13	2	Placenta, fetal kidney
Unknown	11	10	Placenta, decidua

From Centers for Disease Control: Rubella Surveillance, July 1973–December 1975, p. 12. Issued August 1976.

Preblud and colleagues also refer to four children with defects consistent with congenital rubella whose mothers had received rubella vaccine within three months of conception. Subsequent studies by a number of authors, quoted by Preblud et al. (1980), suggested that infection with wild virus may have occurred at about the time of vaccination. In a subsequent report, Preblud et al. (1981) included details of the effect of the RA27/3 vaccine, which had only recently been licensed in the United States. No evidence of fetal infection or fetal damage was encountered in 92 vaccinated pregnant women, 25 of whom were susceptible.

Information is now available on 956 women who have received rubella vaccine during pregnancy, including data on 260 women who were known to be susceptible at the time of vaccination. Details are shown in Table 3–24. In part a of the table, the data are given for those who received Cendehill or HPV-77 duck embryo vaccine. The outcome was known in 500 of 538 cases; 290 (58 per cent) had full-term pregnancies and 24 (4.5 per cent) had spontaneous abortions. None of the 94 infants born alive to susceptible mothers had any detectable abnormality. Eight infants born to susceptible mothers or mothers whose immune status was unknown showed evidence of infection, either rubella-specific IgM in the cord blood or the persistence of HI antibody beyond six months of age. All eight children, now aged two to seven years, are developing normally. The dates of vaccination and the estimated dates of conception were known for 87 of the 94 susceptible women. Of these, 33 (38 per cent) were vaccinated within one week before and four weeks after conception, which would be regarded as a major at-risk period. No abnormalities were detected in infants born at term.

The data on the use of RA27/3 human diploid vaccine have reflected a similar trend. Details of the latest evaluation for the period through December 1982 are shown in Table 3–24b. The pregnancy outcomes have now been recorded for 390 women out of a total of 418 who received this vaccine at some stage in pregnancy. Of the 111 women known to be susceptible at the time of vaccination, 81 (73 per cent, excluding two twin births) carried their pregnancies to term. Fifty-seven women (70 per cent) were vaccinated within six weeks before and six weeks after conception. None of the 346 liveborn children had any defects compatible with congenital rubella at birth, but 11 children were born with one or more congenital defects. Of these, two were born to susceptible mothers and seven to mothers of unknown immune status. The two infants born to susceptible mothers had asymptomatic glandular hypospadias, not a congenital defect normally associated with congenital rubella; both of these infants had negative serology (i.e., IgM or persistence of HI antibody). The clinical and serological evaluation of the 241 live infants born to mothers of unknown immune status did not reveal any evidence of a teratogenic effect of this vaccine or of congenital infection, except in one case.

Additional cases of subclinical congenital infection following rubella vaccination have been reported by Hayden and colleagues (1980). Rubella vaccine had been administered to four young women between conception and the fourteenth week of gestation. Serological evidence of infection was present in all cases, and no abnormalities were detected at birth. Three of the four children remained normal by two to three years of age.

From all these data acquired over the past decade, a number of general conclusions can be drawn.

Table 3–24a. **PREGNANCY OUTCOMES FOR 538 RECIPIENTS OF CENDEHILL OR HPV-77 VACCINE, UNITED STATES, THROUGH DECEMBER 31, 1981**

Prevaccination Immunity Status	Total Cases	Live Births		Spontaneous Abortions and Stillbirths		Induced Abortions		Outcome Unknown	
		No.	%	No.	%	No.	%	No.	%
Susceptible	149	94	17.5	6	1.1	43	8.0	6	1.1
Immune	25	22	4.1	0	–	3	0.5	0	–
Unknown	364	174	32.3	18	3.4	140	26.0	32	6.0
Total	538	290	53.9	24	4.5	186	34.5	38	7.1

From Rubella vaccination during pregancy. United States, 1971–1981. Morbidity Mortality Rep *31*:477–481, 1982.

Table 3–24b. **PREGNANCY OUTCOME FOR 418 RECIPIENTS OF RA27/3 VACCINE, UNITED STATES, THROUGH DECEMBER 31, 1982**

Prevaccination Immunity Status	Total Cases	Live Births		Spontaneous Abortions and Stillbirths		Induced Abortions		Outcome Unknown	
		No.	%	No.	%	No.	%	No.	%
Susceptible	111	83*	19.8	3	0.7	19	4.5	8	1.9
Immune	24	22	5.2	1	0.2	0	–	1	–
Unknown	283	241†	57.6	7	1.6	17	4.0	19	4.5
Total	418	346	82.6	11	2.5	36	8.5	28	6.4

*Includes two twin births.
†Includes one twin birth.
From Rubella vaccination during pregnancy. Morbidity Mortality Rep *32*:429–432, 1983.

a. The risk of fetal *damage* following administration of rubella vaccines in pregnancy appears to be very low indeed. Nevertheless, the data summarized in the CDC report (CDC, 1976) cannot be discounted.

b. The risk of fetal *infection* also appears to be very low, but it certainly exists. Although many of these infected children have been followed up for a number of years and their development has been uneventful, it is essential that all such cases be fully evaluated for at least five years after birth to ensure that no late-onset defects such as deafness have developed.

c. Although *pregnancy* should remain a major contraindication to the use of rubella vaccines and should be avoided for three months after vaccination, the action to be taken when vaccination and pregnancy do coincide needs to be reviewed.

The ACIP in the United States has already stated that rubella vaccination during pregnancy should not be a reason to *routinely* recommend termination. This is reasonable advice, provided it is emphasized that the evidence on which it is based is still limited. The authors concur with the statement of the ACIP that a final decision on the course of action should be discussed between patient and physician. Physicians should continue to be reminded that pregnancy remains a major contraindication to the use of rubella vaccine until many more data are available.

Despite the few instances of fetal *infection* following vaccination already referred to, there have been no reported cases, as far as the authors are aware, of fetal *damage* leading to the birth of an infant with rubella defects. This brings into question the interpretation of the Medical Termination of Pregnancy or Abortion Act in the United Kingdom (ER II Ch. 87). The relevant clause states that it is permissible under statutory law to terminate a pregnancy "if there is a substantial risk that

if the child were born it would suffer from such physical or mental subnormality as to be seriously handicapped." At present the number of pregnancies terminated in the United Kingdom on the grounds that rubella vaccination has been stated to be a contributory factor is excessive. Between 1974 and 1981, 521 legal abortions were carried out associated with rubella vaccination. This represents a figure far in excess of the number of infants with congenital rubella who were born during that period, but on the other hand the number of legal abortions associated with clinical rubella or contact with rubella during the same period was very much higher. If these pregnancies had not been terminated, the number of children born with congenital rubella would almost certainly have been very much higher. This problem emphasizes once again the need to reduce the risk of exposure to rubella, whether by wild virus or by vaccine virus, during pregnancy.

4. Vaccine-induced immunity and its duration

Most investigators have found that vaccine-induced immunity is lower in terms of antibody levels than the immunity following natural infection, but there is as yet no indication of how long protection will last. Horstmann (1975) has found that, broadly speaking, the length of immunity is probably related to the quantitative, as well as the qualitative, initial response to vaccination. In a study of several hundred children vaccinated with HPV-77 DE5 vaccine, they found that the persistence of antibody can be correlated with the initial HI antibody response. Children with an HI antibody response of greater than 1:64 also showed a response to CF antibody and anti-theta persistence, but a significant proportion of children with initial HI antibody levels of less than 1:8 to 1:16 had little or no CF or anti-theta response and were found to be seronegative after vaccination. Approximately 25 per cent of those with a poor or low response had no detectable HI antibody three years after vaccination. Horstmann concluded that if such figures were representative of the immunized population as a whole, children immunized early in life might well become susceptible in adult life, unless even after such a long interval re-exposure were to lead to an asymptomatic reinfection. Quantitative differences in the immune response following vaccination may also serve to explain the high rate of reinfection recorded by Horstmann et al. (1970) among military personnel who had been vaccinated only a few months prior to exposure to epidemic rubella.

Many investigators, however, found that rubella antibody levels were well maintained over periods ranging from four to seven years (Krugman, 1977). Meyer and Parkman (1971) found that antibody had persisted well for seven years after vaccination. Similar findings have been reported by Weibel and colleagues (1975) for 5½ years after HPV-77 duck embryo vaccine and by Herrman and colleagues (1976) in over 4000 children given either Cendehill or RA27/3 vaccine. Data on the RA27/3 vaccine were less extensive, but an initial report by Plotkin and co-workers (1973) showed that immunity was maintained for up to five years.

The crucial question, however, is the long-term effect of vaccine-induced immunity (Horstmann, 1975). Ideally, it should last as long as immunity from the natural disease, and it should certainly last for 40 years to cover the age of childbearing if vaccination is carried out early in childhood. In testing for rubella antibody as a measure of rubella immunity some years after vaccination, it is essential to use laboratory methods that can detect very low levels of antibody. Balfour and Amren (1978) found that 58 of 159 (36 per cent) children had lost detectable HI antibody three to five years after vaccination with HPV-77 duck embryo vaccine. Subsequent tests following challenge with RA27/3 vaccine showed, however, that these children were probably still immune. No viremia could be detected, and the immune response following challenge was a typical secondary-type response with undetectable or very low levels of IgM (Balfour et al., 1981). When the original prechallenge sera were retested by a more sensitive technique, rubella antibody was detected.

The long-term follow-up of the rubella antibody status of 123 nurses vaccinated between six and 16 years previously revealed persistence of antibody in approximately 90 per cent (O'Shea et al., 1982). Antibody levels above the minimum concentration (15 IU/ml) were found in 89.4 per cent, low levels (<15 IU/ml) in 8.9 per cent. Two nurses (1.6 per cent) were seronegative. A further study by the same authors showed that 97 per cent of these nurses were still seropositive eight to 18 years after vaccination, and the eight volunteers who had lost detectable antibody responded to challenge inoculation with RA27/3 vaccine without symptomatic illness. Nevertheless, viremia has been detected in two women with low concentrations of rubella antibody (Balfour et al., 1981; O'Shea et al., 1981), so continued surveillance of vaccinated groups is essential.

The risk to the fetus from reinfection after natural infection, which has already been referred to, is very low indeed. The risk following exposure after vaccination is not known but is also probably very low, assuming that there has been an adequate immune response in the first place. Two cases, however, are of interest in this connection. Forrest and her colleagues (1972) reported a case of clinical rubella 11 months after vaccination. A susceptible 24 year old nurse was vaccinated with Cendehill vaccine. She developed a normal antibody response with detectable IgM antibody. Eleven months later she developed clinical rubella with a rash and pronounced arthralgia that lasted several weeks. An eightfold rise in antibody occurred, but no increase in IgM could be detected.

A case of congenital rubella after successful vaccination has also been reported from Australia (Bott and Eisenberg, 1982). A 24 year old woman who had previously been vaccinated with Cendehill vaccine after her second pregnancy because of a low level of antibody later gave birth to an infant with typical symptoms of congenital rubella. Blood specimens taken before and during her pregnancy showed that antibody was present but had increased eightfold during a two-year period preceding the pregnancy that resulted in the birth of the congenital rubella–infected infant. No symptoms had developed, and serological tests carried out by the HI technique were suggestive of a reinfection in the presence of antibody.

Congenital Rubella and Vaccine Surveillance. Most new immunization programs are based on the theory that the new immunological product will have a protective effect. A certain amount of information can be gained from studies in experimental animals and small-scale clinical trials in human volunteers, but the final test of protective efficacy is in the population as a whole. Analogies made between the protective ability of the new vaccine and that of other viral vaccines are often misleading because of fundamental differences in the pathogenesis of the diseases. Consideration has to be given to the composition of the vaccine, its potency, and, especially, the age at which it should be administered. These theoretical considerations should be backed up by a surveillance program to determine whether protection is being achieved in the field. Such schemes are currently being used to determine vaccine effectiveness in the prevention of measles and poliomyelitis. The same should apply to rubella vaccines. The diagnosis of congenital rubella on clinical grounds can now be made with reasonable certainty, and a definitive diagnosis can be confirmed by laboratory tests. It is reasonable to carry out rubella vaccine surveillance to determine whether the incidence of rubella-type defects is reduced in countries where a rubella vaccination program is in operation.

5. Safety of vaccines

The final requirement mentioned in the criteria for rubella vaccines was safety. This means safety for the recipient and, in pregnant women, safety for the fetus. Experience in the decade since the withdrawal of the dog kidney vaccine has shown that rubella vaccines currently in use are safe and effective in respect of both the vaccine strain and the cell substrate. If these vaccines are properly utilized and effectively monitored, it should be possible within the foreseeable future to prove that congenital rubella is a preventable disease.

Congenital Rubella Surveillance

In the United Kingdom a National Congenital Rubella Surveillance Programme was initiated in 1971. It has two registries: one located in the north of England at Leeds, the other in the south in London. The two registries serve approximately the same size population of between 25 and 27 million persons.

Cases of suspected congenital rubella are reported from two main sources: (1) pediatricians and (2) medical officers of local authorities (who mainly report children with suspected hearing loss detected through screening at a Hearing Center for Speech in the southern region). Cases are reported, blood tests are carried out, and evaluations are made from details supplied by the referring clinicians. Cases are classified as "confirmed" congenital rubella or, if they show one of the stigmata of the syndrome and there is some laboratory evidence to support the diagnosis, as "suspected" congenital rubella. The interpretation of the diagnosis depends to some extent on the age of the child when first investigated. Some cases have been recorded as confirmed congenital infection because laboratory tests were positive, but no defects could be detected (Dudgeon et al., 1973). Since the scheme came into operation in 1971, the referral rate has been extremely good and is being well maintained. From 1971 to 1975, 1239 patients were referred and, of these, 367 patients were classified as having confirmed or suspected congenital rubella (Sheppard et al., 1977). No history of maternal rubella was obtained in 38 per cent of cases. Multiple defects were observed more frequently in the pediatric referrals, and these were of the expected types (Table 3–25). Forty-one per cent of these children were first-born, and 76 per cent were born between the months of October and March.

More recent data that include the 11-year period from 1971 to 1981 (Smithells et al., 1982) are shown in Table 3–26. Considerable

Table 3–25. **MANIFESTATIONS IN 367 CASES OF CONFIRMED OR SUSPECTED CONGENITAL RUBELLA**

	Hospital	(%)	Community	(%)	Total	(%)
Multiple defects	94	(45.2)	37	(23.3)	131	(35.7)
Single defects	59	(28.4)	102	(64.2)	161	(43.9)
Disease in infancy only	27	(13.0)	1	(0.6)	28	(7.6)
Congenital rubella infection only	28	(13.5)	19	(11.9)	47	(12.8)
Total	208	(100)	159	(100)	367	(100)

From Sheppard, S., et al.: National Congenital Rubella Surveillance, 1971–75. Health Trends 9:38–41, 1977.

Table 3–26. CLINICAL DATA FOR 664 CONFIRMED OR SUSPECTED CASES OF CONGENITAL RUBELLA IN THE UNITED KINGDOM

	Pre-1970	1970	1971	1972	1973	1974	1975	1976	1977	1978	1979	1980	Total	Mean
Maternal history														
Rubella-like illness (%)	51	41	45	41	47	52	36	52	40	56	63	58		48
Rubella contact only (%)	10	14	15	22	23	13	18	3	13	16	12	17		15
No history of illness, contact, or rash (%)	26	29	28	30	21	21	27	26	40	16	13	8		24
Total (no.)	94	59	60	78	83	52	55	31	15	43	60	12	642	
Pregnancy order														
1st pregnancy (%)	43	47	43	37	40	23	28	39	33	34	34	50		38
4th pregnancy and over (%)	18	18	13	14	20	21	30	23	13	13	21	17		19
Total (no.)	90	57	61	79	85	47	54	31	15	38	56	12	625	
Birth weight for gestational age														
<10th percentile (%)	58	48	61	54	49	62	45	63	47	48	57	75		54
Total (no.)	78	50	56	74	80	42	44	27	15	40	61	12	579	
Clinical manifestations														
Multiple defects (%)	40	32	33	42	34	35	46	48	68	42	63	58		42
Single defect (%)	57	57	47	41	43	52	25	36	25	23	13	8		40
Neonatal manifestations only (%)	–	2	8	6	7	4	7	–	–	5	2	–		4
None (%)	3	10	13	11	17	10	21	15	6	30	23	33		14
Total (no.)	96	60	64	81	89	52	56	33	16	43	62	12	664	

Data from Smithells, R. W., et al.: National Congenital Rubella Surveillance Programme: 1971–81. Communicable Disease Report 36:3–4, 1982.

Table 3–27. **CASES AND RATES OF CONGENITAL RUBELLA SYNDROME BY SOURCE OF REPORTED DATA IN THE UNITED STATES**

Year of Birth	National Congenital Rubella Syndrome Registry		Birth Defects Monitoring Program	
	No. of Cases	Rate per 10^5 Births	No. of Cases	Rate per 10^5 Births
1969	81	2.7	–	–
1970	91	3.0	42	5.0
1971	50	1.7	20	2.3
1972	42	1.4	32	3.5
1973	39	1.3	38	3.9
1974	27	0.9	29	2.7
1975	41	1.4	45	4.2
1976	31*	1.0	12	1.1
1977	27*	0.9	36	3.4
1978	18*	0.6	33†	3.4
1979	8*	–	–	–

*Reporting for recent years is incomplete, as some cases are not diagnosed until later in childhood.
†Provisional data.
 Data from Centers for Disease Control: Rubella Surveillance, January 1976–December 1980, Table 5. Issued May 1980.

fluctuation in the pregnancy order has been noted since the earlier reports; that is probably accounted for by the fact that the data have been reanalyzed by recording the child's year of birth rather than the year of reporting. The figures also show that 547 (98 per cent of the 569 mothers for whom the year of birth was known were born before 1958 and were therefore not eligible for vaccination (Smithells et al., 1982). Against the apparently low figures for confirmed cases during an epidemic of rubella in 1978 and 1979, which are in any event provisional, it must be borne in mind that there was a large and parallel increase in the number of therapeutic abortions due to rubella or contact with rubella in pregnancy.

These figures for 1978 onward are considered provisional because children with a single defect, such as hearing loss, may not be identified until later in life, and it is clearly important to take into account both the effect of immunization and the number of pregnancies terminated following exposure to rubella in assessing a change in the incidence of congenital rubella. In a study of the consequences of maternal rubella in pregnancy reported by Miller and colleagues (1982), 523 (54 per cent) of the 966 women for whom the outcome of pregnancy was known had therapeutic abortions. Furthermore, it has been estimated that in 1979 and 1980 25 to 30 per cent of all pregnancies terminated because of rubella were ended because of rubella vaccination (Banatvala, 1982).

In the United States congenital rubella became a notifiable disease in 1960. Reports are made from two main sources, the National Congenital Rubella Syndrome Registry (NCRSR) and the Birth Defects Monitoring Program (BDMP) (Centers for Disease Control, 1980; Preblud et al., 1980). The criteria for classification of cases are broadly similar to those used in the United Kingdom, but recently the categories have been extended from three to five to include congenital rubella infection only and to divide uncertain cases into "possible" and "probable" groups. The BDMP monitors the discharge diagnosis of approximately 1 million newborns annually in the United States. Details of cases of confirmed congenital rubella are recorded in Table 3–27 by source of reported data and by year of birth. A decline in the number of cases reported by the NCRSR has been recorded, from 2.7 cases per 100,000 births in 1969 to 1.0 per 100,000 in 1976. Figures for the years 1977 through 1979 must be regarded as provisional, as reporting may be incomplete and a delay in diagnosis must be allowed for in the most recent years. For example, an outbreak of congenital rubella occurred in Chicago in 1978 and was not reported until four years later. Thirty-one infants with congenital rubella (including confirmed, probable, and possible cases) were identified, an incidence of 48.9 per 100,000 live births. None of the mothers had been vaccinated (Lamprecht et al., 1982). It seems unlikely that these cases were reported to the NCRSR or to the BDMP. A decline has also been noted in the BDMP figures, but this is less consistent than that in the NCRSR data. It must be emphasized that the data reported to the NCRSR are not limited to cases in the newborn period, whereas the BDMP data are. Reporting of cases to either the NCRSR or the BDMP has limitations: age of reporting, accuracy of diagnosis, and means of laboratory confirmation. Complete reporting, whether voluntary or compulsory, is impossible, but the present surveillance schemes in the United States and the United Kingdom should allow trends to emerge over a period of time. A further method of surveillance is analysis of records documenting therapeutic abortions and the reasons for which they were performed.

Bibliography

ACIP recommendations. Collected recommendations of the Public Health Services Advisory Committee on Immunization Practices. Morbidity Mortality Rep. *21*:23–24, 1972.

Ainger, J. E., Lawyer, N. G., and Fitch, C. W.: Neonatal rubella myocarditis. Br. Heart J. *28*:691–697, 1966.

Alford, C. A.: Studies on antibody in congenital rubella infections. Am. J. Dis. Child. *110*:455–643, 1965.

Alford, C. A., Neva, F. A., and Weller, T. H.: Virological and serological studies of human products of conception after maternal rubella. N. Engl. J. Med. *271*:1275–1281, 1964.

Alford, C. A., Schaefer, J., Blankenship, W. J., Straumfjord, J. V., and Cassady, G.: A correlative immunologic, microbiologic and clinical approach to the diagnosis of acute and chronic infections in newborn infants. N. Engl. J. Med. *277*:437–449, 1967.

Alford, C. A., Blankenship, W. J., Straumfjord, J. V., and Cassady, G.: The diagnostic significance of IgM-globulin elevations in newborn infants with chronic intrauterine infections. In Bergsma, D., and Krugman, S. (eds.): Intrauterine Infections. Birth Defects. Original Article Series, Vol. IV, No. 7. New York, The National Foundation—March of Dimes, 1968, pp. 5–19.

Al-Nakib, W., Best, J. M., and Banatvala, J. E.: Rubella-specific serum and nasopharyngeal immunoglobulin responses following naturally acquired and vaccine-induced infection. Lancet *2*:182–185, 1975.

Ames, M. D., Plotkin, S. A., Winchester, R. A., and Atkins, T. E.: Central auditory imperception: a significant factor in congenital rubella deafness. J.A.M.A. *213*:419–421, 1970.

Anderson, H., Barr, B., and Wedenberg, E.: Genetic disposition—a prerequisite for maternal rubella deafness. Arch. Otolaryngol. *91*:141, 1970.

Andrewes, C., Pereira, H. G., and Wildy, P.: Viruses of Vertebrates. 4th ed. Baltimore, Williams & Wilkins Company, 1978.

Auruskin, T. W., Brakin, M., and Juan, C.: Congenital myxoedema and congenital rubella. Pediatrics *69*:495–496, 1982.

Avery, G. B., Monif, G. R. G., Sever, J. L., and Leekin, S. L.: Rubella syndrome after inapparent maternal illness. Am. J. Dis. Child. *110*:444–446, 1965.

Axton, J. M. H., Nathoo, K. J., and Mbengeranwa, O. L.: Simultaneous rubella and measles epidemics in an African community. Cent. Afr. J. Med. *25*:242–244, 1979.

Baldursson, G., Bjarnason, O., Hallforsson, S., Juliusdottir, E., and Kjeld, S.: Maternal rubella in Iceland, 1963–64: some observations on 37 children with rubella syndrome. Scand. Audiol. *1*:3–10, 1972.

Balfour, H. H., and Amren, D. P.: Rubella, measles and mumps antibodies following vaccination. A potential rubella problem. Am. J. Dis. Child. *132*:573–577, 1978.

Balfour, H. H., Groth, K. E., Edelman, C. K., Amren, D. P., Best, J. M., and Banatvala, J. E.: Rubella viraemia and antibody responses after rubella vaccination and reimmunization. Lancet *1*:1078–1080, 1981.

Banatvala, J. E.: Immunofluorescence and tissue culture. Proc. R. Soc. Med. *62*:374–378, 1969.

Banatvala, J. E.: Rubella vaccination: remaining problems. Br. Med. J. *284*:1285–1286, 1982.

Banatvala, J. E., and Best, J. M.: Cross-serological testing of rubella virus strains. Lancet. *1*:695–697, 1969.

Banatvala, J. E., Potter, J. E., and Webster, M. J.: Foetal interferon responses induced by rubella virus. In Intrauterine Infections. Ciba Foundation Symposium 10 (new series). Amsterdam, Associated Scientific Publishers, 1973, pp. 77–99.

Barr, B., and Lundström, R.: Deafness following maternal rubella. Retrospective and prospective studies. Acta Otolaryngol. (Stockh.) *53*:413, 1961.

Bart, K. J., Orenstein, W. A., Dostar, S. W., and Hinman, A. R.: Rubella and congenital rubella infections: the history of control efforts. Symposium on Conquest of Agents That Endanger the Brain, Baltimore, October 28–29, 1982. In press, 1983.

Beck, E. S.: Review of studies with inactivated rubella virus. Am. J. Dis. Child. *118*:328–333, 1969.

Bellanti, J. A., Artenstein, M. S., Olson, L. C., Beuscher, E. L., Luhrs, C. E., and Milstead, K. L.: Congenital rubella: clinico-pathologic, virologic and immunologic studies. Am. J. Dis. Child. *110*:464–472, 1965.

Berry, C. L., and Thompson, E. N.: Clinico-pathological study of thymic dysplasia. Arch. Dis. Child. *43*:579–584, 1968.

Best, J. M., Almeida, J. D., and Waterson, A. P.: Morphological characteristics of rubella virus. Lancet *2*:237–239, 1967.

Best, J. M., Banatvala, J. E., and Bowen, J. M.: New Japanese rubella vaccine: comparative trials. Br. Med. J. *2*:221–224, 1974.

Best, J. M., Harcourt, G., and Banatvala, J. E.: Congenital rubella affecting an infant whose mother had rubella antibodies before conception. Br. Med. J. *282*:1235, 1981.

Beswick, R. C., Warner, R., and Warkany, J.: Congenital anomalies following maternal rubella. Am. J. Dis. Child. *78*:334–348, 1949.

Boner, A., Wilmott, R. W. P., Dinwiddie, R., Jeffries, D. J., Matthew, D. J., Marshall, W. C., Mowbray, J. F., Pincott, J. R., and Rivers, R. P.: Desquamative interstitial pneumonia and antigen-antibody complexes in two infants with congenital rubella. Pediatrics *72*:835–839, 1983.

Bott, L. M., and Eisenberg, D. H.: Congenital rubella after successful vaccination. Med. J. Aust., *1*(12):514–515, 1982.

Boué, A., Papiernick-Berkhauer, E., and Lévy-Thierry, S.: Attenuated rubella virus vaccine in women. Clinical trials during the postpartum period. Am. J. Dis. Child. *118*:230–233, 1969.

Boué, A., Nicolas, A., and Montagnon, B.: Reinfection

with rubella in pregnant women. Lancet *1*:1251–1253, 1971.

Brody, J. A., Sever, J. L., McAlister, R., Schiff, G. M., and Cutting, R.: Rubella epidemic on St. Paul Island in the Pribilofs, 1963. I. Epidemiologic, clinical, and serologic findings. J.A.M.A. *191*:619–623, 1965.

Buimovici-Klein, E., Lang, P. B., Ziring, P. R., and Cooper, L. Z.: Impaired cell-mediated immune responses in patients with congenital rubella: correlation with gestational age at time of infection. Pediatrics *64*:620–626, 1979.

Bunnell, C. E., and Monif, G. R. G.: Interstitial pancreatitis in the congenital rubella syndrome. J. Pediatr. *80*:465–466, 1972.

Burnet, F. M., and Fenner, F.: The Production of Antibodies. 2nd ed. London, Macmillan Company, 1949.

Butler, N. R., Dudgeon, J. A., Hayes, K., Peckham, C. S., and Wybar, K. C.: Persistence of rubella antibody with and without embryopathy. Br. Med. J. *2*:1027–1029, 1965.

Buynak, E. B., Hilleman, M. R., Weibel, R. E., and Stokes, J.: Live attenuated rubella virus vaccines prepared in duck embryo cell culture. I. Development and clinical testing. J.A.M.A. *204*:195–200, 1968.

Campbell, P. E.: Vascular abnormalities following maternal rubella. Br. Heart J. *27*:134–138, 1965.

Cantell, K., Strander, H., Saxen, L., and Meyer, B.: Interferon response of human leukocytes during intrauterine and post-natal life. J. Immunol. *100*:1304–1309, 1968.

Carruthers, D. G.: Congenital deaf-mutism as sequela of rubella-like maternal infection during pregnancy. Med. J. Aust. *1*:315–320, 1945.

Centers for Disease Control: Rubella Surveillance. Appendix VI.D., No. 2. Issued August 1970.

Centers for Disease Control: Rubella Surveillance. Appendix VII.D., No. 3, pp. 21–22. Issued October 1971.

Centers for Disease Control: Rubella Surveillance, July 1973–December 1975, p. 11. Issued August 1976.

Centers for Disease Control: Rubella Surveillance, January 1976–December 1978, Appendix I, p. 27, and Appendix II, pp. 29–32. Issued May 1980.

Chang, T. W.: Rubella reinfection and intrauterine involvement. J. Pediatr. *84*:617–618, 1974.

Chang, T. W., Moorhead, P. S., Boué, J. G., Plotkin, S. A., and Hoskins, J. M.: Chromosome studies of human cells infected in utero and in vitro with rubella virus. Proc. Soc. Exp. Biol. Med. *112*:236–243, 1966.

Chess, S.: Autism in children with congenital rubella. J. Autism Child. Schizo. *1*:33–47, 1971.

Chess, S.: Behaviour and learning of school-age rubella children. Final report. Congenital Rubella Behavior Studies (CRBS) Project MC-R-360183-03-0, December 31, 1974.

Chess, S., Korn, S. J., and Fernandez, P. B.: Psychiatric Disorders of Children with Congenital Rubella. New York, Brunner/Mazel, 1971.

Clarke, M., Seagrott, V., Schild, G. C., Pollock, T. M., Miller, C., Finlay, S. E., and Barbara, J. A. J.: Surveys of rubella antibodies in young adults and children. Lancet *1*:667–669, 1983.

Cockburn, W. C.: World aspects of the epidemiology of rubella. Am. J. Dis. Child. *118*:112–122, 1969.

Collis, W. J., and Cohen, D. N.: Rubella retinopathy, a progressive disorder. Arch. Ophthalmol. *84*:33, 1976.

Comas, A. P., and Bentances, R. E.: Congenital rubella and acquired hypothyroidism secondary to Hashimoto thyroiditis. J. Pediatr. *88*:1065, 1976.

Cooper, L. Z.: Rubella: a preventable cause of birth defects. In Bergsma, D., and Krugman, S. (eds.): Intrauterine Infections. Birth Defects. Original Article Series, Vol. IV, No. 7. New York, The National Foundation—March of Dimes, 1968, pp. 23–35.

Cooper, L. Z.: Congenital rubella in the United States. In Krugman, S., and Gershon, A. A. (eds.): Symposium on Infections of the Fetus and Newborn Infant. New York, Alan R. Liss Inc., 1975, pp. 1–22.

Cooper, L. Z., and Krugman, S.: Clinical manifestations of postnatal and congenital rubella. Arch. Ophthalmol. *77*:434–439, 1967.

Cooper, L. Z., Green, R. H., Krugman, S., Giles, J. P., and Mirick, G. S.: Neonatal thrombocytopenic purpura and other manifestations of rubella contracted in utero. Am. J. Dis. Child. *110*:416–427, 1965.

Cooper, L. Z., Ziring, P. R., Ockerse, A. B., Fedun, B. A., Kiely, B., and Krugman, S.: Rubella: clinical manifestations and management. Am. J. Dis. Child. *118*:18–29, 1969.

Cooper, L. Z., Florman, A. L., Ziring, P. R., and Krugman, S.: Loss of rubella hemagglutination-inhibition antibody in congenital rubella. Am. J. Dis. Child. *122*:397–403, 1971.

Coyle, P. K., and Wolinsky, J. S.: Characterisation of immune complexes in progressive rubella panencephalitis. Ann. Neurol. *9*:557–562, 1981.

Coyle, P. K., Wolinsky, J. S., Buimovici-Klein, E., Maucha, R., and Cooper, L. Z.: Rubella-specific immune complexes after congenital rubella infection and vaccination. Infect. Immun. *36*:498–503, 1982.

Cradock-Watson, J. E., Ridehalgh, M. K. S., Pattison, J. R., Anderson, M. J., and Kangro, H. O.: Comparison of immunofluorescence and radioimmunoassay for detecting rubella IgM antibody in infants with the congenital rubella syndrome. J. Hyg. Camb. *83*:413–423, 1979.

Cradock-Watson, J.E., Ridehalgh, M. K. S., Anderson, M. J., Pattison, J. R., and Kangro, H. O.: Fetal infection resulting from maternal rubella after the first trimester of pregnancy. J. Hyg. Camb. *85*:381–390, 1980.

Desmond, M. M., Wilson, G. S., Melnick, J. L., Singer, D. B., Zion, T. E., Rudolph, A. J., Pineda, R. G., Mir-Hashen, Z., and Blattner, R. J.: Congenital rubella encephalitis. J. Pediatr. *71*:311–331, 1967.

Desmyter, J., Rawls, W. E., Melnick, J. L., Yow, M. D., and Barrett, F. F.: Interferon in congenital rubella: response to live attenuated measles vaccine. J. Immunol. *99*:771–777, 1967.

Deutman, A. F., and Grizzard, W. S.: Rubella retinopathy and subclinical neovascularization. Am. J. Ophthalmol. *85*:82–87, 1978.

Doss, A. F.: *In vitro* markers of rubella virus. Ph.D. thesis. University of London, 1972.

Driscoll, S. G.: Histopathology of gestational rubella. Am. J. Dis. Child. *118*:49–53, 1969.

Dudgeon, J. A.: Communication to International Symposium on Pediatrics, Tokyo, 1965a.

Dudgeon, J. A.: Serological studies on the rubella syndrome. Arch. Ges. Virusforsch. *16*:501–505, 1965b.

Dudgeon, J. A.: New rubella syndrome. Br. Med. J. *1*:46, 1966.

Dudgeon, J. A.: Unpublished data, 1967.

Dudgeon, J. A.: Congenital rubella. Pathogenesis and immunology. Am. J. Dis. Child. *118*:35–44, 1969a.

Dudgeon, J. A.: Rubella vaccines. Br. Med. Bull. *25*:159–164, 1969b.

Dudgeon, J. A.: Congenital rubella: a preventable disease. Postgrad. Med. J. *48*(Suppl. 3):7–11, 1972.

Dudgeon, J. A.: Rubella: the U.K. Experience. Immunization—Benefit versus Risk Factors. Developments in Biological Standardization, Vol. 43. Basel, S. Karger, 1979, 327–338.

Dudgeon, J. A.: Current views on the conquest of Rubella. Symposium on Conquest of Agents That Endanger the Brain, Baltimore, October 28–29, 1982. In press, 1983.

Dudgeon, J. A., Butler, N. R., and Plotkin, S. A.: Further serological studies on the rubella syndrome. Br. Med. J. 2:155–160, 1964.

Dudgeon, J. A., Marshall, W. C., Peckham, C. S., and Hawkins, G. T.: Clinical and laboratory studies with rubella vaccines in adults. Br. Med. J. 1:271–276, 1969.

Dudgeon, J. A., Peckham, C. S., Marshall, W. C., Smithells, R. W., and Sheppard, S.: National Congenital Rubella Surveillance Programme. Health Trends 5:75–79, 1973.

Eilard, T., and Strannegard, O.: Rubella reinfection in pregnancy followed by transmission to the fetus. J. Infect. Dis. 129:594–596, 1974.

Esterly, J. R., and Oppenheimer, E. H.: Intrauterine rubella infection. In Rosenberg, H. S., and Bolande, R. P. (eds.): Perspectives in Pediatric Pathology. Vol. 1. Chicago, Year Book Medical Publishers, 1973, pp. 313–338.

Evans, P. R., and Evans, B.: Personal communication, 1966.

Fisch, L.: Causes of congenital deafness. In International Audiology. IX International Congress of Audiology, London, September 15–19, 1969, Vol. 8, No. 1, pp. 85–89.

Fleet, W. F., Benz, E. Q., Karzon, D. T., Lefkowitz, L. B., and Herrmann, K. L.: Fetal consequences of maternal rubella immunization. J.A.M.A. 227:621–627, 1974.

Florman, A. L., Cooper, L. Z., Ziring, P. R., and Krugman, S.: Response to rubella vaccine among seronegative children with congenital rubella. Communication to the American Pediatric Society (abstract). Pediatr. Res. 4:372, 1970.

Fogel, A., and Plotkin, S. A.: Differentiation of rubella virus variants by plaque morphology and antigenic character. Fed. Proc. 26:421, 1967.

Forrest, J. M., and Menser, M. A.: Congenital rubella in school children and adolescents. Arch. Dis. Child. 45:63–69, 1970.

Forrest, J. M., Menser, M. A., and Harley, J. D.: Diabetes mellitus and congenital rubella. Pediatrics 44:445–446, 1969.

Forrest, J. M., Menser, M. A., and Burgess, J. A.: High frequency of diabetes mellitus in young adults with congenital rubella. Lancet 2:332–334, 1971.

Forrest, J. M., Menser, M. A., Stout, M., and Murphy, A. A.: Clinical rubella eleven months after vaccination. Lancet 2:399–400, 1972.

Forrester, R. M., Lees, V. T., and Watson, G. H.: Rubella syndrome: escape of a twin. Br. Med. J. 1:1403–1404, 1966.

Forsgren, M., Carlström, G., and Stranger, C.: Congenital rubella after maternal reinfection. Scand. J. Infect. Dis. 11:81–83, 1979.

Franch, R. H., and Gay, B. B.: Congenital stenosis of the pulmonary artery branches. Am. J. Med. 35:512–529, 1963.

Frank, K. E., and Purnell, E. W.: Subclinical neovascularization following rubella retinopathy. Am. J. Ophthalmol. 86:462–468, 1978.

Frankel, J. W.: Neutralising antibody responses of guinea pigs to inactivated rubella virus vaccine. Nature 204:655–656, 1964.

Fraser, G. R.: Profound childhood deafness. J. Med. Genet. 1:118, 1964.

Friedmann, I.: Cochlear pathology in viral disease. Adv. Otorhinolaryngol. 20:155–177, 1973.

Friedmann, I.: The Pathology of the Ear. Oxford, Blackwell Scientific Publications, 1974, pp. 418–419.

Friedmann, I., and Wright, M. I.: Histopathological changes in the foetal and infantile inner ear caused by maternal rubella. Br. Med. J. 2:20–23, 1966.

Fuccillo, D. A., Steele, R. W., Hensen, S. A., Vincent, M. M., Hardy, J. B., and Bellanti, J. A.: Impaired cellular immunity to rubella virus in congenital rubella. Infect. Immun. 9:81–84, 1974.

Furukawa, T., Plotkin, S. A., Sedwick, W. D., and Profala, M. L.: Studies on hemagglutination by rubella virus. Proc. Soc. Exp. Biol. Med. 126:745–750, 1967.

Garcia, A. G. P., Olinto, F., and Fortes, T. G. O.: Thymic hypoplasia due to congenital rubella. Arch. Dis. Child. 49:181–185, 1974.

Gittenberger-de-Groot, A. C., Moulaert, A. J. M., and Hitchcock, J. F.: Histology of the persistent ductus arteriosus in cases of congenital rubella. Circulation 62:183–186, 1980.

Green, R. H., Balsamo, M. R., Giles, J. P., Krugman, S., and Mirick, G. S.: Studies on the natural history and prevention of rubella. Am. J. Dis. Child. 110:348–365, 1965.

Gregg, N. M.: Congenital cataract following German measles in the mother. Trans. Ophthalmol. Soc. Aust. 3:34–45, 1941.

Gregg, N. M.: Further observations on congenital defects in infants following maternal rubella. Trans. Ophthalmol. Soc. Aust. 4:119–131, 1944.

Gregg, N. M., Beavis, W. R., Heseltine, M., Macklin, A. E., and Vickery, D.: Occurrence of congenital defects in children following maternal rubella during pregnancy. Med. J. Aust. 2:122–126, 1945.

Grillner, L., Forsgren, M., Barr, B., Bottinger, M., Danielsson, L., and de Verdieu, C.: Outcome of rubella during pregnancy with special reference to the 17th and 24th weeks of gestation. Scand. J. Infect. Dis. 15:321–325, 1983.

Gumpel, S. M.: Clinical and social status of patients with congenital rubella. Arch. Dis. Child. 47:330–337, 1972.

Gumpel, S. M., Hayes, K., and Dudgeon, J. A.: Congenital perceptive deafness: role of intrauterine rubella. Br. Med. J. 2:300–304, 1971.

Halonen, P. E., Ryan, J. M., and Stewart, J. A.: Rubella hemagglutinin prepared with alkaline extraction of virus grown in suspension culture of BHK-21 cells. Proc. Soc. Exp. Biol. Med. 125:162–167, 1967.

Hancock, M. P., Huntley, M. P., and Sever, J. L.: Congenital rubella syndrome with immunoglobulin disorder. J. Pediatr. 72:636–645, 1968.

Hanid, T. K.: Hypothyroidism in congenital rubella. Lancet 2:854, 1976.

Hardy, J. B., McCracken, G. H., Gilkeson, M. R., and Sever, J. L.: Adverse fetal outcome following maternal rubella after the first trimester of pregnancy. J.A.M.A. 207:2414–2420, 1969a.

Hardy, J. B., Sever, J. L., and Gilkeson, M. R.: Declining antibody titers in children with congenital rubella. J. Pediatr. 75:213–220, 1969b.

Hastreiter, A. R., Joorabchi, B., Pujatti, G., van der Horst, R., Pataesil, G., and Sever, J. L.: Cardiovascular lesions associated with congenital rubella. J. Pediatr. 71:59–65, 1967.

Haukenes, G., and Haram, K. O.: Clinical rubella after reinfection. N. Engl. J. Med. 287:1204, 1972.

Haukenes, G., Haram, K. O., and Solberg, C. O.: Clinical

rubella after reinfection. False-positive reactions of specific HI antibody. N. Engl. J. Med. *289*:429, 1973.

Hayden, G. F., Herrman, K. L., Buimovici-Klein, E., Weiss, K. E., Nieburg, P. L., and Mitchell, J. E.: Subclinical rubella infection associated with maternal rubella vaccination in early pregnancy. J. Pediatr. *96*:869–872, 1980.

Hayes, K., Dudgeon, J. A., and Soothill, J. F.: Humoral immunity in congenital rubella. Clin. Exp. Immunol. *2*:653–667, 1967.

Heggie, A. D.: Intrauterine infection in maternal rubella. J. Pediatr. *71*:777–782, 1967.

Herrman, K. L., Halstead, S. B., and Brandling-Bennett, A. D.: Rubella immunization. Persistence of antibody four years after large scale trial. J.A.M.A. *235*:2201–2204, 1976.

Hinman, A. R., Preblud, S. R., and Brandling-Bennett, A. D.: Rubella: the U.S. Experience. Immunization—Benefit versus Risk Factors. Developments in Biological Standardization, Vol. 43. Basel, S. Karger, 1979, 315–326.

Hirayama, M.: Paediatria Universitatis, Tokyo *18*:41, 1970.

Holmes, I. H., and Warburton, M. F.: Is rubella an arbovirus? Lancet *2*:1233–1236, 1967.

Holmes, I. H., Wark, M. C., and Warburton, M. F.: Is rubella an arbovirus? II. Ultrastructural morphology and development. Virology *37*:15–25, 1969.

Honeyman, M. C., and Menser, M. A.: Ethnicity of a significant factor in the epidemiology of rubella and Hodgkin's disease. Nature *25*:441–442, 1974.

Hope Simpson, R. E.: Rubella and congenital malformations. Lancet *1*:483, 1944.

Horstmann, D. M.: Controlling rubella: problems and perspectives. Ann. Intern. Med. *83*:412–417, 1975.

Horstmann, D. M., Banatvala, J. E., Riodan, J. T., Payne, M. C., Whittmore, R., Opton, E. M., and Florey, C.: Maternal rubella and the rubella syndrome in infants. Am. J. Dis. Child. *110*:408–415, 1965.

Horstmann, D. M., Pajot, T. G., and Liebhaber, H.: Epidemiology of rubella. Subclinical infection and occurrence of reinfections. Am. J. Dis. Child. *118*:133–136, 1969.

Horstmann, D. M., Liebhaber, H., Le Bouvier, G. L., Rosenberg, D. A., and Halstead, S. B.: Rubella: reinfection of vaccinated and naturally immune persons exposed in an epidemic. N. Engl. J. Med. *283*:771–778, 1970.

Hosking, C. S., Ryman, C., and Wilkins, B.: The nerve deaf child—intrauterine rubella or not? Arch. Dis. Child. *58*:327–329, 1983.

Hovi, T., and Vaheri, A.: Rubella virus–specific ribonucleic acids in infected BHK21 cells. J. Gen. Virol. *42*:1–8, 1970.

International Conference on Rubella Immunization. Am. J. Dis. Child. *118*:1–410, 1969.

International Symposium on Rubella Vaccines, London, 1968. Symposia Series in Immunobiological Standardization, Vol. 11. Basel, S. Karger, 1969.

Jackson, A. D. M., and Fisch, L.: Deafness following maternal rubella: results of a prospective investigation. Lancet *2*:1241–1244, 1958.

Johnson, G. M., and Tudor, R. B.: Diabetes mellitus and congenital rubella infection. Am. J. Dis. Child. *120*:453–455, 1970.

Karmody, C. S.: Subclinical maternal rubella and congenital deafness. N. Engl. J. Med. *278*:809–814, 1968.

Kay, H. E. M., Peppersorn, M. E., Porterfield, J. A., McCarthy, K., and Taylor-Robinson, C. H.: Congenital rubella infection of a human embryo. Br. Med. J. *2*:166–167, 1964.

Kejtorp, M., and Mansa, B.: Rubella IgM antibodies in sera from infants born with maternal rubella later than the 12th week of pregnancy. Scand. J. Infect. Dis. *12*:1, 1980.

Kenrick, K. G., Slinn, R. F., Dorman, D. A., and Menser, M. A.: Immunoglobulins and rubella-virus antibodies in adults with congenital rubella. Lancet *1*:548–551, 1968.

Kiely, B., Cooper, L. Z., Doyle, E. J., Engle, M. A., Farnsworth, P. B., and Moollam, F.: Cardiovascular malformations in children with congenital rubella. Quoted by Cooper, L. Z.: In Krugman, S., and Gershon, A. A. (eds.): Symposium on Infections of the Fetus and Newborn Infant. New York: Alan R. Liss Inc., 1975.

Kistler, G. S.: Discussion: clinical impact of intrauterine rubella. In Intrauterine Infections. Ciba Foundation Symposium 10 (new series). Amsterdam, Associated Scientific Publishers, 1973, p. 16.

Kistler, G. S., Best, J. M., Banatvala, J. E., and Töndury, G.: Elektronenmikroskopische Untersuchungen an rötelninfizierten menschlichen Organkulturen. Schweiz. Med. Wochenschr. *97*:1377–1382, 1967.

Kono, R.: Antigenic structures of American and Japanese rubella virus strains and experimental vertical transmission of rubella virus in rabbits. In International Symposium on Rubella Vaccines, London, 1968. Symposia Series in Immunobiological Standardization, Vol. 11. Basel, S. Karger, 1969, pp. 195–204.

Kono, R., Hayakawa, Y., Hibi, M., and Ishii, K.: Experimental vertical transmission of rubella virus in rabbits. Lancet *1*:343–347, 1969.

Kono, R., Inove, S., Tanaka, S., Itahashi, M., Onishi, E., and Hayakawa, Y.: Experimental vertical transmission of rubella virus in rabbits. II. Observation of placenta and fetuses in utero. In Proceedings of International Conference on the Application of Vaccines Against Viral, Rickettsial and Bacterial Diseases of Man, December 14–18, 1970. WHO Scientific Publication No. 226. Washington, D.C., Pan American Health Organization, 1971, pp. 273–280.

Korones, S. B., Ainger, L. E., Monif, G. R. G., Roane, J., Sever, J. L., and Fuste, F.: Congenital rubella syndrome: study of 22 infants. Myocardial damage and other new clinical aspects. Am. J. Dis. Child. *110*:434–440, 1965.

Krugman, S.: Present status of measles and rubella immunization in the United States: a medical progress report. Review article. J. Pediatr. *90*:1–12, 1977.

Krugman, S., and Ward, R.: The rubella problem. Clinical aspects, risk of fetal abnormality and methods of prevention. J. Pediatr. *44*:489–498, 1954.

Krugman, S., Ward, R., Jacobs, K. G., and Lazer, M.: Studies of rubella immunization: demonstration of rubella without rash. J.A.M.A. *151*:285–288, 1953.

Lamprecht, C., Schauf, V., Warren, D., Nelson, K., Northrop, R., and Christiansen, M.: An outbreak of congenital rubella in Chicago. J.A.M.A. *247*:1129–1133, 1982.

Lancaster, H. O.: The epidemiology of deafness due to maternal rubella. Acta Genet. (Basel) *5*:12, 1954.

Lawrence, G. D., and Gould, J.: Morphology of rubella plaques in RK13 cultures. In International Symposium on Rubella Vaccines, London, 1968. Symposia Series in Immunobiological Standardization, Vol. 11. Basel, S. Karger, 1969, pp. 177–181.

Le Bouvier, G. L.: Precipitinogens of rubella virus–infected cells. Proc. Soc. Exp. Biol. Med. *130*:51–54, 1969.

Leerhöy, J.: Comparison of rubella haemagglutination-inhibition and neutralizing antibody curves in natural infection. Acta Med. Scand. *184*:380–392, 1968.

Lefkowitz, L. B., Rafajko, R. R., Federspiel, C. F., and Quinn, R. W.: A controlled family study of live attenuated rubella virus vaccine. N. Engl. J. Med. *283*:229–232, 1970.

Lejarraga, H., and Peckham, C. S.: Birthweight and subsequent growth in children exposed to rubella infection in utero. Arch. Dis. Child. *49*:50–54, 1974.

Lennette, E. H., and Schmidt, N. J.: Development and application of hemadsorption-inhibition test for rubella virus. In International Symposium on Rubella Vaccines, London, 1968. Symposia Series in Immunobiological Standardization, Vol. 11. Basel, S. Karger, 1969, pp. 109–114.

Liggins, G. C., and Phillips, L. I.: Rubella embryopathy. An interim report on a New Zealand epidemic. Br. Med. J. *1*:711–713, 1963.

Limbacter, J. P., Hill, M. E., and Janicki, P. C.: Hypoplasia of the abdominal aorta associated with rubella syndrome. South. Med. J. *72*:617–619, 1979.

Lingeman, C. H., Schulz, D. M., and Lukemeyer, J. W.: Pneumocystic pneumonia in congenital rubella. Am. J. Dis. Child. *113*:585–587, 1967.

Lipman, P. R.: Immunization of man against rubella. Am. J. Dis. Child. *118*:310–312, 1969.

Lundström, R.: Rubella during pregnancy. A follow-up study of children born after an epidemic of rubella in Sweden, 1951. With additional investigations on prophylaxis and treatment of maternal rubella. Acta Paediatr. *51*(Suppl. 133):1–110, 1962.

Lundström, R., Ahnsjö, S., Berczy, J., Blomqvist, B., and Eklund, G.: Maternal rubella, a long-term follow-up study. XIV Congress Internacional de Pediatria, Buenos Aires, October 3–9, 1974, pp. 1–11.

Magnusson, P., and Skaaret, P.: Purification studies of rubella virus. Distribution of infectivity in equilibrium centrifugation of potassium citrate density gradients and after chromatography on anion exchange. Arch. Ges. Virusforsch. *20*:374–382, 1967.

Manson, M. M., Logan, W. P. D., and Loy, R. M.: Rubella and other virus infections during pregnancy. Rep. Pub. Hlth. Med. Subj. No. 110, 1960.

Marshall, W. C.: Immunological studies of intrauterine rubella. Ph.D. thesis. University of London, 1971.

Marshall, W. C.: The clinical impact of intrauterine rubella. In Intrauterine Infections. Ciba Foundation Symposium 10 (new series). Amsterdam, Associated Scientific Publishers, 1973, pp. 3–12.

Marshall, W. C., Trompeter, R. S., and Risdon, R. A.: Chronic rashes in congenital rubella: isolation of virus from the skin. Lancet *1*:1349, 1975.

McCombs, R. M., and Rawls, W. E.: Density gradient centrifugation of rubella virus. J. Virol. *2*:409–415, 1968.

McCracken, G. H., Jr., Hardy, J. B., Chen, T. C., Hoffman, L. S., Gilkeson, M. R., and Sever, J. L.: Serum immunoglobulin levels in newborn infants. II. Survey of cord and follow-up sera from 123 infants with congenital rubella. J. Pediatr. *74*:383–392, 1969.

Menser, M. A., and Reye, R. D. K.: The pathology of congenital rubella: a review writen by request. Pathology *6*:215–222, 1974.

Menser, M. A., Dorman, D. C., Reye, R. D. K., and Reid, R. R.: Renal-artery stenosis in the rubella syndrome. Lancet *1*:790–792, 1966.

Menser, M. A., Dods, C., and Harley, J. D.: a 25-year follow-up of congenital rubella. Lancet *2*:1347–1350, 1967a.

Menser, M. A., Harley, J. D., Hertzberg, R., Dorman,

D. C., and Murphy, A. M.: Persistence of virus in lens for three years after prenatal rubella. Lancet *2*:387–388, 1967b.

Menser, M. A., Robertson, S. E. J., Dorman, D. C., Gillespie, A. M., and Murphy, A. M.: Renal lesions in congenital rubella. Pediatrics *40*:901–904, 1967c.

Menser, M. A., Dorman, D. C., Kenrick, K. G., Purvis-Smith, S. G., Slinn, R. F., Dods, L., and Harley, J. D.: Congenital rubella. Long-term follow-up study. Am. J. Dis. Child. *118*:32–34, 1969.

Menser, M. A., Forrest, J. M., Honeyman, M. C., and Burgess, J. A.: Diabetes HL-A antigens and congenital rubella. Lancet *2*:1508–1509, 1974.

Menser, M. A., Forrest, J. M., and Bransby, R. D.: Rubella infection and diabetes mellitus. Lancet *1*:57–60, 1978.

Meyer, H. M., and Parkman, P. D.: Rubella vaccination. A review of practical experience. J.A.M.A. *215*:613, 1971.

Meyer, H. M., Parkman, P. D., and Panos, T. C.: Attenuated rubella virus. II. Production of an experimental live-virus vaccine and clinical trials. N. Engl. J. Med. *275*:575–580, 1966.

Meyer, H. M., Parkman, P. D., Panos, T. C., Stewart, G. L., Hobbins, T. E., and Ennis, F. A.: Clinical studies with attenuated rubella virus. In First International Conference on Vaccines Against Viral and Rickettsial Disease in Man. WHO Scientific Publication No. 147. Washington, D.C., Pan American Health Organization, 1967, pp. 390–398.

Michaels, R. H., and Kenny, F. M.: Postnatal growth retardation in congenital rubella. Pediatrics *43*:251–259, 1969.

Miller, E., Cradock-Watson, J. E., and Pollock, T. H.: Consequences of confirmed maternal rubella at successive stages of pregnancy. Lancet *2*:781–784, 1982.

Mims, C. A.: Pathogenesis of viral infections of the fetus. Prog. Med. Virol. *10*:194–237, 1968.

Miyazaki, S., Ohtsuka, M., Ueda, K., Shibota, R., and Goya, N.: Coombs positive hemolytic anemia in congenital rubella. J. Pediatr. *94*:759–760, 1979.

Modlin, J. F., Hermann, K. L., Brandling-Bennett, A. D., Witte, J. J., Campbell, C. C., and Meyers, J. D.: A review of five years experience with rubella vaccine in the United States. Pediatrics *55*:20–29, 1975.

Modlin, J. F., Herrmann, K., Brandling-Bennett, A. D., Eddins, D. L., and Hoyden, G. F.: Risk of congenital abnormality after inadvertent rubella vaccination of pregnant women. N. Engl. J. Med. *294*:972–974, 1976.

Monif, G. R., Avery, G. B., Korones, S. B., and Sever, J. L.: Postmortem isolation of rubella virus from three children with rubella syndrome defects. Lancet *1*:723–724, 1965.

Monif, G. R., and Sever, J. L.: Chronic infection of the central nervous system with rubella virus. Neurology *16*:111–112, 1966.

Morbidity and Mortality Report: Rubella and congenital rubella, United States 1980–1983. *32*:429–432, 1983.

Murphy, A. M., Reid, R. R., Pollard, I., Gillespie, A. M., Dorman, D. C., Menser, M. A., Harley, J. D., and Hertzberg, R.: Rubella cataracts. Further clinical and virological observations. Am. J. Ophthalmol. *64*:1109–1119, 1967.

Naeye, R. L., and Blanc, W.: Pathogenesis of congenital rubella. J.A.M.A. *194*:1277–1283, 1965.

Nagayama, T., et al.: Frequency of rubella antibody among pregnant women in the Fukuoka District of southern Japan. Fukuoka Acta Med. *57*:303–305, 1966.

Nagono, Y., Honda, S., and Goya, N.: Dermatoglyphics in congenital rubella syndrome with congenital heart disease. Jpn. Circ. J. *42*:1192, 1978.

Nieburg, P., and Gardner, L.: Thyroiditis and congenital rubella syndrome. J. Pediatr. *89*:156, 1976.

Northrop, R. L., Gardner, W. M., and Geitmann, W. F.: Low level immunity to rubella. N. Engl. J. Med. *287*:615, 1972a.

Northrop, R. L., Gardner, W. M., and Geitmann, W. F.: Rubella reinfection during early pregnancy. A case report. Obstet. Gynecol. *39*:524–526, 1972b.

Ogra, P., Kerr-Grant, D., Umana, G., Dzlerba, J., and Weintraub, D.: Antibody response in serum and nasopharynx after naturally acquired and vaccine-induced infection with rubella virus. N. Engl. J. Med. *285*:1333–1339, 1971.

Olson, G. B., South, M. A., and Good, R. A.: Phytohaemagglutinin unresponsiveness of lymphocytes from babies with congenital rubella. Nature *214*:695–696, 1967.

Olson, G. B., Dent, P. B., Rawls, W. E., South, M. A., Montgomery, J. R., Melnick, J. L., and Good, R. A.: Abnormalities of in vitro lymphocyte response during rubella virus infections. J. Exp. Med. *128*:47–68, 1968.

Orenstein, W. A., Doster, S. W., Bart, K. J., Sirotkin, B., and Hinman, A. R.: Symposium on Conquest of Agents That Endanger the Brain, Baltimore, October 28–29, 1982. In press, 1983.

O'Shea, S., Parsons, G., and Best, J. M.: How well do low levels of rubella antibody protect? Lancet *2*:1284, 1981.

O'Shea, S., Best, J. M., Banatvala, J. E., Marshall, W. C., and Dudgeon, J. A.: Rubella vaccination: persistence of antibodies for up to 16 years. Br. Med. J. *285*:253–255, 1982.

Parkman, P. D.: Discussion on virology and epidemiology of rubella. Am. J. Dis. Child. *118*:153, 1969.

Parkman, P. D., Beuscher, E. L., and Artenstein, M. S.: Recovery of rubella virus from army recruits. Proc. Soc. Exp. Biol. Med. *111*:225–230, 1962.

Parkman, P. D., Meyer, H. M., Kirschstein, R. L., and Hopps, H. E.: Attenuated rubella virus. I. Development and laboratory characteristics. N. Engl. J. Med. *275*:569–574, 1966.

Partridge, J. W., Flewett, T. H., and Whitehead, J. E. M.: Congenital rubella affecting an infant whose mother had rubella antibodies before conception. Br. Med. J. *282*:187–188, 1981.

Patrick, D. G.: Report of a survey of children born in 1941 with reference to congenital abnormalities arising from maternal rubella. Med. J. Aust. *1*:421, 1948.

Peckham, C. S.: Clinical and laboratory study of children exposed in utero to maternal rubella. Arch. Dis. Child. *47*:571–577, 1972.

Peckham, C. S., Martin, J. A. M., Marshall, W. C., and Dudgeon, J. A.: Congenital rubella deafness: a preventable disease. Lancet *1*:258–261, 1979.

Peckham, C. S., Tookey, P., Nelson, D. B., Coleman, J., and Morris, N.: Ethnic minority women and congenital rubella. Br. Med. J., *287*:129–130, 1983.

Phelan, P., and Campbell, P.: Pulmonary complications of rubella embryopathy. J. Pediatr. *75*:202–212, 1969.

Pitt, D. B.: Congenital malformations and maternal rubella: progress report. Med. J. Aust. *1*:881–890, 1961.

Pitt, D. B., and Keir, E. H.: Results of rubella in pregnancy. I. Med. J. Aust. *2*:647–651, 737–741, 1965.

Plotkin, S. A., and Kaye, R.: Diabetes and congenital rubella. Pediatrics *46*:650–651, 1970.

Plotkin, S. A., and Vaheri, A.: Human fibroblasts infected with rubella virus produce a growth inhibitor. Science *156*:659–661, 1967.

Plotkin, S. A., Dudgeon, J. A., and Ramsay, A. M.: Laboratory studies on rubella and the rubella syndrome. Br. Med. J. *2*:1296–1299, 1963.

Plotkin, S. A., Oski, F. A., Hartnett, E. M., Hervada, A. R., Friedman, S., and Gowing, J.: Some recently recognized manifestations of the rubella syndrome. J. Pediatr. *67*:182–191, 1965a.

Plotkin, S. A., Boué, A., and Boué, J. G.: The in vitro growth of rubella virus in human embryo cells. Am. J. Epidemiol. *81*:71–85, 1965b.

Plotkin, S. A., Klaus, R. M., and Whitely, J. A.: Hypogammaglobulinemia in an infant with congenital rubella syndrome: failure of 1-adamantanamine to stop virus excretion. J. Pediatr. *69*:1085–1091, 1966.

Plotkin, S. A., Farquahar, J. D., and Ogra, P. L.: Immunologic properties of RA 27/3 rubella vaccine. J.A.M.A. *225*:585–590, 1973.

Preblud, S. R., Serdula, M. K., Frank, J. A., Brandling-Bennett, A. D., and Hinman, A. R.: Rubella vaccination in the United States. A ten year review. Epidemiol. Rev. *2*:171–173, 1980.

Preblud, S. R., Stetlen, H. C., Frank, J. A., Greaves, W. L., Hinman, A. R., and Heffman, K. L.: Fetal risk associated with rubella vaccine. J.A.M.A. *246*:1413–1417, 1981.

Preece, M. A., Kearney, P., and Marshall, W. C.: Growth hormone deficiency in the rubella syndrome. Lancet *2*:842, 1977.

Purvis-Smith, S. G., and Menser, M. A.: Dermatoglyphics in adults with congenital rubella. Lancet *2*:141–143, 1968.

Rausen, A. R., Richter, P., Tallal, L., and Cooper, L. Z.: Hematologic effects of intrauterine rubella. J.A.M.A. *199*:75–78, 1967.

Rawls, W. E., Melnick, J. L., Bradstreet, C. M. P., Baily, M., Ferris, A. A., Lehmann, N. I., Nagler, F. P., Furess, J., Kono, R., Ohtawara, M., Haenan, P., Stewart, J., Ryan, J. M., Strauss, J., Zdrazilck, J., Leerhöy, J., Magnus, von H., Sohier, R., and Ferreira, W.: WHO collaborative study on the sero-epidemiology of rubella. Bull. W.H.O. *37*:79–88, 1967.

Rawls, W. E., Desmyter, J., and Melnick, J. L.: Serological diagnosis and fetal involvement in maternal rubella. J.A.M.A. *203*:627–631, 1968.

Recommendations of the Immunization Practices Advisory Committee (ACIP). Morbidity Mortality Rep. *30*:37–42, 1981.

Reid, R. R., Murphy, A. M., Gillespie, A. M., Dorman, D. C., Menser, M. A., Hertzberg, R., and Harley, J. D.: Isolation of rubella virus from congenital cataracts removed at operation. Med. J. Aust. *1*:540–542, 1966.

Robbins, F. C.: A letter. N. Engl. J. Med. *287*:615, 1972.

Rorke, L. B., and Spiro, A. J.: Cerebral lesions in congenital rubella syndrome. J. Pediatr. *70*:243–255, 1967.

Ross, L. J.: Fingerprints in congenital rubella following maternal gammaglobulin. Acta Pediatr. Scand. *681*:71–74, 1979.

Roy, F. H., Hiatt, R. L., Korones, S. B., and Roane, J.: Ocular manifestations of congenital rubella syndrome. Arch. Ophthalmol. *75*:601–607, 1966.

Rubella and congenital malformations (annotation). Lancet *1*:316, 1944.

Rubella Symposium. Am. J. Dis. Child. *110*:345–478, 1965.

Rubella vaccination during pregnancy. United States, 1971–1981. Morbidity Mortality Rep. *31*:477–481, 1982.

Rudolph, A. J., Singleton, E. B., Rosenberg, H. S., Singer, D. B., and Phillips, C. A.: Osseous manifestations of the congenital rubella syndrome. Am. J. Dis. Child. *110*:428–433, 1965.

Scheie, H. G., Schaffer, D. B., Plotkin, S. A., and Kertesz, E. D.: Congenital rubella cataracts. Arch. Ophthalmol. *77*:440–444, 1967.

Schiff, G. M., and Dine, M. S.: Transmission of rubella from newborns. Am. J. Dis. Child. *110*:447–451, 1965.

Schiff, G. M., et al.: Paper presented at the Annual Meeting of the American Pediatric Society, Atlantic City, April 30, 1970.

Schmidt, N. J., and Lennette, E. H.: Antigens of rubella virus. Am. J. Dis. Child. *118*:89–93, 1969.

Selzer, G.: Virus isolation, inclusion bodies and chromosomes in a rubella-infected human embryo. Lancet *2*:336–337, 1963.

Selzer, G.: Rubella in pregnancy. S. Afr. J. Obstet. Gynaecol. *2*:5–9, 1964.

Sever, J. L., and Monif, G.: Limited persistence of virus in congenital rubella. Am. J. Dis. Child. *110*:452–454, 1965.

Sever, J. L., Schiff, G. M., and Huebner, R. J.: Inactivated rubella virus vaccine. J. Lab. Clin. Med. *62*:1015, 1963.

Sever, J. L., Schiff, G. M., and Huebner, R. J.: Frequency of rubella antibody among pregnant women and other human and animal populations. Obstet. Gynecol. *23*:153–159, 1964.

Sever, J. L., Fabiyi, A., McCallin, P. F., et al.: Rubella antibody among pregnant women in Hawaii. Am. J. Obstet. Gynecol. *92*:1006–1008, 1965.

Sever, J. L., Hardy, J. B., Nelson, K. B., and Gilkeson, M. R.: Rubella in the collaborative perinatal research study. Am. J. Dis. Child. *118*:123–132, 1969.

Sheppard, S., Smithells, R. W., Peckham, C. S., Dudgeon, J. A., and Marshall, W. C.: National Congenital Rubella Surveillance, 1971–75. Health Trends *9*:38–41, 1977.

Sheridan, M. D.: Final report of a prospective study of children whose mothers had rubella in early pregnancy. Br. Med. J. *2*:536–539, 1964.

Shishido, A., Hirayama, M., and Kumura, M.: A nationwide epidemic of rubella in Japan. Jpn. J. Med. *32*:253–268, 1979.

Siegel, M., and Fuerst, H. J.: Low birth weight and maternal virus disease. J.A.M.A. *197*:680–684, 1966.

Siegel, M., Fuerst, H. T., and Peress, N. S.: Fetal mortality in maternal rubella. Results of prospective study from 1957 to 1964. Am. J. Obstet. Gynecol. *96*:247–253, 1966.

Siegel, M., Fuerst, H. T., and Guinee, V. F.: Rubella epidemicity and embryopathy. Results of a long-term study. Am. J. Dis. Child. *121*:469–473, 1971.

Siegel, M., and Greenberg, M.: Virus diseases in pregnancy and their effect of the fetus. Am. J. Obstet. Gynecol. *77*:620, 1963.

Simons, M. J., and Fitzgerald, M. G.: Rubella virus and human lymphocytes in culture. Lancet *2*:937–970, 1968.

Singer, D. B., Rudolph, A. J., Rosenberg, H. S., Rawls, W. E., and Boniuk, M.: Pathology of the congenital rubella syndrome. J. Pediatr. *71*:665–675, 1967.

Singer, D. B., South, M. A., Montgomery, J. R., and Rawls, W. E.: Congenital rubella syndrome. Lymphoid tissue and immunologic status. Am. J. Dis. Child. *118*:54–61, 1969.

Singleton, E. B., Rudolph, A. J., Rosenberg, H. S., and Singer, D. B.: The roentgenographic manifestations of the rubella syndrome in newborn infants. Am. J. Roentgenol. *97*:82, 1966.

Smithells, R. W., Sheppard, S., Marshall, W. C., and Peckham, C. S.: Congenital rubella and diabetes mellitus. Lancet *1*:439, 1978.

Smithells, R. W., Sheppard, S., Marshall, W. C., and Stark, O.: National Congenital Rubella Surveillance Programme: 1971–81. Communicable Disease Report *36*:3–4, 1982.

Soothill, J. F., Hayes, K., and Dudgeon, J. A.: The immunoglobulins in congenital rubella. Lancet *1*:1385–1388, 1966.

South, M. A., and Good, R. A.: Hypogammaglobulinemia in a child with congenital rubella syndrome. Communication to the American Pediatric Society (abstract), 1966, p. 63.

Sperling, D. R., and Verska, J. J.: Rubella syndrome. Cardiovascular manifestations and surgical therapy. Calif. Med. *105*:340–344, 1966.

Starkova, O., and Ebrahim, S.: Personal communication, 1972.

Stewart, G. L., Parkman, P. D., Hopps, H. E., Douglas, R. D., Hamilton, J. P., and Meyer, H. M.: Rubella-virus hemagglutination-inhibition test. N. Engl. J. Med. *276*:554–557, 1967.

Strannegard, O., Holm, S. E., Hermodsson, S., Norrby, R., and Lyeke, E.: Case of apparent reinfection with rubella. Lancet *1*:240–241, 1970.

Struckless, E. R.: Impact of congenital rubella infection on the education system. Presented at the International Symposium on the Prevention of Congenital Rubella Infection (to be published).

Swan, C.: Rubella in pregnancy as an aetiological agent in congenital malformations, still births, miscarriage and abortion. J. Obstet. Gynaecol. Br. Emp. *56*:341–363, 1949.

Swan, C., Tostevin, A. L., Moore, B., Mayo, H., and Black, G. H. B.: Congenital defects in infants following infectious diseases during pregnancy. Med. J. Aust. *2*:201–210, 1943.

Swan, C., Tostevin, A. L., and Black, G. H. B.: Final observations on congenital defects in infants following infectious diseases during pregnancy with special reference to rubella. Med. J. Aust. *2*:889, 1946.

Taranger, J.: Vaccination programme for eradication of measles, mumps and rubella. Lancet *1*:915–916, 1982.

Tardieu, M., Grospierre, B., Durandy, A., and Griscelli, C.: Circulating immune complexes containing rubella antigens in late-onset rubella syndrome. J. Pediatr. *97*:370–373, 1980.

Taylor, D. S. I.: Choice of surgical techniques in the management of congenital cataract. Trans. Ophthalmol. Soc. U.K. *101*:114–117, 1981.

Taylor, D. S. I.: The risks and difficulties of the treatment of aphakia in infancy. Trans. Ophthalmol. Soc. U.K. *102*:403–406, 1982a.

Taylor, D. S. I.: Developments in the treatment of cataracts. Trans. Ophthalmol. Soc. U.K. *102*:441–453, 1982b.

Taylor, D. S. I.: Personal communication, 1983.

Thompson, K. M., and Tobin, J. O.: Isolation of rubella virus from abortion material. Br. Med. J. *1*:264–266, 1970.

Thorburn, M. J., and Miller, C. G.: The pathology of congenital rubella in Jamaica. Arch. Dis. Child. *42*:389–396, 1967.

Töndury, G.: Pathologie und Klinik in Einzeldarstellungen: XI Embryopathien. Berlin, Springer-Verlag, 1962.

Töndury, G., and Smith, D. W.: Fetal rubella pathology. J. Pediatr. *68*:867–879, 1966.

Townsend, J. J., Baringer, J. R., Wolinsky, J. A., Malamus, N., Mednick, J. P., Panitch, H. S., Scott, R. A.

T., Oshiro, L. A., and Cremer, N. E.: Progressive rubella panencephalitis. Late onset after congenital rubella. N. Engl. J. Med. *292*:990–993, 1975.

Townsend, J. J., Wolinsky, J., and Baringer, J. R.: The neuropathology of progressive rubella panencephalitis of late onset. Brain *99*:81–90, 1976.

Ueda, K., Nishida, Y., Oshima, K., Yochikawa, H., and Nonaka, S.: An explanation for the high incidence of congenital rubella syndrome in Ryuku. Am. J. Epidemiol. *107*:344–351, 1978.

Ueda, K., Nishida, Y., Oshima, K., and Shephard, T. H.: Congenital rubella syndrome: correlation of gestational age at time of maternal rubella with type of defect. J. Pediatr. *94*:763–765, 1979.

Vaheri, A., Vesikari, T., and Oker-Blom, N.: Isolation of attenuated rubella vaccine virus from human products of conception and uterine cervix. N. Engl. J. Med. *286*:1071–1074, 1972.

Vesikari, T., Vaheri, A., and Leinikki, P.: Antibody response to rubella virion (V) and soluble (S) antigens in rubella infection and following vaccination with live attenuated rubella virus. Archiv fur die Gesambe Virusforschung *35*:25, 1971.

Weibel, R. E., Buynak, E. B., McLean, A. A., and Hilleman, M. R.: Long-term follow-up for immunity after measles, mumps and rubella virus vaccines. Pediatrics *56*:380–387, 1975.

Weil, M. L., Habashim, H. H., Cremer, N. E., Oshiro, L. S., Lennette, E. H., and Carney, L.: Chronic progressive panencephalitis due to rubella virus stimulating SSPE. N. Engl. J. Med. *292*:994–998, 1975.

Weiss, D. I., Cooper, L. Z., and Green, R. H.: Infantile glaucoma, a manifestation of congenital rubella. J.A.M.A. *195*:725–727, 1966.

Weller, T. H., and Neva, F. A.: Propagation in tissue culture of cytopathic agents from patients with rubella-like illness. Proc. Soc. Exp. Biol. Med. *111*:215–225, 1962.

Weller, T. H., Alford, C. A., and Neva, F. A.: Retrospective diagnosis by serologic means of congenitally acquired rubella infections. N. Engl. J. Med. *270*:1039–1041, 1964.

Wesselhoeft, C.: Medical progress; rubella (German measles). N. Engl. J. Med. *236*:943–950, 978–988, 1947.

White, L. R., Leikin, S., Villavicencio, O., Abernathy, W., Avery, G., and Sever, J. L.: Immune competence in congenital rubella: lymphocyte transformation, delayed hypersensitivity, and response to vaccination. J. Pediatr. *73*:229–234, 1968.

Wilkins, J., Leedom, J. M., and Salvatore, M. A.: Clinical rubella with arthritis resulting from reinfection. Ann. Intern. Med. *77*:930–932, 1972.

Witte, J. J., Karchmer, A. W., Case, G., Herrman, K. L., Abrutyn, E., Kassanoff, I., and Neil, J. G.: Epidemiology of rubella. Am. J. Dis. Child. *118*:107–111, 1969.

Wolff, S. M.: The ocular manifestations of congenital rubella. A prospective study of 328 cases of congenital rubella. J. Pediatr. Ophthalmol. *10*:101–141, 1973.

Wolinsky, J. A., Berg, B. O., and Maitland, C. H.: Progressive rubella panencephalitis. Arch. Neurol. *33*:722–723, 2976.

Woods, W. A., Johnson, R. T., Hostetler, D. D., Lepon, M. L., and Robbins, F. C.: Immunofluorescent studies on rubella-infected tissue cultures and human tissues. J. Immunol. *96*:253–260, 1966.

World Health Organization: Prevention of Rubella. Report by a working group convened by the Regional Office for Europe of the World Health Organzation, Budapest, June 12–16, 1972. Copenhagen, WHO, 1973.

Zimmerman, L. E., and Font, R. L.: Congenital malformations of the eye: some recent advances in knowledge of the pathogenesis and histological characteristics. J.A.M.A. *196*:684, 1966.

Zinkham, W. H., Medearis, D. N., and Osbon, J. E.: Blood and bone-marrow findings in congenital rubella. J. Pediatr. *71*:512–524, 1967.

Ziring, P. R., Fedun, B. A., and Cooper, L. Z.: Thyrotoxicosis in congenital rubella. J. Pediatr. *87*:1002, 1975.

Ziring, P. R., Gallo, G., and Firegold, M.: Chronic lymphocytic thyroiditis. Identification of rubella virus antigen in the thyroid of a child with congenital rubella. J. Pediatr. *90*:419–420, 1977.

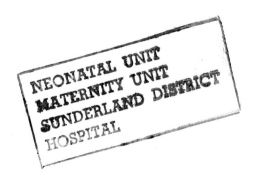

4

Congenital Cytomegalovirus

INTRODUCTION AND HISTORY

When cytomegalovirus (CMV) comes in contact with the unborn infant, the infection may be contained by the several host defense mechanisms of the fetus or disease, ranging from subtle abnormalities not detectable at birth to severe generalized disease in the newborn period, may result. The latter, more recognizable form of the infection has been better documented than the milder manifestations. Classically, cytomegalic inclusion disease (CID) is characterized by hepatosplenomegaly, hyperbilirubinemia, thrombocytopenia with petechiae or purpura, and variable involvement of the central nervous system, including cerebral calcifications, microcephaly, chorioretinitis, deafness, and psychomotor retardation (Weller and Hanshaw, 1962). These features occur in several variations and combinations. Most often, no manifestations of disease are present in early infancy, and the infant is born with a "silent" CMV infection.

The importance of congenital CMV infection as a medical problem is related, in large part, to the long-term development of infants with asymptomatic infection, as well as to that of the less common but more endangered infants with overt CID. It is probable that, for every infant born with symptoms of CID, there are at least 10 infected infants who do not have abnormalities that might suggest this diagnosis to the physician (Melish and Hanshaw, 1973).

Several studies indicate that most infants born with silent CMV infections perform well in the developmental milestones of *early* life (Kumar et al., 1973). Other studies suggest that there is a greater incidence of mental retardation and sensorineural hearing loss among these children than might be expected in control groups (Melish and Hanshaw, 1973; Reynolds et al., 1974; Hanshaw et al., 1976). The long-term studies of Peckham (1972) on silent congenital rubella infection provide sufficient data to make us wary of premature judgments about the benign nature of any viral infection acquired *in utero*. The concept of long-range damage following silent infection is no longer tentative. However, it may take several years of detailed, well-controlled psychometric and neurological examinations to determine the extent of significant sequelae occurring in a brain exposed to a virus in early gestational life.

Diosi and David (1968) and Krech and coworkers (1976) have provided comprehensive historical information concerning the CMVs. Weller (1970) has written an interesting chronicle of the isolation of the first human strains of CMV in the mid 1950's. Strikingly large inclusion-bearing cells were first documented in Germany by Ribbert (1904), who observed them in the kidneys of a stillborn infant with syphilis in 1881. He described the inclusion as a homogeneous body in the nucleus that was separated by a clear area from the nuclear membrane. His observation was not reported until 23 years later, when Jesionek and Kiolemenoglou (1904) published the first illustrations of these "protozoan-like" cells in the kidneys, lungs, and liver of another stillborn infant with syphilis. Lowenstein (1907), an assistant of Ribbert's, found inclusions in four of 30 parotid glands obtained from children two months to two years of age. Subsequently, similar inclusions were described by several investigators from 1909 through 1937.

Considerable difference of opinion existed among the various observers about the source and nature of these peculiar cellular formations. At various times they were regarded as amoebae, coccidia, and sporozoa. Goodpasture and Talbot (1921) were the first to suggest that the cellular alterations were not unlike those seen by Tyzzer (1906) in cutaneous lesions of varicella and that the "cytomegaly" could be due to the indirect effect upon the cell of a similar agent. These authors also observed that the nuclear inclusions were sometimes associated with inclusions in the cytoplasm.

It is of interest that some investigators writing in the 1920's dismissed the possibility of a protozoan origin for these cells because it was inconceivable to them that an organism of such size could cross the placenta.

In the same year that Goodpasture and Talbot alluded to the similarities of the inclusions to those observed in cells infected by Tyzzer's varicella virus, Lipschutz (1921) reported that similar structures were associated with lesions in humans and rabbits infected with herpes simplex. He maintained that the structures constituted a specific reaction on the part of the cell to a living virus. A similar view was taken by Von Glahn and Pappenheimer (1925), Farber and Wolbach (1932), and Cowdry (1934). Farber and Wolbach were the first to employ the term "salivary gland virus disease," chosen because of the propensity of the virus to induce characteristic nuclear inclusions in the lining cells of the salivary gland ductal epithelium.

Experimental evidence confirming the viral etiology of the disease was provided by Cole and Kuttner (1926), who induced the formation of inclusion bodies in guinea pigs with filtered material using a Berkefeld N filter impermeable to bacteria. They found the guinea pig virus to be heat-sensitive and relatively unstable. Andrewes (1930) attempted to propagate rodent salivary gland viruses *in vitro*. Although he was able to demonstrate intranuclear inclusion-body formation in primary cultures, attempts at serial cultivation of the agent were unsuccessful. Smith (1954) succeeded in propagating the salivary gland virus of mice in primary explant cultures of mouse embryonic tissue. Utilization of similar techniques led to the independent isolation of human CMV strains shortly thereafter by Smith (1956), Rowe and co-workers (1956), and Weller (1957).

Weller and colleagues (1960) proposed the term "cytomegalovirus" because the CID–salivary gland virus disease nomenclature was both unwieldy and misleading in that the salivary glands are only one of many possible sites of involvement. Furthermore, the term "salivary gland virus" had been used to designate unrelated agents obtained from bats.

Since the isolation of the virus in tissue culture and the subsequent development of antigens for use in a variety of serological tests, Weller and Hanshaw (1962) and Medearis (1964) have established that human CMVs are significant pathogens of the human fetus, capable of inducing a wide spectrum of oculocerebral defects as well as a variety of extraneural abnormalities. These observations have been extended and confirmed by numerous investigators in the last two decades. (Ho, 1982; Hanshaw, 1983).

EPIDEMIOLOGY

Host Range

The human CMVs have not been established as causes of natural infection in nonhuman hosts. It is difficult to elicit an immune response even when large amounts of infective virus are injected into a variety of laboratory animals. There is no evidence that the few successful immune responses that have been reported are the result of active viral replication in the inoculated nonhuman host. Macfarlane and Sommerville (1969) have reported the growth of human CMV strains in VERO cells derived from cercopithecus kidney. Thus, the possibility exists that nonhuman primates are a source of human infection.

Geographical Distribution

Wherever CMV seroepidemiological studies have been done, there has been evidence to support the concept that CMV infection is ubiquitous. The factors that are responsible for different seroconversion rates at different ages are not completely understood but may be related to socioeconomic level, crowding, breast-feeding, promiscuity, and early child-rearing practices such as day care nurseries (Pass et al., 1982a).

Numazaki and co-workers (1970) found active CMV infection in most infants five and nine months of age but no infection at birth. These infants apparently developed infection while living at home but did not become symptomatic. Table 4–1 indicates the prevalence of CMV complement-fixing (CF) antibody in different populations of children. As might be expected, the lowest incidence of positive reactors was observed in children between the ages of six months and two years. Seroconversion rates are relatively low during middle childhood and tend to rise during adolescence. It should be noted, however, that a CMF-CF antibody titer below 1:8 does not necessarily mean that an individual has not had previous experience with a given CMV strain (Waner et al., 1973).

Incidence of Infection During Pregnancy

Cervical CMV infection has been reported in several studies in Britain (Stern, 1971), the United States (Montgomery et al., 1972), Taiwan (Alexander, 1967), and Japan (Numazaki et al., 1970). All of these investigations confirm the high frequency of cervical infection during pregnancy, which ranged from 3 to 28 per cent of women cultured. As suggested, it is possible that intrapartum transmission is an important route for the vertical transmission of CMV infection. In this respect, the pathogenesis could be similar to that of the type 2 or genital strain of herpes simplex virus. Stagno and co-workers (1975a) have indicated that cervical CMV exertions seem to be suppressed in the early months of pregnancy.

We have found cytomegaloviruria in nine (4.3 per cent) of 209 women cultured in the first half of prengancy (Table 4–2) (Hanshaw et al., 1973). Two of these had CMV-IgM-antibody, suggesting, but not proving, that the infections were primary. None of these women delivered infants with cytomegaloviruria. There was evidence of an increased tendency toward reduced birth weight and premature delivery. One infant had seizures of unknown etiology in early infancy. Nonprimary infection during pregnancy may reach the developing embryo (Embil et al., 1970; Krech et al., 1971a; Stagno et al., 1973, 1977a). According to Stern (1973), approximately 50 per cent of women with primary CMV infections deliver infants with viruria. It is not known whether the remaining 50 per cent are affected in any way by the primary maternal infection. It is possible that the infections studied by Stern were not primary and represented fluctuations in CMV-CF levels such as were observed in longitudinal studies of blood donors by Waner and colleagues (1973). Stagno and co-workers (1982a) have found that approximately 15 per cent of primary maternal infections result in disease in the newborn period and that congenital disease following primary infection is more frequent and more serious than that resulting from recurrent infection. Since

Table 4–1. **PREVALENCE OF CMV COMPLEMENT-FIXING ANTIBODY IN DIFFERENT POPULATIONS OF CHILDREN**

Location	Reference	Age Range Tested	No. Tested	No. Positive	Per Cent Positive
Washington, DC	Rowe et al. (1958)	6 mo–15 yr	139	47	33.8
San Juan, PR	Mendez-Cashion et al. (1963)	1–11 yr	99	20	20.2
Stockholm, Sweden	Carlström (1965)	7 mo–15 yr	108	27	25.0
London, England	Stern and Elek (1965)	6 mo–15 yr	447	73	16.3
Debrecen, Hungary	Baczi et al. (1965)	4–14 yr	120	33	27.5
Albany, NY	Deibel et al. (1965)	0–10 yr	59	4	6.8
Rochester, NY	Hanshaw (1966)	5 mo–17 yr	380	30	7.9
Migrants from Florida	Li and Hanshaw (1967)	1–13 yr	42	21	50.0
St. Gallen, Switzerland	Krech et al. (1971)	6 mo–14 yr	1212	347	28.6
Tanzania	Krech et al. (1971)	6 mo–14 yr	66	60	90.9
Sendai, Japan	Numazaki et al. (1970)	10 mo–13 yr	238	156	65.5
Lyon, France	Jeddi et al. (1970)	6 mo–14 yr	281	52	18.6
Nova Scotia, Canada	Embil et al. (1969)	6 mo–14 yr	225	30	13.3

Table 4–2. **CYTOMEGALOVIRURIA IN UNSELECTED PREGNANT WOMEN**

Location	Reference	No. Tested	No. Positive	Per Cent Positive
Washington, DC	Hildebrandt et al. (1967)	210	7	3.3
Atlanta, GA	Feldman (1969)	185	6	3.2
Pittsburgh, PA	Montgomery et al. (1972)			
Negro		76	2	2.6
Caucasian		28	1	3.6
Rochester, NY	Hanshaw et al. (1973)	209	9	4.3
Birmingham, AL	Reynolds et al. (1973)	463	29	6.3

susceptibility to primary infection increases with socioeconomic status, the incidence of congenital disease resulting from primary infection also rises with economic status. Nevertheless, intrauterine infection was found to be more prevalent in women of low socioeconomic status (1.6 per cent) than in those of higher status (0.6 per cent), since for some unknown reason *immune* women of the former group show higher rates of congenital infection than do those of the latter.

It is possible that the impact of maternal CMV, whether primary or recurrent, upon the fetus, has been overestimated in recent years. At one time it was reported that congenital CMV was almost as common a cause of mental retardation as Down syndrome. Retrospective and prospective studies did not take into account the background element of mental retardation in the study populations. The incidence of mental retardation may vary greatly with socioeconomic status. A recent prospective survey in the United Kingdom indicates that the incidence of neurological handicaps with or without significant deafness is of the order of 195 to 260 per annum, assuming a birth rate of approximately 650,000 per year. This is of the same order of magnitude as the incidence of congenital rubella prior to the implementation of rubella vaccination.

Mothers of congenitally infected infants and asymptomatic adults with CMV infections usually do not excrete virus for more than a year. Pass and co-workers (1982a) have recently reported that shedding of CMV and the incidence of viruria declined less rapidly in the months post partum among infected women who gave birth to congenitally infected children than among those with uninfected infants. Twelve months post partum, 35 per cent of the former group of mothers shed virus, compared with 3 per cent in the latter group. A patient with CMV mononucleosis or a person subject to opportunistic infection secondary to immunosuppression or certain disease states may excrete virus in the urine or throat for one to two years or more (Jacox et al., 1964). Rowe and colleagues (1958), in an early study of CMV infection among institutionalized preschool children, found that many children excreted the virus for several months. In some instances, virus shedding was intermittent.

Seasonal Incidence

There is no clear evidence at this time that congenital or acquired CMV infection has a well-defined seasonal incidence. We were unable to recover the virus from 449 infants cultured from July through October in either 1968 or 1969. During the same years virus was recovered from 12 of 690 infants born outside these months (Hanshaw, 1971). Other investigators have not found evidence of a decreased prevalence of congenital infection during the summer months.

Duration of Virus Excretion in Congenital Infections

A congenitally infected infant may excrete CMV in the urine for months and even years after birth. We have been able to culture the virus of a congenitally infected infant for seven consecutive years. A child who is asymptomatic is less likely to have viruria beyond the third year of life. Although virus excretion may be intermittent (Benyesh-Melnick et al., 1964), it is usually found to be constant if specimens are processed in an optimal manner with respect to time and temperature variation. Stagno and colleagues (1980a) have found that perinatally acquired CMV may also be excreted in the urine and saliva for years. Stagno (1982) states that nearly all congenitally infected infants continue to excrete virus at two years of age, more than 50 per cent excrete virus for four years, and approximately 30 per cent are still virus-positive at eight years. There is little difference in the duration of excretion between infants with congenital and those with perinatal CMV infection.

TRANSMISSION

There is very little direct evidence bearing on the precise method of transmission of CMV from one host to another. There are probably several mechanisms involved, related to sex, age, lactation, state of host resistance, medications, and other treatments such as blood transfusions and hemodialysis.

Seroepidemiological studies suggest that infection is commonly acquired in early infancy in some countries such as Japan (Numazaki et al., 1970) and, to a lesser extent, the United States and the United Kingdom. A second rise in seroconversion rates has been shown to occur after puberty. This is of interest in view of the demonstration by Lang and Kummer (1972) of high titers of CMV in semen and the isolation by others of CMV from cervical swabs (Alexander, 1967; Collaborative study, 1970; Stern, 1971; Montgomery et al., 1972). The prevalence of CMV cervicitis apparently increases with gestational time, suggesting that the hormonal changes of pregnancy may have an immunosuppressive effect (Stagno et al., 1975).

An alternative explanation for increased seroconversion rates following puberty may be the presence of virus in saliva, which is exchanged in kissing (Collaborative study, 1970).

Table 4–3. **ASSOCIATION BETWEEN MATERNAL EXCRETION OF CMV FROM VARIOUS SITES AND SUBSEQUENT INFECTION OF INFANT**

Only Site of Maternal Excretion	No. Infants Infected/No. Exposed*	Percentage
Breast milk		
Breast-fed infant	11/19	58
Bottle-fed infant	0/9	0
Cervix		
3d trimester & postpartum	8/14	57
3d trimester	18/68	26
1st & 2d trimester	1/8	12
Urine†	0/11	0
Saliva†	0/15	0
Nonexcreting women		
Bottle-fed infant	0/125	0
Breast-fed infant	1/11	9

*Late 3d trimester.
†Excretion 1 day postpartum.
From Stagno, S., Reynolds, D. W., Pass, R. F., and Alford, C. A.: Breast milk and the risk of cytomegalovirus infection. N. Engl. J. Med. *302*:1073–1076, 1980.

Prenatal Transmission

Active excretion of CMV by the pregnant women is more common than intrauterine infection (Tables 4–3 and 4–4). Several investigators (Alexander, 1967; Numazaki et al., 1970; Stern, 1971; Montgomery et al., 1972) have found that cervical CMV infections occur in approximately 3 to 28 per cent of women at some time in pregnancy. Approximately 4 to 5 per cent of pregnant women excrete CMV in the urine (Hanshaw et al., 1973).

There is a wide range in the prevalence of congenital CMV infection in different pop-

Table 4–4. **CONGENITAL CMV INFECTION IN SCREENED INFANTS**

Location	No. Tested	No. Positive (%)	Screening Method
Bethesda, MD Birnbaum, et al. (1969)	545	3 (0.55)	Urine culture
Cleveland, OH Starr et al. (1970)	2147	25 (1.21)	Urine culture
Rochester, NY Melish and Hanshaw (1973)	1963	20 (1.01)	Urine culture
Birmingham, AL Stagno et al. (1977a)	939	23 (2.45)	Urine culture
Aarhus and Viborg, Denmark Andersen et al. (1979)	3060	11 (0.36)	Urine culture
Malmo, Sweden Ahlfors et al. (1979)	2200	7 (0.31)	Urine culture
Hamilton, Ontario, Canada Larke et al. (1980)	15,212	64 (0.42)	Urine culture
London, UK Peckham et al. (1983)	14,000	44 (0.30)	Urine culture

ulations. Larke and co-workers (1980) isolated virus from 0.42 per cent of 15,212 infants born in Hamilton, Ontario, Canada. In Rochester, the congenital infection rate was 1.01 per cent (Melish and Hanshaw, 1973). In Birmingham, Alabama, the incidence of congenital infection is 2.45 per cent (Stagno et al., 1977b). The prevalence of congenital CMV infection in various parts of the world is given in Table 4–4.

Stagno and colleagues (1980a) have suggested that CMV in breast milk is probably an important means of vertical transmission of virus. They studied 278 lactating women and isolated CMV from 38 (13 per cent) individuals shortly after delivery. The virus was found more often in milk (36 per cent) than in colostrum (8 per cent). Virus shedding in milk was usually brief but was detectable in some women over a two- to six-month period. Specific IgA antibody was found in 45 per cent of uninfected milk samples, as opposed to 7 per cent of the infected specimens. Although none of nine bottle-fed infants of infected mothers subsequently became virus-positive, 58 per cent of 19 infants fed infected breast milk acquired CMV infections. Dworsky and coworkers (1982b) have confirmed these results in a study indicating that human milk is the most common source of CMV for breast-fed infants. These researchers also found that CMV persisted variably in human milk after various storage and temperature treatments commonly used by milk banks, although pasteurization (62° C for 30 minutes) consistently inactivated the virus. Unless this is done, seronegative infants should receive milk from seronegative donors only. The association between maternal excretion of CMV from various sites and subsequent infection of the infant is given in Table 4–3.

These data suggest that transmission through breast milk explains the rapid and common acquisition of CMV that occurs among breast-fed infants. This should be considered a form of natural immunity in view of the minimal morbidity associated with the infection. Infants born to seronegative mothers who receive infected breast milk from other women may be at risk of disease, however. Effective mechanisms seem to exist that prevent fetal infection even when virus is readily isolated from the mother. Virus may infect the placenta (as in rubella) and not involve the fetus (Hayes et al., 1971). It is also possible for one fraternal twin to be infected with CMV and the other twin to be free from infection.

It has been widely assumed that in order for the virus to gain access to the fetus, the mother must have experienced a primary infection during pregnancy. This is apparently not universally so. Embil and colleagues (1970), Krech and colleagues (1971a), and Stagno and colleagues (1973, 1977a) have independently reported congenital CMV in consecutive pregnancies. Thus, a primary infection with viremia is not requisite for intrauterine infection. Although the possibility exists that repeated congenital infection is due to antigenically different strains of CMV, it is more likely the result of reactivation of CMV with transmission to the fetus (Stagno et al., 1977a). This explanation is supported by the enzyme restriction analysis experiments of Huang and co-workers (1980). It is generally believed that fetal infection is secondary to establishment of the infection in the placenta, which has been demonstrated by several investigators. What is not known, however, is precisely how CMV crosses from the maternal to the fetal circulation. Possibly maternal lymphocytes carry the virus to the placenta, and infection then becomes established in contiguous cells of the fetal circulation. It is quite possible that this transfer is dependent upon other, unknown, environmental factors that change the permeability of the placental vasculature.

The time at which the virus gains access to the fetus may be an important determinant of the prognosis. Monif and colleagues (1972) have reported differences in clinical severity among four patients in whom seroconversion occurred in the second and third trimesters. The two mothers whose serum converted in early pregnancy had symptomatic infants, whereas those born to the mothers whose serum converted in late pregnancy had silent infections. Further observations of this type are required before one can conclude that the time of maternal infection is as important a factor in CMV infection as it is in rubella and toxoplasmosis. Haymayer and co-workers (1954) have postulated that infants with periventricular calcifications acquired CMV encephalitis in the third or fourth month of gestation, because this is the time that the subependymal matrix is most susceptible to viral damage.

Intrapartum Transmission

In view of the relatively frequent infection of the parturient cervix, it is apparent that many infants are exposed to CMV during

Table 4–5. **CYTOMEGALOVIRURIA IN UNSELECTED HOSPITAL ADMISSIONS**

Location	Reference	Age Range Tested	No. Tested	No. Positive	Per Cent Positive
Boston, MA	Weller and Hanshaw (1962)	0–2 years	136	0	0.0
Houston, TX	Benyesh-Melnick et al. (1964)	2–10 years	30	6	20.0
Rochester, NY	Hanshaw et al. (1965)	0–14 years	100	1	1.0
London, England	Stern (1968)	0–4 years	136	13	9.6
St. Gallen, Switzerland	Krech et al. (1968)	0–9 years	224	0	0.0
Manchester, England	Collaborative study (1970)	0–4 years	1333	44	3.3

the descent through the birth canal. This type of exposure is not usually associated with disease. It is more likely to result in disease when the infant weighs less than 1500 gm and has a long oxygen requirement. Yeager and co-workers (1983) found neutropenia, lymphocytosis, thrombocytopenia, and hepatosplenomegaly in 18 of 106 (17 per cent) such infants born to seropositive mothers. Among six infected premature infants, five had undetectable antibody titers when CMV excretion began. Numazaki and colleagues (1970) found that between five and nine months of age, 60 per cent of Japanese infants excreted virus into the urine or upper respiratory tract. Some of these infections may have resulted from intrapartum contact with infected cervical secretions; others were transmitted through ingestion of virus in maternal milk immediately after birth (see Table 4–3) (Hayes et al., 1972; Stagno et al., 1980b). In both instances, IgG antibody should have been present in the maternal serum and transferred to the fetus prior to birth. Specific IgA antibody is excreted with the virus in the milk. The newborn infant may thus be exposed to virus at a time when he or she possesses antibody of maternal origin. This, in effect, could provide "passive active immunization" and account for the usually benign nature of the infection in early infancy.

Transmission During Infancy and Childhood (Tables 4–5 and 4–6)

Although few data are available, there are indications that transmission requires rather intimate contact. With virus in the infant's saliva and urine, there is opportunity for spread from one child to another. That this occurs is suggested by the generally higher rate of CMV viruria and seroconversion among institutionalized children (Hanshaw et al., 1965; Stern and Elek, 1965). As the child becomes older and improves in habits of hygiene and in socialization, there appears to be a diminution in seroconversion rates. If there is one child in the family excreting CMV, the probability is that at least one of several siblings will also have cytomegaloviruria (Hanshaw et al., 1965). Usually all children in such an environment eventually have viruria or demonstrate CMV antibody (Li and Hanshaw, 1967).

Effect of Sanitation and Socioeconomic Group on Transmission

There is a correlation between standard of living and prevalence of CMV infection in young children. The children of migrant farm workers are more likely to be actively

Table 4–6. **INCIDENCE OF CMV INFECTION IN INSTITUTIONALIZED CHILDREN**

Location	Reference	No. Tested	No. Positive	Per Cent Positive
Washington, DC	Rowe et al. (1958)	47	13	27.7
Rochester, NY	Hanshaw et al. (1965)	22	5	22.7
Timisoara, Romania	Diosi et al. (1966)	30	5	16.7
St. Gallen, Switzerland	Krech et al. (1968)	147	46	31.3
Total		246	69	28.0

infected with CMV than are children seen in urban and suburban clinics (Li and Hanshaw, 1967).

Pakistani women in London are infected with CMV more often during pregnancy than are their Caucasian counterparts (Stern, 1971). Almost all children in Tanzania acquire antibody to CMV by the age of 14 (Krech et al., 1971).

Weller (1971) has called attention to the higher seroconversion rates among preschool children living in Stockholm than among their contemporaries in the United States and the United Kingdom. He suggests that the differences may be accounted for by the Swedish child's increased probability of exposure to other children at an early age owing to the prevalence of day care nurseries in that country. Recent data from Pass and co-workers (1982a) support this theory by indicating a high rate of CMV transmission among children in a day care center; the risk to employees and mothers is unknown at this time.

Transmission Between Adults

There is increasing evidence that CMV transmission from one adult to another can be related to sexual activity. As noted, seroconversion rates increase during adolescence and early adult life. This seroepidemiological pattern has also been noted in Epstein-Barr virus (EBV) and herpes simplex virus type 2 infections. Transmission at this time could result from oral or genital infection since it is well established that virus is present in the oral cavity and in the cervix. The presence of the virus in the semen of an adult male convalescing from CMV mononucleosis has been established. The latter observation, by Lang and Kummer (1972), is of particular interest because CMV is one of the few viral agents of humans isolated from this biological fluid. Morrisseau and colleagues (1970) have detected Marburg virus antigen in the semen of a patient recently recovered from infection with this vervet-monkey virus. The patient reported by Lang and Kummer was a 23 year old Vietnam veteran with complaints of low back pain, recurrent tonsilitis, increasing lethargy and depression, fever and chills, splenomegaly, and lymphocytosis whose liver function test results were abnormal. CMV was recovered from urine and semen on six occasions during an 11-week period. The fact

that virus titers from semen samples were significantly higher than those from urine cultures suggested that the virus found in the semen was not simply a contaminant from the urine. This observation raises questions regarding the venereal transmission of CMV during heterosexual and male homosexual activity. The recent association of CMV infection with Kaposi's sarcoma in immunosuppressed male homosexuals is of considerable biological and social importance (Gottlieb et al., 1981; Drew et al., 1982).

Stagno and co-workers (1973) found similar rates of *Neisseria gonorrhoeae* isolation in CMV-excreting and CMV-nonexcreting women. CMV can be associated with systemic disease characterized by chronic fatigue, recurrent sore throats, and atypical lymphocytosis (CMV mononucleosis). It is not known, however, whether infection introduced through cervical contact can result in more than localized illness. Isolation of CMV from the cervix is often not associated with cervicitis. It is possible that many of these inapparent infections are not primary. There is evidence that, once infection becomes established in the cervix, there is a capacity for reactivation, especially during pregnancy (Numazaki et al., 1970; Montgomery et al., 1972; Stagno et al., 1973). This is perhaps not unexpected for a member of the herpesvirus group; certainly the phenomenon has been observed in herpes simplex virus type 2 cervicitis (Nahmias, 1971), which is now regarded as the second most common venereal disease.

Transmission by Blood Transfusion

In the first report by Klemola and Käärräinen (1965) on the association of CMV infection with a disease resembling infectious mononucleosis, it was noted that large amounts of blood had been given to one of their five patients. Subsequently, the same group of investigators in Helsinki presented evidence that subclinical CMV infection or CMV mononucleosis could follow the transfusion of fresh blood (Palotteimo et al., 1968). The same event was frequently observed after open heart surgery. Lang and Hanshaw (1969) studied four patients with the postperfusion syndrome and showed that these infections were transmitted by fresh blood in the fraction rich in leukocytes. Yeager and colleagues (1981) and Ballard and colleagues

(1979) have presented convincing evidence that CMV can be transmitted by blood transfusions. This phenomenon probably occurs commonly. Specimens from small, symptomatic preterm infants requiring care in a neonatal intensive care unit for more than 28 days were cultured for CMV. Of 51 infants, 16 began excreting the virus at 28 to 148 days of age (mean, 55 days). Fourteen of the 16 developed respiratory deterioration, hepatosplenomegaly, a remarkable gray pallor, and both atypical and absolute lymphocytosis. All of the infants had underlying chronic lung disease, such as respiratory distress syndrome, and all had received multiple blood transfusions.

Yeager and colleagues (1981) showed that transfusion-acquired CMV infections in newborn infants can be prevented by screening donor blood for CMV antibody. They found that seropositive blood given to seronegative infants resulted in fatal or serious symptoms in 50 per cent of the infected infants of seronegative mothers and in one of the 32 infected infants of seropositive mothers. The use of seronegative donors reduced virus shedding among hospitalized infants from 12.5 to 1.8 per cent and eliminated CMV infections in infants of seronegative mothers. Freezing and thawing of packed red blood cells will have the same effect (Adler, et al., 1983).

Transmission in the Hospital

There is little evidence that the CMVs have the capacity of rubella to cause hospital outbreaks of infection. Unpublished data from our laboratory indicate that nursing personnel working with newborn infants in premature, intensive care, and regular nurseries are no more likely to have serological evidence of infection than nurses working with children of grade school age. We have experienced one instance in which three infants in the premature nursery were excreting CMV in the urine at the same time. A culture from one of these infants taken shortly after birth was negative. Yeager and co-workers (1972) have reported the acquisition of infection after birth in two infants in a premature nursery. One infant transmitted the infection to her susceptible mother.

Yeager and colleagues (1975) also studied hospital employees for evidence of CMV seroconversion in different settings. Whereas no

seroconversions occurred among 27 seronegative hospital employees with little patient contact, annual seroconversion did occur among 4.1 per cent of 34 neonatal nurses and 7.7 per cent of 31 nurses working with older infants and children.

Haneberg and co-workers (1980) studied antibodies to CMV among personnel at a children's hopsital in Norway. They found approximately twice as many antibody-positive individuals among personnel working closely with patients than among employees with little patient contact. Their results indicate that young personnel, such as student nurses working in close contact with infants and children, are at greater risk for acquiring CMV infection. However, once standard hygienic measures were enforced, no seronegative nurses became seropositive.

There is little convincing evidence to date to indicate that CMV infection is readily disseminated to other patients or personnel in a hospital setting. Dworsky and colleagues (1983) found that the annual attack rate of 2.2 per cent among 175 susceptible nurses and physicians-in-training was lower than the 5.5 per cent attack rate among 372 new mothers in Birmingham, Alabama. They speculate that the high attack rate among new mothers is related to toddler acquisition of CMV outside the home and conclude that there is little occupational risk of CMV infection among pediatric health care workers. Wenzel and his associates (1973) have shown that natural transmission in an adult male population is characterized by limited communicability and the need for intimate contact. As age increases, viruria in the congenitally infected infant diminishes, and presumably the capacity to transfer infection to susceptible contacts is also reduced. Stagno and co-workers (1975b) found that infected infants developed decreasing titers of infectious virus per 0.2 ml of urine over the first several months of life. Asymptomatic infants with congenital infections had virus that was slightly less infectious than that of symptomatic infants. Infants with natally acquired infections shed less virus than those with congenitally acquired infections.

Guidelines for Nursery Personnel

Although CMV infection has not been proven to cause hospital epidemics of infection or disease, the *theoretical* possibility exists that a susceptible woman could acquire the primary infection on exposure to an infant with virus in the urine or upper respiratory tract. It is, therefore, prudent that some precautions be taken. The following guidelines are suggested:

1. Women who work in nurseries, especially intensive care nurseries, who are or may become pregnant should have their antibody status for CMV determined. While a positive titer for CMV-CF antibody ($\geq$ 1:8) does not preclude a subsequent fetal infection, a clinically apparent infection has been reported only once in an infant born to a woman with pre-existing antibody (Ahlfors et al., 1981).

2. Complete data indicating that seronegative pregnant women should not care for infants with known or suspected CMV infection are not yet available. As noted, the study by Dworsky and co-workers (1983) does not support the widely held concern that there is an increased occupational risk for such women.

3. Newborn infants with known or suspected CMV disease should be placed in a separate room or cubicle. If these are not available, an isolette is acceptable.

4. Strict handwashing and gown technique should be enforced.

These recommendations notwithstanding, it should be emphasized that the danger of CMV to health care personnel has not been fully established. Its communicability is clearly not of the same order of magnitude as that of rubella. This important subject is authoritatively discussed by Stagno (1982).

PATHOGENESIS AND PATHOLOGY

There are many uncertainties in our understanding of the pathogenesis of CMV infection. Not only do we not know how the fetus becomes infected, but there are large gaps in our knowledge of how the infection is transmitted to the normal and compromised adult host.

The report by Gurevich and Cunha (1981) of an outbreak of CMV infection among infants in a neonatal intensive care unit is difficult to evaluate because blood from a single donor had been given to several of the infected infants simultaneously. The use of restriction endonuclease analysis of CMV DNA as an epidemiological tool will be of great assistance in determining the true risk for nursery personnel (Wilfert et al., 1982; Yow et al., 1982). Spector (1983) used this method to detect three infants infected with the same virus in the nursery at the same time. Quinnan and colleagues (1982) have presented evidence in older children and adults that recovery from CMV infection is mediated by CMV-specific cytotoxic lymphocyte activity. Bone marrow recipients who die tend to have depressed natural and antibody-dependent killer-cell activities both before and during infection. Survivors do not.

Pathogenesis of Fetal Infection

There are a variety of possible effects that may result from CMV infection of the pregnant woman. Mothers who are infected systemically (as evidenced by cytomegaloviruria) do not necessarily produce infected offspring. Hanshaw and co-workers (1973) did not find infection in any of eight newborns born to mothers with viruria. The surrounding membranes and separate circulation of the fetus provide effective barriers to the passage of most infectious agents. The manner in which CMV is able to circumvent these barriers is not understood. Even if the infection does not pass directly to the fetus, it is conceivable that its intrauterine growth and well-being may be affected by placental or systemic maternal infection. The concept of a possible indirect effect on the fetus of an infected mother requires further study.

Stagno and colleagues (1982a) have presented important new information indicating that the pathogenesis of fetal infection is closely tied to the immune state of the mother at the time of pregnancy. They found that although primary and recurrent CMV infections both resulted in fetal infection, half of the primary infections of the mother reached the fetus and five of 33 (15 per cent) of these infants were diseased at birth. None of the 27 infants born after recurrent maternal infection had clinically apparent disease in the newborn period.

Other studies of primary CMV infections in pregnancy have been done recently by Griffiths and co-workers (1980), Grant and co-workers (1981), Ahlfors and co-workers (1981), and Kumar and co-workers (1983).

CMV and Abortions

There is some question concerning the relationship between inapparent maternal infection and the premature termination of pregnancy. Berenberg and Nankervis (1970) noted an increase in abortions of subsequent pregnancies following the delivery of infants with clinical CID. Kumar and co-workers (1973) observed subsequent pregnancies in mothers who gave birth to infants with inapparent infection and were unable to corroborate this earlier observation. Kriel and colleagues (1970) cultured aborted fetuses and found 10 per cent to be positive for CMV. This finding has not yet been confirmed by other observers. In contrast, Bouè and Loffredo (1970) attempted to isolate virus from the products of spontaneous and surgical abortions and failed to demonstrate latent viruses. The only virus of any type isolated was a type 2 strain of herpes simplex virus. Thus, the hypothesis that CMV is capable of terminating a pregnancy is not based on well-documented evidence at this time.

Recovery of Virus from Amnionic Fluid

There is a case report by Davis and co-workers (1971) of a woman with CMV mononucleosis that was diagnosed in the third month of pregnancy. Fluid from an amniocentesis performed at this time was positive for CMV. On the basis of this finding, the pregnancy was terminated. Yambao and colleagues (1981) found CMV at 36 weeks' gestation in the amnionic fluid of a woman who had CMV hepatitis at 10 weeks' gestation. The infant was born with an undescended testis, right equinovarus, and hypotonia. CMV was isolated from throat, urine and gastric aspirate cultures of the newborn. CMV was also isolated at 32 weeks' gestation from the amnionic fluid in an asymptomatic woman who delivered an infant with microcephaly, hepatosplenomegaly, intracerebral calcifications, and psychomotor retardation. The virus was also found in the infant's urine (Huikeshoven et al, 1982). It is not known if the presence of virus in the amnionic fluid always correlates with disease in the fetus or sequelaè in later life. It is probable that it does not.

CMV Infection of the Human Placenta

There is no known virus that infects the human placenta that cannot infect the fetus. All infectious agents of the fetus have been shown, on the basis of pathological and vi-

rological data, to be capable of establishing infection in placental tissue. Histopathological evidence of CMV placental infection has been described by several investigators. Feldman (1969) has isolated CMV directly from a human placenta. Placental infection can occur without leading to fetal infection. There are no viral counterparts to Q fever, which may heavily infect the placenta but does not infect the fetus directly (Syrucek et al, 1958).

Transmission to Fetus via the Cervix

Although there are numerous studies indicating that CMV commonly infects the human cervix, it is not certain that this is a source of fetal infection. It is considered more probable that fetal infection is secondary to viral infections that become established in the placenta following viremia. Cervical infections may be responsible for postpartum endometritis and cervicitis, however (Diosi et al., 1967). It is probable that CMV cervicitis produces infection in the newborn through contamination by secretions during the second stage of labor. There is little evidence to suggest, however, that infection acquired in this way is usually clinically significant.

Although not clearly established, the probability is high that the more significant fetal CMV infections occur early in pregnancy (Monif et al., 1972) and that virus reaches the fetus through the placenta or through infection of endometrial vessels, fetal mesenchyma, or trophoblast cells in the period prior to placental development. There is no precise information that explains how this might occur. The placental junction is comparable to the blood-brain barrier. Virus can leak across or be carried across by cells composing the barrier or by mobile cells. It is also possible that virus may succeed in reaching the fetus by infecting contiguous cells until it passes from the maternal to the fetal side (Mims, 1968). The replication or nonreplication of a given virus in the cells that compose the barrier may be an important determinant in successful transmission of a particular virus. The establishment of a focus of infection at the placental junction would probably be a particularly efficient pathway to the fetus. There are many viruses that are known to replicate at this site in animals, including lymphocytic choriomeningitis virus (Mims, 1968), hamster osteolytic virus (Ferm and Kilham, 1964), and infectious bovine rhinotracheitis virus (Molello et al., 1966).

If the fetus is infected prior to the development of circulating blood or lymph, the spread of virus must be by contiguous infection. After five to six weeks' gestation, with the development of a placenta and the fetal cardiovascular system, the spread of infection is probably similar to that seen postnatally. Unlike rubella virus, which is thought to spread by infection of the lining cells of blood vessels, resulting in pulmonary stenosis and patent ductus arteriosus (Rowe, 1963), there is no evidence that CMV is capable of affecting the development of the cardiovascular system in this way. It may be that CMV is less able to replicate in vascular endothelial cells. The possibility also exists that the differences in the teratogenic potential of the two agents with respect to the cardiovascular system are chiefly a function of the gestational age of the fetus at the time of virus exposure. The most typical abnormalities involving the central nervous system in infants with CMV infection (such as microcephaly and intracranial calcifications) are thought to result from the destructive effects of virus operating during the third and fourth gestational months. The classic defects in rubella embryopathy are thought to occur before this time.

Just as CMV is able to cross the placental barrier, it is able to gain access to the central nervous system across the blood-brain barrier. There is recent evidence that this occurs in the adult central nervous system as well as in the more readily penetrated fetal central nervous system (Chin et al., 1973; Dorfman, 1973). It is possible that once the virus gains access to the central nervous system, it replicates most actively in the subependymal tissue lining the ventricle. The preference may be related to the fact that this tissue is particularly undifferentiated. The involvement of subependymal cells (which subsequently migrate into the brain) is thought to have a secondary effect on subsequent brain growth and the development of microcephaly. The presence of periventricular (or subependymal) calcifications of the brain is always associated with a failure of brain development and severe neurological sequelae.

Infection of the Fetus Without Apparent Effect

In animal virology there are several examples of congenital viral infection with no adverse effect on the fetus. These include lymphocytic choriomeningitis in mice, hog cholera, equine infectious anemia, and infection with Aleutian virus. These viruses usually produce disease when introduced later in life. Rubella and CMV are examples of viral agents that may cause fetal infection without necessarily producing fetal disease.

Fetal Lesions Secondary to CMV Infection

Abnormalities resulting from early interference with organogenesis should be differentiated from those arising from infection of fully formed tissues. Most of the clinical abnormalities seen in CMV are the result of inflammatory changes occurring relatively late in pregnancy. These include hepatosplenomegaly, thrombocytopenia with petechiae and purpura, hepatitis associated with icterus, pneumonitis, and chorioretinitis. Abnormalities resulting from faulty organogenesis secondary to infection include microcephaly, optic atrophy, aplasia of various parts of the brain, and microphthalmus.

There is only indirect evidence that congenital CMV infection is responsible for malformations outside the central nervous system. Several investigators have reported an association with congenital heart lesions, but because of their rarity and diversity it is uncertain whether these abnormalities are more than coincidental. Clubfoot deformities, indirect inguinal hernias, high-arched palate, and hypospadias are some extraneural abnormalities that have been associated with congenital infection. Lists of central nervous system and extraneural defects associated with congenital CMV infections have been published (Hanshaw, 1970)

PATHOLOGICAL FINDINGS

Acute Fulminant Infection

Most infants who die in the neonatal period are premature or small for dates, indicating that intrauterine growth retardation has taken place. Of the organs affected, the kidney, liver, and lung are common sites of involvement. Less often the pathologist may find inclusion-bearing cells in the pancreas, thyroid, and brain. Rarely, inclusions are found in the intestine, ovary, pituitary, parathyroid, and thymus. Foci of extramedullary hematopoiesis are seen in the liver, spleen,

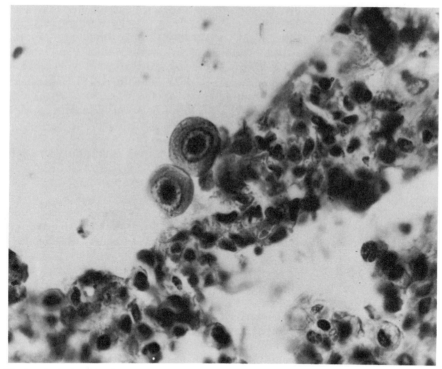

Figure 4–1. Nuclear inclusion–bearing cells exfoliated into alveolar space in patient with cytomegalovirus pneumonitis. (From Hanshaw, J. B., and Weller, T. H.: Urinary excretion of cytomegaloviruses by children with generalized neoplastic disease. Correlation with clinical and histopathologic observations. J. Pediatr. 58:305–311, 1961.)

and kidneys. The gross and microscopic appearance of the liver may be identical with that in neonatal giant cell hepatitis. It is not uncommon for this pathologic appearance to occur in the absence of the typical inclusion-bearing cells.

Kidneys. The kidneys show no gross alterations. Microscopically, inclusion-containing cells are seen, especially in the epithelium of the proximal convoluting tubules. They may also be present in the distal and collecting tubules, the interstitial tissue, and the glomeruli. Affected cells may desquamate into the lumina of the tubules and appear in the urinary sediment. This phenomenon was the basis for a diagnostic test used prior to the development of methods for the isolation of virus. Some tubular cells may show cloudy swelling. Mononuclear cell infiltration may be present in the peritubular zones of the kidney.

Lungs. Pulmonary CMV lesions are similar in the adult and the newborn. The pneumonitis may be bilateral or unilateral and generally involves the lower lobes. On gross examination there may be well-defined rounded areas, 2 mm to 6 cm in diameter, located just beneath the pleura. Their nod-

ular character may be lost as the disease process advances and becomes more confluent. Microscopically, the alveolar cells appear large, and some contain intranuclear inclusions (Fig. 4–1). An asphyxial barrier to gas exchange may be present in the form of periodic acid–Schiff (PAS)-positive hyaline membranes adjacent to the septal wall. These membranes are found less often in young infants than in older children and adults. Numerous mononuclear and plasmacytic inflammatory cells may appear focally or more diffusely throughout the septal walls.

Pneumocystis carinii and bacterial infections frequently coexist with CMV infection. This usually occurs in older patients who have been on immunosuppressive therapy.

Liver. The gross changes in the liver are variable. Some patients dying in early infancy have yellow fatty changes; others have evidence of cirrhosis. Microscopically, there may be disintegration of the normal lobular architecture with areas of necrosis in the parenchyma, peripherally as well as in the center of the lobule. When inclusions are present, they are often in the parenchyma, Kupffer's cells, and biliary duct epithelium. Observations of inclusions in the biliary duct epithelium have led to the speculation that intrauterine CMV infection may be one cause of biliary duct reduplication. Regenerative activity of the hepatic cells is often present.

Brain. The most extensive changes in the brain involve the subependymal mantle and the adjacent periventricular areas. The ependyma can appear rust-colored and become irregularly thickened to form either coarse rugae or fine granulations. Calcifications occur in discrete clusters in the subependymal mantle and adjacent white mantle. Rarely, aqueductal stenosis leading to hydrocephalus occurs, presumably owing to obstruction of the fourth ventricle.

CLINICAL MANIFESTATIONS

There are many clinical variants in congenital CMV infection, ranging from silent infection to the more severe classic CID. The more adversely affected infants represent less than 5 per cent of all infected newborns. Typical clinical features include hepatomegaly, splenomegaly, jaundice, petechial or purpuric rash, microcephaly, chorioretinitis, and cerebral calcifications. Each of these manifestations will be considered separately.

Hepatomegaly

This sign, along with splenomegaly, is probably the most common abnormality noted in the newborn period. The liver edge is smooth and nontender and usually extends 3 to 7 cm below the right costal margin. The larger the liver, the greater the probability that hyperbilirubinemia will be present. Liver function test results are often abnormal but usually not markedly so. The serum glutamic oxalacetic transaminase (SGOT) level rarely exceeds 800 and is usually below 500 units. Histopathological examination of the neonatal liver may reveal multinucleated giant cells not unlike those of the so-called giant cell hepatitis of neonates that is associated with other known and unknown disease states. The presence of large inclusion-bearing cells may permit a distinction between CMV infection and other causes of giant-cell transformation. Additional changes in the liver include nuclear swelling, focal infiltration or necrosis, and bile stasis. Giant-cell transformation may be associated with disorganization of the liver architecture, early regeneration and scarring, focal necrosis, and

extramedullary hematopoiesis. Weller and Hanshaw (1962) isolated CMV from the urine or liver of five of 10 infants with the histological changes of "neonatal hepatitis." In most instances, other findings characteristic of CID were also present.

It is believed that enlargement of the liver and the spleen is a reticuloendothelial response to chronic infection.

The association of CMV with liver abnormalities has been established in both congenital and acquired CMV infection. In an institutional study, Rowe and co-workers (1958) noted hepatomegaly in some children with CMV infection. In 1965, Hanshaw and colleagues reported hepatomegaly or abnormal liver function test results (particularly alkaline phosphatase and SGOT), or both, in 19 of 20 children with asymptomatic viruria. Although some patients with congenital CMV infection have developed cirrhosis of the liver (Lysaught, 1962), there is no good evidence that chronic active hepatitis is associated with acquired CMV infection (Toghill et al., 1969). Reller (1973) has presented evidence that acquired CMV infection may be responsible for granulomatous hepatitis.

In the great majority of patients with congenital or acquired CMV infection involving the liver, the abnormalities noted are mild and reversible. Patients with CMV mononucleosis frequently have some liver enlargement and liver function abnormalities, such as elevation of the SGOT. In this respect these patients are not unlike those with infectious (EBV) mononucleosis.

The persistence of hepatomegaly is variable. In some infants, enlargement disappears by the end of the second month of life. In others, significant hepatomegaly persists throughout the second year. Viruria may continue long after the diminution in liver size. Massive hepatomegaly extending beyond the first 12 months of life is quite uncharacteristic of CID.

Splenomeglay

Enlargement of the spleen is found to a greater or lesser degree in all the common congenital infections of humans and is especially frequent in congenital CMV infections. It may be the only abnormality present at birth. In some instances, splenomegaly and a petechial rash coexist as the prime manifestations of the disease. Occasionally the spleen size is greater than 5 to 6 cm. Rupture of the

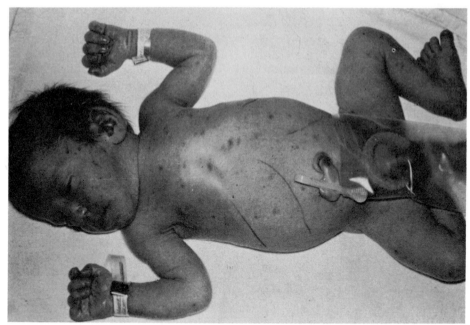

Figure 4–2. Generalized purpura and hepatosplenomegaly in a newborn infant with cytomegalic inclusion disease. (See the color frontispiece illustration.) (Courtesy of Dr. Joseph L. Butterfield, Denver, Colorado.)

spleen, a complication of EBV-induced infectious mononucleosis in older persons, has not been reported in CMV mononucleosis or in congenital disease.

In some patients dying of CID, there may be direct evidence of CMV infection of splenic tissue. Virus is often directly isolated from this organ, and large inclusion-bearing cells may be seen.

Hyperbilirubinemia

This is a common manifestation of congenital CMV infection, occurring in more than half of symptomatic infants in the first week of life. The pattern of hyperbilirubinemia may take several forms: levels on the first day may be high enough to require exchange transfusion; or there may be undetectable jaundice on day 1, with gradual elevation of the bilirubin level to clinically apparent jaundice (Weller and Hanshaw, 1962). There may be considerable fluctuation in the level of jaundice in the early weeks of life. In some instances, icterus is a transient phenomenon, beginning on the first day of life and disappearing by the end of the first week. More often, however, the jaundice tends to persist beyond the time usual for physiological jaundice. Occasionally patients may have transient jaundice in early infancy followed by marked

hyperbilirubinemia during the third month. The bilirubin levels are elevated in both the direct and indirect components. Characteristically, the direct component increases after the first few days of life and may constitute as much as 40 to 50 per cent of the total bilirubin level. It is unusual for the indirect bilirubin to rise to levels requiring exchange transfusion, but this has been reported (Weller and Hanshaw, 1962).

Petechiae, Purpura, and Thrombocytopenia

There is evidence that CMV has a direct effect on the megakaryocytes of the bone marrow, resulting in a depression of the platelets and a localized or generalized petechial rash. In some patients, the rash is purpuric in character, similar to that described in the expanded rubella syndrome (Fig. 4–2 and the frontispiece, Fig. B). Unlike the latter infection, however, fine pinpoint petechiae are a common manifestation of congenital CMV infection. The petechial rash may be transient, disappearing within 48 hours. It is rarely present at birth, but often appears a few hours thereafter. The petechiae may be the only clinical manifestation of CMV infection. More often, however, there is associated enlargement of the liver and the spleen. The petechiae may persist for weeks after birth and, in some instances, are present well into the first year of life. Crying, coughing, the application of a tourniquet, a lumbar puncture, or restraints of any kind may result in the appearance of petechiae. Although purpuric phenomena have not been clearly established as manifestations of acquired CMV infection, we have observed one sibship of two brothers who had cytomegaloviruira and chronic recurrent petechiae.

Platelet counts in the first week of life vary from less than 10,000 to 125,000, with a majority in the range from 20,000 to 60,000. Some infants with petechial rashes do not have associated thrombocytopenia.

Microcephaly

Prior to 1962, it was not fully appreciated that reduced head circumference was a major manifestation of CID. As virologically documented patients were followed into the first and second years of life, the diminution in head circumference with respect to crown-rump length, chest circumference, and weight became more apparent. Microcephaly (Fig. 4–3), usually defined as a head circumference of less than the third percentile, was found to be present in 14 of the 17 patients reported by Weller and Hanshaw (1962) and in all seven patients studied by Medearis

(1964). With expanded use of tissue culture methods and increased clinical awareness of the infection, microcephaly became a less prominent symptom in subsequent study series, which were composed mainly of infants born with less severe disease. Although there are reports of infants with microcephaly who later were judged to have normal intelligence (Berenberg and Nankervis, 1970), the great majority of infants with disproportionate growth in head circumference have associated psychomotor retardation. Not all infants with microcephaly continue to have head circumferences less than the third percentile. This is especially true if the head measurement is close to the third percentile in an infant of low birth weight. If intracranial calcifications are present, the growth of the brain is invariably impaired. The presence of calcifications is an indication that the infant will have severe psychomotor retardation.

In the 1960's, CMV-infected patients with microcephalic mental deficiency, periventricular calcifications, and severe psychomotor retardation were observed who did not have a neonatal history of hepatosplenomegaly, petechiae, or jaundice. The characteristic calcifications alone distinguished them from the many patients referred for severe developmental retardation. These observations suggested that if CMV could induce severe damage localized in the central nervous system, then more subtle yet clinically significant

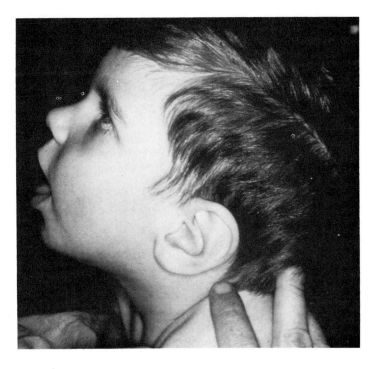

Figure 4–3. Three year old boy with microcephaly and severe psychomotor retardation.

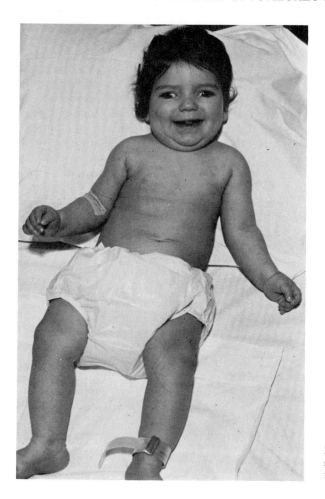

Figure 4–4. Nine month old female infant with strabismus associated with cytomegalovirus chorioretinitis.

forms of cerebral dysfunction might also occur. On the basis of this hypothesis, microcephalic patients were compared with normocephalic children with respect to the prevalence of CMV-CF antibody. Nine of 25 (36 per cent) children six months to eight years old were antibody-positive, in contrast to seven of 157 (5 per cent) normocephalic control children (Hanshaw, 1966). Subsequently, younger patients (6 to 24 months of age) with microcephaly were studied, and a similar percentage (35 per cent) was found to be seropositive (Hanshaw, 1968). Baron and co-workers (1969) found a higher prevalence of CMV-CF antibody in microcephalic than in normocephalic children five months to five years of age. These differences were not significant, however. Stern and colleagues (1969) found antibody in 14 of 64 (22 per cent) microcephalic mentally retarded children and in 6.5 per cent of 154 normal controls. These differences are statistically significant.

These studies were all done retrospectively and therefore do not provide accurate estimates of the true prevalence of damage to the central nervous system caused by *congenital* CMV. In prospective studies of 47 infected infants by Stern (1968), Birnbaum and co-workers (1969), Starr and co-workers (1970), and Hanshaw and co-workers (1973), eight were found to have some kind of central nervous system abnormality. Of these, four were microcephalic. These data strongly suggest that most congenitally infected infants detected in surveys of general deliveries do not subsequently develop disease severe enough to reduce the head circumference significantly.

Ocular Defects

The principal abnormalities related to the eye are chorioretinitis, strabismus (Fig. 4–4), and optic atrophy, although microphthalmus, cataracts, retinal necrosis and calcification, blindness, anterior chamber and optic disc malformations, and pupillary membrane vestige have been described in association with generalized congenital CID (Hanshaw, 1970). Nonetheless, the presence of unusual abnormalities such as microphthalmus and cataracts is evidence that the disease process is probably *not* due to CMV.

CMV chorioretinitis cannot be differentiated on the basis of location or appearance from the lesions produced by toxoplasmosis. Both *Toxoplasma gondii* and CMV can induce central retinal lesions. If the lesion involves the macula or there is optic atrophy, there may be an associated diminution or distortion of vision; blindness is rare. Occasionally strabismus necessitating referral to an ophthalmologist is the means by which CMV or toxoplasma chorioretinitis is detected. Once present the lesions persist, but they may become inactive in early infancy.

Cerebral Calcifications

Areas of periventricular calcification in the subependymal region are characteristic but not pathognomonic of severe congenital CMV encephalitis (Fig. 4–5). Severe microcephaly is frequently associated with calcium deposition. Rarely, obstruction of the fourth ventricle follows and hydrocephalus develops, a condition that is usually fatal (Fig. 4–6). Chorioretinitis, optic atrophy, and strabismus are frequently seen in patients with cerebral calcifications. Although fewer than 1 per cent of all CMV-infected infants have calcifications, their appearance in a periventricular distribution is strong evidence of the severest form of congenital CID.

Deafness

Medearis (1964) was the first investigator to call attention to the presence of deafness in congenitally infected patients with documented viruria. Subsequently, other reports have appeared that establish CMV as one of several known causes of deafness (Williamson et al., 1982, Saigal et al., 1982). There is evidence that the deafness is the result of a direct viral effect on the inner ear. Davis

Figure 4–5. Linear periventricular calcifications in a patient with microcephaly secondary to congenital cytomegalovirus infection.

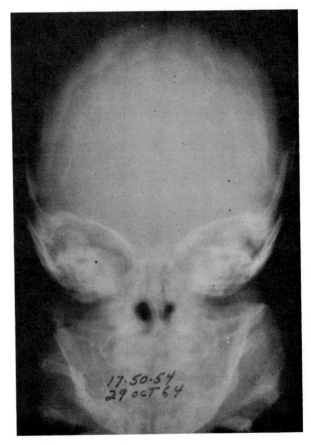

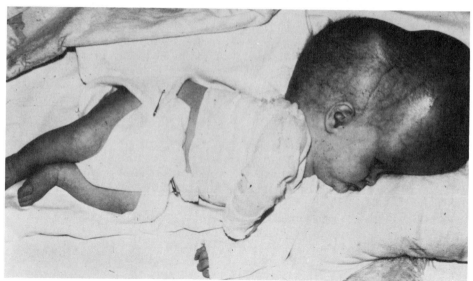

Figure 4–6. Obstructive hydrocephalus in an infant with periventricular calcifications secondary to congenital cytomegalovirus infection.

(1969) found cytomegalic cells in the stria vascularis, Reissner's membrane, and semicircular canals. In 1979 Davis and his associates isolated CMV from the inner ear. The effect of virus on the inner ear may be a continuing one, as suggested by the observation that hearing loss may not be suspected until the second year of life (Melish and Hanshaw, 1973). In some infants the sensorineural loss is unilateral. Evidence suggests that from 10 to 20 per cent of infants born with clinically apparent or silent infection will have hearing loss in one or both ears (Hanshaw, 1982a).

Other Clinical Manifestations of Acute Infection

Hemolytic anemia has occasionally been described in association with CMV infection. The Coombs' test results have been both negative and positive in the few reported cases (Zuelzer et al., 1970).

Pneumonitis, a common clinical manifestation of CMV infection following renal allograft (Craighead et al., 1967), is also seen in the newborn period. We observed one premature infant who was well except for peaceful tachypnea. In the third month of life she returned to the hospital with sudden and severe respiratory distress and died within 24 hours. Occasionally older infants, three to five months of age, with diffuse interstitial pneumonitis, pertussis-like cough, and enlargement of the liver or spleen are

seen. The illness may last several weeks. Virus can be recovered from the upper respiratory tract and the urine. It may be difficult to determine whether these infections are CMV-induced or simply associated with the disease process.

Stagno and co-workers (1981) found 21 of 104 infants with pneumonitis to be infected with CMV, while noting that pneumonitis syndromes associated with chlamydia, pneumocystis, and CMV were clinically indistinguishable. Dworsky and Stagno (1982) have reported that symptoms of the disease had a longer duration when associated with CMV infection and that paroxysmal cough was often observed in CMV-related pneumonitis. Since pneumonitis is found in fewer than 1 per cent of newborns with congenital CMV infection, the condition may result from infection acquired during birth or from breast milk. The study found significantly more black infants with CMV-related pneumonitis than white infants.

There are no characteristic radiographic changes caused by CMV pneumonitis in the newborn. The patient with silent tachypnea already described had a diffuse interstitial infiltrate appearing late in the course of the illness. Infants with pertussis-like illnesses have had peribronchial infiltrates not unlike those seen in other viral infections of the lower respiratory tract. It should be emphasized that pulmonary abnormalities are not usually part of the CID clinical presentation in the neonatal period, and an etiological

Table 4–7. **CARDIOVASCULAR ABNORMALITIES ASSOCIATED WITH CONGENITAL CMV INFECTION**

Atrial septal defect
Congenital mitral stenosis
Ventricular septal defect
Tetralogy of Fallot
Enlarged ductus
Accessory semilunar fold of foramen ovale
Hyperplasia of elastica in abnormal arteries
Anomalous venous return

Table 4–8. **GASTROINTESTINAL ABNORMALITIES ASSOCIATED WITH CONGENITAL CMV INFECTION**

Biliary atresia
Esophageal atresia
Megacolon
Omphalocele
Cleft palate
Stenosis of the ileum and colon
Intestinal perforation
Malformed pylorus
Ascites
Peritonitis

relationship between CMV infection and a pertussis-like illness has not been fully established. Kim and colleagues (1982) have reported a case in which perinatal CMV infection appeared to result in bilateral diffuse nodular pulmonary infiltration.

Congenital Anomalies

Extraneural Anomalies. Abnormalities involving many organs have been associated with congenital CMV infection. It is doubtful that all of these associations are the result of congenital infection.

Cardiovascular Abnormalities. A list of cardiovascular abnormalities is given in Table 4–7. Although cardiovascular defects are associated with congenital CMV infection, there is no consistent pattern to these abnormalities, and the great majority of infected infants have normally functioning hearts. Prospective studies of unselected newborns do not suggest that CMV has the same cardiovascular teratogenicity that rubella possesses. Indeed, it is questionable whether CMV can be considered a cardiovascular teratogen.

Genitourinary Abnormalities. Although cytomegaloviruria is a consistent finding in congenital CMV infection and there is evidence of glomerular, proximal, and distal tubule infection, there is little evidence to support the thesis that CMV is a cause of genitourinary tract anomalies. Occasional reports of hypospadias suggest a possible causal effect (Hildebrandt et al., 1967). It is interesting to note that this abnormality has also been observed in congenital rubella.

Gastrointestinal Abnormalities. There are several reports associating gastrointestinal defects with congenital CMV infection. These abnormalities are listed in Table 4–8. The association with biliary atresia (Oppenheimer and Esterly, 1973) is of particular interest because this anomaly has also been seen in congenital rubella. The atretic bile ducts could be the result of chronic CMV infection of the bile duct epithelium *in utero*, but there is no evidence to support this concept at present. It is of interest that gastrointestinal ulcerations involving the esophagus, the stomach, and the small and large bowel have been associated with histological evidence of CMV infection. CMV has been cultured from the gastrointestinal tract (Cox and Hughes, 1973). Rosen and co-workers (1973) have reported three cases of gastrointestinal CMV infection in adults with malignant disease. These authors consider the infection an aggravating factor in immunosuppressed patients who develop ulcerative lesions of the gastrointestinal tract. They postulate that the virus may be carried to the ulcer site by circulating macrophages that are coincidentally infected with CMV.

Musculoskeletal Abnormalities. Medearis (1964) and Lang (1966) called attention to the association of indirect inguinal hernia and congenital CMV infection. Numerous investigators have noted a variety of abnormalities, ranging from mild spasticity to spastic quadriplegia. Abnormalities involving the musculoskeletal system are listed in Table 4–9.

Dental Abnormalities. Stagno and co-workers (1982b) have documented yellowish

Table 4–9. **MUSCULOSKELETAL ABNORMALITIES ASSOCIATED WITH CONGENITAL CMV INFECTION**

Flabby abdominal musculature
Clubfoot
Bilateral dislocation of hip
Deformity of right ankle
Diastasis recti
Inguinal hernia
Spastic diplegia and quadriplegia
Generalized hypotonia
Myocardial aneurysm

discoloration and hypocalcification of enamel in the teeth of 40 per cent of children with severe congenital CMV infection and 5.4 per cent of infected but asymptomatic children. The subjects of the study were too young for prognosis concerning enamel in permanent teeth.

Late Clinical Manifestations

As indicated, there is growing evidence that most infants with congenital CMV infection may have few or no early clinical manifestations but develop subtle neurological abnormalities that become apparent in the late preschool or early school years. If CMV has a late effect, it should be detectable during the early school years. However, in some instances a slow child is also culturally disadvantaged, and no thought is given to the possibility of an organic cause for poor school performance. This concept is a relatively new one in the evaluation of the child who fails to do well in a school setting, and it deserves further study. The possibility exists that a significant proportion of children who do not do well in school are, in fact, handicapped because of chronic CMV infection that began *in utero* (Reynolds et al., 1974; Hanshaw et al., 1976). OF 44 such children evaluated by our group at three and one-half to seven years of age, 16 (36 per cent) had neurological sequelae severe enough to predict school failure. The abnormalities included one or more of the following: mental retardation, minimal cerebral dysfunction, speech and hearing defects, and behavioral disturbances. In contrast, six of 44 (14 per cent) matched control children had abnormalities predictive of school failure (Hanshaw et al., 1976).

Immune Complexes in Congenital Disease

Stagno and co-workers (1977b) found immune complexes in three of four symptomatic patients whose deaths were due to severe congenital CMV infection. These patients had granular deposits of immunoglobulins and C3 in a pattern typical of immune complexes along the glomerular basal membrane of the glomeruli. It is not known whether these heavy immune complexes contributed to the adverse clinical outcome.

These complexes were apparently filtered from the circulation and trapped in the glo-merulus. Their presence in this location suggests the probability of abnormal renal function. It is conceivable that a slow and insidious process could take place over months and years in children who are not clinically ill with CMV disease.

Comments

The manifestations of congenital CMV infection are highly variable, but it is apparent that most infected infants are not identifiable on the basis of the clinical presentation. Probably fewer than 5 per cent of neonates have manifestations typical enough to suggest the diagnosis. Some infants may be small for dates with evidence of intrauterine growth retardation. Others simply do not do well, and their condition is labeled "failure to thrive." Such infants may have a head circumference and weight less than the third percentile with normal height. Associated with these measurements may be evidence of psychomotor retardation, spasticity, hypotonia, premature closure of the anterior fontanelle, equinus varus, strabismus, high-arched palate, and indirect inguinal hernia. The degree of psychomotor retardation or other neurological dysfunction (especially minimal cerebral dysfunction and specific learning disabilities) may take several years to identify. Many infected infants are hyperactive, have a short attention span, and exhibit abnormalities in gross and fine motor movements. The measured IQ may be above 70, but school achievement is often below the level of that of other family members.

LABORATORY ASPECTS

Classification of the Organism

As suggested by the earliest pathological observations, the cellular changes in CMV-infected tissue resemble those seen with herpes simplex virus and herpesvirus varicella infections. With the evolution of the system of viral classification proposed by Andrewes (1962) and Lwoff and co-workers (1962), it has become clear that, on the criteria of nucleic acid type, symmetry, presence of an envelope, and numbers of capsomeres, the CMVs are herpesviruses. Thus, in 1965 the Provisional Committee for Nomenclature of Viruses proposed that CMV be considered a separate genus within the Herpesviridae family. This genus also included the nonhuman CMV isolated by Smith (1954) from mice and the guinea pig strains isolated by Hartley and colleagues (1957), as well as the strains isolated from African green monkeys (Black et al., 1963), pigs (L'Ecuyer and Corner, 1966), rats (Rabson et al., 1969), and horses (Hsiung et al., 1969). There is cytological evidence that many other species can be infected with viruses capable of producing the cytomegaly characteristic of the CMVs. These include dogs (Jackson, 1921), hamsters (Kuttner and Wang, 1934), moles (Rector and Rector, 1934), chimpanzees (Vogel and Pinkerton, 1955), and sheep (Hartley and Done, 1963).

CMV is one of five known herpesviruses of humans. In addition to the two herpes simplex viruses and herpesvirus varicellae, EBV has also been found to have the ultrastructure and physicochemical properties of a herpesvirus. On the basis of cross-reactions observed in indirect fluorescent antibody tests (Hanshaw et al., 1972), there is evidence that CMV, EBV, and varicella-zoster (V-Z) viruses are antigenically related. In addition, herpes simplex and V-Z viruses show antigenic similarities in cross-neutralization tests.

Although species specificity is generally characteristic of human strains, the host range of viruses from nonhuman sources may be less restricted (Raynaud et al., 1969).

Morphology

A large intranuclear inclusion is the most striking morphological feature of the CMV-infected cell (see Fig. 4–1). The inclusion is approximately 8 to 10 μ in diameter, with an overall cellular diameter of 25 to 40 μ. Thus, the large cellular size is the result of an increase in the volume of both the nucleus and the cytoplasm. The nuclear inclusion is located centrally and corresponds to the shape of the cell. It is composed of aggregates of chromatin and three types of virus particles. With hematoxylin and eosin staining, the nuclear inclusion is seen to be more eosinophilic than the nuclear membrane and the cytoplasmic contents. The nuclear membrane consists of beads of nuclear chromatin. The nucleolus of CMV-infected cells is usually displaced peripherally within the nucleus, in contrast to the nucleolus in uninfected cells, which is more centrally located. There are no viral particles in the nucleolus. After negative staining with potassium

phosphotungstate, the virion can be seen to consist of a 110-mμ icosahedron capsid with 162 capsomeres. The enveloped particle ranges in size from 180 to 250 mμ. Particles measuring 95 to 100 mμ are formed in the nuclear inclusion and consist of a central core surrounded by a single membrane. A second coat is acquired from the inner nuclear membrane as the particle moves into the cytoplasm. Within the cytoplasm and after extrusion from the cell, the enveloped particles usually measure 150 to 170 mμ in diameter.

In 1965, Patrizi and colleagues described three virus particles in the nucleus. One is a spherical particle 65 to 95 mμ in diameter with a limiting membrane; a second form is spherical and consists of an electron-lucent or electron-opaque core surrounded by an outer and inner membrane. These virus particles are associated with aggregates of chromatin in the nuclear inclusion. A third virus particle (diameter 115 to 145 mμ) has an additional outer coat with an electron-opaque core. It is surrounded by an electron-lucent area 60 to 74mμ in diameter. The particles may be seen in clusters between the outer and inner nuclear membranes and near the nuclear periphery.

Unlike other herpesviruses of humans, with the rare exception of V-Z virus, the CMV-infected cells frequently have cytoplasmic inclusions measuring 2 to 4 μ in diameter. These inclusions are seen only in cells that also have nuclear inclusions. They are usually basophilic and react positively with PAS stain. The cytoplasmic inclusions contain mature virus particles surrounded by larger, nonviral particles that are thought to be lysosomes. Horn and co-workers (1967) have postulated that lysosomes engulf and surround the virus particles in a manner comparable to the phagocytosis of bacteria. It is possible that this mechanism accounts for the low infectivity of CMV *in vitro*. A low lysosomal content may be a factor in the persistence of CMV in salivary glands (Ruebner et al., 1966).

Electron microscopic studies have shown that CMV differs in some respects from some of the other members of the herpesvirus group. Smith and Rasmussen (1963) have observed a large number of partially or completely empty nucleoids in CMV particles. These authors have postulated that their observation may explain the high particle-infectivity ratio of CMV (approximately 10^7 to 10^8). In this respect, CMV resembles V-Z virus, which produces very little virus in tissue culture media despite the fact that as many as 10^9 V-Z virus particles may be seen per milliliter of medium.

Irregular masses of homogeneous dense material have been noted in the cytoplasm of cells infected with human CMV. According to Craighead and colleagues (1972), this substance appears to be produced by microtubular membranes and the Golgi apparatus. It "buds" into cytoplasmic tubules, forming circumscribed bodies with an investing membrane that has antigenic determinants in common with the viral envelope. The biological role of this homogeneous dense material is not yet known. It has not been observed in viruses other than human CMV.

The morphology of cultured human fibroblasts infected with "wild" and "adapted" strains of CMV differ with regard to the number of morphological types of inclusions and their appearance. Kanich and Craighead (1972) have found that the nuclei of cells infected with an adapted strain retain their oval configuration. The nuclear inclusions in cells supporting the growth of the two strains of virus are structurally similar. Cytoplasmic inclusions of five ultrastructural types have been described. Wild virus strains tend to produce extensive cell lysis early in the course of infection in association with the release of incomplete viral components of low infectivity. This is in contrast to an adapted strain (AD 169) that produces a more chronic infection of cells and is associated with the release of large amounts of infectious virus.

Kanich and Craighead have also noted electron microscopic differences in wild and adapted strains of CMV. Whereas adapted virus particles characteristically have electron-dense cores of irregular outline, the wild strain produces semitranslucent cores with "doughnut" configurations. These authors postulate that abnormal core synthesis and assembly may be responsible for the low yield of infectious virus by cells inoculated with the wild strain of CMV. The possibility exists that premature interruption of the replicative sequence by early cell lysis may prevent the complete assembly of infectious virions.

Staining Reactions

The DNA core of CMV can be distinguished with uranyl acetate when particles are observed at electron microscopic magnification (Benyesh-Melnick et al., 1966a). The DNA structure is also indicated by acridine orange staining (Niven, 1959). Although the nuclear and cytoplasmic inclusions of CMV-infected murine cells were found to be Feulgen-positive and PAS-negative by Ruebner and co-workers (1964), cytoplasmic inclusions in human CMV-infected cells have been found to be PAS-positive (Smith, 1959).

McAllister and colleagues (1963) have correlated cytochemical observations of intracellular lesion development with viral synthesis and release. They employed May-Gruenwald-Giemsa, methyl green–pyronine, fluorescent Feulgen, and PAS stains in their study. Twenty-four hours after infection, basophilic, lipid-containing, PAS-positive bodies surrounded by a halo containing RNA appeared in the cytoplasm near the nucleus. DNA and viral antigen appeared in the nucleus in 48 hours. DNA was present in the cytoplasmic lesion, and the nucleus was significantly enlarged in 72 hours. At this time, infectious virus was found in the cell, and it was released into the medium shortly thereafter.

Growth in Tissue Culture

Although human CMV infection *in vivo* primarily involves epithelial cells, human fibroblastic cells are required for *in vitro* growth. This paradox has not been explained. Many kinds of fibroblastic cells can support the growth of CMV. These include embryonic skin and muscle, lung, testis, myometrium, and foreskin. Diploid cells, such as WI-38, are widely used because of their susceptibility to viral replication and their availability through commercial sources.

The cytopathic changes characteristic of CMV appear more slowly in tissue culture than do those of most other viruses. Adapted strains and some wild strains, however, may produce cell rounding within 24 hours. Since infectious CMV is mainly cell-associated, infection usually spreads from cell to cell, producing foci, or clusters, of rounded, refractile cells. These foci increase in number throughout the cell sheet, develop central degeneration, and eventually involve the entire monolayer. This progression may take two to four weeks. In well-adapted strains, complete cellular involvement may occur in 10 days or less.

Virus strains may be passed serially in tissue culture by trypsin dispersion of the infected monolayer or with passage of the cells to an uninfected monolayer. Trypsin dispersion of cell cultures with early viral cytopathic effect (CPE) can be employed to promote more rapid progression of the CPE. This may be related to the effect of trypsin on membrane permeability. Benyesh-Melnick (1969) has presented in detail the methodology for virus passage and storage, preparation of cell-free virus stocks, and virus assay. Huang and co-workers (1974) have described a method for procurement of large amounts of extracellular virus.

Antigenic Structure

Antigenic heterogeneity among various human CMV strains was first suggested by cross-neutralization tests reported in 1960 by Weller and colleagues. Similarly, complement-fixing (CF) antibody tests performed by Medearis (1964) have also suggested an antigenic mosaic within the CMV subgroup. These differences appear to be less apparent in older children and adults. Waner and co-workers (1973) performed longitudinal CF antibody tests on normal adults and found that when sera are tested at monthly intervals against antigens prepared from three prototype strains, complement may be preferentially fixed with one or two strains, or all three strains may fix at the same level. The AD 169 strain, widely used in serodiagnostic tests, is broadly reactive but not uniquely so. Although multiple serotypes of CMV are not yet clearly established or officially adopted by the Provisional Committee for Nomenclature of Viruses, Weller et al. (1960) tentatively proposed that the Davis strain be classified as type 1 and the AD 169 strain as type 2. The Kerr and Esp strains are possibly a third serotype.

It is not certain whether neutralizing and CF antibodies are stimulated by different antigens. Benyesh-Melnick and colleagues (1966b) have provided evidence that half of the CF antigen from infected CMV cells is soluble and can be separated from the viral particles by differential ultracentrifugation. Very little or no CF activity is found in supernatant fluids of CMV-infected cells. The CF antigen is more stable at 4° C than at 37° C. This is in contrast to the viral infectivity of CMV.

Hemolysis has not been associated with CMV cell infection, and hemadsorption has not been demonstrated.

In general, there is no CF cross-reactivity between human and nonhuman CMV strains. It has been found, however, that serum from cercopithecus monkeys may react in a unidirectional CF cross-reaction with the AD 169 strain of CMV. This does not occur with other strains such as the Davis strain, which may react weakly or not at all (Dreesman and Benyesh-Melnick, 1967). Human sera react only with human CMV-CF antigens. In contrast, monkey sera *neutralize* only human CMV. On the basis of variable CF reactivities of human CMV-CF antigens, it is probable that human CMV strains possess overlapping mosaics of CF antigens. These can be differentiated with sera from monkeys naturally infected with CMV.

The existence of distinct CMV serotypes has not been confirmed by studies in animals. In an attempt to differentiate CMV strains using rabbit sera, Andersen and co-workers (1971) have provided experimental support for the existence of antigenic differences between a field strain for CMV and the AD 169 strain. They noted, however, a pronounced cross-reactivity between these two strains in experiments with fresh guinea pig serum, suggesting that the serotypes are not entirely distinct. Clearly, more investigations employing hyperimmune sera obtained from animals are needed to define the antigenic relationship among human CMV strains. The degree of homology existing among human CMV strains is greater than that between herpes simplex virus types 1 and 2, which is about 47 to 50 per cent (Kieff et al., 1972). Although no two human isolates have completely identical DNA fragment-mapping patterns, study of interstrain nucleic acid homology revealed that human CMV strains had at least 80 per cent DNA sequence homology with prototype AD 169 (Huang et al., 1976).

Genetic Relatedness

Huang and co-workers (1980) employed restriction endonuclease analysis of purified DNA to distinguish one strain of CMV from another. This method has been useful in determining whether a given infection is a reactivation of endogenous virus or a reinfection with a newly introduced strain. These investigators found that viruses from unrelated workers were always genetically different, whereas strains from congenitally infected babies were usually identical with or closely related to those from their mothers. Strains from subsequently infected siblings were also concordant. The authors reported major differences in viral DNA in strains recovered from the same woman or from a mother-baby pair in two instances. Thus it would appear that both reinfection and reactivation do occur—the former less commonly.

DIAGNOSIS

There are several methods that may be used to make a diagnosis of congenital CMV infection.

Stagno and colleagues (1980b) have published a comparative study of diagnostic procedures. They did a prospective study of 1412 neonates and found viruses in 31 (2.2 per cent). Among immunoserological methods used to screen these neonates, the rheumatoid factor test, although nonspecific, proved to be the most convenient. The test was positive in 35 to 45 per cent of CMV-positive infants and in none of the CMV-negative infants. Indirect fluorescent CMV IgM antibody was present in 76 per cent of the virus excreters but also in 21 per cent of the virus-negative infants. Tests for specific and nonspecific IgA antibody were not useful. Electron microscopic examination of urine was positive in less than one hour in 92 per cent of virus-positive specimens. The detection of early induced CMV nuclear antigens by anticomplement immunofluorescence was diagnostic in 91 per cent of cases within one day of the inoculation of urine specimens in tissue culture. The authors noted that urine refrigerated for seven days at 4° C retains its infectivity. This is useful information, as sometimes transport of specimens to a distant virus laboratory is necessary.

Clinical

The diagnosis can almost never be made with certainty on purely clinical grounds. This would require a classic presentation, and a conclusive diagnosis should not be made even in the presence of periventricular calcifications. It is improbable that this type of calcification would be found in toxoplasmosis, rubella, or congenital syphilis, although perhaps a similar radiological finding could be observed in the very rare patient with congenital herpes simplex virus infection. In the few examples of the latter disease, the calcifications are not restricted to the periven-

tricular areas. Even in the most typical case of CID, it is advisable to confirm the diagnosis through one or more laboratory tests.

Computerized tomography (CT) has been used to define central nervous system involvement in a manner more sensitive than conventional skull films. Anders and co-workers (1980) described a newborn infant who had a normal neurological examination and a normal roentgenogram of the skull. The CT scan showed a mild hydrocephalus of the entire ventricular system and voluminous subarachnoid space, and extensive periventricular calcium was identified. Thus it would appear that a CT scan should be considered if plain films are normal in infants with suspected or proven CMV disease.

Virological

Isolation of virus from a fresh urine specimen, a throat swab, a liver biopsy specimen, or another organ at autopsy will establish that CMV infection is present but does *not* establish that the disease observed is due to CMV. This is particularly true when the virus is isolated three weeks after birth, a time when an asymptomatic infection could have been acquired. The probability is high (over 90 per cent) that if an infant has a systemic CMV infection, urine cultures for CMV will be positive. The cells required for cultivation of the virus are human fibroblasts. These can be embryonic lung fibroblasts, such as WI-38 cells, or cell lines derived from foreskin or embryonic skin and muscle. A variety of other cell culture types may support the growth of the virus, but, in general, no cytopathic effect is obtained in most nonhuman tissues or in epithelial cell types. (This is in contrast to the *in vivo* predilection of the virus for epithelial cells.)

The urine obtained for culture should be a clean-voided specimen. If transfer to the virus laboratory is not immediate, the specimen should be refrigerated or held in wet ice to prevent bacterial overgrowth and the fall in virus titer caused by warmer temperatures.

Before inoculation of the urine it is advisable to centrifuge the specimen at 2500 rpm for 20 to 30 minutes. An aliquot of 0.25 ml of urine supernatant is then pipetted into two or more tissue culture tubes containing 1.5 ml of minimal essential medium with 10 per cent newborn calf serum. Antibiotics (penicillin, gentamicin, and amphotericin B) are added to the medium to avoid bacterial contamination. There are a variety of satisfactory methods for virus isolation (Benyesh-Melnick, 1969). Some workers allow the urine to be absorbed onto the cell sheet for 30 minutes, remove the urine, and then add the medium. Satisfactory results have been obtained with both techniques described.

Once the cultures are inoculated, the tubes are placed in an incubator at 35 to 36° C. Cultures may be rolled or incubated in stationary racks. The appearance of viral CPE is accelerated by the rotation of the tubes. Tubes are observed under the light microscope one or two times per week and compared with control tubes prepared at the same time. Cultures may become positive as early as the first day or, more commonly, between days 7 and 14. Most positive cultures show a CPE by the end of the third week. Rarely, cultures become positive after a 30-day observation period. An early CPE (within 24 hours) is often generalized; a more delayed CPE is typically focal in character, with small clusters of five to 10 rounded, refractile, elongated fibroblasts appearing in a sheet of less conspicuous fibroblastic cells. This appearance is characteristic enough in most cultures to warrant specific identification of the agent as a CMV (Hanshaw, 1969). The progression of the CPE is usually slow. Some cultures do not go on to involve the entire cell sheet. Complete involvement is likely to occur, however, in a culture that becomes positive within seven to 10 days. In some instances, the failure to progress toward generalization to the CPE throughout the cell sheet is a reflection of the declining vigor of aging cells supporting the growth of the virus.

Chou and Merigan (1983) have reported the rapid detection (24 hours) and quantification of CMV in urine through DNA hybridization. CMV-positive urine usually had an infective titer in fresh samples of 2.5 log $TCID_{50}/0.2$ ml or higher. It is quite possible that tests of this type will eventually replace the more time-consuming tissue culture method of diagnosis.

Inoculation of Other Specimens. In addition to urine and the upper respiratory tract, CMV has been recovered from many organs, particularly liver, lung, spleen, kidney, and brain, as well as leukocytes, feces, tears (Cox and Hughes, 1973), milk (Hayes et al., 1972), and semen (Lang and Kummer, 1972). Virus can occasionally be isolated from cerebrospinal fluid. If the specimen is a piece of tissue,

it should be ground in a mortar containing medium with an abrasive substance such as sterile alundum. A 10 per cent suspension of the ground tissue should be allowed to settle in the mortar before it is inoculated with 0.2 ml of the supernatant.

Rapid Detection of Antigen with Specific Monoclonal Antibodies. Volpi and co-workers (1983) have described a method for the rapid detection of CMV antigen in infected cells. They employed monoclonal antibodies specific to CMV in an immunofluorescence test to diagnose CMV infection in lung tissue taken from patients with suspected CMV pneumonitis. Fluorescent cells were seen in all seven specimens from which CMV was isolated.

Serological

There are several methods available for measuring CMV antibody.

Complement-Fixation (CF) Test. This test, first developed by Rowe and colleagues (1956), was modified by Medearis (1964) and Sever and co-workers (1963). Most laboratories now employ the micromethod, which is accurate, requires small amounts of serum, and is convenient for large-scale testing. The variable antigenic composition of the CMVs may account for the fact that as many as 10 to 20 per cent of infants with cytomegaloviruria may not have antibody to any one CMV antigen, such as the commonly used AD 169 strain. The percentage of seropositive specimens can be increased if other strains, such as Kerr and Davis, are also used. This is not usually done, however, in routine diagnostic work because of the greater technical effort required to detect a relatively small number of "false negatives" and because of a general lack of appreciation of the antigenic heterogeneity in the CF test. Although the CF test may be relatively insensitive, it can distinguish between persons who are seropositive and those who are seronegative to CMV as readily as can more sensitive assays, provided that the alkaline glycine–extracted CF antigen is used (Betts et al., 1976; Griffiths et al., 1978; Booth et al., 1979).

There is evidence that CF antibody is predominantly IgG immunoglobulin. This is based on the absence of CF antibody in some patients with CMV-IgM antibody, the failure to lose titer when sera from infants with known macroglobulin are treated with 2-mercaptoethanol, and the close correlation with the CMV-IgG immunofluorescent tests (Hanshaw, 1969).

The CF test may be used alone or in conjunction with virus isolation or CMV-IgM tests to determine whether an infant is congenitally infected. More important than the presence of IgG antibody in a young infant with suspected infection is the persistence of a titer of 1:8 or greater during the four to six months after birth. An infant two months of age with a CF titer greater than the maternal titer is probably actively infected. Transplacentally acquired maternal CF antibody does not persist beyond six months. It has been estimated that the half-life of most maternally derived IgG antibody is approximately 23 days. Thus, a relatively high cord CF serum titer of 1:64 shortly after birth might be expected to decline to 1:8 or less at three months of age. Approximately 30 to 60 per cent of cord serum sample obtained in the United States have CF titers of 1:8 or greater. Of these, one might expect fewer than 10 per cent of the total to be greater than 1:64. Although a titer of 1:16 in an infant four to five months of age is strongly suggestive of active CMV infection, it is possible that this infection could have been acquired during or after birth. If such were the case, it would probably be three to six weeks after the exposure before viruria could be detected and at least six to eight weeks before active CMV-CF antibody appeared. Yeager and co-workers (1972) have observed an infant who received a blood transfusion in the neonatal period and began excreting virus at 37 days of age. The patient developed a fourfold increase in antibody titer at three months. This infection occurred in the presence of a passively transferred CMV-CF titer of 1:32.

Waner and colleagues (1973) followed the CMV-CF antibody titers in 50 adult patients over an 18-month period. The AD 169, Davis, and Esp strains were used as antigens. Their data suggest that CMV-host relationships are more dynamic than had been appreciated. Some patients responded to one antigen at certain times and to all three at others. Wide fluctuations were noted in 20 of the 39 CF-reactive donors. Some previously positive sera declined to levels below 1:8 and subsequently rose to titers of 1:64 or higher. These observations suggest that CMV-CF titers must be interpreted with caution, especially in the diagnosis of primary infection in adults. The CMV-IgG immunofluorescent test will detect lower titers of antibody than the CF method, thus avoiding the diagnostic pitfalls that might be encountered with the latter.

Fluorescent Antibody (FA) Tests. Hanshaw and co-workers (1968) developed the CMV-IgM test following the demonstration of toxoplasma-IgM antibody by Remington and co-workers (1968). The main advantage of the immunofluorescent method is the ability to measure *specific* immunoglobulins by using conjugates directed against IgM, IgG, and IgA. This is particularly useful in the detection of congenital infection because of the large amount of masking IgG antibody of maternal origin. Thus, specific CMV-IgM and CMV-IgA antibodies in the neonate can be interpreted as evidence of congenital CMV infection. This must be done with caution, however, because of false-positive results due to rheumatoid factor and Fc receptors. Absorption of the neonatal serum with staphylococcal protein A will eliminate false-negative reactions due to rheumatoid factor or IgG antibody (Tuomanen and Powell, 1980). As noted, rheumatoid factor per se is a convenient, though nonspecific, method of screening for congenital CMV infection. It is about 35 to 45 per cent sensitive and gives no false-positive results (Stagno et al., 1980b). The presence of significant and persisting CMV-CF antibody or, preferably, isolation of the virus from the newborn patient is further proof that the IgM antibody is specific to CMV. As noted, there is evidence that herpesvirus varicellae and EBV are antigenically related to CMV and that infections with these agents may produce a positive CMV-IgM test (Hanshaw et al., 1972). It is unlikely, however, that V-Z infections in the newborn would be confused with CMV disease. Since there is now evidence to indicate that EBV can cause congenital infection, this rare possibility cannot be discarded.

If the CMV-IgM test is employed as the only means of identifying CMV infection in *symptomatic* infants, it will be approximately 95 per cent accurate. We were able to demonstrate this antibody in all of 50 children (ages 0 to 20 years) with virologically documented CID (Hanshaw et al., 1968). In one case we are unable to find CMV-IgM antibody in a virus-positive infant with congenital CID. The test was positive, however, when the Kerr CMV virus was substituted for the AD 169 agent as the CMV antigen source. The FA method is less efficient than virus isolation techniques used to detect excretors. The prevalence of viruria in routinely delivered infants in Rochester, New York, is 1 per cent, whereas the prevalence of CMV-IgM antibody in the cord serum is approximately 0.6 to 0.7 per cent. These differences may be somewhat spurious because the surveys employing virus isolation as the means of detection have been done on a population from a somewhat lower socioeconomic group than that studied in the CMV-IgM survey. There is evidence to suggest, in addition, that the asymptomatic, IgM-negative infants are either unaffected or affected in a minimal way by the congenital infection. The level at which the CMV-IgM antibody persists tends to correlate with the degree of clinical disease associated with the infection.

Once CMV-IgM is detected, the level may remain elevated for weeks or months after birth. Although there is widespread belief that the presence of IgM antibody is strong evidence of a primary infection, IgM antibody may fluctuate in patients tested over a period of several months (Hanshaw, J.B., unpublished observations, 1973), suggesting that one cannot always equate the presence of specific macroglobulin with recently acquired primary infection.

Hemagglutination Inhibition (IHA) Test. A specific indirect microhemagglutination test described for herpes simplex virus types 1 and 2 by Fuccillo and co-workers (1970) has been applied successfully to the detection of CMV indirect hemagglutinating antibody by the same group of workers (Fuccillo et al., 1971), as well as by Bernstein and Stewart (1971). The specificity of the CMV antibody response detected by the IHA test correlates well with results of the standard neutralization test. The method is somewhat more sensitive than the CF test in detecting antibody in congenitally infected newborns, although this difference is minimized if potent CF antigens are prepared. Bernstein and Stewart found the test to be highly sensitive and reproducible. Both IgM and IgG antibodies are detected by this method. For this reason it is less valuable in early infancy than specific FA tests for CMV-IgM. Because the hemagglutination reaction can be inhibited by small amounts of homologous antigen, it is possible to use this technique to identify virus isolated from diagnostic specimens.

Enzyme-Linked Immunosorbent Assay (ELISA). Cappel and colleagues (1978) described a rapid method for the detection of IgG and IgM antibodies for CMV by the ELISA technique. This procedure is sensitive and can be done rapidly and inexpensively. Castellano and co-workers (1977) found that the method compares favorably with the IHA test. Yolken and Stopa (1980) compared

seven enzyme immunoassay systems using different enzyme-labeled immunoreactants and antigen detection systems. The sensitivity, and ease of operation of ELISA suggest that this method will be used widely to diagnose CMV infection.

Neutralization Tests. The neutralization procedures, which include the traditional virus-serum tube-dilution method (Weller et al., 1957) and the plaque-reduction neutralization test (Plummer and Benyesh-Melnick, 1964), are not used for routine CMV diagnostic serology because they are cumbersome and tend to accentuate antigenic differences in various strains. They also may give misleading results, because antibody may be adsorbed by noninfectious particles.

If neutralization tests are used to measure antibody, it should be recognized that some patients will become positive for CMV-CF antibody four to eight weeks before neutralizing antibody becomes detectable. Higher titers might be expected if the CMV strain isolated from the patient is employed as the test antigen.

Radioimmunoassay (RIA). Griffiths and colleagues (1982a) have reported that significantly higher IgM titers measured by RIA, were observed in infants infected by primary maternal CMV infections than in those whose mothers had recurrent CMV infection. One study by this group (1982b) has shown that RIA could detect IgM antibodies in 55 per cent of women for up to four months following primary CMV infection, whereas specific antibodies were not found by this test in the sera of women with recurrent infections. It appears that a reliable diagnosis of primary infection during the first trimester of pregnancy, a time for which data concerning congenital transmission are now lacking, is possible through RIA. The CMV RIA test does not defect herpes simplex or V-Z antibody. Kimmel and colleagues (1980) consider the test convenient, rapid, and characterized by an objective end-point. Its disadvantage is the expense of the reagents and equipment used. For accurate measurement of specific IgM, rheumatoid factor, if present, must be absorbed with glutaraldehyde-insolubilized IgG. This procedure requires a relatively large serum specimen.

Histopathological

Prior to the development of *in vitro* techniques for the isolation of CMV, Fetterman (1952) proposed that inclusion-bearing cells

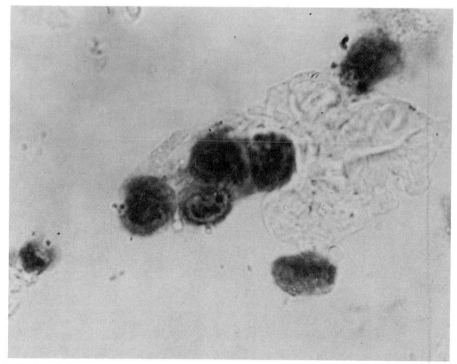

Figure 4–7. Nuclear inclusion–bearing cell in renal epithelial cells of the urinary sediment. (From Hanshaw, J. B.: Clinical significance of cytomegalovirus infection. Postgrad. Med. *35:*472–480, 1964. Copyright 1964, McGraw-Hill, Inc.)

might be found in the urine sediment (Fig. 4–7). This was found to be the case in approximately 50 per cent of the most severely affected newborns (Weller and Hanshaw, 1962). It is in the symptomatic group that the test is of moderate usefulness. It should be employed when the more sensitive virological or serological methods are not available. Inclusions can be seen with Papanicolaou, Giemsa, and hematoxylin and eosin stains of the urinary sediment. Whereas a negative urine sediment preparation has little significance, a smear showing large nuclear inclusion–bearing cells is strongly suggestive of CID. Only exceedingly rare reports of herpes simplex virus infection involving the renal tubular epithelium cells may cause some problem in the differential diagnosis. It is unlikely that measles, adenovirus infection, V-Z, mumps, or an infection with any of the enteroviruses would cause confusion in the interpretation of the smear. The urinary sediment is of minimal value in the diagnosis of acquired CMV infection.

Histopathological findings for any one of several tissues may be sufficiently characteristic to warrant a diagnosis of CMV infection. Since the nuclear inclusions are similar to those seen with other herpesviruses, the size

of the cell is of particular importance in ruling out these closely related agents. Only CMV infection appears to be capable of inducing an overall cell diameter of 25 to 40 μ with an inclusion diameter of approximately 8 to 10 μ. Unlike other herpesviruses, CMV may have a cytoplasmic inclusion as well as an intranuclear inclusion body. These inclusions are usually less well delineated than the nuclear inclusions. In many tissue specimens, cytoplasmic inclusions are not present at all. Similar variability is also noted among various strains under *in vitro* conditions.

DIFFERENTIAL DIAGNOSIS

CMV infection in the young infant must be distinguished from a large number of diseases that are capable of causing hyperbilirubinemia, petechiae or purpura, hepatosplenomegaly, respiratory infections, and a variety of oculocerebral and extraneural abnormalities. The list of diseases that must be considered in the differential diagnosis becomes predictably broader and less well defined as the clinical manifestations diminish in severity (see Chapter 13).

Congenital Rubella

Both CMV and rubella infections can cause petechiae and purpuric rashes, jaundice, hepatosplenomegaly, thrombocytopenia, microcephaly, deafness, and mental retardation. Both diseases may be associated with prematurity and intrauterine growth retardation. Although an association has been reported, it is questionable whether CMV can cause central cataracts. The association with congenital heart defects is distinctly less common than that seen with rubella. Rubella is somewhat less likely to induce a fine petechial rash; the lesions may be raised and are usually concentrated around the face and neck. CMV chorioretinitis is focally distributed and quite unlike the more generalized "salt and pepper" pattern seen in infants with congenital rubella syndrome.

Whereas periventricular calcifications may occur in 10 to 30 per cent of infants with *typical* CID, calcifications in any distribution are not part of the rubella syndrome.

Little confidence can be placed in the history of maternal rubella disease. Although rubella may be strongly suspected in some instances, particularly in epidemic years, it is usually necessary and advisable to confirm the clinical impression by virological and serological tests.

Congenital Toxoplasmosis

It is remarkable that two infectious agents as diverse as CMV and toxoplasma should share so many signs and symptoms. Almost all of the clinical manifestations seen in CID have been described in toxoplasmosis. Table 4–10 lists abnormalities common to the two infections.

Table 4–10. CLINICAL MANIFESTATIONS COMMON TO BOTH CYTOMEGALIC INCLUSION DISEASE AND TOXOPLASMOSIS*

Microcephaly	Splenomegaly
Hydrocephalus	Cerebral calcifications
Deafness	Petechiae/purpura
Chorioretinitis	Lymphadenopathy
Strabismus	Pneumonitis
Blindness	Cerebral palsy
Jaundice	Microphthalmus
Anemia	Heptomegaly
Convulsions	Abnormal cerebrospinal fluid
"Failure to thrive"	

*Infection proven by urine or respiratory tract cultures.

Some differences in the two conditions are worthy of note. The calcifications in toxoplasmosis tend to be scattered throughout the cerebral cortex. This does not occur in CID. The infant with calcifications due to toxoplasmosis may not be severely brain damaged, whereas he or she almost certainly would be with CID calcifications. A maculopapular rash may appear in toxoplasmosis, but it does not necessarily have a petechial or purpuric component. The chorioretinitis seen in the two diseases cannot be differentiated on the basis of appearance or distribution. Whereas chorioretinitis is likely to be associated with microcephaly in CID, it frequently occurs in the absence of microcephaly and other major manifestations of disease in toxoplasmosis. Chorioretinitis may be a late manifestation of both CMV and *T. gondii* infections. It is the most common abnormality associated with clinical toxoplasmosis and is often the only abnormality present.

The diagnosis of toxoplasmosis may be made by serial antibody determinations using fluorescent or Sabin-Feldman dye-test antibody procedures. The toxoplasma-IgM test developed by Remington (1968) is a useful indirect FA test when positive in early infancy as well as in later life. Unfortunately, many newborns with congenital toxoplasmosis do not have detectable IgM antibody.

It should be noted that congenital toxoplasmosis and CMV infection have been known to co-exist in the same patient (Demian et al., 1973).

Disseminated Herpes Simplex Infection

There have been several cases of congenital herpes simplex virus infection reported that resemble CID (Schaffer, 1965; South et al., 1969; Montgomery et al., 1973). These patients have had microcephaly and cerebral calcifications as well as systemic symptoms suggestive of congenital CID. The presence of vesicular lesions containing herpes simplex virus on the skin is of value in the differential diagnosis. Present information suggests that *congenital* herpes simplex infection is very rare. The more usual neonatal infection results from exposure during or just prior to parturition and does not usually present as an acute disease until the fifth to tenth day of life. Unlike the patient with neonatal CID, the infant is well during most of the first week. When illness does occur, it is frequently severe, with seizures, encephalitis, respiratory distress, and disseminated intravascular coagulation. Vesicular lesions that tend to cluster, especially on the scalp in vertex deliveries and on the buttocks in breech presentations, have been noted by Hodgman and co-workers (1971).

Sepsis of the Newborn

Infants with bacterial sepsis usually appear more seriously ill than infants with CID. They are lethargic and unresponsive, and approximately one-third have evidence of meningitis. Both conditions can be associated with jaundice, and a petechial rash may be present. Jaundice is particularly common in gram-negative infections but may also occur in group B streptococcal infections. Although a petechial rash is not characteristic of bacterial sepsis, it has been described. The suspicion of sepsis rests primarily on the clinical manifestations. Confirmation is dependent upon a positive blood culture. Many infants with CID and other nonbacterial congenital infections must be treated with antibiotics because of the uncertainty of the diagnosis during the period when the cultures are pending. The white cell count may be of assistance but in itself is usually not reliable enough to form the basis for a decision to withhold antibiotics. It is unusual for CID to be complicated by bacterial sepsis in the newborn period.

Congenital Syphilis

The most consistent signs of early congenital syphilis are osteochondritis and epiphysitis on the roentgenogram of the long bones. These findings occur in approximately 90 per cent of patients and are likely to appear in symptomatic infants in the first week of life. Rhinitis, sometimes associated with laryngitis, is another common accompaniment of congenital syphilis. It is often followed by a dark red, maculopapular, spotted rash. Lesions of the skin and mucous membranes are also seen. Hepatosplenomegaly occurs but is less common in early syphilis than in CID. Calcifications of the brain are not characteristic of congenital syphilis. Choroiditis may be seen, however.

Laboratory tests for syphilis include dark-field examination of the spirochete-laden nasal discharge, and one of several standard tests (treponemal or reagin) should be done on both the mother and the infant.

PROGNOSIS

Patients with Central Nervous System Symptoms at Birth

The prognosis in congenital CMV infection is difficult to determine with accuracy. Patients who have a reduced head circumference at birth or cerebral calcifications during the first two months of life will usually experience moderate to severe psychomotor retardation. The development of hydrocephalus, indicating fourth ventricle obstruction, is usually followed by death within six to 12 months. Pass and colleagues (1980) recently reported on the outcome for 34 symptomatic patients with congenital CMV infection. Ten of these patients died, and all but two of the 23 survivors had evidence of CNS or auditory handicaps. Microcephaly was present in 16 (70 per cent), mental retardation in 14 (61 per cent), hearing loss in seven (30 per cent), neuromuscular disorders in eight (35 per cent), and chorioretinitis or optic atrophy in five (22 per cent). Thus, any child with CMV who is symptomatic in the neonatal period is at very high risk for a handicap that will impair development significantly.

Symptomatic Newborns Without Central Nervous System Abnormalities

Infants who do not have symptoms referable to the central nervous system during the neonatal period are less likely to have severe neurological sequelae, but they may develop microcephaly that does not become apparent until the later part of the first year of life. They also may fail to thrive, and they may develop spastic quadriplegia, deafness, and many of the symptoms that occur in patients with central nervous system disease in the neonatal period. As noted, (Pass et al., 1980), fewer than 10 per cent of *symptomatic* newborns are either mildly affected or unaffected by the infection when carefully examined at four to five years of age. The extraneural manifestations, such as purpura, jaundice, hepatomegaly, splenomegaly, and pneumonitis, are usually reversible. The long-term effects are primarily related to the progression of the infection in the central nervous system, including the inner ear, or to irreversible damage sustained *in utero* and not detected at birth.

Infants Asymptomatic in the Newborn Period

Studies of several thousand routine deliveries have permitted the identification of large numbers of infants born with unsuspected CMV infection. Fewer than 10 per cent of these infants have been symptomatic in the newborn period; the remainder have not been significantly different from normal infants, with the exception of a lower mean birth weight (Starr et al., 1970). Reynolds and co-workers (1974) have follow-up data on 18 CMV-infected infants observed for an average of 38 months. They found that two infected children developed moderate to severe brain damage, nine had sensorineural hearing loss, and two with concomitant brain damage required hearing aids.

In Rochester, New York, Hanshaw and colleagues (1976) have tested cord sera from 8644 infants of CMV-IgM antibody. One in 163 (0.6 per cent) was positive. Of 44 children followed for three and one-half to seven years after birth, 16 (36 per cent) had neurological sequelae severe enough to predict school failure. In contrast, seven of the 88 (8.8 per cent) random and matched control children had abnormalities predictive of school failure.

Kumar and colleagues (1984) were not able to demonstrate an adverse cognitive outcome in their long-term follow-up of 17 virus-positive neonates with asymptomatic congenital CMV. Four of the 17 children, however, had impaired auditory thresholds.

CMV persists as a chronic but active viral infection for at least several years after birth. The possibility exists that virus, acting within the inner ear or in other central nervous system locations, may exert a detrimental effect on neurological function over a period of several years. Peckham's (1972) experience with long-term follow-up of asymptomatic congenital rubella–infected children suggests that school failures and, particularly, hearing loss may be explicable on the basis of the persistence of infection. An alternative explanation for this observation is that the damage was undetectable at an earlier age by the methods commonly employed to detect neurological sequelae.

THERAPY

Specific Therapy

There is no specific therapy for congenital CMV infection that has been shown to be clearly helpful. Although several drugs and biologicals, such as acyclovir, adenine arabinoside, cytosine arabinoside, idoxuridine (IDU), floxuridine, interferon, transfer factor, and interferon-inducers, have been used experimentally in patients, there is no evidence that these agents have any lasting effect on the progression of congenital disease. Both arabinosides and IDU can induce a transient diminution in virus excretion in some patients, but there is no evidence that this effect alters the clinical course or long-term prognosis. In view of their uncertain efficacy and possible toxicity, especially that related to bone marrow depression, these drugs cannot be recommended. They especially should not be employed in hospitals that do not have ready access to platelet transfusions.

Although the use of acyclovir as an antiviral agent has been favored owing to its specific reaction with thymidine kinase, Burns and co-workers (1982) have found the drug to be effective against mouse CMV, which does not encode for thymidine kinase. Balfour and colleagues (1982) have indicated that acyclovir may improve the status of CMV-infected renal allograft recipients, while Wade and colleagues (1982) reported less encouraging data on the treatment of CMV pneumonia with the drug. Plotkin and co-workers (1982) have reported a wide variation in resistance to acyclovir among several strains *in vitro* and little clinical improvement in congenitally infected infants given acyclovir intravenously.

Cheng and colleagues (1983) found an acyclovir analogue, DHPG, more active *in vitro* against CMVs than acyclovir. It has not been clinically tested as yet.

Hirsch and co-workers (1983) have shown that interferon alpha affords effective prophylaxis against serious CMV infections in adults receiving kidney transplants.

Nonspecific Therapy

Most infants with symptomatic infection do not require therapy. Exchange transfusion is rarely indicated for hyperbilirubinemia, much of which is direct. Neonatal sepsis, an unusual complication of CID, may be due to enteric organisms or a streptococcal infection. Thus, the therapy would not be different from that used in other newborns with sepsis. Since CID can be a cause of cerebral palsy, mental retardation, and obstructive hydrocephalus, long-range measures for dealing with these specific chronic problems must be planned on an individual basis.

PREVENTION

CMV infection can be transmitted to a susceptible pregnant woman or a newborn infant by the transfusion of fresh blood. This possibility may be diminished by using CMV antibody–negative blood (Yeager et al., 1981). Others have recommended the use of frozen deglycerolized red blood cells (Adler et al., 1983). Patients with mononucleosis-like diseases during pregnancy and negative heterophile agglutination tests should be suspected of having CMV mononucleosis. If this suspicion is documented by virus isolation and appropriate serological tests in a woman who is less than 20 weeks pregnant, the question arises whether the pregnancy should be terminated because the infection is probably primary and there is a 15 per cent chance of symptoms appearing in the newborn period (Stagno et al., 1982a).

In most instances, however, the symptoms of maternal CMV infection are not clinically recognizable Even when they are, the decision about termination is more difficult than that faced by the woman who has rubella in the first trimester because there are fewer data available with which to assess accurately the risk to the fetus. Recovery of CMV from the cervix of a pregnant woman has not been shown to be a risk to the fetus. We have recovered virus from the urine of eight pregnant women in the first 20 weeks of pregnancy. All delivered infants were free of detectable CMV infection.

The problems of developing a CMV vaccine have been considered by several workers (Dudgeon, 1973; Hanshaw, 1982b; Phillips, 1977; Lang, 1980). The present prospective studies on the frequency and long-term sequelae of congenital CMV provide justification for a CMV vaccine. The development of a satisfactory immunizing agent presents many problems. Elek and Stern (1974) gave up to 10^4 $TCID_{50}$ of CMV to seronegative volunteers by an intradermal route. No antibody response was noted. On rechallenge six to eight weeks later, an accelerated skin lesion suggesting sensitization was produced, but no antibody response was detected. When two volunteers were given 10^5 $TCID_{50}$ of virus, a striking local indurated lesion became apparent, the glands in the axilla enlarged slightly, and a few reactive lymphocytes appeared in the peripheral blood. These volunteers did develop a response with CF and neutralizing antibodies. During a two-month follow-up period, no virus appeared in the throat or the urine. The same dose of virus, 10^5 $TCID_{50}$, did not produce a local lesion in volunteers with pre-existing antibody.

Neff and co-workers (1979), in M. R. Hilleman's laboratory, inoculated 20 seronegative clergymen with a cell-free preparation of AD 169 virus and observed essentially the same results as did Elek and Stern. All subjects seroconverted, did not shed virus, were not ill and did not transmit the infection to seronegative contacts. Just and colleagues (1975) in Switzerland and Plotkin and colleagues (1976) in the United States tested the Towne 125 strain in a total of 14 seronegative subjects with results similar to those of the AD 169 trials.

The questions that have been raised concerning the vaccine involve its possible oncogenicity and the consequences of persistent infection. Questions of efficacy cannot be answered at this time because we do not know if the host will be protected and what degree of cross-protection exists between CMV strains. It is hoped that it may be possible to "dampen down" the severity of disease to an inconsequential level clinically. As noted, the recent observations by Stagno and co-workers (1982a) give promise of a modulating effect of pre-existing antibody. None of the infected offspring of women with reinfection were symptomatic in the newborn period, whereas 15 per cent of infants born to women with primary infection had symptoms. We know that the most devastating effects of the virus are seen in the latter group of infants. The main thrust of vaccination will be to protect the fetus, although it may be possible also to protect the immunocompromised host.

It should be noted that the vaccine strains are attenuated in the sense that they have not produced disease to date, are not contagious, and are not shed following vaccination. It is possible to distinguish vaccine from wild strains of virus by restriction enzyme analysis of DNA fragments of virus (Plotkin et al., 1979).

The question of oncogenicity has been raised because it is possible to transform human cells with the slow-growing Major strain of CMV (Geder et al., 1976). These transformed cells can, in turn, produce tumors in athymic nude mice. One cannot conclude, however, that such laboratory-induced oncogenesis can occur in nature or following vaccination with laboratory-adapted strains of virus. The Towne strain has been inoculated into nude and thymectomized mice and does not produce tumors. It has also been noted that restriction enzyme analysis of high- and low-passage virus does not show a change in the characteristic Towne pattern (Plotkin et al., 1979).

This information notwithstanding, certain minimum conditions should be met before larger trials are undertaken. We need to know if infected infants born to immune mothers have sequelae apparent several years after birth. We also must extend present investigations of candidate strains (Towne and AD 169) for their possible oncogenicity. This should be studied exhaustively using the most sophisticated methods of modern molecular biology.

Bibliography

Adler, S. P., Chandrika, T., Lawrence, L., Baggett, J., and Biro, V.: Hospital-acquired cytomegalovirus infections in neonates (abstract). Conference on Pathogenesis and Prevention of Human Cytomegalovirus, Philadelphia, 1983.

Ahlfors, K., Ivarsson, S. A., Johnsson, T., Svanberg, L.: A prospective study on congenital and acquired cytomegalovirus infections in infants. Scand. J. Infect. Dis. *11*:177–178, 1979.

Ahlfors, K., Harris, S., Ivarsson, S. A., and Svanberg, L.: Secondary maternal cytomegalovirus infection causing symptomatic congenital infection (letter). N. Engl. J. Med. *305*:284, 1981.

Ahlfors, K., Ivarsson, S. A., Johnsson, T., Svanborg, L.: Primary and secondary maternal cytomegalovirus infections and their relation to congenital infection. Acta Paediatr. Scand. *71*:104–113, 1982.

Albrecht, T., and Rapp, F.: Malignant transformation of hamster embryo fibroblasts following exposure to ultraviolet-irradiated human cytomegalovirus. Virology *55*:53–61, 1973.

Alexander, E. R.: Maternal and neonatal infection with cytomegalovirus in Taiwan. Pediatr. Res. *1*:210–211, 1967.

Anders, B. J., Lauer, B. A., and Foley, L. C.: Computerized tomography to define CNS involvement in congenital cytomegalovirus infection. Am. J. Dis. Child. *134*:795–797, 1980.

Andersen, H. K., Godtfredsen, A., and Spencer, E. S.: Studies on the specificity of the complement fixation test to cytomegalovirus infections. With special reference to possible cross-reactions with other herpesvirus antigens. Scand. J. Infect. Dis. *3*:183–197, 1971.

Andersen, H. K., Brostrom, K., Hansen, K. B., Leerhoy, J., Pedersen, M., Osterballe, O., Felsager, U., Mogensen, S.: A prospective study on the incidence and significance of congenital cytomegalovirus infection. Acta Paediatr. Scand. *68*:329–336, 1979.

Andrewes, C. H.: Immunity to' the salivary galnd virus of guinea pigs studied in the living animal and in tissue culture. Br. J. Exp. Pathol. *11*:23–34, 1930.

Andrewes, C. H.: Classification of viruses of vertebrates. Adv. Virus Res. *9*:271–296, 1962.

Baczi, L., Conczol, E., Leehel, F., and Geder, L.: Isolation of cytomegalovirus and incidence of complement-fixing antibodies against cytomegalovirus in different age groups. Acta Microbiol. Acad. Sci. Hung. *12*:115–121, 1965.

Balfour, H. H., Bean, B., Mitchell, C. D., Sachs, G. W., Boen, J. R., and Edelman, C. K.: Acyclovir in immunocompromised patients with cytomegalovirus disease. Acyclovir Symposium. Am. J. Med. *73A*:241–248, 1982.

Ballard, R. A., Drew, W. L., Hufnagle, K. G., and Reidel, P. A.: Acquired cytomegalovirus infection in preterm infants. Am. J. Dis. Child. *133*:482–485, 1979.

Baron, J., Youngblood, L., Siewers, C. M. F., and Medearis, D. N., Jr: The incidence of cytomegalovirus, herpes simplex, rubella, and toxoplasma antibodies in microcephalic mentally retarded and normocephalic children. Pediatrics *44*:932–939, 1969.

Benyesh-Melnick, M.: Cytomegaloviruses. In Lennette, E. H., and Schmidt, N. J. (eds.): Diagnostic Procedures for Viral and Rickettsial Infections. 4th ed. New York, American Public Health Association, Inc., 1969, pp. 701–732.

Benyesh-Melnick, M., Dessey, S. I., and Fernbach, D. J.: Cytomegaloviruria in children with acute leukemia and in other children. Proc. Soc. Exp. Biol. Med. *117*:624–630, 1964.

Benyesh-Melnick, M., Probstmeyer, F., McCombs, R., Brunschwig, J. P., and Vonka, V.: Correlation between infectivity and physical viral particles in human cytomegalovirus. J. Bacteriol. *92*:1555–1561, 1966a.

Benyesh-Melnick, M., Vonka, V., Probstmeyer, F., and Wimberly, I.: Human cytomegalovirus: properties of the complement-fixing antigen. J. Immunol. *96*:261–267, 1966b.

Berenberg, W., and Nankervis, G.: Long-term follow-up of cytomegalic inclusion disease of infancy. Pediatrics *46*:403–410, 1970.

Bernstein, M. T., and Stewart, J. A.: Indirect hemagglutination test for detection of antibodies to cytomegalovirus. Appl. Microbiol. *21*:84–89, 1971.

Betts, R. F., George, S. D., Rundell, B. B., Freeman, R. B., and Douglas, R. G.: Comparative activity of immunofluorescent antibody and complement-fixing antibody in cytomegalovirus infection. J. Clin. Microbiol. *4*:151–156, 1976.

Birnbaum, G., Lynch, J. I., Margileth, A. M., Lonergan,

W. M., and Sever, J. L.: Cytomegalovirus infections in newborn infants. J. Pediatr. 75:789–795, 1969.

Black, P. H., Hartley, J. W., and Rowe, W. P.: Isolation of a cytomegalovirus from an African green monkey. Proc. Soc. Exp. Biol. Med. 112:601–605, 1963.

Booth, J. C., Hannington, G., Aziz, T. A. G., and Stern, H.: Comparison of enzyme-linked immunosorbent assay (ELISA) technique and complement fixation test for estimation of cytomegalovirus IgG antibody. J. Clin. Pathol. 32:122–127, 1979.

Boué, A., and Loffredo, V.: Avortement causé par le virus de l'virus de l'herpés type II. Isolement du virus à partir de cultures de tissues zygotiques. Presse Méd. 78:103–106, 1970.

Burns, W. H., Wingard, J. R., Sandford, G. R., Bender, W. J., and Saral, R.: Acyclovir in mouse cytomegalovirus infections. Acyclovir Symposium. Am. J. Med. 73A:118–124, 1982.

Cappel, R., DeCuyper, F., and Debraekeleer, J.: Rapid detection of IgG and IgM antibodies for cytomegalovirus by the enzyme-linked immunoabsorbent assay (ELISA). Arch. Virol. 58:253–258, 1978.

Carlstrom, G.: Virologic studies on cytomegalic inclusion disease. Acta Paediatr. Scand. 54:17–23, 1965.

Castellano, G. A., Hazzard, G. T., Madden, D. L., and Sever, J. L.: Comparison of the enzyme-linked immunosorbent assay and the indirect hemagglutination test for detection of antibody to cytomegalovirus. J. Infect. Dis. 136:337–340, 1977.

Cheng, Y'.-C., Huang, E.-S., Lin, J.-C., Mar, E.-C., and Pagano, J. S.: Unique spectrum of 9-(1,3-dihydroxy-2-propoxy) methyl—guanine against herpesvirus in vitro and its mode of action against herpes simplex virus type 1. Proc. Soc. Natl. Acad. Sci. U.S.A. 80:2767–2770, 1983.

Chien, L. T., Cannon, N. J., Charamella, L. J., Dismokes, W. E., Whitely, R. J., Buchanan, R. A., and Alford, C. A., Jr.: Effect of adenine arabinoside on severe Herpesvirus hominis infections in man. J. Infect. Dis. 128:658–663, 1973.

Chin, W., Magoffin, R., Frierson, J. G., and Lennett, E. H.: Cytomegalovirus infection: a case with meningoencephalitis. J.A.M.A. 225:740–741, 1973.

Chou, S., and Merigan, T. C.: Rapid detection and quantification of human cytomegalovirus in urine through DNA hybridization. N. Engl. J. Med. 308:921–925, 1983.

Cole, R., and Kuttner, A. G.: Filterable virus present in the salivary glands of guinea pigs. J. Exp. Med. 44:855–873, 1926.

Collaborative study. Cytomegalovirus in the northwest of England: a report on a two-year study. Arch. Dis. Child. 45:513–522, 1970.

Cowdry, E. V.: The problem of intranuclear inclusions in virus diseases. Arch. Pathol. 18:527–542, 1934.

Cox, F. E., and Hughes, W. T.: Isolation of cytomegalovirus from feces and tears (abstract). Pediatr. Res. 7:146, 1973.

Craighead, J. E., Hanshaw, J. B., and Carpenter, C. J.: Cytomegalovirus infection after renal allotransplantation. J.A.M.A. 120:725–728, 1967.

Craighead, J. E., Kanich, R. E., and Almeida, J.: Nonviral microbodies produced by cytomegalovirus infected cells. J. Virol. 10:766–775, 1972.

Davis, G. L.: Cytomegalovirus in the inner ear: case report and electron microscopic study. Ann. Otol. Rhinol. Laryngol. 78:1179–1188, 1969.

Davis, L. E., Tweed, G. V., and Stewart, J. A.: Cytomegalovirus mononucleosis in a first trimester pregnant female with transmission to the fetus. Pediatrics 48:200–206, 1971.

Deibel, R., Fairley, R. J., and Ducharme, C.: Serological studies with the cytomegalovirus. Annual report, 1965. Division of Laboratories and Research, New York State Department of Health, Albany, New York, 1965.

Demian, W., Donnelley, J. F., and Monif, G. R. G.: Coexistent congenital cytomegalovirus and toxoplasmosis in a stillborn (abstract) Am. J. Pathol. 71:2a, 1973.

Diosi, P., and David, C.: Cytomegalic inclusion disease: a historical outline. Clin. Med. 3:149–166, 1968.

Diosi, P., Babusceac, L., Neviglovschi, O., and Kun-Stoicu, G.: Cytomegalovirus infection associated with pregnancy. Lancet 2:1063–1066, 1967.

Diosi, P., Babusceac, L., Neviglovschi, O., and Stoicanescu, A.: Duration of cytomegaloviruia in nursery children. Pathol. Microbiol. (Basel) 29:513–518, 1966.

Dorfman, L. J.: Cytomegalovirus encephalitis in adults. Neurology 23:136–144, 1973.

Dreesman, G. R., and Benyesh-Melnick, M.: Spectrum of human cytomegalovirus complement-fixing antigens. J. Immunol. 99:1106–1114, 1967.

Drew, W. L., Miner, R. C., Ziegler, J. L., Gullett, J. H., Abrams, D. T., Conant, M. A., Huang, E. S., Groundwater, J. R., Volberding, P., and Mintz, L.: Cytomegalovirus and Kaposi's sarcoma in young homosexual men. Lancet 2:125–127, 1982.

Dudgeon, J. A.: Future developments in prophylaxis. In Intrauterine Infections. Ciba Foundation Symposium 10 (new series). Amsterdam, Associated Scientific Publishers, 1973, pp. 179–189.

Dworsky, M. E., and Stagno, S.: Newer agents causing pneumonitis in early infancy. Pediatr. Infect. Dis. 1:188–195, 1982.

Dworsky, M., Yow, M., Stagno, S., Pass, R. F., and Alford, C. A.: Cytomegalovirus in breast milk and transmission in infancy. Pediatrics 72:295–299, 1983.

Dworsky, M., Stagno, S., Pass, R. F., Cassady, G., Alford, C.: Persistence of cytomegalovirus in human milk after storage. J. Pediatr. 101:440–443, 1982b.

Dworksy, M., Welch, K., Cassady, G., and Stagno, S.: Occupational risk for primary cytomegalovirus infection. N. Engl. J. Med. 309:950–953, 1983.

Elek, S. D., and Stern, H.: Development of a vaccine against mental retardation caused by cytomegalovirus infection. Lancet 1:1–4, 1974a.

Elek, S. D., and Stern, H.: Vaccination against cytomegalovirus? Letter to the editior. Lancet 1:171, 1974b.

Embil, J. A., Haldane, E. V., MacKenzie, R. A. E., and van Roozen, C. E.: Prevalence of cytomegalovirus infection in a normal urban population in Nova Scotia. Can. Med. Assoc. J. 101:730–733, 1969.

Embil, J. A., Ozere, R. L., and Haldane, E. V.: Congenital cytomegalovirus infection in two siblings from consecutive pregnancies. J. Pediatr. 77:417–421, 1970.

Farber, S., and Wolbach, S. B.: Intranuclear and cytoplasmic inclusions ("protozoan-like bodies") in the salivary glands and other organs of infants. Am. J. Pathol. 8:123–135, 1932.

Feldman, R. A.: Cytomegalovirus during pregnancy (a prospective study and report of six cases). Am. J. Dis. Child. 117:517–521, 1969.

Ferm, V. H., and Kilham, L.: Congenital anomalies induced in hamster embryos with H-1 virus. Science 145:510–511, 1964.

Fetterman, G. H.: New laboratory aid in clinical diagnosis of inclusion disease of infancy. Am. J. Clin. Pathol. 22:424–425, 1952.

Foy, H. M., Kenny, G. E., Wentworth, B. B., Johnson, W. L., and Grayston, J. T.: Isolation of Mycoplasma hominis, T-strains, and cytomegalovirus from the cervix of pregnant women. Am. J. Obstet. Gynecol. 106:635–643, 1970.

Fuccillo, D. A., Moder, F. L., Catalano, L. W., Jr.,

Vincent, M. M., and Sever, J. L.: Herpesvirus hominis types I and II: a specific microindirect hemagglutination test. Proc. Soc. Exp. Biol. Med. *133*:735–739, 1970.

Fuccillo, D. A., Moder, F. L., Traub, R. G., Hensen, S., and Sever, J. L.: Microindirect hemagglutination test for cytomegalovirus. Appl. Microbiol. *21*:104–107, 1971.

Geder, L., Lausen, R., O'Neill, F., and Rapp, F.: Oncogenic transformation of human embryonic lung cells by cytomegalovirus, Science *192*:1134–1137, 1976.

Goldberg, G. N., Fulginetti, V. A., Ray, G., Ferry, P., Jones, J. F., Cross, H., and Minnich, L.: In utero Epstein Barr virus (infectious mononucleosis) infection, J.A.M.A. *246*:1579–1581, 1981.

Goodpasture, E., and Talbot, F. B.: Concerning the nature of "protozoan-like" cells in certain lesions of infancy. Am. J. Dis. Child. *21*:415–425, 1921.

Gottlieb, M. S., Schroff, R., Schanker, H. M., Weisman, J. D., Fan, P. T., Wolf, R. A., and Saxon, A.: *Pneumocystis carinii* pneumonia and mucosal candidiasis in previously healthy homosexual men: evidence of a new acquired immunodeficiency. N. Engl. J. Med. *305*:1425–1431, 1981.

Grant, S., Emond, E., and Syme, J.: A prospective study of cytomegalovirus infection in pregnancy. I. Laboratory evidence of congenital infection following maternal primary and reactivated infection. J. Infect. *3*:24–31, 1981.

Griffiths, P. D., Buie, K. J., and Heath, R. B.: A comparison of complement fixation, indirect immunofluorescence of viral late antigens, and anti-complement immunofluorescence tests for the detection of cytomegalovirus specific serum antibodies. J. Clin. Pathol. *31*:827–831, 1978.

Griffiths P. D., Campbell-Benzie, A., and Heath, R. B.: A prospective study of primary cytomegalovirus infection in pregnant women. Br. J. Obstet. Gynecol. *87*:308–314, 1980.

Griffiths, P. D., Stagno, S., Pass, R. F., Smith, R. J., and Alford, C. A., Jr.: Congenital cytomegalovirus infection: diagnostic and prognostic significance of the detection of specific immunoglobulin M antibodies in cord serum. Pediatrics *69*:544–549, 1982a.

Griffiths, P. D., Stagno, S., Pass, R. F., Smith, R. J., and Alford, C. A., Jr.: Infection with cytomegalovirus during pregnancy: specific IgM antibodies as a marker of recent primary infection. J. Infect. Dis. *145*:647–653, 1982b.

Gurevich, I., and Cunha, B. A.: Non-parenteral transmission of cytomegalovirus in a neonatal intensive care unit. Lancet *2*:222–224, 1981.

Haneberg, B., Bertnes, E., and Haukens, G.: Antibodies to cytomegalovirus among personnel at a children's hospital. Acta Paediatr. Scand. *69*:407–409, 1980.

Hanshaw, J. B.: The clinical significance of CMV infection. Postgrad. Med. *35*:472–480, 1964.

Hanshaw, J. B.: Cytomegalovirus complement-fixing antibody in microcephaly. N. Engl. J. Med. *275*:476–479, 1966.

Hanshaw, J. B.: Congenital cytomegalovirus infection. In Bergsma, D., and Krugman, S. (eds.): Intrauterine Infections. Birth Defects. Original Article Series, Vol. IV, No. 7. New York, The National Foundation-March of Dimes, 1968, pp. 37–46.

Hanshaw, J. B.: Congenital cytomegalovirus infection: laboratory methods of detection. J. Pediatr. *75*:1179–1185, 1969.

Hanshaw, J. B.: Developmental abnormalities associated with congenital cytomegalovirus infection. Adv. Teratol. *4*:64–93, 1970.

Hanshaw, J. B.: Congenital cytomegalovirus infection: a fifteen year perspective. J. Infect. Dis. *123*:555–561, 1971.

Hanshaw, J. B.: Congenital cytomegalovirus infection. N. Engl. J. Med. *288*:1406–1407, 1973.

Hanshaw, J. B.: On deafness, cytomegalovirus, and neonatal screening. Am .J. Dis. Child. *136*:886–887, 1982a.

Hanshaw, J. B.: The launching of a cytomegalovirus vaccine. Am. J. Dis. Child. *136*:291–292, 1982b.

Hanshaw, J. B.: Cytomegalovirus. *In* Remington, J. B., and Klein, T. D. (eds.): Infectious Diseases of the Fetus and Newborn Infant, 2nd ed. Philadelphia, W. B. Saunders Company, 1983.

Hanshaw, J. B., and Weller, T. H.: Urinary excretion of cytomegaloviruses by children with generalized neoplastic disease: correlation with clinical and histopathologic observations. J. Pediatr. *58*:305–311, 1961.

Hanshaw, J. B., Betts, R. F., Simon, G., and Boynton, R.: Acquired cytomegalovirus infection: association with hepatomegaly and abnormal liver function tests. N. Engl. J. Med. *272*:602–609, 1965.

Hanshaw, J. B., Steinfeld, H. J., and White, C. J.: Fluorescent antibody test for cytomegalovirus macroglobulin. N. Engl. J. Med. *279*:566–570, 1968.

Hanshaw, J. B., Niederman, J. C., and Chessin, L. N.: Cytomegalovirus macroglobulin in cell-associated herpesvirus infection. J. Infect. Dis. *125*:304–306, 1972.

Hanshaw, J. B., Schultz, F. W., Melish, M. M., and Dudgeon, J. A.: Congenital cytomegalovirus infection. In Intrauterine Infections. Ciba Foundation Symposium 10 (new series). Amsterdam, Associated Scientific Publishers, 1973, pp. 23–32.

Hanshaw, J. B., Scheiner, A. P., Moxley, A., Gaev, L., Abel, V., and Scheiner, B.: CNS effects of "silent" cytomegalovirus infection. N. Engl. J. Med. *295*:468–470, 1976.

Hartley, J. W., and Done, J. T.: Cytomegalic inclusion body disease in sheep. A report of two cases. J. Comp. Pathol. *73*:84–87, 1963.

Hartley, J. W., Rowe, W. P., and Huebner, R. J.: Serial propagation of the guinea pig salivary gland virus in tissue cultures. Proc. Soc. Exp. Biol. Med. *96*:281–285, 1957.

Hayes, K., and Gibas, H.: Placental cytomegalovirus infection without fetal involvement following primary infection in pregnancy. J. Pediatr. *79*:401–405, 1971.

Hayes, K., Danks, D. M., Gibas, H., and Jack, I.: Cytomegalovirus in human milk. N. Engl. J. Med. *287*:177–178, 1972.

Haymaker, W., Girdany, B. R., Stephens, J., Lillle, R. D., and Fetterman, G. H.: Cerebral involvement with advanced periventricular calcification in generalized cytomegalic inclusion disease in the newborn. J. Neuropathol. Exp. Neurol. *13*:562–586, 1954.

Hildebrandt, R. J., Sever, J. L., Margileth, A. M., and Callagan, D. A.: Cytomegalovirus in the normal pregnant woman. Obstet. Gynecol. *98*:1125–1128, 1967.

Hirsch, M. S., Schooley, R. T., Cosimi, A. B., Russell, P. S., Delmonico, F. L., Tolkoff-Rubin, N. E., et al.: Effect of interferon-alpha on cytomegalovirus reactivation syndromes in renal transplant recipients. N. Engl. J. Med. *308*:1489–1493, 1983.

Ho, M.: Cytomegalovirus: Biology and Infection. New York, Plenum Publishing Corp., 1982.

Hodgman, J. E., Freedman, R. I., and Leonan, N. E.: Neonatal dermatology. Pediatr. Clin. North Am. *18*:713–756, 1971.

Hoekelman, R. A., and Anderson, V. M.: Congenital thrombocytopenia, hepatosplenomegaly, and growth retardation. Am. J. Dis. Child. *136*:258–264, 1982.

Horn, R. G., Spicer, S. S., and Wetzel, B. K.: Phagocytosis of bacteria by heterophil leukocytes. Acid and alkaline phosphatase cytochemistry. Am. J. Pathol. 45:327–335, 1967.

Hsiung, G. D., Fischmann, H. R., Fong, C. K. Y., and Green, R. H.: Characterization of a cytomegalo-like virus isolated from spontaneously degenerated equine kidney culture. Proc. Soc. Exp. Biol. Med. 130:80–84, 1969.

Huang, Y. T., Huang, E. S., and Pagano, J. S.: Antisera to human cytomegalovirus prepared in the guinea pig: specific immunofluorescence and complememt fixation tests. J. Immunol. 2:528–532, 1974.

Huang, E. S., Kilpatrick, B. A., Huang, Y. T., and Pagano, J. S.: Detection of human cytomegalovirus and strain variation. Yale J. Biol. Med. 49:29–43, 1976.

Huang, E. S., Alford, C. A., Reynolds, D. W., Stagno, S., Pass, R. F.: Molecular epidemiology of cytomegalovirus infections in women and their infants. N. Engl. J. Med. 303:958–962, 1980.

Huikeshoven, F. J. M., Wallenburg, H. C. S., and Jahoda, M. G. J.: Diagnosis of severe fetal cytomegalovirus infection from amniotic fluid in the third trimester of pregnancy. Am. J. Obstet. Gynecol. 142:1053–1054, 1982.

Jackson, L.: A protozoan parasite in the salivary gland of the dog. J. Infect. Dis. 29:302–305, 1921.

Jacox, R. F., Mongan, E. S., Hanshaw, J. B., and Leddy, J. P.: Hypo-gammaglobulinemia with thymoma and probable pulmonary infection with cytomegalovirus. N. Engl. J. Med. 271:1091–1096, 1964.

Jeddi, M., Gandin, O. G., and Sohier, R.: Prevalence of cytomegalovirus in France. International Conference on Cytomegalovirus Infections, St. Gall. April 1–3, 1970.

Jesionek, A., and Kiolemenoglou, B.: Ueber einen Befund von protozoën-antigen Gebilden in den Organen eines hereditar-luestiochen Fötus. Munch. Med. Wochenschr. 51:1905–1907, 1904.

Joncas, J. H., Alfieri, C., Leyritz-Wills, M., Brochu, P., Jasmin, G., Boldogh, I., and Huang, E. S.: Simultaneous congenital infection with Epstein-Barr virus and cytomegalovirus. N. Engl. J. Med. 304:1399–1403, 1981.

Just, M., Buergin-Wolff, A., Emoedi, G., Hernandez, R.: Immunization trials with live attenuated cytomegalovirus Towne 125. Infection 3:111–114, 1975.

Kanich, R. E., and Craighead, J. E.: Human cytomegalovirus infection of cultured fibroblasts. I. Cytopathologic effects induced by an adapted and a wild strain. Lab. Invest. 27:263–282, 1972.

Kieff, E. D., Hayes, B., Bachenheimer, S. L., Roizman, B.: Genetic relatedness of type 1 and 2 herpes simplex viruses. J. Virol. 9:738–745, 1972.

Kim, Y. J., Gururaj, V. J., and Mirkovic, R. R.: Concomitant diffuse nodular pulmonary infiltration in an infant with cytomegalovirus infection. Pediatr. Infect. Dis. 1:173–176, 1982.

Kimmel, N., Friedman, M. G., and Sarov, I.: Detection of human CMV-specific IgG antibodies by a sensitive solid-phase radioimmunoassay and by a rapid-screening test. J. Med. Virol. 5:195–203, 1980.

King-Lewis, P. A., and Gardner, S. D.: Congenital cytomegalic inclusion disease following intrauterine transfusion. Br. Med. J. 2:603–605, 1969.

Klemola, E., and Kääriäinen, L.: Cytomegalovirus as a possible cause of a disease resembling infectious mononucleosis. Br. Med. J. 2:1099–1102, 1965.

Krech, U., Jung, M., Jung, F., and Singeisen, C.: Virologische und klinische Untersuchungen bei konnatelen und postnatalen Cytomegalien. Schweiz. Med. Wochenschr. 98:1459–1469, 1968.

Krech, U., Konjajev, Z., and Jung, M.: Congenital cytomegalovirus infection in siblings from consecutive pregnancies. Helv. Paediatr. Acta 26:355–362, 1971a.

Krech, U., Jung, M., and Jung, F.: Cytomegalovirus Infections of Man. Basel, S. Karger, 1971b, pp. 1–5.

Kriel, R. L., Gates, G. A., Wulff, H., Powell, N., Poland, J. D., and Chin, T. D. Y.: Cytomegalovirus isolations associated with pregnancy wastage. Am. J. Obstet. Gynecol. 106:885–892, 1970.

Kufe, D., Margrath, I. T., Ziegler, J. L., and Spiegelman, S.: Burkitt's tumors contain particles encapsulating RNA-instructed DNA polymerase and high molecular weight virus related RNA. Proc. Natl. Acad. Sci. U.S.A. 70:737–741, 1973a.

Kufe, D., Hehlmann, R., and Spiegelman, S.: RNA related to that of a murine leukemia virus in Burkitt's tumor and nasopharyngeal carcinomas. Proc. Natl. Acad. Sci. U.S.A. 70:5–9, 1973b.

Kumar, M. L., Nankervis, G., and Gold, E.: Inapparent congenital cytomegalovirus infection: a follow-up study. N. Engl. J. Med. 28:1370–1372, 1973.

Kumar, M. L., Gold, E., Jacobs, I. B., Ernhart, C. B., and Nankervis, G. A.: Primary cytomegalovirus infection in pregnancy. J. Pediatr. 104: 669–673, 1984.

Kumar, M. L., Mankervis, G. A., Jacobs, I. B., Ernhart, C. B., Glasson, C. E., McMillan, P. M., and Gold, E.: Congenital and postnatally acquired cytomegalovirus infections: Long-term follow-up. J. Pediatr. 104:674–679, 1984.

Kuttner, A. G., and Wang, S.: The problem of the significance of the inclusion bodies found in the salivary glands of infants, and the occurrence of inclusion bodies in the submaxillary glands of hamsters, white mice, and wild rats. J. Exp. Med. (Peiping) 60:773–791, 1934.

Lang, D. J.: The association of indirect inguinal hernia with congenital cytomegalic inclusion disease. Pediatrics 38:913–915, 1966.

Lang, D. J., and Hanshaw, J. B.: Cytomegalovirus infection and the postperfusion syndrome: recognition of primary infections in four patients. N. Engl. J. Med. 280:1145–1149, 1969.

Lang, D. J., and Kummer, J. F.: Demonstration of cytomegalovirus in semen. N. Engl. J. Med. 287:756–758, 1972.

Larke, R. P. B., Wheatley, E., Saroj, S., and Chernesky, M.: Congenital cytomegalovirus infection in an urban Canadian community. J. Infect. Dis. 142:647–653, 1980.

L'Ecuyer, C., and Corner, A. H.: Propagation of porcine cytomegalic inclusion disease virus in cell cultures. Can. J. Comp. Med. Vet. Sci. 30:321–326, 1966.

Lee, L. F., Kieff, E. D., Bachenheimer, S. L., Roizman, B., Spear, P. G., Burmester, B. R., and Nazerian, K.: Size and composition of Marik's disease virus deoxyribonucleic acid. J. Virol. 7:289–294, 1971.

Li, F. P., and Hanshaw, J. B.: Cytomegalovirus infection among migrant children. Am. J. Epidemiol. 86:137–147, 1967.

Lipschutz, B.: Untersuchungen uber die Aetiologoc der Krankheitem d. herpes genitalis, etc. Arch. Dermatol. Syphilol. 136:428–482, 1921.

Lowenstein, C.: Ueber protozenartige Gebilde in den organen von Kindern. Zentralbl. Allg. Pathol. 18:513–518, 1907.

Lwoff, A., Horne, R., and Tournier, P.: A system of viruses. Cold Spring Harbor Symp. Quant. Biol. 27:51–55, 1962.

Lysaught, J. N.: Cytomegalic inclusion disease. A suggested method of more rapid diangnsis. South. Med. J. 55:1246–1250, 1962.

Macfarlane, D. E., and Sommerville, R. G.: VERO cells

(Cercopithecus aethiops kidney)—growth characteristics and vital susceptibility for use in diagnostic virology. Arch. Ges. Virusforsch. *27*:379–385, 1969.

Martin, G. A., and Schmidt, H. A.: Spermatogene Übertragung des "Virus Marburg" (Erreger der "Marburger Affenkrankheit"). Klin. Wochenschr. *46*:398–400, 1968.

McAllister, R. M., Straw, R. M., Filbert, J. E., and Goodheart, C. R.: Human cytomegalovirus. Cytochemical observations of intracellular lesion development correlated with viral synthesis and release. Virology *19*:521–531, 1963.

McDougal, J. K., and Harnden, D. G.: Vaccination against cytomegalovirus? Letter to the Editor. Lancet *1*:135, 1974.

Medearis, D. N., Jr.: Observations concerning human cytomegalovirus infection and disease. Bull. Johns Hopkins Hosp. *114*:181–211, 1964.

Melish, M. E., and Hanshaw, J. B.: Congenital cytomegalovirus infection: developmental progress of infants detected by routine screening. Am. J. Dis. Child. *126*:190–194, 1973.

Mendez-Cashion, D., Valcarcel, M. I., De Arelleno, R. R., and Rowe, W. P.: Salivary gland virus antibodies in Puerto Rico: report of a serologic survey with clinical notes. Bol. Asoc. Med. P.R. *55*:447–455, 1963.

Mims, C. A.: Pathogenesis of viral infections of the fetus. Prog. Med. Virol. *10*:194–237, 1968.

Molello, J. A., Chow, T. L., Owen, N., and Jensen, R.: Placental physiology. V. Placental lesions of cattle experimentally infected with infectious bovine rhinotracheitis virus. Am. J. Vet. Res. *27*:907–915, 1966.

Monif, R. G., Egan, E. A., Held, B., and Eitzman, D. V.: The correlation of maternal cytomegalovirus infection during varying stages in gestation with neonatal involvement. J. Pediatr. *80*:17–20, 1972.

Montgomery, J. R., Youngblood, L., and Medearis, D. N., Jr.: Recovery of cytomegalovirus from the cervix in pregnancy. Pediatrics *49*:525–531, 1972.

Montgomery, J. R., Flander, R. W., and Yow, M. D.: Congenital herpesvirus infection with possibly related anomalies. Am. J. Dis. Child., *125*:364–366, 1973.

Morrisseau, P. M., Phillips, C. A., and Leadbetter, G. W., Jr.: Viral prostatitis. J. Urol. *103*:767–769, 1970.

Nahmias, A: Perinatal risk associated with maternal genital herpes simplex virus infection. Am. J. Obstet. Gynecol. *110*:835–837, 1971.

Neff, B. J., Weibel, R. E., Buynak, E. B., McLean, A. A., and Hilleman, M. R.: Clinical and laboratory studies of live cytomegalovirus vaccine AD-169. Proc. Soc. Exp. Biol. Med. *160*:32–37, 1979.

Niven, J. S. F.: Fluorescence microscopy of nucleic acid changes in virus-infected cells. Ann. N.Y. Acad. Sci. *81*:84–88, 1959.

Numazaki, Y., Yano, N., Morizuka, T., Takai, S., and Ishida, N.: Primary infection with human cytomegalovirus: virus isolation from healthy infants and pregnant women. Am. J. Epidemiol. *91*:410–417, 1970.

Oppenheimer, E. H., and Esterly, J. R.: Cytomegalovirus infection: a possible cause of biliary atresia. Am. J. Pathol. *71*:2a, 1973.

Pagano, J. S., Huang, C. H., and Levine, P.: Absence of Epstein-Barr viral DNA in American Burkitt's lymphoma. N. Engl. J. Med. *289*:1395–1399, 1973.

Paloheimo, J. A., VonEssen, R., Klemola, E., Kääriäinen, L., and Siltanen, P.: Subclinical cytomegalovirus infections and cytomegalovirus mononucleosis after open heart surgery. Am. J. Cardiol. *22*:624–630, 1968.

Pass, R. F., Stagno, S., Myers, G. J., Alford, C. A.: Outcome of systematic congenital cytomegalovirus infection: result of long-term longitudinal follow-up. Pediatrics *66*:758–762, 1980.

Pass, R. F., August, A. M., Dworsky, M. E., and Reynolds, D. W.: Cytomegalovirus infection in a day care center. N. Engl. J. Med. *307*:477–479, 1982a.

Pass, R. F., Stagno, S., Dworsky, M. E., Smith, R. J., and Alford, C. A.: Excretion of cytomegalovirus in mothers: observations after delivery of a congenitally infected and normal infants. J. Infect. Dis. *146*:1–6, 1982b.

Patrizi, G., Middlekamp. J. N., Herweg, J. C., and Thornton, H. K.: Human cytomegalovirus electron microscopy of a primary viral isolate. J. Lab. Clin. Med. *65*:925–938, 1965.

Peckham, C. S.: A clinical and laboratory study of children exposed *in utero* to maternal rubella. Arch. Dis. Child. *47*:571–577, 1972.

Peckham, C. S., Preece, P. M., and Chin, K. S.: Cytomegalovirus in pregnancy and its consequences. Abstract. Conference on Pathogenesis and Prevention of Human Cytomegalovirus Infection, Philadelphia, 1983.

Penttinen, K., Kääriäinen, L., and Myllyla, G.: Cytomegalovirus antibody assay by platelet aggregation. Arch. Ges. Virusforsch. *29*:189–194, 1970.

Peters, W. P., Kufe, D., Schlom, J., Frankel, J. W., Prickett, C., Groupe, V., and Spiegelman, S.: Biological and biochemical evidence for an interaction between Marek's disease, herpesvirus and avian leukosis virus *in vitro*. Proc. Natl. Acad. Sci. U.S.A. *70*:3175–3178, 1973.

Plotkin, S. A.: Cytomegalovirus vaccine: Towne Strain. In Proceedings of the Experimental Herpesvirus Vaccine Workshop, National Institutes of Health, Bethesda, Maryland, *February 7–9, 1979*. Washington, D.C., U.S. Government Printing Office.

Plotkin, S. A., Farquahar, J., Hornberger, E.: Clinical trials with the Towne 125 strain of human cytomegalovirus. J. Infect. Dis. *134*:470–475, 1976.

Plotkin, S. A., Starr, S. E., and Bryan, C. K.: In vitro and in vivo responses of cytomegalovirus to acyclovir. Acyclovir Symposium. Am. J. Med. *73A*:257–261, 1982.

Plummer, G., and Benyesh-Melnick, M.: Plaque reduction neutralization test for human cytomegalovirus. Proc. Soc. Exp. Biol. Med. *117*:145–150, 1964.

Quinnan, G. V., Kirmani, N., Rook, A. H., Manischewitz, J. F., Jackson, L., Moreschi, G., Santos, G. W., Saral, R., and Burns, W. H.: Cytotoxic T cells in cytomegalovirus infection. N. Engl. J. Med. *307*:6–13, 1982.

Rabson, A. S., Edgcomb, J. H., Legallais, F. Y., and Tyrrell, S. A.: Isolation and growth of rat cytomegalovirus *in vitro*. Proc. Soc. Exp. Biol. Med. *131*:923–927, 1969.

Raynaud, J., Atanasiu, P., Barreau, C., and Jahkola, M.: Adaptation d'un virus cytomégalique provenant du mulot *(Apodemus sylvaticus)* sur différentes cellules hétérologues, y compris les cellules humaines. C R. Acad. Sci. [D] (Paris) *269*:104–106, 1969.

Rector, E. J., and Rector, L. E.: Intranuclear inclusions in the salivary glands of moles. Am. J. Pathol. *10*:629–636, 1934.

Reller, L. B.: Granulomatous hepatitis associated with acute cytomegalovirus infection. Lancet *1*:20–22, 1973.

Remington, J. S., Miller, M. J., and Brownlee, I.: IgM antibodies in acute toxoplasmosis. I. Diagnostic significance in congenital cases and a method for their rapid demonstration. Pediatrics.*41*:1082–1091, 1968.

Reynolds, D. W., Stagno, S., Hosty, T. S., Tiller, M., and Alford, C. A.: Maternal cytomegalovirus excretion and perinatal infection. N. Engl. J. Med. *289*:3–7, 1973.

Reynolds, D. W., Stagno, S., Stubbs, K. G., Dahle, A. J., Livingston, M. M., Saxon, S. S., and Alford, C. A.: Congenital cytomegalovirus infection: relation to auditory and mental deficiency. N. Engl. J. Med. *290*:291–296, 1974.

Ribbert, H.: Veber protozoenartige Zellen in der Niereeines syphilitischen Negeborenenund in der Parotis von Kindern. Zentralbl. Allg. Pathol. *15*:945–948, 1904.

Rosen, P., Armstrong, D., and Rice, N.: Gastrointestinal cytomegalovirus infection. Arch. Intern. Med. *132*:274–276, 1973.

Rowe, R. D.: Maternal rubella and pulmonary artery stenosis. Pediatrics *32*:180–185, 1963.

Rowe, W. P., Hartley, J. W., Waterman, S., Turner, H. C., and Huebner, R. J.: Cytopathogenic agent resembling salivary gland virus recovered from tissue cultures of human adenoids. Proc. Soc. Exp. Biol. Med. *92*:418–424, 1956.

Rowe, W. P., Hartley, J. W., Cramblett, H. G., and Mastrota, F. M.: Detection of human salivary gland virus in the mouth and urine of children. Am. J. Hyg. *67*:57–65, 1958.

Ruebner, B. H ., Miyai, K., Shisser, R. J., Wedermeyer, P., and Medearis, D. N., Jr.: Mouse cytomegalovirus infection: an electron microscopic study of hepatic parenchymal cells. Am. J. Pathol. *44*:799–821, 1964.

Ruebner, B. H., Hirand, T., Slusser, R., Osborn, J., and Medearis, D. N., Jr.: Cytomegalovirus infection: viral ultrastructure with particular reference to the relationship of lysosomes to cytoplasmic inclusions. Am. J. Pathol. *48*:971–989, 1966.

Saigal, S., Lunyk, O., Larke, R. P. B., and Chernesky, M. A.: The outcome of children with congenital cytomegalovirus infection: a longitudinal follow-up study. Am. J. Dis. Child. *136*:896–901, 1982.

Schaffer, A. J.: Diseases of the Newborn. 2nd ed. Philadelphia, W. B. Saunders Company, 1965, p. 733.

Sever, J. L., Huebner, R. J., Castellano, G. A., and Bell, J. A.: Serological diagnosis "en masse" with multiple antigens. Am. Rev. Respir. Dis. *88*(Suppl.):342–359, 1963.

Smith, K. O., and Rasmussen, L. E.: Morphology of cytomegalovirus (salivary gland virus). J. Bacteriol. *95*:1319–1325, 1963.

Smith, M. G.: Propagation of salivary gland virus of the mouse in tissue culture. Proc. Soc. Exp. Biol. Med. *86*:435–440, 1954.

Smith, M. G.: Propagation in tissue cultures of a cytopathogenic virus from human salivary gland virus (SGV) disease. Proc. Soc. Exp. Biol. Med. *92*:424–430, 1956.

Smith, M. G.: The salivary gland viruses of man and animals (cytomegalic inclusion disease). Prog. Med. Virol. *2*:1171–1202, 1959.

South, M. A., Tompkins, W. A. F., Morris, C. R., and Rawls, W. E.: Congenital malformations of the central nervous system associated with genital type (type 2) herpesvirus. J. Pediatr. *75*:13–18, 1969.

Spector, S. A.: Transmission of cytomegalovirus among infants in hospital documented by restriction-endomuclease digestion analyses. Lancet *1*:378–381, 1983.

Stagno, S.: Isolation precautions for patients with cytomegalovirus infections. Pediatr. Infect. Dis. *1*:145–147, 1982.

Stagno, S., Reynolds, D. W., Lakeman, A. W., Charamella, L. J.,and Alford, C. A.: Congenital cytomegalovirus infection: consecutive occurrence due to viruses with similar antigenic compositions. Pediatrics *52*:788–794, 1973.

Stagno, S., Reynolds, D. W., Tsiantos, A., Fuccillo, D. A., Smith, R., Tiller, M., and Alford, C. A., Jr.: Cervical cytomegalovirus excretion in pregnant and nonpregnant women: suppression in early gestation. J. Infect. Dis. *131*:522–527, 1975a.

Stagno, S., Reynolds, D. W., Tsiantos, A., Fuccillo, D. A., Long, W., and Alford, C. A., Jr.: Comparative serial virologic and serological studies of symptomatic and subclinical congenitally and natally acquired cytomegalovirus infections. J. Infect. Dis. *132*:568, 1975b.

Stagno, S., Reynolds, D. W., Huang, E., Thames, S. D., Smith, R. J., and Alford, C. A., Jr.: Congenital cytomegalovirus infection: occurrence in an immune population. N. Engl. J. Med. *296*:1254–1258, 1977a.

Stagno, S., Volanakis, J. E., Reynolds, D. W., Strand, R., and Alford, C. A.: Immune complexes in congenital and natal cytomegalovirus infections of man. J. Clin. Invest. *60*:838–845, 1977b.

Stagno, S., Reynolds, D. W., Pass, R. F., and Alford, C. A.: Breast milk and the risk of cytomegalovirus infection. N. Engl. J. Med. *302*:1073–1076, 1980a.

Stagno, S., Pass, R. F., Reynolds, D. W., Moore, M, A., Nahmias, A. M., and Alford, C. A.: Comparative studies of diagnostic procedures for congenital cytomegalovirus infection. Pediatrics *62*:251–257, 1980b.

Stagno, S., Brasfield, D. M., Brown, M. B., Cassell, G. H., Pifer, L. L., Whitley, R. J., and Tiller, R. E.: Infant pneumonitis associated with cytomegalovirus, Chlamydia, Pneumocystis, and Ureaplasma: a prospective study. Pediatrics *68*:322–329, 1981.

Stagno, S., Pass, R. F., Dworsky, M. E., Henderson, R. E., Moore, E. G., Walton, P. D., and Alford, C. A.: Congenital cytomegalovirus infection: the relative importance of primary and recurrent maternal infection. N. Engl. J. Med. *306*:945–949, 1982a.

Stagno, S., Pass, R. F., Thomas, J. P., Navia, J. M., and Dworsky, M. E.: Defects of tooth structure in congenital cytomegalovirus infection. Pediatrics *69*:646–648, 1982b.

Starr, J. G., Bart, R. D., Jr., and Gold, E.: Inapparent congenital cytomegalovirus infection: clinical and epidemiologic characteristics in early infancy. N. Engl. J. Med. *282*:1075–1078, 1970.

Stern, H.: Isolation of cytomegalovirus and clinical manifestations of infection at different ages. Br. Med. J. *1*:665–669, 1968.

Stern, H.: Cytomegalovirus and mental deficiency. In Infectious Diseases. Proceedings XIII International Congress of Paediatrics, Vol. 6. Vienna, Wiener Medizinische Akademie, 1971, pp. 301–306.

Stern, H.: Discussion. Intrauterine Infections. Ciba Foundation Symposium 10 (new series). Amsterdam, Associated Scientific Publishers. 1973, pp. 32–43.

Stern, H., and Elek, S. D.: The incidence of infection with cytomegalovirus in a normal population (a serological study in Greater London). J. Hyg. (Camb.) *63*:79–87, 1965.

Stern, H., Elek, S. D., Booth, J. C., and Fleck, D. G.: Microbial causes of mental retardation. The role of prenatal infections with cytomegalovirus, rubella virus, and toxoplasmosis. Lancet *2*:443–448, 1969.

Syrucek, L., Sobelslavsky, O., and Gutvirth, I.: Isolation of *Coxiella burneti* from human placentas. J. Hyg. Epidemiol. *2*:29–35, 1958.

Toghill, P. J., Williams, R., and Stern, H.: Cytomegalovirus infection in chronic liver disease. Gastroenterology *56*:936–937, 1969.

Tuomanen, E. I., and Powell, K. R.: Staphylococcal

protein A adsorption of neonatal serum to facilitate early diagnosis of congenital infection. J. Pediatr. *97*:238–243, 1980.

Tyzzer, E. E.: The histology of skin lesions in varicella. Philippine J. Sci. *1*:349–372, 1906.

Vogel, F. S., and Pinkerton, H.: Spontaneous salivary gland virus disease in chimpanzees. Arch. Pathol. *60*:281–288, 1955.

Volpi, A., Whitley, R. J., Ceballos, R., and Stagno, S.: Rapid diagnosis of pneumonia due to cytomegalovirus with specific monoclonal antibodies. J. Infect. Dis. *147*:1119–1120, 1983.

Von Glahn, W. C., and Pappenheimer, A. M.: Intranuclear inclusions in visceral disease. Am. J. Pathol. *1*:445–466, 1925.

Wade, J. C., Hintz, M., McGuffin, R. W., Springmeyer, S. C., Connor, J. D., and Meyers, J. D.: Treatment of cytomegalovirus pneumonia with high-dose acyclovir. Acyclovir Symposium. Am. J. Med. *73A*:249–256, 1982.

Waner, J., Weller, T. H., and Kevy, S. V.: Patterns of cytomegaloviral complement-fixing antibody activity: a longitudinal study of blood donors. Pediatr. Res. *127*:538–543, 1973.

Weller, T. H.: The cytomegaloviruses: the difficult years. J. Infect. Dis. *122*:532–539, 1970.

Weller, T. H.: The cytomegaloviruses: ubiquitous agents with protean clinical manifestations. N. Engl. J. Med. *285*:203–214, 267–274, 1971.

Weller, T. H., and Hanshaw, J. B.: Virological and clinical observations of cytomegalic inclusion disease. N. Engl. J. Med. *266*:1233–1244, 1962.

Weller, T. H., Macauley, J. C., Craig, J. M., and Wirth, P.: Isolation of intranuclear inclusion producing agents from infants with illnesses resembling cytomegalic inclusion disease. Proc. Soc. Exp. Biol. Med. *94*:4–12, 1957.

Weller, T. H., Hanshaw, J. B., and Scott, D. E.: Serological differentiation of viruses responsible for cytomegalic inclusion disease. Virology *12*:130–132, 1960.

Wenzel, R. P., McCormick, D. P., Davies, J. A., et al.: Cytomegalovirus infection: a seroepidemiologic study of a recruit population. Am. J. Epidemiol. *97*:410–414, 1973.

Wilfert, C. M., Huang, E.-S., and Stagno, S.: Restriction endonuclease analysis of cytomegalovirus deoxyribonucleic acid as an epidemiologic tool. Pediatrics *70*:717–721, 1982.

Williamson, W. D., Desmond, M. M., Lafevers, N., Taber, L., Catlin, F. I., and Weaver, T. G.: Symptomatic congenital cytomegalovirus: disorders of language, learning, and hearing. Am. J. Dis. Child. *136*:902–905, 1982.

Yambao, T. J., Calrk, D., Weiner, L., and Aubry, R. H.: Isolation of cytomegalovirus from the amniotic fluid during the third trimester. Am. J. Obstet. Gynecol. *139*:937–938, 1981.

Yeager, A. S.: Transfusion-acquired cytomegalovirus infection in newborn infant. Am. J. Dis. Child. *128*: 478–483, 1974.

Yeager, A. S.: Longitudinal serological study of cytomegalovirus infections in nurses and in personnel without patient contact. J. Clin. Microbiol. *2*:448–452, 1975.

Yeager, A. S., Jacobs, H., and Clark, J.: Nursery-acquired infection in two premature infants. J. Pediatr. *81*:332–335, 1972.

Yeager, A. S., Hafleigh, M. T., Arvin, A. M., Bradley, J. S., and Prober, C. G.: Prevention of transfusion-acquired cytomegalovirus infections in newborn infants. J. Pediatr. *98*:281–287, 1981.

Yeager, A. S., Palumbo, P. E., Malachowski, N., Ariagno, R. L., and Stevenson, D. K.: Sequelae of maternally derived cytomegalovirus infections in premature infants. J. Pediatr. *102*:918–922, 1983.

Yolken, R. H., and Stopa, P. J.: Comparison of seven enzyme immunoassay systems for measurement of cytomegalovirus. J. Clin. Microbiol. *11*:546–551, 1980.

Yow, M. D., Lakeman, A. D., Stagno, S., Reynolds, R. B., and Plavidal, F. J.: Use of restriction enzymes to investigate the source of a primary cytomegalovirus infection in a nurse. Pediatrics *70*:713–716, 1982.

Zuelzer, W. W., Mastrangelo, R., Stulberg, C. S., Poulik, M. D., Page, R. H., and Thompson, R. I.: Autoimmune hemolytic anemia: natural history and viral immunologic interactions in childhood. Am. J. Med. *49*:80–93, 1970.

5

Herpes Simplex Infection of the Fetus and Newborn

Although herpes simplex virus (HSV) has been known as a cause of infection in the newborn period since Batignani (1934) observed an infant with isolated keratoconjunctivitis and Hass (1935) described hepatoadrenal necrosis, the condition has not received a great deal of attention in the literature. Information obtained in the last decade concerning the spectrum of disease, improved methods of diagnosis, the heterogeneity of HSV strains, and the possibility of antiviral therapy has quickened the interest of medical virologists, pediatricians, and obstetricians in this condition. It is now known that at least some neonates with HSV infections may be asymptomatic and that others have localized forms of the disease that may be followed by late central nervous system sequelae. Two strains of the virus have been identified: type 1 is primarily a nongenital virus, type 2 is often a genital one, although this distinction is less clear than it once seemed (Kalinyak et al., 1977). It is recognized that although most infections in neonates are due to the type 2 agent, approximately 30 per cent are due to type 1 strains of the virus.

EPIDEMIOLOGY

Herpes simplex infections are among the most common infections of humans. Although approximately 90 to 95 per cent of infected persons are asymptomatic, clinical disease may be severe under certain conditions. The newborn infant (especially the premature infant), the malnourished child or adult, and the patient with a defect in cellular immune function are all particularly vulnerable to the effects of this infection. There does not appear to be a significant clinical difference between newborns infected with type 1 and those affected with type 2 strain of the virus.

Virological and cytological swabs taken from the cervix or vagina indicate that maternal herpes infection is three times more common during pregnancy than at other times and that approximately 1 per cent of women in the lowest socioeconomic group have evidence of infection (Nahmias et al., 1971).* The incidence of infection is less in

*The use of cotton swabs and storage of specimens at refrigerator temperature have been shown to be significantly more successful in isolating virus than the use of calcium alginate swabs and storage at freezing temperatures (Bettoli et al., 1982).

private obstetrical patients than among women attending clinics, ranging from 0.02 to 0.1 per cent (Ng et al., 1970). As in cytomegalovirus (CMV) cervicitis, the incidence of infection apparently increases as pregnancy progresses (Nahmias et al., 1971). Pettay and co-workers (1972) did a preliminary survey of 100 women at the time of delivery using a direct immunofluorescent method to detect herpesvirus antigen in cervical smears. They found that cervical cells from 10 of the 100 women reacted with HSV antigen when stained with rabbit antiherpes antiserum. In a survey done a few weeks after delivery, only one of the mothers still had herpes antigen.

Sever and colleagues (1963) were able to demonstrate fourfold complement-fixing antibody responses of unspecified herpesvirus type in 2.5 per cent of 198 pregnant women residing in Boston and Philadelphia. If most of these responses can be interpreted as evidence of active infection, the prevalence of infection in the mother during pregnancy is considerably higher than that found in the offspring and is certainly higher than the number of newborns with manifestations of herpetic disease. Although precise figures are not available on the frequency of herpetic disease in the newborn, the probability is that it is relatively rare in its clinically recognizable form. On the basis of observations made in Atlanta and in Brooklyn, it has been estimated that symptomatic herpetic infection in the newborn occurs approximately once in 7500 deliveries (Nahmias, 1970b). Both of the populations studied consisted of women from lower socioeconomic groups, 80 to 90 per cent of whom were seropositive for HSV type 2. This rate is in contrast to that in more affluent populations, in which about half would be expected to be seropositive for type 2 antibody. It is quite probable that a significant number of newborn patients with herpetic infection are not diagnosed. This may be because the characteristic skin lesions are not present, the disease is not as severe as most physicians expect neonatal HSV infection to be, or the infection is asymptomatic. With an annual birthrate of about 3.6 million per year in the United States, there would be 180 infants with herpes simplex infection born annually if infection occurred only once in 20,000 deliveries. It is of interest that there are eight reports in the literature in which three to eight cases of herpetic disease occurred in the same hospital within a two- to three-year period. We observed five cases of disseminated disease in a four-year period, for a prevalence of approximately one in 8000 newborns.

In assessing the probability of infection in a given infant, it should be noted that Nahmias and co-workers (1967b) found neonatal *disease* in only 1 of 28 infants born to women who had had herpetic infections sometime during pregnancy. The time at which the infection occurs, whether it is primary or recurrent, the type of delivery, and, possibly, the antibody level of the mother are factors that may influence the outcome for the infant. The overall risk of neonatal infection is approximately 10 per cent in women with cytological, serological, or clinical evidence of genital HSV infection (primary or recurrent) after 32 weeks' gestation. If the virus is present at delivery, the risk of infection in the infant is 40 to 50 per cent, unless the infant is delivered by cesarean section before or within four hours of rupture of the membranes (Nahmias et al., 1971).

St. Geme and colleagues (1975) observed five women with genital herpes simplex infection beyond 32 weeks' gestation. Two of the women had fresh vesicular lesions at parturition. The five infants were delivered per vaginam at term and escaped subsequent overt infection. One infant had a nonvesicular crusted lesion on the occiput at birth, which was thought to represent the trauma of forceps. Examination of the infants two months to four years after birth failed to detect sequelae of possible subclinical infection.

PATHOGENESIS

The main route of transmission of HSV from one individual to another is thought to be by close contact with virus in cutaneous lesions of infected persons. Transmission to the fetus and the newborn may occur by maternal viremic-transplacental spread or by the ascending cervical amniotic route (Fig. 5–1).

Possibility of Venereal Transmission

Nahmias and co-workers (1969b) have presented evidence for the venereal transmission of HSV. This includes the observation that seven of eight female contacts of seven males

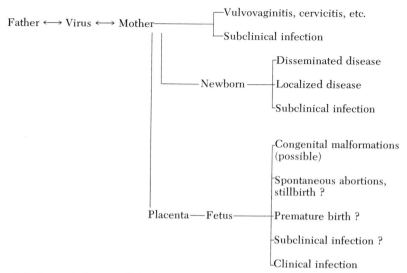

Figure 5–1. Transmission and clinical manifestations of herpes simplex infection in pregnancy.

with herpetic infection showed evidence of active HSV infection. They also found that 6 per cent of female patients and 0.3 per cent of male patients attending a venereal disease clinic had virologically confirmed herpes.

Antepartum Transmission to the Fetus

There is evidence that HSV may reach the fetus at different stages of gestational life. Transplacental transmission is not as well documented in humans as it is in certain animals, such as the rabbit. The evidence that it occurs is based in part on a small number of case reports of first-trimester maternal herpetic infection followed by congenital abnormalities of a similar type in the newborn. The cases reported by Schaffer (1965) and by South and co-workers (1969) are strikingly similar. Montgomery and colleagues (1973) observed a third patient with less central nervous system involvement. These observations, plus those of several other investigators that have not been documented in the literature, lend support to the thesis that HSV can infect the fetus during the period of organogenesis and induces anomalies such as microcephaly and microphthalmos. It is probable that infection *in utero* is not compatible with continued life in some instances and that abortion occurs. Boué and Loffredo (1970) have isolated HSV from fetal tissue obtained following spontaneous abortion, and Naib and co-workers (1970) have found

an association between cytologically detected genital herpes and a significantly higher than normal abortion rate. Nahmias and colleagues (1971) observed an increased abortion rate during the first 20 weeks of pregnancy among 39 women with cytologically detected HSV infection. After this period an increased prematurity rate was noted in 101 women studied. These rates were especially high among women with clinical or serological evidence of primary infection. No fetal or neonatal effects were found among 43 women with cytological evidence of HSV infection in the postpartum period.

Presumably, as in most other congenital infections, it is necessary for maternal viremia to occur and for the virus to become established as a placental infection before successful transmission to the fetus can take place. There is little available information about how transmission occurs. On the basis of the case reports recorded thus far, the probability is that survival after fetal infection is a relatively uncommon event. It is known, however, that maternal genital infection is more likely to be inapparent than overt; thus, the possibility exists that more fetuses are exposed to HSV than are currently recognized. Fifteen years ago it was not suspected that CMV reached the protected environment of the fetus with the frequency that it does. In view of reports of congenital malformations following the appearance of maternal infection in early pregnancy, it will be particularly important to follow the long-term development of infants born to mothers with herpetic infections in the first half of pregnancy.

Intrapartum Transmission to the Newborn Infant

The transmission of infection and disease to the neonate during the second stage of labor is more important and far more frequent than transplacental infection. The majority of reported cases concern severely ill infants who presumably acquired the infection on exposure to the virus-containing secretions of the maternal genital tract. Nahmias and his associates (1967b) found that most isolates recovered from infected newborns were type 2. It is of interest that one of their type 1 infections was associated with a type 1 genital infection in the mother. During passage through the vagina there is contamination of the infant's scalp, eyes, skin, umbilical cord, and upper respiratory tract. Although transmission of infection by exposure to nongenital herpetic infection and to nursery personnel infected with a variety of herpetic lesions does occur, the risk to the infant appears, on the basis of the very few cases reported in the literature, to be decidedly small. It is important, however, not to assume that only maternal herpetic lesions constitute a risk to the infant. The greater risk in maternal genital infections is probably related to a combination of factors, such as a high titer of virus inoculum, the enhanced vulnerability of exposed surfaces of the infant during the trauma of the first and second stages of labor, and the type and severity of maternal infection. The infection per se may be a factor in inducing premature labor. If the infection is of the recurrent type, maternal IgG antibody will be transferred to the newborn. The protective value of this antibody is probably not as great as that of cell-mediated immunity in herpesvirus infections (St. Geme et al., 1965; Wilton et al., 1972). On the basis of recorded experience, the greatest predictable hazard to the newborn occurs in those whose mothers have experienced a primary genital infection in the two to four weeks prior to delivery.

Neonatal herpes simplex infection has been associated with fetal scalp monitoring. Presumably inapparent CMV infection is better able to become established as a pathogen during this kind of monitoring and should be considered as a possible complication of such invasive procedures (Katz et al., 1980).

Transmission from Paternal Source

The case report by Zavoral and co-workers (1970) is of interest because it illustrates the importance of timing in transmission and the venereal nature of the genital infection. This report involves the exposure of a wife to her husband, who had been given a special leave from military service one week prior to delivery of their child. During the preceding period overseas, the husband had experienced a herpetic infection of the penis that was recurrent at the time of his return. His wife had a primary genital herpetic lesion at the time of delivery. The infant, born by cesarean section six hours after rupture of the membranes, contracted a disseminated herpetic infection and died at eight days of age.

Dini and colleagues (1980) have described a fatal HSV infection in an infant whose mother showed no signs of genital lesions but whose father developed multiple lesions of the penis two weeks before the infant's birth. Delivery was by cesarean section three days after membrane rupture, and HSV was found post mortem in the adrenal glands, liver, lungs, and brain.

Time of Transmission

Although the time of onset of neonatal disease supports the concept that most infections in the newborn period are acquired during the first and second stages of labor, this may not always be true. Witzleben and Driscoll (1965) have found evidence of herpetic infection in the placenta of a newborn infant who did not have systemic disease until the sixth day of life. Similar findings have been reported by Gagnon (1968), who isolated herpes simplex from the placenta of an infant who became ill on the fifth day of life. Since it is estimated that the incubation period of HSV infection may vary from two to 12 days, lesions appearing on the first day of life are probably the result of infection acquired before birth.

Postpartum Transmission to the Newborn Infant

Postpartum acquisition of HSV by a neonate is a rare but serious condition; 16 of 24 cases reported were fatal (Light, 1979). Suspected sources of infection include mothers, nursery personnel, and other infants. Confirmation of these suspicions is made possible by DNA "fingerprinting"—the gel electrophoresis of viral DNA broken up by specific endonucleases. A comparison of electrophoretic banding patterns allows distinction

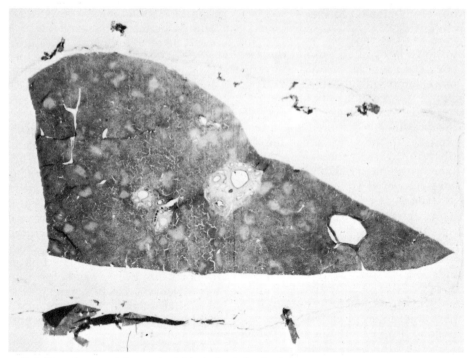

Figure 5–2. Hepatic necrosis is grossly visible in focal distribution in fatal case of neonatal HSV infection.

among strains of virus; this technique has been employed in epidemiological investigations of possible nosocomial transmission of HSV. Linnemann and co-workers (1978) have reported two newborns infected with the same strain of HSV type 1 within one month at one nursery, whereas Halperin (1980) used the process to show that adjacent infants within a nursery were infected with two distinct viruses.

PATHOLOGY

Once infection becomes established in disseminated form, the liver and the adrenals are almost universally involved, as is noted in the early description by Hass (1935). Focal coagulative necrosis is the characteristic lesion (Fig. 5–2). There is usually no associated inflammatory infiltration. The fact that nuclear inclusions are best seen in the periphery of the focal lesions and may be present in many organs other than the liver and the adrenals suggests that the term "hepato-adrenal necrosis" (Zuelzer and Stulberg, 1952) frequently does not fully describe the pathological findings. In addition to the liver and the adrenals, virus has been cultured from numerous other organs.

It is now well recognized that the absence of inclusions in a given type of tissue does not necessarily mean that HSV is not present in an organ. The nuclear changes that are seen are similar to those of the other herpesvirus infections of man, with beading at the nuclear membrane due to margination of nuclear chromatin. The inclusions are indistinguishable from those of varicella-zoster but are not as large as those seen in CMV infection.

SUSCEPTIBILITY TO INFECTION

It is well established that the incidence of herpetic infection in the newborn period is proportionately greater among premature infants than among full-term infants. It has been suggested that the premature infant is more vulnerable because he or she lacks the full complement of maternal IgG antibody and the capacity to respond immunologically in one of several ways.

The susceptibility of the premature infant, which is four to five times that of a full-term infant, may also be explained by the impairment of immunological functions other than the humoral response. Sterzl and Silverstein (1967) have shown that the humoral immune response by the fetal lamb to different antigens occurs at different times, beginning as early as 20 weeks' gestation. Overall and Glasgow (1970a) found that the capacity of the fetal lamb to produce interferon is remarkably efficient. It is possible that the critical deficit in the premature infant is in his or her ability to provide an adequate cellular immune response. This is suggested by the increased susceptibility to herpes simplex infection noted in older infants with severe protein deficiency syndromes or with the Wiskott-Aldrich syndrome (St. Geme et al., 1965) and in animals treated with antilymphocytic globulin (Nahmias et al., 1969a). It has also been observed that newborn mice are relatively inefficient in their macrophage responses compared with older animals (Hirsch et al., 1971). The observations by Wilton and co-workers (1972) suggest that susceptibility to recurrent herpesvirus infections may be due to a cell-mediated immunodeficiency involving macrophage migration inhibition factor and lymphocyte toxicity. It is of interest that infections with other herpesvirus infections of humans, including Epstein-Barr virus, CMV, and varicella-zoster viruses, occur more frequently in patients with defects in cellular immune function.

Preliminary studies indicate that women who show cytological evidence of HSV infections in later pregnancy have a higher prevalence of premature deliveries (Nahmias et al., 1971), suggesting that the maternal infection may be the key factor in producing the prematurity. Whitley and colleagues (1980a) have concurred with this view of HSV infection as a cause of premature labor, noting that prematurity, in addition to viral infection, may explain the high morbidity and mortality associated with this neonatal disease. Other complications found with HSV infection include respiratory distress, bacterial sepsis, and hypoglycemia; etiological connections among the conditions are currently speculative.

The cause of the infant's susceptibility to disseminated HSV infection may be more complicated than mere immunodeficiency. Sullivan-Bolyai and co-workers (1982) have found that cord blood mononuclear cells not adherent to plastic are permissive for HSV infection, which may indicate predisposition to dissemination.

CLINICAL MANIFESTATIONS

Maternal Disease

The diagnosis of HSV infection during pregnancy may be easily missed. Approximately one-third of the patients will have characteristic vesicular or ulcerative lesions or both (Nahmias et al., 1971). The cervix is the most common site of infection, with the vulva only secondarily involved.

In primary vulvovaginitis, the lesions are not unlike the primary vesicles and ulcerations seen in the oral mucosa primary in herpetic stomatitis (Slavin and Gavett, 1946). The vesicles tend to rupture soon after formation to produce a few shallow erosions that are extremely painful. The ulcers develop in different areas of the labia, progress, and then coalesce, until the entire labial mucosa is involved (Fig. 5–3). They are covered with a membranous grayish-yellow exudate with an erythematous base. Unlike the typical syphilitic chancre, the lesions are not indurated. Occasionally the ulceration leads to secondary bacterial infection. Manifestations of the primary disease may range in intensity from minimal symptoms to a 10-day period of fever, headache, malaise, anorexia, and moderate to severe toxicity. A vaginal discharge is frequently present. The painful lesions result in dysuria and dyspareunia. At the end of four or five days, the peripheral ulcers usually begin to heal by secondary intention without scar formation. Complete healing usually requires 10 to 20 days. In some patients the recurrent form of the disease compares in discomfort with the primary infection. Usually, however, the regional lymph nodes are not involved as they are in the primary disease, and systemic symptoms are absent. Some women have recurrent episodes, which may be associated with menstruation, extending over several years.

Intrauterine Infection

Mitchell and McCall (1963), reporting an infant with vesicular lesions appearing on the day of birth, were the first to suggest that transplacental HSV infection occurs. Subsequently, Witzleben and Driscoll (1965) presented evidence indicating that the disseminated, fulminant form of HSV infection may begin prior to birth. They demonstrated intranuclear inclusions in the placenta of an infant dying of disseminated disease at 10 days of age.

The clinical manifestations of an HSV infection acquired *in utero* depend on the time at which the infection became established in the fetus. However, unlike the severity of intrauterine infections with rubella, that of HSV cannot at present be clearly correlated

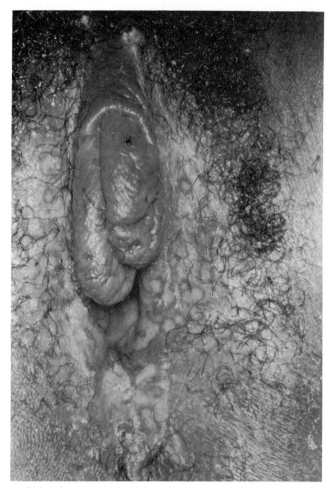

Figure 5–3. Primary vulvovaginitis. (Courtesy of Dr. Marvin S. Amstey.)

with the time of onset of the disease (Komorous et al., 1977). The patient reported by South and co-workers (1969) was born at 33 weeks' gestation to a mother with a history of vaginal discharge associated with recurrent lesions preceding and during the first two weeks of pregnancy. The infant was severely retarded, with marked microcephaly, microencephaly, microphthalmos, intracranial calcifications conforming to atrophic cerebral hemispheres, and retinal dysplasia. HSV type 2 was isolated from vesicles present at birth. Schaffer (1965) described a case with strikingly similar intracranial calcifications, microcephaly, microphthalmos, and cutaneous vesicles from which HSV was isolated. The similarity of these two cases is strong presumptive evidence that HSV is capable of causing developmental anomalies. Montgomery and colleagues (1973) described a patient with vesicular lesions at birth who had chorioretinitis, patent ductus arteriosus, short digits with soft, poorly formed nails, and psychomotor retardation. HSV was isolated from the skin lesions at birth. At least

two other cases have been observed with microcephaly, intracranial calcification, and herpetic vesicles appearing on the first day of life. In one of these HSV type 1 was isolated from the cerebrospinal fluid and the urine (Florman et al., 1972). This patient also had inclusion-bearing cells in the urine sediment. There was no evidence of CMV infection. The other patient had cerebral calcifications (Fig. 5–4) similar to those reported by South et al. (1969) and Schaffer (1965). Komorous and co-workers (1977) have documented two more cases of transplacental herpes simplex infection, describing congenital anomalies of microcephaly, intrauterine growth retardation, encephalitis, chorioretinitis, psychomotor retardation, and skin vesicles.

Infection Acquired at Birth

Infection acquired during birth may have several manifestations (Fig. 5–5), such as a papulovesicular rash, episodes of cyanosis, a

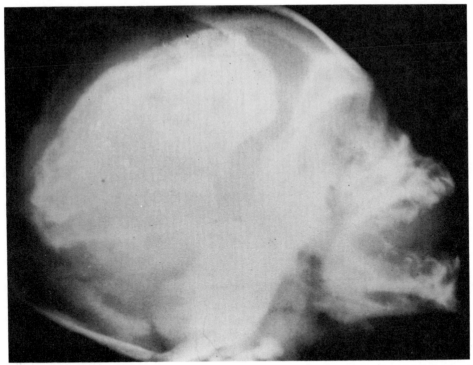

Figure 5–4. Intracranial calcifications on skull film of infant with intrauterine herpesvirus hominis infection. (Courtesy of Dr. Murray Kappleman.)

seizure, or bleeding from the gastrointestinal tract. Slightly more than half of the infants will have some surface manifestation of the disease, usually in the form of a vesicle or bullous skin lesion. These may appear anywhere on the skin, especially on the scalp in vertex presentations (see Frontispiece) and the perianal area in breech presentations (Hodgman et al., 1971). Conjunctivitis followed by keratitis may be the first abnormality noted. This may remain localized or, more commonly, may progress to systemic infection. The appearance of the first vesicle or cluster of vesicles is frequently not associated with evidence of generalized infection for the first few days. The vesicles break down and become encrusted. Occasionally they are secondarily infected with bacteria, which can lead to the mistaken impression that they are primarily bacterial lesions, such as neonatal impetigo. It is usually not until the skin lesions become associated with constitutional

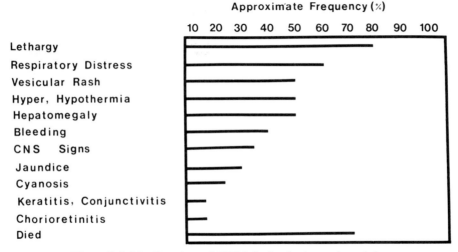

Figure 5–5. Manifestations of HSV infection in the newborn infant.

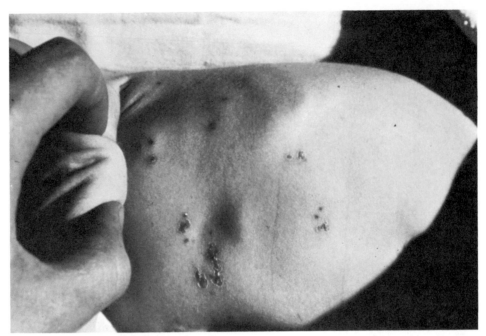

Figure 5–6. Case 1: Rash on trunk of infant with neonatal herpesvirus infection. (Courtesy of Dr. Robert R. Chilcote.)

symptoms of an ill-defined nature, such as fever, vomiting, failure to feed, irritability, and lethargy, that the physician considers the diagnosis of neonatal herpes simplex infection. These symptoms then lead to the manifestations of disseminated disease with a variety of possible clinical patterns, such as are presented in the following case summaries.

Seizures and a Rash

Case 1

This 14 day old infant was admitted to the hospital with a six-day history of vesicular rash on the trunk and a two-day history of "jittery movements" after having several frank seizures. Pregnancy and delivery were uneventful. The birth weight was 3620 gm. At the time the rash appeared it was thought to be bullous impetigo (Fig. 5–6) and was treated with antibiotics. On admission the infant has frequent seizures, and the Moro, suck, and grasp reflexes were absent. A spinal tap revealed 100 lymphocytes per cubic centimeter. The cerebrospinal fluid protein was 40 mg/100 ml, the glucose 60 mg/100 ml. HSV was recovered from a vesicle and the nasopharynx. The infant was placed on idoxuridine (IDU), 100 mg/kg/day for five days. In three days the patient was more alert, the seizures has stopped, and the skin lesions were drying. Within one week after the completion of the IDU therapy, the infant again became lethargic, the seizures recurred, and he displayed marked respiratory distress with pulmonary infiltrates. Repeat cerebrospinal fluid pro-

tein was 250 mg/100 ml with persistent pleocytosis. A second course of IDU at the same dosage level was administered, resulting in the return of normal respiration, alertness, and normal reflexes and in the cessation of seizures. At one year of age, however, the infant showed evidence of severe psychomotor retardation and was microcephalic.

Respiratory Distress

Case 2

This white male infant was admitted to the hospital at 10 days of age with a history of "turning blue and not eating." The patient weighed 3010 gm at birth. The pregnancy had been complicated during its first half by several bouts of "flu-like illness," a kidney infection, and "fever blisters" of the lip. The mother was well during the last trimester of pregnancy. The delivery was uncomplicated, and mother and child were discharged on the fourth day. From that day on, the infant did not feed well, and 12 hours prior to admission he began to have episodes of cyanosis, particularly around the lips and hands. No other symptoms were noted by the mother at the time of admission. On admission to the hospital the infant appeared acutely ill, with irregular respirations at 48 per minute and slight retractions. Examination of the skin revealed a 0.5-cm bullous lesion between the scapulae (Fig. 5–7) and a 1- × 1-cm, slightly erythematous and edematous lesion of the right parietal-occipital area of the scalp. The liver was noted to extend 2½ cm below the right costal margin, and a neurological examination revealed a poor sucking reflex and a fair grasp reflex. The

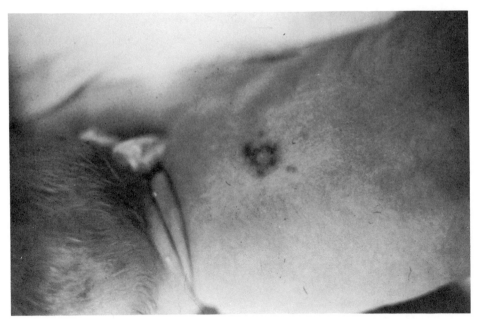

Figure 5–7. Case 2: Cluster of lesions on back of infant with neonatal herpesvirus infection. (Courtesy of Dr. Robert R. Chilcote.)

Moro reflex was normal. A roentgenogram of the chest revealed diffuse, fluffy infiltrates bilaterally (Fig. 5–8). On the second hospital day the skin lesions were cultured for virus and examined histopathologically. Both procedures confirmed the clinical impression of herpes simplex infection, and IDU therapy was instituted at a dosage of 80 mg/kg/day for the first day, followed by four more days at a dosage of 50 mg/kg/day. The patient continued to do poorly during the therapy but did not worsen. Thrombocytopenia, with a platelet count of 10,000, developed on the fifth day of therapy. On the day following the completion of IDU therapy the patient was more alert. His pulmonary status improved gradually, but he was subject to recurrent respiratory infections characterized by coughing spells and a persistent infiltrate involving both the right and left lobes of the lung. At 20 weeks of age the vesicle reappeared in the area of the back between the scapulae. Although herpesvirus hominis was recovered from the respiratory tract at 11 days of age and again at 36 days of age, virus was not recovered from the throat 20 weeks after birth. His development during the first year of life has been slow.

Bleeding

Case 3

This 10 day old white male was admitted to the hospital because of hematemesis and bleeding from the umbilicus and the penis. The birth weight was 3900 gm. The pregnancy had been uneventful. He was circumcised without incident. Six hours before admission hematemesis and loose, nonbloody stools were noted, followed shortly thereafter by bleeding from the umbilicus and the penis. A few petechiae were noted on the scalp, and flat, reddish, pustular lesions were observed on the trunk, right axilla, and lower extremities. Two ulcerations were seen on the upper lip. The liver extended 5 cm below the right costal margin. Coagulation studies revealed prolonged partial thromboplastin time, prothrombin time, and thrombin time, absent fibrinogen, and increased fibrin degradation products. Despite therapy with intravenous fluids, phytonadione (AquaMEPHYTON), kanamycin, methicillin, fresh citrated blood, and fresh-frozen plasma, the infant became cyanotic, had a cardiac arrest, and died 11 hours after admission. Postmortem examination revealed vacuolar nuclear degeneration and nuclear inclusions in the liver, lungs, adrenals, kidneys, spleen, and gastrointestinal tract. Occasional fibrin deposits were noted in the thymus, lungs, liver, and gastrointestinal tract, suggesting disseminated intravascular coagulation. HSV was isolated from the liver.

Although the presenting complaints in these patients are quite different—seizures and a rash, respiratory distress with cyanosis, and bleeding—they do share some common features. The three infants were all very seriously ill by the time they were hospitalized. All had skin lesions, but in only one instance was the rash noted before systemic symptoms developed. The progression of the disease was rapid, with one infant dying on the first hospital day. None of the mothers

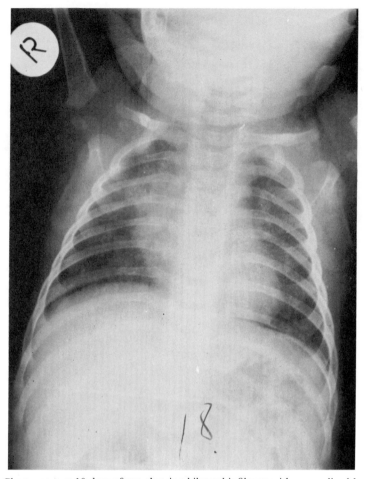

Figure 5–8. Case 2: Chest x-rays at 10 days of age showing bilateral infiltrate with generalized herpesvirus infection.

had genital herpes, although one mother was said to have had "fever blisters" of the lip in early pregnancy.

Central Nervous System Manifestations. In HSV infections of the newborn, involvement of the central nervous system is often the dominant clinical feature or is part of a multisystem disease. As in Case 1, this usually presents with frank seizures with a bulging fontanelle and opisthotonos—evidence of increased intracranial pressure. These signs frequently progress rapidly to nearly continuous seizure activity—which is difficult to control with anticonvulsant therapy—and eventual coma. HSV is occasionally present in the cerebrospinal fluid of the neonate with herpes encephalitis but rarely in that of older persons with the same disease. This may be related to the increased permeability of the central nervous system to infectious agents during the neonatal period. The cerebrospinal fluid protein is usually elevated by the time symptoms of encephalitis become man-

ifest, but this is not invariably so. Similarly, the pleocytosis characteristic of most types of viral encephalitis may not be present on first examination of the spinal fluid. This is true of herpes encephalitis in older persons as well. The predominant cell is mononuclear. It is unusual to have a total cerebrospinal fluid cell count in excess of 400 per cubic millimeter.

On the electroencephalogram, repetitive complexes are seen but are not specific, since they may be observed in anoxia and other forms of encephalitis (Pettay et al., 1972).

Hepatoadrenal Necrosis. In 1935 Hass described the first case of disseminated herpetic infection in the newborn and called attention to the high susceptibility of the liver and the adrenals to the effects of the virus. The involvement of the liver is characterized by grossly visible areas of focal necrosis like those shown in Figure 5–2. In some instances, the degree of liver parenchymal involvement may be extreme, with little functioning liver tissue. Miller and co-workers (1970) have presented evidence indicating that HSV can be the inciting agent for the development of disseminated intravascular coagulation. Although fibrinogen is synthesized entirely in the liver, it is not clear whether extensive liver destruction is a prerequisite for the development of intravascular coagulation. The possible mechanisms involved are shown in Figure 5–9.

The liver is affected in almost all fatal cases of neonatal herpes simplex infection, although not all such infants are jaundiced during life. When hyperbilirubinemia does occur, it is likely to be associated with a rise in the direct as well as the indirect bilirubin. The elevation of the direct component may not become manifest until the icterus has been present for 24 hours or more. Nahmias (1970b) found that only 10 of 148 patients with neonatal herpes had both hepatomegaly and jaundice and that 30 per cent of these patients had neither of these two manifestations of liver involvement. Splenomegaly is less common than hepatomegaly, but it was noted in 22 of 43 patients with disseminated herpes simplex reviewed by Overall and Glasgow (1970b). In their series of patients with disseminated disease, jaundice was present in 13 of 43 subjects.

Eye Involvement. The eye is occasionally the primary site of involvement for herpetic infection in the neonate; this is less frequently so in the adult. The eye may be the portal of entry, with infection remaining localized there or progressing to the central nervous system. It is interesting that the first case of neonatal herpetic infection recorded in the literature was that of a patient with localized keratoconjunctivitis, a relatively unusual form of the disease (Batignani, 1934). Herpes simplex has been associated with chorioretinitis, retinal dysplasia, conjunctivitis, and keratitis. Patients have been described who had relatively benign herpetic infections in the newborn period followed by chorioretinitis with significant visual impairment (Hagler et al., 1969). This observation may have considerable significance and suggests the need for further studies of the relationship between herpes simplex type 2 infections and chorioretinitis in childhood. At present many, perhaps most, patients with chorioretinitis remain undiagnosed. They do not have antibody titers to Toxoplasma, CMV, Histoplasma, or Brucella. The relative rarity of herpes simplex type 2 antibody in persons under the age of 14 suggests that a study to determine the prevalence of specific type 2–IgM antibody in patients with undiagnosed chorioretinitis might be of interest.

DIAGNOSIS

The diagnosis of neonatal herpes infection can be made in some instances by the clinician alone. More often, the assistance of the virologist or the pathologist is required for confirmation of the clinical impression.

Clinical

If an infant manifests typical vesicular lesions of the skin in the first week of life, it

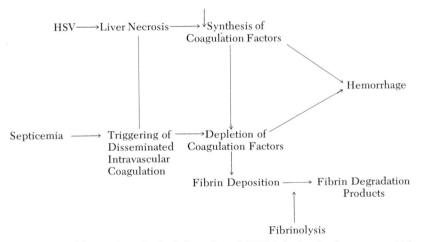

Figure 5–9. Pathogenesis of hemorrhage in fatal disseminated HSV infection in the neonate. (After Miller et al.: Fatal disseminated herpes simplex virus infection and hemorrhage in the neonate. J. Pediatr. 76:409–417, 1970.)

may be possible to diagnose a neonatal HSV infection on the basis of the appearance of the lesions alone. Such was the case for the patient shown in Figure 5–7. The presence of herpetic lesions or a history of such lesions in the mother greatly strengthens the clinical diagnosis. The location of the skin vesicles is varied; the tendency to cluster is typical but inconstant. Approximately half of the infants in whom disseminated infection develops do not have vesicles in the early stages of their disease. Arvin and co-workers (1982) reported several infants lacking mucocutaneous lesions with disseminated HSV infection who demonstrated lethargy, poor feeding, apnea, acidosis, and hepatomegaly, all of which are signs of bacterial sepsis. Eight cases of neonatal HSV encephalitis, without lesions of the skin, eyes, or mucous membranes, were also documented. Arvin et al. have suggested that neonatal HSV encephalitis in the absence of lesions may be distinguished from enteroviral infections by the frequent presence of high fever in the latter and focal, often intractable seizures in the former. Nahmias (1970b) found external herpetic lesions—that is, lesions of the skin, eye, and oral cavity—in 80 of 148 (54 per cent) patients they reviewed. The diagnosis can be confirmed by the laboratory within a few hours by histopathological examination of the cells scraped from the base of the local lesion and usually within 24 to 48 hours by isolation of HSV in tissue culture. It is becoming increasing apparent that early diagnosis and therapy are of critical importance for the outcome of the disease.

Histopathological

HSV and varicella-zoster virus are rarely distinguishable from one another with certainty on the basis of their histopathological appearances. A diagnosis of the latter, however, can usually be dismissed on epidemiological grounds. In order for the newborn infant to have varicella in the first days of life, the mother must have had varicella or herpes zoster during pregnancy. Thus, in the absence of such a history, it can be presumed that intranuclear inclusions, margination of the nuclear chromatin, "ballooning" degeneration, and multinucleated cells that are found in smears made from vesicles from the infant or from the mother's genital area are caused by HSV. CMV infection has not been

known to produce vesicles, although both rubella and CMV have been associated with generalized hemorrhagic-purpuric eruption, termed "dermal erythropoiesis" by Brough and colleagues (1967).

The cells for histopathological examination should be taken from the base of the vesicles and also from the mother's cervix, even when the tissue appears normal. The slides may be stained with a variety of methods, including Papanicolaou, Giemsa, and hematoxylineosin stain and eosin stains. The Papanicolaou method is especially satisfactory for identifying inclusion-bearing cells of the cervical mucosa (Fig. 5–10).

Characteristically, the HSV vesicle is in the prickle cell layer and does not involve the corium of the skin. At the edge of the vesicle, ballooning degeneration may be observed, with many cells bearing nuclear inclusions. Unlike CMV-infected cells, which are larger, cytoplasmic eosinophilic inclusions have not been associated with HSV-infected cells. The vesicle fluid itself is composed of a mixture of epidermal cells, leukocytes, and multinucleated giant cells suspended in fibrinous fluid. The base of the vesicle consists of the naked papillae of the corium.

The histopathological changes of the brain in patients with herpetic encephalitis have been described by Wolf and Cowen (1959) and Hughes (1969). MacCallum and co-workers (1964) have found the early use of brain biopsy of value in the diagnosis of herpetic encephalitis in adult patients. The justification for the procedure rests primarily in the expectation that the early administration of an antiviral drug may be life-saving. There has been less use of brain biopsy in patients with the neonatal form of the disease because of the greater morbidity expected in the very young from a procedure of this type and also because a larger percentage of neonates than adults present with a recognizable form of the disease.

In an infant who is examined post mortem, there is usually no difficulty in establishing the fact that HSV infection, or some complication thereof, was the cause of death. As noted, however, in a given specimen of infected tissue there may be few or no inclusions present. This is true even of the liver, which is so characteristically involved with microscopic and gross areas of focal necrosis. Such tissue, when inoculated into tissue culture, may yield HSV. This must be kept in mind if liver biopsy is performed during life

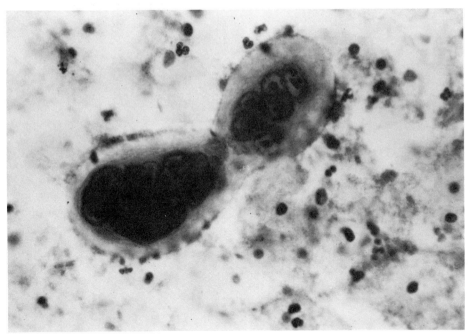

Figure 5–10. Papanicolaou smear of herpetic cervicitis showing cluster of nuclear inclusion–bearing cells. (Courtesy of Dr. Marvin S. Amstey.)

in an effort to establish a diagnosis in an infant without the typical external lesions. The recovery of virus in the absence of inclusions has also been noted in CMV infection (Weller and Hanshaw, 1962) and in adult patients who have undergone brain biopsy for suspected HSV encephalitis (Nolan et al., 1970).

A direct fluorescent antibody test described originally by Biegeleisen and colleagues (1959) and later by Gardner and colleagues (1968) has been applied successfully in the histopathological diagnosis of corneal and skin smears and biopsy material. The test can be performed quickly. The essential reagents needed are conjugated antibodies to HSV types 1 and 2 produced in rabbits.

Serological. There are several methods for measuring antibody. These include the indirect fluorescent antibody, complement-fixation, indirect hemagglutination-inhibition, and neutralization tests. None of these tests is valuable in the early diagnosis of neonatal HSV disease. The measurement of specific IgM antibody (Nahmias et al., 1969b)—which is done by an immunofluorescent assay that is often unreliable—is of limited usefulness in this condition because infection is usually acquired at the time of birth, and the progression of the disease is often so rapid that antibody is not present when the infant pre-

sents with fulminating disease. It may be two to eight weeks before neutralizing or complement-fixing antibody becomes detectable in the infant's serum. The interpretation of specific antibody to type 1 or type 2 virus is dependent upon the antibodies that may have been acquired from the mother and the length of time the antibodies persist in the infant's serum. Type 2 antibodies can be differentiated by neutralization tests (Rawls et al., 1970) and microindirect hemagglutination tests (Fuccillo et al., 1970). Gallo and co-workers (1981) have investigated a microimmunofluorescent test that provides a quick indication of IgM antibodies to agents capable of causing congenital disease, including CMV, rubella virus, and HSV.

Virological. HSV is one of the most readily cultivated viruses. It produces typical cytopathic changes within 24 to 48 hours after inoculation of cultures (Fig. 5–11). Many tissue culture systems are suitable for isolation, including WI-38 cells, primary rabbit kidney cells, chick embryo tissue, HeLa cells, and primary amnion cells. The best source of virus is usually a vesicle, preferably prior to rupture. Other sites include ulcerative lesions, conjunctiva, cornea, throat, or nasopharynx. Occasionally the virus is isolated from the blood, cerebrospinal fluid, feces, or urine. Virus strains can be typed by a neu-

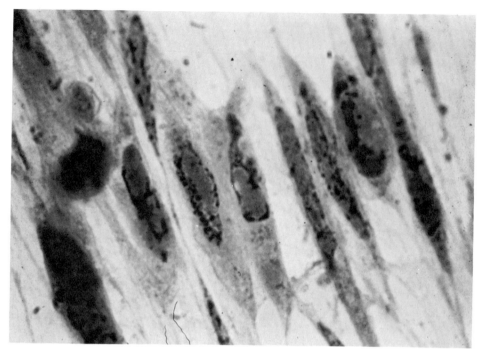

Figure 5–11. Hematoxylin and eosin stain of HSV-infected WI-38 cells showing beading of nuclear chromatin and intranuclear inclusion formation.

tralization test described by Plummer (1964) or by a direct immunofluorescent technique reported by Nahmias and colleagues (1969b).

Electron Microscopic. Electron microscopy is receiving increasing attention from clinical microbiologists as a feasible technique in the diagnosis of herpetic and other viral infections. As in varicella-zoster, the vesicular fluid of HSV lesions is a rich source of identifiable herpesvirus particles. Smith and Melnick (1962), Harland and co-workers (1967), and Rose and Becker (1972) have described techniques for the recognition of herpesvirus particles in human vesicular lesions and in acute necrotizing encephalitis. (See the chapter on Laboratory Diagnosis.)

Cytological. Kobayashi and colleagues (1982) have documented the first non-necropsy cytological detection of HSV infection in a neonate and have suggested that cytological studies be made in suspected cases to allow early treatment with antiviral agents.

MANAGEMENT

Prevention by Cesarean Section

For the woman who is subject to recurrent herpetic lesions of the genitalia, a question arises concerning the risk of the infection to the newborn infant. On the basis of present epidemiological data, the risk of *intrauterine* infection is too small to be considered a serious deterrent to pregnancy, but the risk of exposure of the infant during the second stage of labor is sufficiently real for determination of the presence of HSV in the female genital tract in the last six weeks of gestation to be recommended. Brunell (1980) has noted that since premature labor often occurs in women with congenital herpes infection, viral testing should begin sufficiently early in the pregnancy to allow an informed decision concerning delivery route. If virus is present, even though inapparent clinically, a cesarean section should be considered. If there are actual lesions present, primary or recurrent, most authorities would recommend avoiding exposure of the infant to HSV during vaginal delivery. Although it has been claimed that recurrent maternal infection poses less of a risk to the newborn than does primary infection, the difficulty in clinically distinguishing the two, the high frequency of asymptomatic infection, and the uncertainty in estimating the acquisition of maternal antibodies in cases of recurrent infection make the thesis useless for clinical purposes (Nahmias et al., 1977; Kibrick,

1980). In contrast to a study by Yeager and co-workers (1980) indicating that complete neutralization of the virus may be effected by maternal antibody, Whitley and colleagues (1980a) found no correlation between the presence of maternally acquired antibodies and the severity of neonatal HSV infection. Amstey and co-workers (1979) have pointed out that transplacentally acquired antibodies often do not prevent neonatal herpes of the skin, mouth, eyes, or central nervous system. A workshop at the National Institute of Allergy and Infectious Diseases concurred with these latter views in studying the feasibility of a herpes vaccine (Allen and Rapp, 1982).

If the membranes have already been ruptured for up to four to six hours, the expectation that cesarean section will achieve anything useful is unwarranted. Similarly, Kibrick's study considers cesarean section unlikely to prevent neonatal infection if HSV is found in the amniotic fluid (although Zervoudakis et al. [1980] reported such a case with a healthy and apparently uninfected infant). Nahmias and co-workers (1975) compared the cases of 19 infants delivered by cesarean section four or more hours after membrane rupture with those of 28 infants similarly delivered before or within four hours of rupture. While 18 of the 19 became infected, only two of the 28 did. Firm data on the question of membrane status are not available, however, and one study recommends cesarean section for all mothers with genital HSV infection at labor regardless of time elapsed since membrane rupture (Grossman et al., 1981).

It is recommended that cesarean section be performed prior to rupture of the membranes in any pregnancy in which HSV infection is known to have occurred in the last month. This should be done unless membrane rupture has occurred four hours prior to surgery. If herpetic penile lesions are present in the father, the mother's cervix and vaginal secretions should be cultured in the last month of gestation even if there are no symptoms of infection. Delivery plans for each pregnancy should be based on several factors, including membrane status, gestational age, and risks of HSV infection and cesarean section (American Academy of Pediatrics Committees on Fetus and Newborn and Infectious Diseases, 1980). Table 5–1 gives a breakdown of management strategies in 10 situations associated with HSV infection.

Immunoglobulin

Recommendations concerning the administration of isoimmune globulin have been varied. The results following its administration have been generally unrewarding. Certainly, it can be stated that its efficacy has not been demonstrated. It is possible that this may be a function of the variable potency of type 2 HSV antibody in the various preparations administered. It is more probable, however, that humoral antibody is not sufficiently protective. The route of administration, the time at which the antibody is given, whether the antibody is administered to the mother before delivery, and the amount given are possible variables that could conceivably affect the outcome of the infection in the infant. In spite of the almost uniformly poor results to date, some investigators recommend that large doses of commercial isoimmune globulin (20 to 40 ml) be given to the infant at birth because of the possibility that this might prevent dissemination of virus (Nahmias, 1970b). Once dissemination has occurred, there is little justification for the use of isoimmune globulin.

Antiviral Drugs

Idoxuridine (IDU) and cytosine arabinoside are no longer used in the treatment of disseminated neonatal HSV infection. They have been superseded by adenine arabinoside (ara-A, vidarabine) and the experimental drug acyclovir.

Acyclovir, or 9-[(2-hydroxyethoxy)methyl] guanine, is an acyclic analogue of the nucleoside guanine. Phosphorylation by viral thymidine kinase (an enzyme not found in uninfected cells) and other kinases produces acycloguanosine triphosphate, which preferentially inhibits the specific viral DNA polymerase and is used as a template that terminates the viral DNA chain.

Effective antiherpesvirus action by acyclovir has recently been documented in several studies. Saral and co-workers (1981) have reported acyclovir to be efficacious in preventing reactivated HSV infection in bone marrow transplant patients. Mindel and colleagues (1981) showed that intravenous acyclovir reduced healing time, duration of vesicles, new lesion formation, viral shedding, and other symptoms in patients with primary genital herpes, whereas Corey (1982) found

Table 5–1. RECOMMENDATIONS FOR CESAREAN SECTION AT TERM IN WOMEN WITH PRIOR OR CONCURRENT HERPES

Genital Herpetic Lesions Present at Term	Group	Primary Genital Lesions	Recurrent Genital Lesions (or Genital Reinfection)	Status of Membranes*	Recommended Route of Delivery†	Isolation of Mother	Isolation of Newborn
Yes	1	+		Intact or ruptured < 4–6 hr	Cesarean section	Yes	Yes
	2	+		Ruptured > 4–6 hr	Per vaginam	Yes	Yes
	3	+	or +	Baby has been delivered per vaginam		Yes	Yes
	4		+	Intact or ruptured < 4–6 hr	Cesarean section	Yes	Yes
	5		+	Ruptured > 4–6 hr	Per vaginam	Yes	Yes
No, but cervicovaginal culture or cytology is positive for herpes	6			Intact or ruptured < 4–6 hr	Cesarean section	Yes	Yes
	7			Ruptured > 4–6 hr	Per vaginam	Yes	Yes
No, but there is past history of genital herpes, presently inactive or status unknown	8			Intact or ruptured	Per vaginam	No	No
No, but nongenital herpes is present at term	9			Intact or ruptured	Per vaginam	Yes	No at birth (yes, after newborn goes out to mother)
No, but there is past history of nongenital herpes	10			Intact or ruptured	Per vaginam	No	No

*The shorter the interval between rupture of the membranes and cesarean section, the less the risk of fetal infection. The critical period appears to be four to six hours.

†Dependent on evaluation of individual risks and benefits.

From Kibrick, S.: Herpes simplex infection at term. J.A.M.A. 243:157–160, 1980.

that topical acyclovir shortened healing time and duration of viral shedding in a similarly infected group. Spruance and co-workers (1982) reported that treatment of recurrent herpes simplex labialis with topical acyclovir led to a decrease in median titers of virus, although no clinical benefit was seen. The danger of virus strains developing resistance to acyclovir, via a loss of viral thymidine kinase activity or a change in viral DNA polymerase, has resulted in several authors recommending caution in the drug's large-scale use (Burns et al., 1982; Crumpacker et al., 1982; Field and Wildy, 1982).

Owing to the experimental nature of the drug, few data exist concerning its effectiveness against neonatal HSV infection. One study by Yeager (1982) showed encouraging results and lack of drug toxicity to neonates, and one premature infant with HSV infection showed marked improvement when vidarabine was replaced with intravenous acyclovir in the treatment regimen (Offit et al., 1982). Hintz (1982) indicated that neonatal acyclovir pharmacokinetics is analogous to that found in adults. The proceedings of an extensive symposium on acyclovir have been published (Acyclovir Symposium, 1982).

Adenine arabinoside, or vidarabine, is an analogue of the nucleosides adenine and deoxyadenosine and also exerts its antiviral effect by inhibiting viral DNA polymerase and other specific enzymes. It lacks the preferential reaction with thymidine kinase, however, that makes acyclovir such a highly selective drug.

Whitley and co-workers (1977) found vidarabine to reduce mortality significantly in cases of herpes simplex encephalitis, and in 1981 they provided further evidence that brain biopsies are warranted for early diagnosis and treatment of the disease in adults. A controlled study of neonatal HSV infection by Whitley et al. (1980b) also showed a reduction in mortality with vidarabine therapy. Among infants with localized central nervous system disease, mortality ranged from 10 per cent in those given drug treatment to 50 per cent in those given placebos. Disseminated disease mortality was reduced from 74 per cent to 38 per cent, regardless of gestational age.

Interferon Inducers

Catalano and Baron (1970) have demonstrated a protective effect of the double-stranded RNA, polyinosinic-cytidilic, in HSV infection. A report using the same interferon inducer in a young male infant with herpetic encephalitis resulted in uncertain clinical benefit (Catalano et al., 1971). In contrast to previous findings in animals, high levels of interferon were produced in the serum and the cerebrospinal fluid. The drug showed mild toxicity after 11 days of therapy, with elevation of the blood urea nitrogen, serum glutamic pyruvic transaminase, lactic dehydrogenase, and alkaline phosphatase. Myers and co-workers have suggested that interferon may help increase killer cell response, which is usually low in neonates, as well as having an anitviral effect itself. It is conceivable that the interferon inducers may be of some therapeutic use in the future—perhaps more in anticipation of disease than as therapeutic agents. This possibility is far from a clinical reality at this time, however.

General Measures

Once skin lesions appear and disseminated infection has taken place, there is an increased risk of bacterial sepsis, particularly with gram-negative infections and hemolytic *Staphylococcus aureus*. Thus, blood cultures should be taken and antibacterial therapy given. Steroid therapy has been shown to be ineffective and probably harmful in experiments carried out in animals by Nahmias (1970b).

Evidence has accumulated that heparin is indicated in the treatment of acute disseminated intravascular coagulation. The rationale for the use of heparin is that it blocks consumption of coagulation factors. The use of heparin presupposes that adequate amounts of coagulation factors are being synthesized by the liver and other tissues. In HSV infection of the neonate with extensive liver involvement, synthesis of clotting factors may be abnormally depressed. Therefore, replacement therapy with heparinized whole blood, fibrinogen, and fresh plasma is necessary when heparin is used (Miller et al., 1970).

As in all severely ill infants, monitoring of electrolyte levels is essential. Seizures are often difficult to control. Phenobarbital, paraldehyde, phenytoin (Dilantin), and diazepam (Valium) have all been employed with variable success. In patients with severe liver disease, phenobarbital is contraindicated.

The possibility of nosocomial HSV infection has led several authors to recommend separation of personnel with active and exposed lesions from newborns (Light, 1979; Kibrick, 1980; Valenti et al., 1980).

Recommendations for the management of mother and child were made in 1980 by committees of the American Academy of Pediatrics. Proper hand-washing and covering of active lesions by the mother upon handling the infant are strongly recommended; breast-feeding has not been conclusively implicated as a route of infection. If vaginal delivery occurs in a woman with genital HSV infection, it should be followed by isolation and viral, liver function, and cerebrospinal fluid studies of the infant. One can make a strong case for starting antiviral therapy at birth. If a cesarean section before membrane rupture is performed as recommended, isolation and weekly observation of the infant should follow. The probability of neonatal disease is less than 10 per cent (Nahmias et al., 1975). Detailed recommendations for the management of mother and newborn have been suggested by Kibrick (1980) and are summarized in Table 5–1.

The guidelines for nursery personnel with exposed active lesions, such as herpetic whitlow or "cold sores," are ambiguous and confusing. Valenti and co-workers (1980) have recommended that such personnel should not work with newborn infants (term or preterm). The American Academy of Pediatrics Committee on Infectious Diseases (1980) states: "Compromising patient care by excluding personnel with 'cold sores' who are essential for the operation of the unit must be weighed against the potential risk of infecting newborn infants." Needless to say, nursery staff with "cold sores" should not kiss newborn babies. This is a good rule for all nursery personnel because of the relatively high percentage of asymptomatic individuals (5 to 10 per cent) shedding HSV into the oral cavity.

It is recommended that personnel with "cold sores" not work with newborn infants.

PROGNOSIS

The prognosis for herpetic infection is largely dependent upon whether the infection is disseminated and whether central nervous system involvement is present (Table 5–2). Although the immediate outlook may be better when disease is limited to the central nervous system than when it is present in disseminated form in one or more viscera, the long-term prognosis is poor. Of 25 such patients reported by Nahmias and co-workers (1967b), 11 died, and of the 14 survivors only two were without sequelae. The prognosis for life in patients with localized disease of the skin, eye, or oral cavity is more favorable. All of 29 such patients studied by Nahmias et al. (1967b) survived. Eleven of these patients, however, had neurological sequelae. Thus, one should be cautious in making long-term predictions of normal intellectual development in any child with any form of symptomatic herpesvirus infection in the newborn period. Little is known at the present time of the implications of asymptomatic infection, since few patients have been reported to date. It may be shown eventually that, as in congenital rubella and CMV infection, subtle but definite neurological sequelae occur even in asymptomatic patients when the period of observation is extended over several years. HSV is almost certainly capable of reaching the developing central nervous system in the critical first trimester without causing the death of the fetus. This event could have more importance in the causation of certain forms of brain damage than is now recognized.

Table 5–2. **MANIFESTATIONS AND PROGNOSES IN 169 CASES OF HSV INFECTION IN NEWBORNS**

Type of Infection	No. of Cases	No. of Deaths	Survivors with Sequelae	Survivors without Sequelae
Generalized disease	138	114	19	5
Localized disease				
Skin	20	0	8	12
Eye	7	0	3	4
Oral cavity	2	0	0	2
Asymptomatic	2	0	0	2
Total	169	114 (67%)	30 (18%)	25 (15%)

Bibliography

Acyclovir Symposium Am. J. Med. *73*:1–392, 1982.

Allen, W. P., and Rapp, F.: Concept review of genital herpes vaccines. J. Infect. Dis. *145*:413–421, 1982.

Amstey, M. S., Monif, G. R. G., Nahmias, A. J., and Josey, W. E.: Cesarean section and genital herpesvirus infection. Editorial. Obstet. Gynecol. *53*:641–642, 1979.

Arvin, A. M., Yeager, A. S., Bruhn, F. W., and Grossman, M.: Neonatal herpes simplex infection in the absence of mucocutaneous lesions. J. Pediatr. *100*:715–721, 1981.

Ashwal, S., Finegold, M., Fish, I., and Brunell, P.: Effect of the antiviral drug cytosine arabinoside on the developing central nervous system. Pediatr. Res. *8*:945–950, 1974.

Batignani, A.: Congiunctivite da virus erpetico in neonata. Boll. Ocul. (Bologna) *13*:1217–1220, 1934.

Bell, W. R., Whang, J. J., Carbone, P. P., Brecher, G., and Block, J. B.: Cytogenetic and morphologic abnormalities in human bone marrow cells during cytosine arabinoside therapy. Blood *27*:771–781, 1966.

Bettoli, E. J., Brewer, P. M., Oxtoby, M. J., Zaidi, A. A., and Guinan, M. E.: The role of temperature and swab materials in the recovery of herpes simplex virus from lesions. J. Infect. Dis. *145*:399, 1982.

Biegeleisen, J. Z., Jr., Scott, L. V., and Lewis, V., Jr.: Rapid diagnosis of herpes simplex virus infections with fluorescent antibody. Science *129*:640–641, 1959.

Boué, A., and Loffredo, V.: Avortement causé par le virus de l'herpes type II. Isolement du virus à partir de cultures de tissues zygotiques. Presse Med. *78*:103–106, 1970.

Brough, A. J., Jones, D., Page, R. H., and Mizukami, I.: Dermal erythropoiesis in neonatal infants. A manifestation of intrauterine viral disease. Pediatrics *40*:627–635, 1967.

Brunell, P. A.: Prevention and treatment of neonatal herpes. Pediatrics *66*:806–808, 1980.

Burke, P. J., Serpick, A. A., Carbone, P. P., and Tarr, N.: A clinical evaluation of dose and schedule of administration of cytosine arabinoside. Cancer Res. *28*:274–279, 1968.

Burns, W. H., Saral, R., Santos, G. W., Laskin, O. L., Lietman, P. S., McLaren, C., and Barry, D. W.: Isolation and characterisation of resistant herpes simplex virus after acyclovir therapy. Lancet *1*:421–423, 1982.

Catalano, L. W., Jr., and Baron, S.: Protection against herpes virus and encephalomyocarditis virus encephalitis with a double-stranded RNA inducer of interferon. Proc. Soc. Exp. Biol. Med. *133*:684–687, 1970.

Catalano, L. W., Jr., Safley, G. H., Muscles, M., and Harzynski, D. J.: Disseminated herpesvirus infection in a newborn infant. J. Pediatr. *79*:383–400, 1971.

Ch'ien, L. T., Cannon, N. J., Charmella, L. J., Dismukes, W. E., Whitley, R. J., Buchanan, R. A., and Alford, C. A., Jr.: Effect of adenine arabinoside in severe Herpesvirus hominis infections in man. J. Infect. Dis. *128*:658–663, 1973.

Committees on Fetus and Newborn and Infectious Diseases of the American Academy of Pediatrics: Perinatal herpes simplex virus infections. Pediatrics *66*:147–149, 1980.

Corey, L., Nahmias, A. J., Guinan, M. E., Benedetti, J. K., Critchlow, C. W., and Holmes, K. K.: A trial of topical acyclovir in genital herpes simplex virus infections. N. Engl. J. Med. *306*:1313–1319, 1982.

Crumpacker, C. S., Schnipper, L. E., Marlowe, S. I., Kowalsky, P. N., Hershey, B. J., and Levin, M. J.: Resistance to antiviral drugs of herpes simplex virus isolated from a patient treated with acyclovir. N. Engl. J. Med. *306*:343–346, 1982.

Dini, M., Alrenga, O. P., and Freese, U.: Perinatal herpes virus infection: report of a case indicating the paternal role. J. Natl. Med. Assoc. *72*:1193–1196, 1980.

Field, M. J., and Wildy, P.: Clinical resistance of herpes simplex virus to acyclovir (letter). Lancet *1*:1125, 1982.

Florman, A. L., et al.: Intrauterine infection with herpes simplex virus. Resultant congenital malformations (abstract). Pediatr. Res. *442*:162, 1972.

Fuccillo, D. A., Moder, F. L., Catalano, L. W., Jr., Monroe, M. V., and Sever, J. L.: Herpesvirus hominis types I and II: a specific microindirect hemagglutination test. Proc. Soc. Exp. Biol. Med. *133*:735–739, 1970.

Gagnon, A.: Transplacental inoculation of fatal herpes simplex in the newborn. Obstet. Gynecol. *31*:682, 1968.

Gallo, O., Riggs, J. L., Schacter, J., and Emmons, R. W.: Multiple-antigen slide test for detection of immunoglobulin M antibodies in newborn and infant sera by immunofluorescence. J. Clin. Microbiol. *13*:631–636, 1981.

Hagler, W. S., Walters, P. V., and Nahmias, A. J.: Ocular involvement in neonatal herpes simplex virus infection. Arch. Ophthalmol. (Chicago) *82*:169–176, 1969.

Halperin, S. A., Hendley, J. O., Nosal, C., and Roizman, B.: DNA fingerprinting in investigation of apparent nosocomial acquisition of neonatal herpes simplex. J. Pediatr. *97*:91–93, 1980.

Hanshaw, J. B.: Idoxuridine in herpesvirus encephalitis. Editorial. N. Engl. J. Med. *282*:47, 1970.

Hanshaw, J. B.: Herpesvirus hominis infections of the fetus and the newborn. Am. J. Dis. Child. *126*:546–557, 1973.

Harland, W. A., Adams, T. H., and McSeveney, D.: Herpes-simplex particles in acute necrotising encephalitis. Lancet *2*:581–582, 1967.

Hass, G. M.: Hepato-adrenal necrosis with intranuclear inclusion bodies: report of a case. Am. J. Pathol. *11*:127–142, 1935.

Hintz, M., Connor, J. O., Spector, S. A., Blum, M. R., Keeney, R. E., and Yeager, A. S.: Neonatal acyclovir pharmacokinetics in patients with herpes virus infections. Acyclovir Symposium. Am. J. Med. *73*:210–214, 1982.

Hirsch, M. S., Zisman, B., and Allison, A.: Macrophages and age-dependent resistance to herpes simplex virus in mice. J. Immunol. *104*:1160–1165, 1971.

Hodgman, J. E., Freedman, R. I., and Levan, N. E.: Neonatal dermatology. Pediatr. Clin. North Am. *18*:713–756, 1971.

Hughes, J. T.: Pathology of herpes simplex encephalitis. In Whittier, C. W., Hughes, J. T., and MacCallum, F. O. (eds.): Virus Diseases of the Central Nervous System. Oxford, Blackwell Scientific Publications, 1969, p. 29.

Jordan, J., and Rytel, M. W.: Detection of herpes simplex virus (HSV) type 1 I_gG and I_gM antibodies by enzyme-linked immunosorbent assay (ELISA). Am. J. Clin. Pathol. *76*:467–471, 1981.

Kalinyak, J. E., Fleagle, G., and Docherty, J. J.: Incidence and distribution of herpes simplex virus types 1 and 2 from genital lesions in college women. J. Med. Virol. *1*:175–181, 1977.

Karchmer, A. W., and Hirsch, M. S.: Cytosine arabinoside versus virus or man? Editorial. N. Engl. J. Med. *289*:912–913, 1973.

Katz, M., Greco, M. A., Antony, L., and Young, B. K.:

Neonatal herpesvirus sepsis following internal monitoring. Int. J. Gynaecol. Obstet. *17*:631–633, 1980.

Kibrick, S.: Herpes simplex infection at term. J.A.M.A. *243*:157–160, 1980.

Kobayashi, T. K., Umezawa, Y., Uemura, M., Kurosaka, F., Matsunaga, Y., Tanaka, B., and Chiba, S.: Cytodiagnosis of herpes simplex virus infection in the newborn infant. Acta Cytol. *26*:65–68, 1982.

Komorous, J. M., Wheeler, C. E., Briggaman, R. A., and Caro, I.: Intrauterine herpes simplex infections. Arch. Dermatol. *113*:918–922, 1977.

Lerner, A. M.: Acyclovir reaches clinical trial. Editorial. Ann. Intern. Med. *96*:370–372, 1982.

Light, I. J.: Postnatal acquisition of herpes simplex virus by the newborn infant: a review of the literature. Pediatrics *63*:480–482, 1979.

Linnemann, C. C., Jr., Buckmann, T. G., Light, I. J., Ballard, J. L., and Roizman, B.: Transmission of herpes simplex type 1 in a nursery for the newborn: identification of viral isolates by DNA "fingerprinting." Lancet *1*:964–966, 1978.

MacCallum, F. O., Potter, J. M., and Edwards, D. H.: Early diagnosis of herpes-simplex encephalitis by brain biopsy. Lancet *2*:332–334, 1964.

Miller, D. R., Hanshaw, J. B., O'Leary, D. S., and Hnilicka, J. V.: Fatal disseminated herpes simplex virus infection and hemorrhage in the neonate. J. Pediatr. *76*:409–415, 1970.

Mindel, A., Adler, M. W., Sutherland, S., and Fiddian, A. P.: Intravenous acyclovir treatment for primary genital herpes. Lancet *1*:697–703, 1982.

Mitchell, C. D., Bean, B., Sachs, G. W., and Balfour, M. M., Jr.: Acyclovir therapy in 129 immunocompromised patients with herpesvirus infections (abstract). Pediatr. Res. *16*:246A, 1982.

Mitchell, J. E., and McCall, F. C. Transplacental infection by herpes simplex virus. Am. J. Dis. Child. *106*:207–209, 1963.

Mitchell, M., Wade, M., Bertino, J., and Calabresi, P.: Effects of cytosine arabinoside and methotrexate upon antibody synthesis and delayed hypersensitivity in man (abstract). Proc. Am. Assoc. Cancer Res. *9*:50, 1968.

Montgomery, J. R., Flanders, R. W., and Yow, M. D.: Congenital herpesvirus infection with possibly related anomalies. Am. J. Dis. Child. 125:364–366, 1973.

Myers, M. W., Glasgow, L. A., and Galasso, G. J.: Summary of a workshop on antiviral agents for genital herpesvirus infections. J. Infect. Dis. *145*:774–782, 1982.

Nahmias, A. J.: Herpesvirus hominis types 1 and 2 in humans. I. Antibodies to genital infections. Am. J. Epidemiol. *91*:539, 1970a.

Nahmias, A. J.: Unpublished observations. Cited in Nahmias, A. J., Alford, C. A., and Korones, S. B.: Infection of the newborn with herpesvirus hominis. Adv. Pediatr. *17*:185–226, 1970b.

Nahmias, A. J., and Dowdle, W. R.: Antigenic and biologic differences in herpesvirus hominis. Prog. Med. Virol. *10*:110–159, 1968.

Nahmias, A. J., Naib, Z. M., Josey, W. E., and Clapper, A. C.: Genital herpes simplex infection. Virologic and cytologic studies. Obstet. Gynecol. *29*:395–400, 1967a.

Nahmias, A. J., Josey, W. E., and Naib, Z. M.: Neonatal herpes simplex infection. Role of genital infection in mother as the source of virus in the newborn. J.A.M.A. *199*:164–168, 1967b.

Nahmias, A. J., Hirsch, M. S., Kramer, J. H., and Murphy, F. A.: Effect of antithymocyte serum on herpesvirus hominis (type 1) infection in adult mice. Proc. Soc. Exp. Biol. Med. *132*:696–698, 1969a.

Nahmias, A. J., Chiang, W. T., Del Buono, I., and Duffey, A.: Typing of Herpesvirus hominis strains by a direct immunofluorescent technique. Proc. Soc. Exp. Biol. Med. *132*:386–390, 1969b.

Nahmias, A. J., Josey, W. E., Naib, Z. M., Freeman, M. G., Fernandez, R. J., and Wheeler, J. H.: Perinatal risk associated with maternal genital herpes simplex virus infection. Am. J. Obstet. Gynecol. *110*:835–837, 1971.

Nahmias, A. J., Visintine, A. M., Reimer, C. B., Del Buono, I. D., Shore, S. L., and Starr, S. E.: Herpes simplex virus infection of the fetus and newborn. In Krugman, S., and Gershon, A. E. (eds.): Infections of the Fetus and the Newborn Infant. New York, Alan R. Liss, 1975, pp. 63–77.

Nahmias, A. J., Visintine, A. M., and Josey, W. E.: Cesarean section and genital herpes (letter). N. Engl. J. Med. *296*:1359, 1977.

Naib, Z. M., Nahmias, A. J., Josey, W. E., Facog, M. D., and Wheeler, J. H.: Association of maternal genital herpetic infection with spontaneous abortion. Obstet. Gynecol. *35*:260–263, 1970.

Ng, A. B. P., Reagan, J. W., and Yen, S. S. C.: Herpes genitalis: clinical and cytopathologic experience with 256 patients. Obstet. Gynecol. *36*:645–651, 1970.

Nolan, D., Carruthers, M., and Lerner, A. M.: Herpesvirus hominis encephalitis in Michigan. Report of 13 cases, including six treated with idoxuridine. N. Engl. J. Med. *283*:10–13, 1970.

Offit, P. A., Starr, S. E., Zolnick, P., and Plotkin, S. A.: Acyclovir therapy in neonatal herpes simplex virus infection. Pediatr. Infect. Dis. *1*:253–255, 1982.

Overall, J. C., Jr., and Glasgow, L. A.: Fetal response to viral infection: interferon production in sheep. Science *167*:1139–1141, 1970a.

Overall, J. C., Jr., and Glasgow, L. A.: Virus infections of the fetus and newborn infant. J. Pediatr. *77*:315–333, 1970b.

Pettay, O., Leinikki, P., Donner, M., and Lapinlemu, K.: Herpes simplex virus infection in the newborn. Arch. Dis. Child. *47*:97–103, 1972.

Plummer, G.: Serological comparison of the herpesviruses. Br. J. Exp. Pathol. *45*:135–141, 1964.

Rawls, W. E., Iwamoto, K., Adam, E., and Melnuck, J. L.: Measurement of antibodies to herpesvirus types 1 and 2 in human sera. J. Immunol. *104*:599–606, 1970.

Robinson, M. G., and Kauffman, S.: Disseminated herpes simplex—a case of consumption coagulopathy. Cited in Nahmias, A. J., Alford, C. A., and Korones, S. B.: Infection of the newborn with herpesvirus hominis. Adv. Pediatr. *17*:185–226, 1970.

Rose, A. G., and Becker, W. B.: Disseminated Herpesvirus hominis (herpes simplex) infection: retrospective diagnosis by light and electron microscopy of paraffin wax–embedded tissues. J. Clin. Pathol. *25*:79–87, 1972.

Saral, R., Burns, W. H., Laskin, O. L., Santos, G. W., and Lietman, P. S.: A randomized, double-blind, controlled trial in bone-marrow-transplant recipients. N. Engl. J. Med. *305*:63–67, 1981.

Schaffer, A. J.: Diseases of the Newborn. 2nd ed. Philadelphia, W. B. Saunders Company, 1965, p. 733.

Sever, J. L., Huebner, R. J., Castellano, G. A., and Bell, J. A.: Serological diagnosis "en masse" with multiple antigens. Am. Rev. Respir. Dis. *88*:342, 1963.

Slavin, H. B., and Gavett, E.: Primary herpetic vulvovaginitis. Proc. Soc. Exp. Biol. Med. *63*:345–347, 1946.

Smith, K. O., and Melnick, J. L.: Recognition and quantitation of herpesvirus particles in human vesicular lesions. Science *137*:543–544, 1962.

South, M. A., Tompkins, W. A. F., Morris, C. R., and Rawls, W. E.: Congenital malformation of the central nervous system associated with genital type (type 2) herpesvirus. J. Pediatr. 75:13–18, 1969.

Spruance, S. L., Schnipper, L. E., Overall, J. C., Jr., Kern, E. R., Wester, B., Modlin, J., Wernerstrom, G., Burton, C., Arndt, K. A., Chiu, G. L., and Crumpacker, C. S.: Treatment of herpes simplex labialis with topical acyclovir in polyethylene glycol. J. Infect. Dis. 146:85–90, 1982.

St. Geme, J. W., Jr., Prince, J. T., Burke, B. A., Good, R. A., and Krivit, W.: Impaired cellular resistance to herpes-simplex virus in Wiskott-Aldrich syndrome. N. Engl. J. Med. 273:229–234, 1965.

St. Geme, J. W., Jr., Bailey, S. R., Koopmen, J. S., Oh, W., Hobel, C., and Imagawa, D.: Neonatal risk following late gestational genital herpesvirus hominis infection. Am. J. Dis. Child. 129:342–343, 1975.

Sterzl, J., and Silverstein, A. M.: Developmental aspects of immunity. Adv. Immunol. 6:337–459, 1967.

Stevens, D. A., Jordan, G. W., Waddell, T. F., and Merigan, T. C.: Adverse effect of cytosine arabinoside on disseminated zoster in a controlled trial. N. Engl. J. Med. 289:873–878, 1973.

Sullivan-Bolyai, J. Z., Wilson, C. B., Brewer, L., and Corey, L.: Permissiveness of neonatal cells for infection by herpes simplex virus (HSV) type 2 (abstract). Pediatr. Res. 16:236A, 1982.

Valenti, W. M., Betts, R. F., Hall, C. B., Hruska, J. F., and Douglas, R. G., Jr.: Nosocomial viral infections. II. Guidelines for prevention and control of respiratory viruses, herpes viruses and hepatitis viruses. Infect. Contr. 1:165–178, 1980.

Weller, T. H., and Hanshaw, J. B.: Virologic and clinical observations on cytomegalic inclusion disease. N. Engl. J. Med. 266:1233–1244, 1962.

Whitley, R. J., Soong, S., Dolin R., Galasso, G. J., Ch'ien, L. T., Alford, C. A., and the NIAID Collaborative Antiviral Study Group: Adenine arabinoside therapy of biopsy-proven herpes simplex encephalitis. N. Engl. J. Med. 297:289–294, 1977.

Whitley, R. J., Nahmias, A. J., Visintine, A. M., Fleming, C. L., and Alford, A. L.: The natural history of herpes simplex virus infection of mother and newborn. Pediatrics 66:489–494, 1980a.

Whitley, R. J., Nahmias, A. J., Soong, S., Galasso, G. J., Fleming, C. L., and Alford, A. L.: Vidarabine therapy of neonatal herpes simplex virus infection. Pediatrics 66:495–501, 1980b.

Whitley, R. J., Soong, S., Hirsch, M. S., Karchmer, A. W., Dolin, R., Galasso, G. J., Dunnick, J. K., Alford, C. A., and the NIAID Collaborative Antiviral Study Group: Herpes simplex encephalitis: vidarabine therapy and diagnostic problems. N. Engl. J. Med. 304:313–315, 1981.

Wilton, J. M. A., Ivanyi, L., and Lehner, T.: Cell-mediated immunity in Herpesvirus hominis infections. Br. Med. J. 1:723–726, 1972.

Witzleben, C. L., and Driscoll, S. G.: Possible transplacental transmission of herpes simplex infection. Pediatrics 36:192–199, 1965.

Wolf, A., and Cowen, D.: Perinatal infections of the central nervous system. J. Neuropathol. Exp. Neurol. 18:191–243, 1959.

Yeager, A. S.: Use of acyclovir in premature and term neonates. Acyclovir Symposium. Am. J. Med. 73:205–209, 1982.

Yeager, A. S., Arvin, A. M., Urbani, L. J., and Kemp, J. A.: Relationship of antibody to outcome in neonatal herpes simplex virus infections. Infect. Immun. 29:532–538, 1980.

Yeager, A. S., Arvin, A. M., and Sweeney, M. C.: Absence of history of genital herpes simplex virus (HSV) infections in mothers of infected infants: source—asymptomatic shedding vs. primary infection (abstract). Pediatr. Res. 16:254A, 1982.

Zavoral, J., Ray, W., Kinnard, P., and Nahmias, A. J.: Neonatal herpetic infection—a fatal consequence of penile herpes in a serviceman. Unpublished data. Cited in Nahmias, A. J., Alford, C. A., and Karones, S. B.: Infection of the newborn with herpesvirus hominis. Adv. Pediatr. 17:185–266, 1970.

Zervoudakis, I. A., Silverman, F., Senterfit, L. B., Strongin, M. J., Read, S., and Cederquist, L. L.: Herpes simplex in the amniotic fluid of an unaffected fetus. Obstet. Gynecol. 55(Suppl.):16S–17S, 1980.

Zuelzer, W. W., and Stulberg, C. S.: Herpes simplex virus as the cause of fulminating visceral disease and hepatitis in infancy. Am. J. Dis. Child. 83:421–439, 1952.

6

Enteroviral Infections

The enteroviruses consist of three main groups, the polioviruses, the Coxsackie viruses, and the ECHO viruses. Poliovirus was first identified in 1909 by inoculation of monkeys with central nervous system material from a person with paralytic poliomyelitis. It was not until 1949, however, following the discovery by Enders, Weller, and Robbins that the virus could be grown in tissue cultures, that the importance of the enteroviruses as a cause of human disease came to be appreciated. In 1948 Dalldorf and Sickles recovered a new group of agents by inoculation of fecal extracts from two children with paralytic disease into newborn mice. These agents, later shown to be viruses, were named Coxsackie viruses after the township of Coxsackie in New York State, where the isolations were made. Two types, A and B, were identified on the basis of the histopathological changes they produced in newborn mice and their capacity to grow in cell cultures. Later a third group, the ECHO viruses, was identified. Associated from time to time with human diseases, these were found to be nonpathogenic for subhuman primates and newborn mice but produced cytopathic changes in cell cultures. Within the space of a few years it was found that all three groups of virus were antigenically distinct and consisted of several and, in some cases, numerous serological subtypes. Their main characteristics are shown in Table 6–1.

The enteroviruses have a worldwide distribution and appear in both sporadic and epidemic forms, particularly in the summer and warmer months of the year. Despite their global distribution and their high frequency of infection, there is no firm evidence to suggest that any of them cause congenital defects, although maternal infection acquired late in pregnancy may lead to perinatal infection and disease.

POLIOMYELITIS INFECTION

Since the introduction of polio vaccine, both inactivated and live attenuated, poliomyelitis has ceased to be a major public health problem in many countries. In the United States, from a peak of 57,000 cases in 1952, the number of reported infections has fallen to well under 100 per annum. In the United Kingdom the number of reported cases of paralytic disease has averaged three to four per annum from 1970 to 1974. In Finland, where the inactivated vaccine is still used, no indigenous cases of paralytic disease have been observed since 1964 (Oker-Blom, et al., 1984). Nevertheless, poliomyelitis remains a problem in many countries, particularly in tropical and subtropical areas.

Congenital and Perinatal Infection

Congenital poliomyelitis was very rare before the days of immunization. It is now a matter of historical interest. Between 1897

154

Table 6–1. **SOME PROPERTIES OF THE ENTEROVIRUSES**

| | | Pathogenicity | | | | |
Main Type	Serological Subtypes	Man	Subhuman Primates	Newborn Mice	Cell Cultures	Predominant Disease in Humans
Poliovirus	**3** types 1, 2, 3	+	+	–	+	Paralysis, aseptic meningitis
Coxsackie A	**23** types 1–24*	+	±	+	±	Aseptic meningitis, herpangina, undifferentiated febrile disease
Coxsackie B	**6** types 1–6	+	–	+	+	Aseptic meningitis, disseminated neonatal disease, myocarditis, encephalitis, Bornholm disease, myalgia
ECHO viruses	**31** types 1–34†	+	±	–	+	Aseptic meningitis, with or without rash, undifferentiated febrile disease

*Type A-23 now classified as ECHO 9.

†Three types now reclassified as a reovirus, a rhinovirus, Coxsackie A-24.

and 1955 only 58 cases of neonatal poliomyelitis had been reported in the literature (Bates, 1955). All of these occurred in infants born to infected mothers, but in view of the variable incubation periods, not all could have been true congenital infections.

There is sound evidence that poliovirus can cross the placenta, causing the onset of paralytic symptoms prior to the fifth day of life (Aycock, 1941; Baskin et al., 1950; Johnson and Stimson, 1952; Pugh and Dudgeon, 1954; Bates, 1955; Elliott and McAllister, 1956). In addition to paralytic disease, congenital infection has been associated with spontaneous abortion (Schaffer et al., 1954; Siegel and Greenberg, 1956) and stillbirth (Barsky and Beale, 1957; Kibrick, 1961). In some instances of abortion or stillbirth, the fact that virus cannot be recovered from the fetus or placenta suggests that some fetal wastage may be an indirect effect of the maternal disease.

The majority (approximately 65 per cent) of pregnant women who have clinically apparent poliomyelitis will deliver normal, full-term infants, but the fatality rate among infected infants is approximately 50 per cent (Wyatt, 1979). There is little evidence that the congenital defects occasionally found in infants born to mothers with poliomyelitis are etiologically related to fetal poliovirus infection.

When poliomyelitis does develop in a neonate, the symptoms are not unlike those seen in mature persons, but they may be more severe. The illness may be characterized by fever, diarrhea, malaise, and signs of diminished muscle function. Muscle weakness occurs in approximately 50 to 60 per cent of

such cases. Some infants show signs of meningeal irritation, with pleocytosis and increased protein in the spinal fluid. The rate of mortality from poliomyelitis is higher in newborns than it is in older infants (approximately 25 per cent).

COXSACKIE VIRUS INFECTION

It is noteworthy that the newborn mouse was the first animal known to support the growth of this subgroup of enteroviruses. Although these agents (later identified as type A strains) were recovered from two children with mild paralysis, poliovirus was later found to be present in the feces as well, so it is difficult to ascertain whether Coxsackie A virus or poliovirus or both were responsible for the paralytic symptoms. The special susceptibility of the newborn to Coxsackie viruses also occurs in humans and is especially evident in the case of the B strains. However, Archibald and Purdham (1979) were the first to document postnatal transmission of Coxsackie type A-16 from the mother to the neonate; this was shown by the occurrence of hand-foot-and-mouth disease in the infant. Later, Ogilvie and Tearne (1980) noted spontaneous abortion after coxsackievirus A-16 infection in the first trimester of pregnancy.

Evidence incriminating Coxsackie B virus as a pathogen for the neonate was provided by Gear and Measroch (1953) and by Javett and co-workers (1956) during the course of a study of an outbreak of an infection in 1952 in a Johannesburg maternity home. The first report involved 10 newborn infants who had fever and signs of acute myocarditis and, in some cases, of acute meningoencephalitis. Six died after fulminating illness ending in circulatory collapse. Focal lesions involving the myocardium, brain, and liver, as well as other organs, were found on postmortem examination. Since these early experiences there have been numerous reports of Coxsackie B infection in the newborn infant (Gear and Measroch, 1973). Barson and co-workers (1981) reported the rare complication of myocardial calcification after Coxsackie B-4 infection. Necrotizing enterocolitis possibly related to B-2 viral infection was described by Johnson and colleagues (1977). Damage to the pancreatic islet cells in four newborns with coxsackievirus encephalomyocarditis suggests that the B virus may be involved in the causation of diabetes mellitus (Ujevich and Jaffe, 1980). A retrospective study by Madden and co-workers (1978), however, failed to demonstrate a correlation between history of juvenile diabetes and level of coxsackievirus B1-6 antibody in matched control subjects. There is also evidence that asymptomatic infection occurs more often than overt infection (Hall and Miller, 1969). This point must be kept in mind when studying the effect of an infection on the fetus and newborn.

Epidemiology and Source of Infection

Coxsackie viruses are usually prevalent in the warmer months of the year. In Rochester, New York, approximately 90 per cent of enterovirus isolations occur from July to November. There is a tendency for specific types to occur in waves in any given season, and the same virus type may be prevalent for more than one season. Epidemics of Coxsackie B-5 in New York State have resulted in aseptic meningitis in newborn infants, as well as in older infants and children.

Newborn infants acquire coxsackievirus infections from one of three sources: their own mothers; nursing or other hospital personnel; and possibly, indirectly from other infected infants. Rarely, the infection may be transmitted across the placenta to the fetus during the latter part of pregnancy.

Clinical Manifestations

Congenital Coxsackie B virus infection has been described but occurs only rarely, ap-

pearing as an overt disease within 48 hours after birth. O'Shaughnessey and Buechner (1962) reported a case of maternal Coxsackie B-5 infection with hepatitis and encephalomyocarditis occurring in the third trimester. The infant born during the convalescent phase of the illness appeared to be unaffected at birth but showed developmental retardation at 10 months of age. Cherry and colleagues (1968) have recovered Coxsackie virus group B type 2 from an asymptomatic newborn investigated as part of a prospective survey of viral infections in the newborn period. Baker and Phillips (1980) described four cases of fatal coxsackievirus infection in the newborn, as well as several possible congenital defects: heart disease, diabetes, mental retardation, and urogenital, digestive, and cardiovascular anomalies. Severe problems may arise in the newborn despite what are most often subclinical symptoms in the mother.

Infants infected with Coxsackie B virus have been noted to have some or all of the symptoms listed in Table 6–2.

Some infants have illness with a diphasic course. The first phase is mild, characterized by slight elevation of the temperature, anorexia, and possibly coryza and diarrhea. After an apparent recovery lasting one to seven days, symptoms may return and may be more severe than those in the initial phase. Earlier case reports from South Africa (Gear and Measroch, 1953) describe this second phase as often characterized by fever, tachycardia (as high as or in excess of 200 per minute), tachypnea, cyanosis, and mottling, followed by the gray, ashen pallor of circulatory collapse.

On examination of the hearts of the most severely affected infants, cardiac enlargement, a systolic murmur over the entire precordium, arrhythmia, and gallop rhythm were often noted. The infants frequently

Table 6–2. **CLINICAL MANIFESTATIONS OF NEONATAL COXSACKIE B INFECTION**

Incubation period 3–5 days (range, 1–14 days)
Fever
Failure to feed
Irritability
Listlessness
Vomiting
Hypotonia
Apnea
Convulsions
Diarrhea
Occasional diphasic course
Circulatory collapse

lapsed into heart failure with hypotension, edema, atelectasis, abdominal distention, and hepatic enlargement. Some patients had hepatitis, and a few had disseminated intravascular coagulation.

It has been suggested by Brown and Evans (Evans and Brown, 1963; Brown, 1965; Brown and Evans, 1967) that Coxsackie B infections acquired in pregnancy may be etiologically related to congenital heart disease in the offspring. In a long-term prospective study (Brown and Evans, 1967), they determined the incidence of Coxsackie B virus infection, as defined by either a fourfold or greater increase in neutralizing antibody titer or a fourfold or greater decrease in titer, which indicates a recent infection, in the mother. They concluded that Coxsackie types B-3 and B-4 in mothers were more frequently associated with congenital heart disease in the children than occurred in a matched control series. They also observed that this trend of an association between maternal infection and infant malformations continued with remarkable consistency over several years. Although the predominant type of heart defect encountered was tetralogy of Fallot, the other cardiac defects included many seen in children who had congenital heart disease without any evidence of maternal infection. Furthermore, there was no predominance of lesions such as a persistent ductus arteriosus or pulmonary stenosis, which are encountered in congenital rubella. A further prospective study on the relationship between the infective agents and embryopathy in a study carried out by Ross and co-workers (1972) failed to substantiate the theory that Coxsackie B infections are a cause of congenital heart disease. Unpublished studies by Starkova and colleagues (1972) on several hundred patients with congenital heart disease admitted to the Hospital for Sick Children, Great Ormond Street, London, for corrective surgery failed to show any evidence of an association between maternal Coxsackie B infection and cardiac defect in the child.

ECHO VIRUS INFECTIONS

There is serological and virological evidence that ECHO viruses can cross the placenta to reach the developing fetus. Berkovich and Smithwick (1968) have reported a newborn infant with inapparent congenital infection due to ECHO type 22 that initiated an outbreak of respiratory infection in a premature infant nursery. Cherry and co-workers (1968) recovered ECHO type 17 from the placenta and throat of an asymptomatic newborn.

Epidemics of ECHO 9 virus infections were widespread throughout the world in the late 1950's and were particularly extensive in Europe and parts of the United States. Rawls and colleagues (1964) documented fatal infection in a 10 day old infant, isolating ECHO 9 virus from the brain, lung, and spinal fluid. A study by Cho and co-workers (1973) described a three day old infant with clinical signs of neonatal sepsis and meningoencephalitis linked with ECHO 9 virus. A fatal neonatal infection, notable for its lack of hepatic involvement and hemorrhage and its severe pneumonia, was reported by Cheeseman and colleagues (1977). Prospective surveys, including clinical and virological studies, failed to reveal unequivocal evidence that ECHO 9 infection in pregnancy was associated with congenital defects in the offspring (Rantasalo et al., 1960). Kleinman and co-workers (1962) studied the effect of an extensive epidemic in Minnesota and could find no evidence of an association between maternal infection and infant defects. A similar study carried out by Landsman and colleagues (1964) in Scotland also failed to incriminate ECHO 9 as a cause of congenital defects.

Enteroviral meningitis has been linked with several ECHO virus types. Jarvis and Tucker (1981) reported a greater degree of cerebrospinal fluid pleocytosis in newborns with ECHO 7 meningitis than in patients several months old. Wilfert and co-workers (1981) used the Peabody Picture Vocabulary Test to suggest that enteroviral meningitis during the first three months of life could lead to decreased receptive language functioning.

ECHO 11 virus infections have been the subject of several recent studies. Nagington and colleagues (1978) documented a fatal epidemic in a special care baby unit, noting renal hemorrhage and small vessel thrombi in the medulla, among other pathological effects. Davies and co-workers (1979) reported a similar wide range of clinical symptoms in an outbreak at a maternity ward. Both of these studies implicated hospital personnel in the spread of disease. Modlin (1980) investigated fatal ECHO 11 perinatal infection in four infants, suggesting that they lacked maternal antibody as a result of premature birth. A later study by Modlin and colleagues (1981) indicated that passive acquisition of maternal antibody does not preclude mucosal infection of the perinatally infected newborn. Disseminated intravascular coagulation was the primary pathological finding in the work of Kurnetz and co-workers (1981) and Berry and Nagington (1982). The latter study supported Modlin et al.'s (1981) suggestion that maternal antibody may prevent symptomatic but not necessarily asymptomatic infection. Intrauterine ECHO 11 infection was suggested by a case of Skeels and colleagues (1981) and positively demonstrated by Jones and colleagues (1980). Malfon and Spector (1981) reported the first fatal nonparalytic case of ECHO 11 infection beyond the neonatal period.

DIAGNOSIS

The diagnosis of enteroviral infection can be suspected on the basis of the clinical symptoms, the tendency for outbreaks of Coxsackie and ECHO virus infections to occur, and epidemiological evidence of their prevalence in the community. If symptoms appear within 48 hours of birth, infection probably occurred during intrauterine life. More commonly, symptoms appear toward the end of the first week of life, and one can conclude that the infant probably acquired the infection during or after birth. In general, a diagnosis can be made only retrospectively, and in view of the number of antigenic subtypes of the enteroviruses, serological tests have a limited value in diagnosis. Attempts should therefore be made to isolate the causative organism by virus culture. Recovery of the viral agent in tissue culture or suckling mice requires its subsequent identification as a member of one of the three main groups of enteroviruses.

TREATMENT

The treatment of an infant with suspected perinatal poliomyelitis is similar to that of a child or adult with the disease.

If an infant has evidence of myocarditis and congestive heart failure as a result of Coxsackie B infection, digoxin, oxygen, diuretics, and sodium restriction should be employed. There is no evidence that corticosteroids are helpful, and an appreciable number of data in laboratory animals suggest that the use of this class of drugs may be detrimental, interfering with normal host defense mechanisms and enhancing viral replication.

There are no sound data in support of the use of specific antiviral therapy.

Impaired heart function as a late sequela of neonatal Coxsackie B virus infection has not been reported, although this possibility exists. When meningoencephalitis occurs in the newborn period, it is not usually followed by adverse effects on development (Rantakallio et al., 1970).

PREVENTION

As poliomyelitis can now be controlled by immunization, congenital poliomyelitis no longer presents a significant problem. However, there is a potential risk of fetal infection following administration of live polio vaccine to the mother during pregnancy. In most instances, immunization against poliomyelitis is an elective procedure, so this risk should be reduced to an absolute minimum. Although there are no reports of adverse effects on the fetus following administration of polio vaccine in pregnancy, it is reasonable to assume that virus transmission to the fetus could occur. It is also well known that virus shedding follows vaccination and that there is a risk of recipient-associated and contact-associated poliomyelitis, but the risk is of the order of 0.5 per million doses administered.

If poliovirus vaccine is inadvertently administered to a pregnant woman, the risk to the fetus is insufficient to recommend termination of the pregnancy. In the event that a pregnant woman is exposed to a poliovirus infection, an inactivated vaccine is recommended rather than a live attenuated vaccine. Wild strains of poliovirus are still widespread in Africa, Asia, and Latin America, and these virulent strains present a greater hazard to the unimmunized pregnant woman than do the attenuated strains.

It is important for physicians responsible for the care of newborns to be aware of the presence in the community of Coxsackie B virus infection because of its potential virulence for these patients. This requires surveillance for enteroviruses during the warmer months by regional public health laboratories, as well as continuing awareness of the potential danger to the fetus and newborn from maternal disease and from infected members of staff of maternity units around the time of delivery. If there is known infection in the community, most especially in the maternity ward, every effort should be made to enforce enteric precautions. Should infection occur in the nursery, closing the unit to new admissions is strongly advised.

Suggestions have been made that interruption of infection in a nursery population can be achieved by interference with monovalent poliovirus vaccine (type II). Insufficient evidence exists to permit a firm recommendation for this approach. Although recent outbreaks of Coxsackie B virus have tended to be associated with disease of less severity than that described in earlier reports, this is always subject to change with variation in strain as well as with individual differences in host susceptibility.

At the present time there does not appear to be sufficient morbidity or mortality associated with Coxsackie B infection to warrant a vaccine development program. The impetus for such development is further weakened by the antigenic heterogeneity of the Coxsackie viruses. The same hindrances to a vaccine development program apply even more strongly to the Coxsackie A and ECHO viruses.

Bibliography

Archibald, E., and Purdham, D. R.: Coxsackievirus type A 16 infection in a neonate (letter). Arch. Dis. Child. *59*:649, 1979.

Aycock, W. L.: The frequency of poliomyelitis in pregnancy. N. Engl. J. Med. *225*:405–408, 1941.

Baker, D. A., and Phillips, C. A.: Maternal and neonatal infection with coxsackievirus. Obstet. Gynecol. *55*:125–153, 1980.

Balduzzi, P., and Glasgow, L. A.: Paralytic poliomyelitis in a contact of a vaccinated child. N. Engl. J. Med. *279*:796–797, 1967.

Barsky, P., and Beale, A. J.: Transplacental transmission of poliomyelitis. J. Pediatr. *51*:207–211, 1957.

Barson, W. J., Craenen, J., Mosier, D. M., Brawley, R. L., and Milty, M. D.: Survival following myocarditis and myocardial calcification associated with infection by Coxsackie virus B 4. Pediatrics *68*:79–81, 1981.

Baskin, J. L., Soule, E. H., and Mills, S. L.: Poliomyelitis in the newborn. Pathology changes in two cases. Am. J. Dis. Child. *80*:10–21, 1950.

Bates, T.: Poliomyelitis in pregnancy, fetus, and newborn. Am. J. Dis. Child. *90*:189–195, 1955.

Berkovich, S., and Smithwick, E. M.: Transplacental infection due to ECHO virus type 22. J. Pediatr. *72*:94–96, 1968.

Berry, P. J., and Nagington, J.: Fatal infection with echovirus II. Arch. Dis. Child. *57*:22–29, 1982.

Brown, G. C.: Serological studies on the viral etiology of congenital heart disease. Circulation *32*:59–60, 1965.

Brown, G. C., and Evans, T. N.: Serologic evidence of coxsackievirus etiology of congenital heart disease. J.A.M.A. *199*:183–187, 1967.

Burch, G. E., Sun, S., Chu, K., Sohal, R. S., and Colclough, H. L.: Interstitial and coxsackie virus group B myocarditis in infants and children. J.A.M.A. *203*:1–8, 1968.

Cheeseman, S. H., Hirsch, M. S., Keller, E. W., and Keim, O. E.: Fatal neonatal pneumonia caused by echovirus type 9. Am. J. Dis. Child. *131*:1169, 1977.

Cherry, J. D., Soriano, F., and John, C. L.: Search for perinatal viral infection: a prospective clinical, virological and serological study. Am. J. Dis. Child. *116*:245–250, 1968.

Cho, C. T., Janelle, J. G., and Behlehani, A.: Severe neonatal illness associated with ECHO 9 virus infection. Clin. Pediatr. *12*:304–305, 1973.

Dalldorf, G., and Sickles, G. M.: An unidentified filterable agent isolated from the feces of children with paralysis. Science *108*:61–62, 1948.

Davies, D. P., Hughes, C. A., MacVicar, J., Hawkes, P., and Mais, H. J.: Echovirus II infection in a special-care baby unit (letter). Lancet *1*:96, 1979.

Elliott, G. B., and McAllister, J. E.: Fetal poliomyelitis. Am. J. Obstet. Gynecol. *72*:896–902, 1956.

Enders, J. F., Weller, T. H., and Robbins, F. C.: Cultivation of Lansing strain of poliomyelitis virus in cultures of human embryonic tissues. Science *109*:85–87, 1949.

Evans, T. N., and Brown, G. C.: Congenital anomalies and virus infections. Am. J. Obstet. Gynecol. *87*:749–758, 1963.

Gear, J. H. S., and Measroch, D.: South African Institute Medical Research Annual Report for 1952. 1953, pp. 38–39.

Gear, J. H. S., and Measroch, D.: Coxsackie infections in the newborn. Prog. Med. Virol., *15*:42, 1973.

Hall, C. B., and Miller, D. G.: The detection of silent Coxsackie B-5 virus perinatal infection. J. Pediatr. *75*:124–127, 1969.

Jarvis, W. R., and Tucker, G.: Echovirus type 7 meningitis in young children. Am. J. Dis. Child. *135*:1009–1012, 1981.

Javett, S. N., Hymann, S., Mundel, B., Pepler, W. J., Lurie, H. I., Gear, J., Measroch, D., and Kirsch, Z.: Myocarditis in the newborn infant: a study of an outbreak associated with Coxsackie group B virus in a maternity home in Johannesburg. J. Pediatr. *48*:1–22, 1956.

Johnson, F. E., Crnic, D. M., Simmons, M. A., and Lilly, J. R.: Association of fatal coxsackie B-2 viral infection and necrotizing enterocolitis. Arch. Dis. Child. *52*:802–804, 1977.

Johnson, J. F., and Stimson, P. M.: Clinical poliomyelitis in the early neonatal period: report of a case. J. Pediatr. *40*:733–737, 1952.

Jones, M. J., Kolb, M., Votara, H. J., Johnson, R. L., and Smith, T. F.: Intrauterine echovirus type II infection. Mayo Clin. Proc. *55*:509–512, 1980.

Kibrick, S.: Virus infections of the fetus and the newborn. Perspect. Virol. *2*:140–157, 1961.

Kleinman, H., Prince, J. T., Mathey, W. E., Rosenfield, A. B., Bearman, J. E., and Syverton, J. T.: Echo 9 virus infection and congenital abnormalities: a negative report. Pediatrics *29*:261–269, 1962.

Kurnetz, R., Cacciarelli, A., Egere, R., and Yang, S. S.: Neonatal infection. J. Pediatr. *99*:822–826, 1981.

Landsman, J. B., Grist, N. R., and Ross, C. A. C.: Echo 9 virus infection and congenital malformations. Br. J. Prev. Soc. Med. *18*:152–156, 1964.

Madden, D. L., Fuccillo, D. A., Travo, R. G., Ley, A. C., Sever, J. L., and Beadle, E. L.: Juvenile or respiratory syncytial virus infections. J. Pediatr. *92*:959–960, 1978.

Malfon, N., and Spector, S. A.: Fatal echovirus type 11 infections. Am. J. Dis. Child. *135*:1017–1020, 1981.

Modlin, J. F.: Fatal echovirus II disease in premature neonates. Pediatrics *66*:775–780, 1980.

Modlin, J. F., Polk, B. F., Morton, P., Elkind, P., Crane, E., and Spiliotes, A.: Perinatal echovirus infection: risk of transmission during a community outbreak. N. Engl. J. Med. *305*:368–371, 1981.

Nagington, J. Wreghitt, T. G., Gandy, G., Roberton, N. R. C., and Berry, P. J.: Fatal echovirus II infections in outbreak in special care baby unit. Lancet *2*:725–728, 1978.

Ogilvie, M. M., and Tearne, C. F.: Spontaneous abortion after hand-foot-and-mouth disease caused by coxsackie virus A 16. Br. Med. J. *281*:1527–1528, 1980.

Oker-Blom, N., Penttinen, K. and Weckström, P.: Inactivated Poliovirus Vaccine in Finland. Rev. Infect. Dis. *6*:Supplement 2, S461–462, 1984.

O'Shaughnessey, W. J., and Buechner, H. S.: Hepatitis associated with a Coxsackie B5 virus during late pregnancy. J.A.M.A. *179*:71–72, 1962.

Pugh, R. C. B., and Dudgeon, J. A.: Fatal neonatal poliomyelitis. Arch. Dis. Child. *29*:381–384, 1954.

Rantakallio, P., Saukkonen, A., Krause, U., and Lapinleimu, K.: Follow-up study of 17 cases of neonatal Coxsackie B meningitis and one with suspected myocarditis. Scand. J. Infect. Dis. *2*:25–28, 1970.

Rantasalo, I., Penttinen, K., Saxen, L., and Ojala, A.: Echo 9 virus antibody status after an epidemic period and the possible teratogenic effect of the infection. Ann. Paediatr. Fenn. *6*:175–184, 1960.

Rawls, W. E., Shorter, R. G., and Herrmann, E. C.: Fatal neonatal illness associated with ECHO 9 (Coxsackie A 23) virus. Pediatrics *33*:278–279, 1964.

Ross, C. A. C., Bell, E. J., Kerr, M. M., and Williams, K. A. B.: Infective agents and embryopathy in the west of Scotland, 1966–70. Scott. Med. J. *17*:252–258, 1972.

Schaffer, M., Fox, M. J., and Li, C. P.: Intrauterine poliomyelitis infection. J.A.M.A. *155*:248–250, 1954.

Siegel, M., and Greenberg, M.: Polio in pregnancy: effect on the fetus and the newborn infant. J. Pediatr. *49*:280–288, 1956.

Skeels, M. R., Williams, J. J., and Ricker, F. M.: Perinatal echovirus infection (letter). N. Engl. J. Med. *305*:1529, 1981.

Starkova, O., Ebrahim, S., and Dudgeon, J. A.: Unpublished data. 1972.

Ujevich, M. M., and Jaffe, R.: Pancreatic islet cell damage. Arch. Pathol. Lab. Med. *104*:438–441, 1980.

Wilfert, C. M., Thompson, R. J., Sunder, T. R., O'Quinn, A., Zeller, J., and Blacharsh, J.: Longitudinal assessment of children with enteroviral meningitis during the first three months of life. Pediatrics *67*:811–815, 1981.

Wyatt, H. V.: Poliomyelitis in the fetus and newborn. Clin. Pediatr. *18*:33–38, 1979.

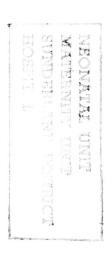

7

Varicella-Zoster Infections

Varicella (chickenpox) and zoster (shingles) are caused by the same virus, varicella-zoster (V-Z) virus. The two conditions differ only in their clinical manifestations and pathogenesis. Varicella is a disseminated infection resulting from primary infection with V-Z virus in a susceptible person, whereas zoster results from reactivation of a latent infection in a person who acquired varicella earlier in life. Varicella in pregnancy is comparatively rare because infection is normally acquired in childhood. Zoster, on the other hand, is more likely to occur in pregnancy because it occurs more frequently in adult life, but fetal infection is less likely after zoster than after varicella because of differences in pathogenesis. If primary infection does occur in pregnancy, the effect on the fetus is largely dependent on the gestational age at which maternal infection occurs. Maternal infection acquired in the first and second trimesters very rarely leads to congenital defects. Infection acquired close to term may lead to varicella and, less commonly, to zoster in early life.

NATURAL HISTORY OF POSTNATAL INFECTION

Varicella is a disease of childhood; its main incidence is in the first decade of life. The incubation period is usually between 14 and 18 days, but it is extremely variable and may be as short as 10 days or as long as 21 days.

The characteristic papular-vesicular rash appears after a short prodromal illness, but this rash may be absent altogether. The cutaneous lesions, appearing characteristically in crops, mature rapidly from papule to vesicle. After crusting, the skin lesions are usually healed within a week of onset. Varicella is highly contagious and has a very high clinical attack rate. Complications are rare, and apart from a hemorrhagic eruption, pneumonitis, and a postinfectious type of encephalomyelitis, they are seldom serious. In children with leukemia and on immunosuppressive therapy, however, a severe disseminated form of the disease may occur (Krugman and Katz, 1981).

Recovery is followed by long-term immunity, so second attacks of varicella are very rare. They have been reported occasionally—some occurring in children suffering from some form of immunodeficiency—but the likelihood of errors in diagnosis of the first attack should be taken into account. Nevertheless, because V-Z virus is a member of the herpes group of viruses, infection may remain latent, to become reactivated later in life in the form of zoster. Hence, the use of the term "immunity" in the generally accepted sense needs qualification in the case of latent infections.

Zoster is essentially a disease of adults, with a peak incidence between the ages of 20 and 60 years (Hope-Simpson, 1965). Miller and Brunell (1970) found that, of 108 patients with zoster, 69 per cent were 50 years of age

161

or older and only 10 per cent were children. When zoster does occur in children, it usually follows a definite history of varicella earlier in life. Brunell and co-workers (1968) have described 15 cases of zoster in children whose ages ranged from 3½ months to 14 years. The mother of the youngest patient had acquired varicella during the seventh month of pregnancy. The infant showed no evidence of V-Z complement-fixing CF antibody during convalescence. Similar cases of early childhood zoster consequent to exposure to the virus *in utero* have been reported by David and Williams (1979) and Dworsky and colleagues (1980). Cases of neonatal zoster have also been seen following maternal varicella in late pregnancy (Dudgeon, 1975).

The incubation period of zoster is unknown because it is difficult to determine the time at which reactivation is initiated. The skin lesions in zoster are similar to those seen in varicella but differ in their distribution. They are usually confined to an area supplied by one or more nerve roots. The fifth cranial nerve and the midthoracic, cervical, and lumbar regions are affected more frequently than other areas of the body. Zoster may occur without a rash, being characterized by pain, tenderness, and paresthesiae along the course of the nerves involved. The cutaneous scars observed in infants with congenital varicella also have a zoster-like distribution. Occasionally a patient with zoster may develop a generalized varicella-like eruption three to four days later. Zoster varicellosus is a rare event—for which there may be an immunological explanation—since it is generally assumed that in zoster the lesions are probably limited in their distribution by the presence of circulating antibody.

PATHOGENESIS AND PATHOLOGY

The pathogenesis of varicella is similar in many respects to that of variola. The portal of entry of virus is probably the respiratory tract, although this has never been proven. Infection is spread by close contact. Local multiplication of virus is followed by a viremic phase with dissemination of virus and the appearance of cutaneous lesions. It is difficult to isolate virus from nasopharyngeal secretions, but there is no difficulty in recovering it from skin lesions during the ve-

sicular stage of the eruption. It becomes progressively more difficult to isolate virus as the lesions become crusted. Virus can also be recovered from the lungs and other viscera in fatal cases of disseminated varicella.

In zoster, the mode of virus spread is different. Although the possibility of reinfection cannot be dismissed, it seems probable that reactivation of latent virus is the more likely explanation. In this respect, V-Z and herpes simplex infection are similar, except that recurrent attacks of zoster are extremely rare. Miller and Brunell (1970) have produced convincing evidence in support of the theory of reactivation in an epidemiological study of 108 patients with zoster. Only four patients had had a possible recent exposure to zoster or varicella, and the cases of zoster showed no seasonal incidence, whereas varicella occurred more frequently in the first few months of the year. Following varicella, the virus remains latent in a noninfectious form in the posterior root ganglia. Following some trigger mechanism that causes irritation, damage, or infiltration of the ganglia involved, virus is reactivated and travels along the nerve roots to produce lesions on the skin supplied by those nerves. It is unlikely, but difficult to prove, that there is a viremic phase in zoster, except in the rare case of zoster varicellosus, in which viremia is probably of short duration if it occurs at all.

EPIDEMIOLOGY

Both varicella and zoster have a worldwide distribution. Although the seasonal incidence of varicella is less regular than that of measles and rubella, cases tend to occur with greater frequency in the winter and spring. Cases of zoster occur sporadically throughout the year. Epidemics of varicella are less frequent than epidemics of measles and rubella, but within a family or hospital ward the disease is highly contagious. Infection is usually spread by close contact, but indirect transmission by the airborne route cannot be ruled out in some instances. Outbreaks of varicella in children may result from contact with an adult with zoster, a finding first made many years ago by Von Bokay (1909) and repeatedly confirmed. Zoster may also occur following exposure to varicella and vice versa (Brunell et al., 1968).

IMMUNITY

The duration of immunity to varicella is similar to that observed in measles, rubella, and many other common viral infections of children, the main features of which are a long incubation period, viremia, infection by a virus with a single antigenic type, and long-term immunity. Following primary infection antibody develops, reaching a peak titer between 21 and 28 days after the onset of the rash. Whether the long-term immunity in varicella results from the initial antigenic stimulus, reinfection, or both is not known. It is evident from serological studies in patients with zoster that antibody, as measured by the complement-fixation test, can persist for many years.

In zoster the antibody response is of the characteristic anamnestic type associated with a secondary stimulus. Antibody may be present, usually in low titer, at the time of onset; it rises rapidly during the next seven days. Miller and Brunell (1970) found that all 108 patients showed a fourfold or greater rise in CF antibody within eight days of onset.

PERINATAL VARICELLA

The comparative rarity of varicella in the newborn period is almost certainly due to the fact that most women have acquired varicella before pregnancy and thus confer passive protection to their infants by antibody transmitted across the placenta. In a study of viral infections in 30,000 pregnancies in the United States, Sever and White (1968) found that the incidence of varicella was 0.7 per 1000 pregnancies. Thus, infection of the fetus or newborn would not be expected to be a common occurrence. Since a case of congenital varicella was first recorded over 100 years ago by Hubbard (1878), some 50 or more cases have been reported in the literature. Freud (1958) encountered only one case of varicella in the newborn out of 220 cases of varicella in a New York hospital over a three-year period and only 46 cases (2.1 per cent) in infants aged two weeks to six months.

The clinical course of perinatal varicella is more variable than that of postnatal infections. The fetus or newborn may escape infection altogether, despite clinical disease in the mother. A typical attack of varicella may ensue, or there may be a fatal disseminated infection with visceral involvement. Freud (1958) reviewed a series of 19 cases reported in the literature from 1878 to 1958. The onset of varicella was between the first and ninth days of life. A history of maternal varicella in the last two weeks of pregnancy was obtained in 17 cases, and in two there was a history of varicella in siblings of the newborn one to two weeks prior to delivery. Since all these cases of neonatal varicella occurred within the first 10 days of life, it is probable that they were congenital in origin. Three infants died; recovery in the remainder was uneventful.

In a typical case following varicella in the mother in late pregnancy, the infant may appear completely normal at birth. Depending on the time of onset of the maternal eruption, fever may develop within a few days of life, and a few "teardrop" vesicles will appear anywhere on the infant's skin. During the next few days, crops of new vesicles that mature in exactly the same way as those in postnatal infections may develop. The lesions may be limited to a few crops, or there may be an extensive eruption covering the skin. Healing is usually complete in seven to 10 days. Newman (1965) reported an outbreak of varicella in a maternity unit in a London hospital in which nine mothers had varicella between 11 weeks before delivery and 14 days postpartum. Although illness in the mothers was moderately severe in eight cases, only one infant became ill. The appearance of this infant's lesions on the tenth day of life is shown in Figure 7–1. None of the other children showed any signs of clinical disease or serological evidence of infection.

Similarly, in a study on neonatal varicella in a New York hospital, Abler (1964) observed 15 cases over a seven-year period. All of the mothers acquired varicella one to 10 days prior to delivery. The clinical course was benign in the mothers, and only 4 of the 15 infants showed any sign of varicella within the first 20 days after birth. In 10 other infants, no varicella was noted at the age of 16 to 35 days. One infant, born after 30 weeks' gestation, survived only four hours. The incubation period of the illness in nine infants was extremely variable, lesions developing between nine and 35 days after birth.

Varicella in the newborn can be a severe and fatal illness, with widespread disseminated cutaneous and visceral lesions. There is usually a sudden rise in temperature and

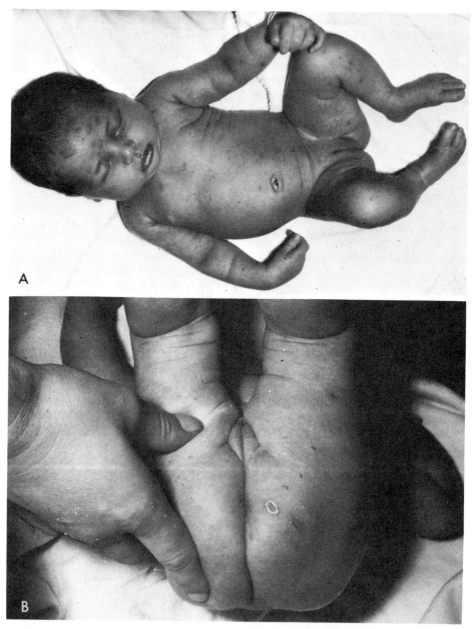

Figure 7–1. Vesicular lesions in the case of neonatal varicella reported by Newman. (B, from Newman, C. G. H.: Perinatal varicella. Lancet 2:1159, 1965.)

refusal to take feedings, followed by the appearance of a macular-vesicular rash. This may become confluent and hemorrhagic, and at the same time the infant may show signs of cyanosis and respiratory distress. Death may ensue within four to six days. Details of fatal neonatal cases that have been studied histopathologically have been reported by Luchessi and co-workers (1947) and by Garcia (1963). These cases were characterized by a fulminating onset, a disseminated vesicular-hemorrhagic rash, and the presence of necrotic lesions in the lungs, liver, brain, kidney adrenals, and, in one case, myocardium.

The most important factor that predisposes to severity of the disease in the neonate is the time of onset of the maternal illness in relation to delivery; the severity of the maternal disease does not appear to be an important factor. Gershon (1975) reviewed the outcome of 50 such cases, including a number previously reported in the literature (Pearson, 1964; Newman, 1965; Myers, 1974) and a few at Bellevue Hospital, New York City. Details of these are shown in Table 7–1, from which it can be seen that in cases where maternal infection occurred five days or more before delivery and varicella occurred in the newborn within the first four days of life, the outcome was good. In contrast, maternal infection acquired just *before* birth frequently led to severe disease in the infant. A possible explanation for this difference is that if there is time for maternal antibody to be produced and reach the fetus, the infection may be modified. Brunell (1967) studied a number of cases of V-Z in pregnancy, including four infants whose mothers had developed varicella within one week of delivery. All four infants received human immunoglobulin (0.3 to 0.6 ml per pound of body weight) on the first day of life. Three of the infants acquired mild varicella and had no detectable V-Z CF antibody before or after administration of the immunoglobulin. The fourth infant with V-Z CF antibody did not have symptoms. Gershon (1975) has also produced further serological evidence in support of this concept by means of the more sensitive fluorescent antibody membrane antigen (FAMA) technique developed by Williams and colleagues (1974). Two infants born to mothers who had had varicella two to three weeks prior to delivery were found to have V-Z IgG antibody titers of 1:32 and 1:64, respectively, in the cord blood. Vesicles were present at birth, but the disease was mild. In a similar case, antibody in the cord blood was detected four days before the onset of varicella.

CONGENITAL V-Z AS A CAUSE OF DEFECTS

In 1947 Laforet and Lynch published a report of a case of "multiple congenital defects following maternal varicella." The mother had had varicella in the eighth week of pregnancy and the infant was delivered at term. While the infant was in the hospital the following defects were observed: paralysis and muscular atrophy of the right leg, rudimentary digits, and defined reddish pigmented areas on the medial side of the left thigh. Cortical atrophy was also present, with hypoplasia of the cerebellum, chorioretinitis, and nystagmus. The skin lesions were later described as postvaricella cicatrices. The infant survived. Since that date additional cases of congenital V-Z have been reported from many different parts of the world. Details of these are summarized in Table 7–2. The

Table 7–1. **MATERNAL VARICELLA NEAR TERM—EFFECT ON THE FETUS (50 CASES)**

	Effect			
Onset	Fatal	Survived	Total	Case Fatality Rate
Maternal varicella, 5 days or more before delivery Baby's varicella, age 0 to 4 days	0	27	27	Nil
Maternal varicella, 4 days or less before delivery Baby's varicella, age 5 to 10 days	7	16	23	30%

From Myers, J. D.: Congenital varicella in term infants: risk reconsidered. J. Infect. Dis. *129*:215–217, 1974; Newman, C. B. H.: Perinatal varicella. Lancet *2*:1159–1161, 1965; and Pearson, H. E.: Parturition varicella-zoster. Obstet. Gynecol. *22*:21–27, 1964. Cited in Gershon, A. A.: Varicella in mother and infant: problems old and new. In Krugman, S., and Gershon, A. A. (eds.): Progress in Clinical and Biological Research. Vol. 3. New York, Alan R. Liss, Inc., 1975, pp. 79–95.

Table 7–2. CONGENITAL V-Z DEFECTS*

Case, Year, and Country	Maternal History and Week of Pregnancy	Clinical Details	Laboratory Findings		
			V-Z CF	Child	Mother
Case 1 1947 U.S.A.	Varicella at 8 weeks	Born at term; poorly developed; reddish pigmented areas on L thigh and leg; hypoplasia, muscular atrophy, and paresis of R leg; rudimentary digits of R foot; talipes; ? postvaricella cicatrices on L leg; cortical atrophy; hypoplasia of cerebellum; chorioretinitis; nystagmus; optic atrophy. Remained inactive. *Survived.*		NT	
Case 2 1969 Norway	Varicella at 15 weeks	2560gr at 41 weeks; R valgus deformity with hypoplasia of R leg and foot; muscular atrophy. Pox-like scars on forehead and long zig-zag scar on posterior aspect of thigh. Hypoplastic rudimentary toes or R foot. Severe convulsions; cortical atrophy; chorioretinitis; nystagmus. Slow development. *Survived.*	Day 12 Day 52	16 32	64 8
Case 3 1973 United Kingdom	Varicella at 11 weeks	2166gr at 41 weeks; reduction deformity and hypoplasia of L arm with rudimentary digits. Scars on hypoplastic limb; denervation of limb; L Horner's syndrome. Recurrent pneumonia. *Died at 9 weeks.*	6 weeks	40 IgM, 70 mg/dl	320
Case 4 1973 Canada	Varicella at 11 weeks	2200gr at term. Hypoplasia of R arm; muscular atrophy and paresis. Denuded skin on same side. Scars on scalp, knee, and L hip. Respiratory distress. Seizures; chorioretinitis; nystagmus. Repeated chest infections. Severely retarded. *Died at 20 weeks.*	5/12 FA 8/12 FA	32 128 8 64	NT NT
Case 5 1973 Belgium	Varicella between 14 and 19 weeks	3000gr at term. Scar on R cervical area spreading to chin and occipital and retroauricular area. Adherence of R ear to scalp. Ulceration of skin in innervation zones of superficial cervical plexus. Paralysis of R facial nerve. R hearing deficit. Difficulty in swallowing. Repeated aspiration pneumonia and vomiting. Muscular atrophy; psychomotor retardation. Zoster at 2½ months. *Died at 14 months.*	Birth 3/12 8/12 IgM, 100 mg/dl V-Z particles detected in zoster lesion	32 2 32	32 8
Case 6 1974 Canada	Contact with child. Varicella between 13 and 15 weeks	2000gr at 41 weeks. Cutaneous scars on distribution of L 4th dermatome. Hypoplastic L leg. Muscular atrophy. Micrognathia. Bilateral microphthalmus and cataracts; nystagmus. Cortical atrophy; nonresponsive; apathetic. *Died at 6 months.* At autopsy, necrotizing encephalitis; reticulitis; chorioretinitis; scars in pancreas and adrenals. Varicella pneumonitis.	Day 2 5/12 Extensive viral cultures negative No virus isolated from eye or brain	256 12	128 64
Case 7 1967 United Kingdom	Varicella at 12 weeks	2700gr at 38 weeks. Cutaneous scars on face and R frontoparietal area. Obliteration of nose. Microstomia. Gross deformity of both eyes and face. Opaque R cornea. Gross panencephaly. Cleft palate. *Died at 3 months.*	3/12	320 IgM, 108 mg/dl	80

Case	Maternal history	Clinical features	Test timing	Titer	Titer	Other
Case 8 1971 United Kingdom	Varicella as a child. Zoster varicellosus at 12 weeks	Birth weight not stated. Healed scars on L leg and buttocks. Hypoplasia of L limb. Muscular atrophy. Extensive scarring with keloid formation. Surgery required to promote full extension. *Survived.*	5/12 9/12	32 32	64 32	
Case 9 1976 United Kingdom	Varicella at 20 weeks	1580gr at term. Respiratory distress. Crusted vesicles on L hand and forearm. Scar on abdomen. L microphthalmus and enophthalmus. Slow initial development at 7 weeks. Skin lesions healed with scarring. L microphthalmus with central cataract. Development normal by 6 months. *Survived.*	Day 14 Day 28 Day 42 Day 56	16 32 16 32	< 8+ < 8 < 8 < 8	
Case 10 1977 U.S.A.	Varicella at 14 to 16 weeks	2988gr at term. Diffuse red papular rash at birth. Nystagmus. Severe hypoplastic L eye. Blind in L eye. Facial asymmetry. At 13 months numerous cicatrices on trunk and legs. Nystagmus. Microphthalmus. L eye opaque pupil. R eye chemosis. Marked chorioretinitis. Enucleation of L eye for cosmetic reasons. Slow development initially, later improved. *Survived.*	FAMA: Day 5 2 months 13 months 18 months	8 8 8 ⎱ 16 ⎰	NT V-Z CMI positive	V-Z IgM negative V-Z IF, EM, and culture negative
Case 11 1977 U.S.A.	Varicella at 16 weeks	1505gr at term. Diffuse nonvesicular rash at birth. Blind in L eye. At 12 months in 3rd percentile. Scars on legs. Hypoplastic L eye. No vision. Opaque cornea; L eye enucleated. *Survived.*	FAMA: 12 months 18 months	8 16	V-Z CMI positive	V-Z IgM cord negative V-Z EM and culture on L eye negative
Case 12 1978 G.D.R.	Varicella at 10 to 12 weeks	2050gr at term. Multiple defects; diffuse scarring and hypoplasia of upper and lower limbs. Severe keloid prevented full extension. Rudimentary digits of L hand. Psychomotor retardation. L Horner's syndrome. Reduced visual acuity. Recurrent chest infections. Exposed to varicella twice, no symptoms. Development improved. *Survived.*	Indirect HI: 21 months	256	NT	
Case 13 1979 United Kingdom	Varicella at 16 to 17 weeks	2400gr at 36 weeks (induced). Dilated L pupil. Skin defect extending from R iliac crest to R lumbar region. Defective skin of L ear. Flaccid paralysis of L arm. *Died at 56 hours.* At autopsy, atresia of the sigmoid colon; diffuse necrotic lesions on surface and in parenchyma of liver. Evidence of calcified varicella lesions in the lung, spleen, and diaphragm.		NT	NT	
Case 14 1981 United Kingdom	Varicella at 12 weeks	3350gr at term. Deficiency of skin and muscle on L 5th and 6th thoracic dermatomes. Hypoplasia of L 5th and 6th ribs. Lax Neurogenic bladder. Bilateral dilated calyces and ureters. At 12 months developed zoster 10 days postoperation for ureteric reimplantation. Normal development at 20 months. *Survived.*	3 months	16	64	
Case 15 1981 United Kingdom	Varicella at 10 weeks	1320gr at 37 weeks. Second of identical twins. Severely retarded. Hypoplasia of L upper arm. Deficiency of skin and muscle of hand to arm and thorax in region of C 7th and 8th and T 1st and 2nd dermatomes. Severe scarring. Paralysis of L arm at 12 months. L Horner's syndrome. Development improved by 3 years. 1st identical twin unaffected. *Survived.*	3 years	16 (Twin) < 8	< 8 < 8	

Table 7–2. CONGENITAL V-Z DEFECTS* (Continued)

Case, Year, and Country	Maternal History and Week of Pregnancy	Clinical Details	Laboratory Findings		
			V-Z CF	Child	Mother
Case 16 1977 United Kingdom	Zoster at 10 weeks	3350gr at term. Microcephalic. Bilateral microphthalmus and dense corneal opacities. Delayed development. No evidence of scars or hypoplasia of limbs. *Survived.*	After onset of zoster	NT	640
			At birth	10	160
			2 months	10	NT
			3 months	NT	40
			IgM Cord	NT	
			IgM at 2/12	<8	
			IgG at 2/12	256	
Case 17 1955 U.S.A.	Zoster at 4th month	Full term. R talipes. Bilateral microphthalmus and cataracts. Severe mental retardation. *Died (of meningitis) at 25 months.*	NT	NT	
Case 18 1955 U.S.A.	"Shingles" at 3rd month	6 lb, 6 oz at term. Defective vision noted at 4 months. Bilateral microphthalmus and dense cataracts. Good response to surgery. *Survived.*	NT	NT	

*Dates refer to dates of publication except for Cases 7 and 8, where they refer to dates of hospital admission. CF = complement-fixing; NT = not tested; FA = fluorescent antibody technique; FAMA = fluorescent antigen membrane antibody technique; CMI = cell-mediated immunity; EM = electron microscopy.
†CF < 8 stated by author to be low titer in the mother compatible with infection 15 weeks earlier.

References
Case 1: Laforet, E. G., and Lynch, C. L.: Multiple congenital defects following maternal rubella. N. Engl. J. Med. 236:534–537, 1947.
Case 2: Rinvik, R.: Congenital varicella encephalomyelitis in surviving newborn. Am. J. Dis. Child. 117:231–235, 1969.
Case 3: Savage, M. O., Moosa, A., and Gordon, R. R.: Maternal varicella infection as a cause of fetal malformations. Lancet 1:352–354, 1973.
Case 4: McKendry, J. B. J., and Bailey, J. D.: Congenital varicella associated with multiple defects. Can. Med. Assoc. 108:66–68, 1973.
Case 5: Dodion-Fransen, J., Dekegel, D., and Thire, L.: Congenital varicella-zoster infection related to maternal disease in early pregnancy. Scand. J. Infect. Dis. 5:149–153, 1973.
Case 6: Srabstein, J. C., et al.: Is there a congenital varicella syndrome? Pediatrics 84:239–243, 1974.
Case 7: Broomhead, I., and Dudgeon, J. A.: Unpublished observations, 1967.
Case 8: Broomhead, I., and Dudgeon, J. A.: Unpublished observations, 1971.
Case 9: Brice, J. E. H.: Congenital varicella resulting from infection during second trimester of pregnancy. Arch. Dis. Child. 51:474–476, 1976.
Case 10: Frey, H. M., Bialkin, G., and Gershon, A.: Congenital varicella: case report of a serologically proved long-term survivor. Pediatrics 59:110–112, 1977.
Case 11: Charles, N. C., Bennett, T. W., and Margolis, S.: Ocular pathology of the congenital varicella syndrome. Arch. Ophthalmol. 95:2034–2037, 1977.
Case 12: Dietzsch, H. J., Rabenhalt, P., and Trlifajova, J.: Varizellen-Embryopathie. Dt. Gesundh.-Wesen, Berlin 33:410, 1978.
Case 13: Alexander, I.: Congenital varicella. Br. Med. J. 2:1074, 1979.
Cases 14 and 15: Borzyskowski, M., Harris, R. F., and Jones, R. W. A.: The congenital varicella syndrome. Eur. J. Pediatr. 137:335–338, 1981.
Case 16: Webster, M. H., and Smith, C. S.: Congenital abnormalities and maternal zoster. Br. Med. J. 2:1193, 1977.
Cases 17 and 18: Duehr, P. A.: Herpes zoster as a cause of congenital cataracts. Am. J. Ophthalmol. 39:157–161, 1955.

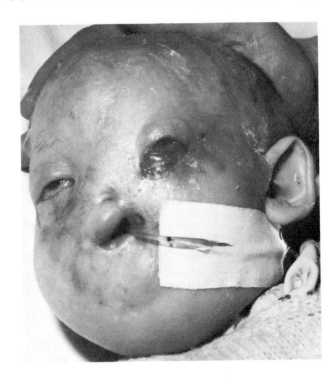

Figure 7–2. Case 7: Cutaneous lesions on the face of an infant seen by Broomhead and Dudgeon (1967), showing severe damage to both eyes, deformed mouth, and remains of scars of the face. (Courtesy of Mr. Ivor Broomhead.)

lesions described in Cases 7 and 8 are shown in Figures 7–2 and 7–3, respectively.

A summary of the main clinical findings in the 18 fully documented cases is shown in Table 7–3. It is emphasized that in all cases multiple defects were present, but in a few (Cases 16, 17, and 18) the lesions tended to be confined to a single organ, such as the eye. A history of maternal varicella was obtained in 14 cases, of zoster in three cases, and of zoster varicellosus in one case (Case 8). This is not altogether surprising, since V-Z infections are invariably associated with symptomatic disease, in contrast to rubella and cytomegalovirus (CMV) infections. There was nothing in the recorded history

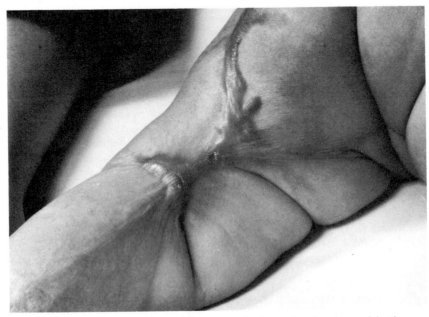

Figure 7–3. Case 8: Severe scar. The healed vesicles seen at birth can just be observed in the surrounding skin. (Courtesy of Mr. Ivor Broomhead.)

Table 7–3. **SUMMARY OF DETAILS IN 18 CASES OF CONGENITAL V-Z**

Illness or Defect	No.
Maternal varicella in pregnancy	14
Maternal zoster in pregnancy	3
Maternal zoster varicellosus in pregnancy	1
Gestational age at maternal illness	8–20 weeks
Infants born "small for gestational age"	8
Cutaneous scars	13
Hypoplasia of a limb	10
Muscular atrophy	9
Rudimentary digits	5
Psychomotor retardation	7
Seizures	3
Muscular paralysis	4
Other CNS signs or symptoms Cortical atrophy Microcephaly Horner's syndrome	7
Microphthalmus	8
Chorioretinitis	4
Cataracts and nystagmus	8
Facial asymmetry	3
Recurrent chest infections	4
Delayed development in infancy	7
Deaths	7
Survivors	11

of the mothers' illnesses to suggest that any unusual event had occurred that might have played a contributory role, except perhaps in Case 11, where there was a bad obstetrical history and indirect evidence of immunodeficiency.

The most commonly encountered manifestations were those affecting the skin and musculoskeletal systems, the eye, and the brain. As already mentioned, frequently these occurred in combination. Another common feature was that eight of these infants were small for gestational age and two more infants were just in the tenth percentile. Multiple defects with evidence of retarded intrauterine growth are characteristic of other virus infections affecting the fetus, notably rubella and CMV. The gestational age at which varicella or zoster developed in the mother varied from eight to 20 weeks, and it may be significant that many of the defects were of a type different from those observed in congenital rubella, except for the cataracts. These occurred, often with associated microphthalmus, following maternal varicella from the twelfth week to the fourth month of gestation. Not unnaturally with such a combination of severe defects, many of the infants had severe developmental problems,

but it is significant that several picked up and developed reasonably well later in childhood with the assistance of surgery for a hypoplastic eye or cataracts and speech therapy.

The description and distribution of the scars, which are more accurately termed "cicatrices" because of their dense fibrous or keloid nature (Cases 8 and 12), are important. Most of these showed a zoster-like distribution at birth and resembled zoster vesicles. The fact that the cicatrices were often present on the hypoplastic limb and were consistent with unilateral involvement of several dermatomes, either cervical, thoracic, or lumbar, suggests that maternal varicella had resulted in fetal zoster. As already stated, this occasionally occurs in the newborn when maternal varicella is acquired close to term. Three of the infants (Cases 1, 10, and 11) had reddish, papular rashes at birth, but these were nonvesicular. In two infants (Cases 6 and 13), both of whom died, there was evidence of a disseminated infection with varicella-like lesions in the liver, a varicella pneumonitis, and scars in the pancreas, adrenals, and spleen.

In the first edition of this book it was noted that five of the eight patients described in the original Table 7–2 had died. Of the 18 patients now recorded, eleven have survived, and among the seven that died, one death (case 17) was probably unconnected with the original fetal insult. In three of the fatal cases, recurrent chest infection was a prominent feature; in the others, a fatal outcome appeared to be associated with the severity and multiplicity of the defects. Frey and co-workers (1977) have suggested that congenital varicella may be manifested as a spectrum of disease, varying from a severe form with extensive somatic neurological and ophthalmological involvement incompatible with life, to a severe form with gross deformities such as facial asymmetry, to a less severe form in which only the eye is involved. This was a feature of the three cases associated with maternal zoster. Several cases are of special interest. Case 15 was the second-born of identical twins and was severely affected. The first-born twin was unaffected and showed no serological evidence of having been infected, although it is feasible that a test for V-Z antibody more sensitive than the CF test might have detected antibody at the age of three years. Fetal infection in twin pregnancies has also been observed following maternal rubella (Dudgeon, 1965) (see Chapter 3). In some instances, in both identical and non-identical twins, both infants have been infected and damaged, but in others, one twin has escaped both damage and fetal infection. It is difficult to explain why this should occur, particularly with uniovular twins, as in Case 15. Zoster developed in two cases (5 and 14), indicating that the virus was latent in the infant as a result of fetal infection. Case 12 was exposed to varicella on two occasions in childhood but developed no symptoms, suggesting resistance to infection.

Confirmatory laboratory evidence of fetal infection was obtained in 14 of the 18 cases, although the strength of this evidence varied from case to case. In most instances confirmation depended on the persistence of V-Z antibody—usually as measured by the CF test, which is not as sensitive as the FAMA test—beyond the age at which maternal antibody should be expected to have disappeared.

A cell-mediated immune response was detected in Cases 10 and 11, but despite tests by the most sensitive and exhaustive methods no evidence of viral antigen or infectious virus could be detected. It is conceivable that fetal infection may occur following maternal V-Z without there being fetal damage, but this has yet to be proven.

These cases have now been observed in many parts of the world (see Table 7–2), and it would seem that the criteria referred to in Chapter 2 (see Table 2–1) for establishing a causal relationship between a maternal infection and fetal damage have been met. It is reasonable to include the defects described under the term "congenital varicella syndrome," as suggested by Srabstein and colleagues (1974), or simply "congenital varicella" (Dudgeon, 1976) or "congenital varicella-zoster," in order to conform to the terminology used for cases of congenital rubella and CMV infection.

It is almost inevitable that other cases will come to light as awareness of this syndrome increases. One such case has recently been observed by Gisela Enders in the Federal Republic of Germany. The major stigmata of scarred skin lesions and hypothraphic limbs were typical of congenital varicella, and the scars closely resembled those observed in Case 8 (see Table 7–2). The infant did not survive (Enders, 1982a, 1982b).

The effect of maternal V-Z infection on the fetus is not simply a matter of academic interest, it is one of practical importance because of the advice that is sought when a woman contracts varicella or is in contact with the disease in pregnancy. There are probably several reasons why so few cases have been reported: the comparative rarity of varicella in the child-bearing years, the lack of recognition of an association between an *event* and an *effect*, and, possibly, a low propensity of the virus to cross the placenta and infect the fetus. This is not altogether conjectural—Gershon (1975) has commented upon the low clinical attack-rate (only 20 per cent) of the virus in infants whose mothers have had varicella close to term. Newman (1965) has also commented on this variability of the attack-rate and on the fact that the fetus frequently escapes clinical disease when the mother is infected. But does the fetus always escape infection? This we do not know.

The outcome of maternal varicella in pregnancy has been the subject of several prospective studies carried out in the United Kingdom and the United States between 1950 and 1964 that were referred to in Chapter 2. In the U.K. report on "Rubella and other virus infections during pregnancy," Manson and her colleagues (1960) were notified of 293 cases of chickenpox in pregnancy. Seventy-three had occurred in the first trimester, 142 in the second, and 78 during subsequent stages. Of the 288 liveborn infants, six had major defects and five suspicious defects. None of these 11 infants had defects bearing any resemblance to those associated with congenital varicella, as they were first described (Table 7–4).

The prospective study carried out by Bradford Hill and co-workers (1958) documented 31 cases of varicella in pregnancy, of which six were preconceptional and 17 were contracted during the first and second trimesters. No evidence of the type of defects referred to as *"congenital varicella-zoster"* defects was encountered. The long-term cohort study carried out by Siegel (1973) in New York City revealed no evidence of malformations or defects. It can only be concluded that there is a risk of severe fetal damage following maternal varicella in the first and second trimesters and that the size of the risk is not known, although it is probably very small. Only by detailed observations combined with laboratory investigations can the size of the problem be determined.

A SYNTHESIS OF MATERNAL V-Z INFECTION AND ITS EFFECT ON THE FETUS

For the fetus or newborn to be *affected* by maternal V-Z infection, it must be assumed

Table 7–4. **MAJOR AND SUSPICIOUS DEFECTS IN LIVEBORN CHILDREN: VARICELLA GROUP (MANSON SERIES, 1950–1952)***

Case Number	Week of Pregnancy	Week of Gestation	Birth Weight in Lb	Type of Defect
Major defects				
1	7	40	6.00	Mental retardation
2	26	41	5.14	CDH
3	22	44	7.1	CDH
4	34	42	8.1	CDH (dextrocardia)
5	17	31	3.12	Hemorrhagic disease
6	30	39	7.0	Stenosis of pelvic rectal junction
Suspicious defects				
7	31	41	6.12	Backward in talking
8	15	43	8.11	Apical systolic bruit
9	23	38	7.2	? Heart lesion
10	36	41	8.8	Murmur ? defect
11	2	40	6.8	Softened 1st sound at apex, slight talipes

*CDH = Congenital disease, heart.

From Manson, M. M., et al.: Rubella and other virus infections during pregnancy. Rep. Public Health Med. Subj. No. 101. London, Her Majesty's Stationery Office, 1960.

that the fetus becomes *infected* through the transplacental route or, in a few cases occurring in the newborn period, by contact during or soon after birth. Although viremia has not been demonstrated in varicella, it is reasonable to assume that it occurs before the onset of the rash and probably ceases abruptly thereafter as antibody is produced. The time relationship is important because, if this concept is correct, viremia should precede the development of antibody. In theory, if virus reaches the fetus, it could initiate fetal infection before maternal antibody is produced and before it crosses the placenta. From the reports of Brunell (1967) and Gershon (1975) already referred to, one can only conclude that even if virus reaches the fetus first, maternally transmitted antibody can modify the effect of the disease in the newborn.

MANAGEMENT OF V-Z IN PREGNANCY AND IN THE NEWBORN

Advice is frequently sought from physicians concerning the risk of a congenital defect following maternal varicella in early pregnancy. At one time one could say without hesitation, on the basis of the available evidence, that no such risk existed. Yet in view of the evidence referred to in this chapter, one can only state that there is probably a very remote risk, one that most families would most likely be prepared to take. Despite the occasional report of zoster as a cause

of congenital defects (Duehr, 1955), the risk is so small as to be discounted.

If a woman comes into contact with varicella or zoster in early pregnancy, consideration should be given to passive immunization with immunoglobulin (IG). Brunell (1966) has shown that V-Z antibody crosses the placenta, and it has been established in clinical trials with zoster immune globulin (ZIG) that infection can be prevented, whereas normal pooled immunoglobulin (IG, ISG) may only modify the disease even if given in very large doses (Brunell et al., 1969, 1972; Gershon et al., 1974). ZIG is an expensive product and is usually in short supply because it is required for protection of immunosuppressed patients or children with leukemia who are exposed to varicella. Its use must, therefore, be limited, and each case should be treated on its merits. The dose of ZIG is 0.05 ml per pound of body weight; it should be administered by the deep intramuscular route within three days of contact. If ZIG is not available, normal IG at a dose of 0.5 ml per pound of body weight can be used, although prevention, as opposed to modification, of infection cannot be guaranteed.

The management of varicella in late pregnancy and the protection of the susceptible newborn present similar problems, particularly for the high-risk group of infants born to mothers who contract the disease within five days of delivery.

The incidence of infection in this group is high—17 per cent according to Myers

(1974)—and the case-fatality ratio reported varies from 14 per cent (Gershon, 1975) to 31 per cent (Myers, 1974). The administration of ZIG should be considered with the reservations already mentioned, in the same dose (0.05 ml/lb), but since ZIG should be given within three days of contact (Gershon et al., 1974), there may be some inevitable delay in achieving passive protection of those infants whose mothers have contracted varicella five days before delivery.

Another situation that may arise is that of an infant whose mother contracts varicella either at or within the first few days of his birth. The infant is at risk, whether the infection has been acquired transplacentally or by direct contact with the mother's cutaneous lesions. It is advisable to isolate the child from the mother, to adopt protective precautions within the maternity unit, and to administer ZIG to the infant. If in any of the above circumstances ZIG is not available, it is reasonable to use large doses of normal IG (ISG) (0.5 ml/lb) because, although it will probably not prevent infection, it may modify the disease.

THE VIRUS

Herpes varicellae or V-Z virus is a DNA virus of the herpesvirus group. Viruses obtained from varicella and zoster have been found to be identical by all available serological tests and by electron microscopy (Andrewes and Pereira, 1972). Viral antigen can be detected by complement fixation, by gel diffusion, and by immunofluorescence. The virus can be propagated in cell cultures prepared from human embryo skin and muscle and human embryo lung fibroblasts (Weller, 1969).

LABORATORY DIAGNOSIS

Microscopy

Examination of vesicle fluid from a cutaneous lesion in varicella or zoster will often reveal multinucleate epithelial cells resulting from the amitotic division of cells in the epidermis.

A rapid diagnosis can also be made by electron microscopy (EM). This method is of particular value in helping to differentiate between varicella and variola-vaccinia.

Virus Culture

V-Z virus can be cultured in primary cultures of human skin, muscle, human embryo lung fibroblasts, human amnion, and HeLa cells. The virus will not grow in the RK13 continuous line of rabbit kidney cells, thus helping to distinguish V-Z virus from herpes simplex virus.

Serology

Antibody can be measured by the complement-fixation test using a CF antigen prepared from infected tissue cultures. CF antibody persists for a long period but may decline to undetectable levels in some patients after many years. A booster response is encountered in zoster as CF antibody rises rapidly after the appearance of the eruption (Miller and Brunell, 1970). Schmidt and colleagues (1969) have demonstrated some cross-reaction between V-Z virus and herpes simplex virus by complement fixation. Antibody can also be measured by gel-precipitin, neutralizing antibody, and fluorescent antibody tests. An improved fluorescence test in which antibody is measured by using a membrane antigen of V-Z infected cells has been described by Williams and co-workers (1974). The FAMA test is a rapid and more reliable method of detecting V-Z antibody than the CF test. Antibody can be detected earlier by the FAMA than by the CF technique. More recently, a radioimmunoassay for V-Z antibody has been described that is as sensitive as the FAMA test and easier to perform. An additional very sensitive test for antibody, the enzyme-linked immunoabsorbent assay, has now been developed. These are described in Chapter 14.

Bibliography

Abler, C.: Neonatal varicella. Am. J. Dis. Child. *107*:492–494, 1964.

Alexander, I.: Congenital varicella. Br. Med. J. *2*:1074, 1979.

Andrewes, C. H., and Pereira, H. G.: In Viruses of Vertebrates, 3rd ed. Baltimore, Williams & Wilkins Company, 1972.

Borzyskowski, M., Harris, R. F., and Jones, R. W. A.: The congenital varicella syndrome. Eur. J. Pediatr. *137*:335–338, 1981.

Bradford Hill, A., Doll, R., Galloway, T. M., and Hughes, J. P.: Virus diseases in pregnancy and congenital defects. Br. J. Prev. Soc. Med. *12*:1–7, 1958.

Brice, J. E. H.: Congenital varicella resulting from infection during second trimester of pregnancy. Arch. Dis. Child. *51*:474–476, 1976.

Broomhead, I., and Dudgeon, J. A.: Unpublished observations, 1967.

Broomhead, I., and Dudgeon, J. A.: Unpublished observations, 1971.

Brunell, P. A.: Placental transfer of varicella-zoster antibody. Pediatrics *38*:1034–1038, 1966.

Brunell, P. A.: Varicella-zoster infections in pregnancy. J.A.M.A. *199*:315–317, 1967.

Brunell, P. A., Miller, L. H., and Lovejoy, F.: Zoster in children. J.A.M.A. *115*:432–437, 1968.

Brunell, P. A., Ross, A., Miller, L. A., and Kuo, B.: Prevention of varicella by zoster immune globulin. N. Engl. J. Med. *280*:1191–1194, 1969.

Brunell, P. A., Gershon, A. A., Hughes, W. T., Riley, H. D., and Smith, J.: Prevention of varicella in high risk children. A collaborative study. Pediatrics *50*:718–722, 1972.

Charles, N. C., Bennett, T. W., and Margolis, S.: Ocular pathology of the congenital varicella syndrome. Arch. Ophthalmol. *95*:2034–2037, 1977.

David, T. J., and Williams, M. J.: Herpes zoster in infancy. Scand. J. Infect. Dis. *11*:186–188, 1979.

Dietzsch, H. J., Rabenhalt, P., and Trlifajova, J.: Varizellen-Embryopathie. Dt. Gesundh.-Wesen, Berlin *33*:410, 1978.

Dietzsch, H. J., Rabenhalt, P., and Trlifajova, J.: Varizellen-Embryopathie. Kinderarztliche Praxis *3*:138–145, 1980.

Dodion-Fransen, J., Dekegel, D., and Thire, L.: Congenital varicella-zoster infection related to maternal disease in early pregnancy. Scand. J. Infect. Dis. *5*:149–153, 1973.

Dudgeon, J. A.: Communication to 5th International Conference on Paediatrics, Tokyo, 1965.

Dudgeon, J. A.: Unpublished observations, 1975.

Dudgeon, J. A.: Infective causes of human malformations. In Human Malformations. Br. Med. Bull. *32*:77–83, 1976.

Duehr, P. A.: Herpes zoster as a cause of congenital cataracts. Am. J. Ophthalmol. *39*:157–161, 1955.

Dworsky, M., Whitley, R., and Alford, C.: Herpes zoster in early infancy. Scand. J. Infect Dis. *11*:186–188, 1980.

Enders, Gisela: Herpes virus of man and animal. In Biological Standardisation. Basel, S. Karger, *52*:221–236, 1982a.

Enders, Gisela: Personal communication, 1982b.

Freud, P.: Congenital varicella. Am. J. Dis. Child. *96*:730–733, 1958.

Frey, H. M., Bialkin, G., and Gershon, A.: Congenital varicella: case report of a serologically proved long-term survivor. Pediatrics *59*:110–112, 1977.

Garcia, A. G. P.: Fetal infection in chickenpox and alastrim with histopathological studies of the placenta. Pediatrics *32*:895–901, 1963.

Gershon, A. A.: Varicella in mother and infant: problems old and new. In Krugman, S., and Gershon, A. A. (eds.): Infections of the Fetus and Newborn. Progress in Clinical and Biological Research. Vol. 3. New York, Alan R. Liss, Inc. 1975, pp. 79–95.

Gershon, A. A., Steinberg, S., and Brunell, P. A.: Zoster immune globulin: a further assessment. N. Engl. J. Med. *290*:243–245, 1974.

Hope-Simpson, R. E.: The nature of herpes zoster: a long-term study and a new hypothesis. Proc. Soc. Med. *58*:9, 1965.

Hubbard, T. W.: Varicella occurring in an infant twenty-four hours after birth. Br. Med. J. *1*:822, 1878.

Krugman, S., and Katz, S.: Infectious Diseases of Children and Adults. 7th ed. St. Louis, C. V. Mosby Company, 1981.

Laforet, E. G., and Lynch, C. L.: Multiple congenital defects following maternal varicella. N. Engl. J. Med. *236*:534–537, 1947.

Luchessi, P. F., La Boccetta, A. C., and Peale, A. R.: Varicella neonatorum. Am. J. Dis. Child. *73*:44–54, 1947.

Manson, M. M., Logan, W. P. D., and Loy, R. M.: Rubella and other virus infections during pregnancy. Rep. Public Health Med. Subj. No. 101. London, Her Majesty's Stationery Office, 1960.

McKendry, J. B. J., and Bailey, J. D.: Congenital varicella associated with multiple defects. Can. Med. Assoc. J. *108*:66–68, 1973.

Miller, L. H., and Brunell, P. A.: Zoster, reinfection or activation of latent virus? Am. J. Med. *49*:480–483, 1970.

Myers, J. D.: Congenital varicella in term infants: risk reconsidered. J. Infect. Dis. *129*:215–217, 1974.

Newman, C. G. H.: Perinatal varicella. Lancet *2*:1159–1161, 1965.

Pearson, H. E.: Parturition varicella-zoster. Obstet. Gynecol. *23*:21–27, 1964.

Rinvik, R.: Congenital varicella encephalomyelitis in surviving newborn. Am. J. Dis. Child. *117*:231–235, 1969.

Savage, M. O., Moosa, A., and Gordon, R. R.: Maternal varicella infection as a cause of fetal malformations. Lancet *1*:352–354, 1973.

Schmidt, N. J., Lennette, E. H., and Magoffin, R. L.: Immunological relationship between herpes simplex and varicella-zoster viruses demonstrated by complement-fixation, neutralization and fluorescent antibody tests. J. Gen. Virol. *4*:321–328, 1969.

Sever, J., and White, L. R.: Intrauterine viral infections. Annu. Rev. Med. *19*:471–486, 1968.

Siegel, M.: Congenital malformations following chickenpox, measles, mumps and hepatitis. J.A.M.A. *226*:1521–1524, 1973.

Srabstein, J. C., Morris, N., Bryle Larke, R. P., deSa, D. J., Castelino, B. B., and Sum, E.: Is there a congenital varicella syndrome? J. Pediatr. *84*:239–243, 1974.

Von Bokay, J.: Uber den atioligischen Zusammenhang der Varizellen mit gewissen Fällen von Herpes zoster. Wien. Klin. Wochenschr. *22*:1323, 1909.

Webster, M. H., and Smith, C. S.: Congenital abnormalities and maternal zoster. Br. Med. J. *2*:1193, 1977.

Weller, T. H.: Varicella-zoster virus. In Lenette, E. H., and Schmidt, N. J. (eds.): Diagnostic Procedures for Viral and Rickettsial Infections. 4th ed. New York, American Public Health Association, 1969, pp. 733–754.

Williams, V., Gershon, A. A., and Brunell, P. A.: Serologic response to varicella-zoster membrane antigens measured by indirect immunofluorescence. J. Infect. Dis. *130*:669–672, 1974.

8

Smallpox and Vaccinia

Smallpox is a highly contagious disease with a high mortality rate caused by a virus of the poxvirus group. The disease exists in three forms: *variola major*, or classic epidemic smallpox; *variola minor*, or alastrim, a much milder form of the disease that occurs more often in sporadic form; and *varioloid*, which is a manifestation of either form of smallpox in a partially immune subject.

Edward Jenner (1798) showed that previous infection with cowpox protected against smallpox. *Vaccinia* is the name given to the infection purposely induced by Jennerian vaccination to prevent smallpox. The precise origin of some strains of vaccinia virus is not known, but some undoubtedly arose from the virus of cowpox (Dudgeon, 1963). Cowpox is a natural disease of cows that was endemic in many farming areas in eighteenth-century England but is seen today only rarely. For a full account of the origin of smallpox vaccine and its relationship to cowpox, the reader should consult *Jenner's Smallpox Vaccine* (Baxby, 1981). Both variola and vaccinia viruses can cause fetal infection, but in view of the completely altered picture resulting from the successful campaign for the eradication of smallpox, which was achieved by the World Health Organization (WHO) in 1979 (WHO, 1979), neither virus now presents a hazard to the fetus. There is no longer any need for smallpox vaccination, so no risk to the fetus exists from inadvertent vaccination in pregnancy. Nevertheless, the details of the risks that once existed are discussed here for reference purposes and for the bearing they have on the pathogenesis of fetal infections.

SMALLPOX

Clinical Manifestations

Full, detailed descriptions of the clinical manifestations of smallpox and alastrim can be found in standard textbooks on the subject (Dixon, 1962; Krugman and Katz, 1981), so only a few aspects pertinent to the consequences of fetal infection are discussed in this chapter.

The incubation period of smallpox is 12 days, with little variation. The disease presents in two phases: a prodromal phase associated with fever and general constitutional symptoms that lasts three or four days; and an eruptive phase with a further rise in temperature. The rash, which may be discrete or confluent, matures through various stages from macules to vesicles to pustules that finally develop into crusts. The mortality rate in confluent smallpox is high (50 per cent), even more so in the hemorrhagic form (80 per cent). Recovery is associated with immunity, since second attacks of smallpox are rare.

Pathogenesis and Pathology

The portal of entry is almost certainly the respiratory tract, where virus multiplies locally before spreading to the regional lymph nodes. There are probably two viremic phases, an assumption based on the analogy between the pathogenesis of smallpox and that of ectromelia, or mousepox, studied by Fenner (1949). The first coincides with the prodromal phase and the second with the onset of the eruptive phase. Infection of the placenta and fetus is presumably the consequence of viremia. Virus is also present in large amounts in the skin and nasopharyngeal washings and can be recovered from the viscera of fatal cases.

The histopathological lesions in the skin are marked by extensive intracellular and extracellular edema of the epithelial cells and cytoplasmic degeneration. The combination of focal necrosis and polymorphonuclear cell infiltration leads to vesicle and pustule formation. Focal necrotic lesions may also be seen in the adrenals, liver, and spleen. Diffuse necrotic lesions in the placenta and viscera have been reported by Garcia (1963) in two fatal cases of fetal alastrim following maternal infection contracted during the fourth and fifth months of pregnancy, respectively.

VACCINIA

Clinical Manifestations

Vaccinia is an acute infectious disease caused by purposeful inoculation of vaccine lymph or by accidental exposure to a recently vaccinated person. Depending on the vaccination technique employed, a local vesicle usually appears within four or five days, matures through a pustular stage, becomes crusted, and then heals, usually between the second and third weeks. During the first week the patient may have a mild fever, and the regional lymph nodes are frequently enlarged. A generalized eruption may also develop between the first and second weeks following primary vaccination, but this is a rare event except in children with atopic eczema (eczema vaccinatum). A more severe form of generalized vaccinia, progressive vaccinia gangrenosa, may occur in persons with some forms of immune deficiency. Many cases of eczema vaccinatum used to occur in children as a result of accidental infection from contact with a recently vaccinated person in the household.

Pathogenesis

Although viremia has never been conclusively demonstrated in primary vaccinia, it almost certainly occurs, albeit for a short period. Generalized vaccinia in the eczematous child results from viremia and from surface spread from infected areas of skin. In uncomplicated primary vaccinia, antibody appears about seven to 10 days after inoculation and reaches a peak during the third week postvaccination. Cell-mediated immunity plays an important part in protection. Revaccination of an immune or partially immune person usually results in a shorter interval before development of the skin lesion. This is probably due to a delayed-type hypersensitivity reaction. Immunity from vaccinia is not as long-lasting as immunity from variola; smallpox can occur in persons who have previously been successfully vaccinated.

CONGENITAL VARIOLA

Documented evidence on the incidence and clinical manifestations of congenital variola following maternal smallpox is scarce. Smallpox, especially variola major, results in a marked increase in fetal death in the first half of gestation and premature delivery in the latter half (Lynch, 1932). Lynch refers to a five-month macerated fetus born of a woman exposed to variola in pregnancy. The mother had been vaccinated in childhood. The infant's skin was covered with an extensive pustular eruption. Premature delivery has been attributed to an increased tendency toward uterine hemorrhage; endometrial bleeding has been recorded by Dixon (1962) in nonpregnant females infected with variola. Most authorities agree that smallpox in pregnant females is more severe and has a higher mortality rate (approximately 50 per cent) than in males and nonpregnant females. The virulence of the strain of variola plays a contributory part; in a study of smallpox over a six-year period (1929 to 1934) at the Smallpox Hospitals in London, Marsden and Greenfield (1934) observed only two women who aborted among many hundreds who contracted smallpox at all stages of pregnancy. These authors noted that during this period more than 13,000 patients admitted to the hospitals were infected with a benign strain of virus and suffered only a modified form of smallpox. This was presumably alastrim or variola minor.

Although congenital infection has ceased to be a matter of concern, the few documented cases are of importance in understanding the mechanisms and pathways of viral infections in the fetus. Marsden and Greenfield (1934) observed 33 women who contracted a mild form of smallpox in the latter stages of pregnancy. Of the 36 infants (there were three twin pregnancies) born to these women, 22 became infected with congenital or "inherited" smallpox; the remaining 14 escaped infection. On closer analysis of these cases, the details of which are shown in Table 8–1, it can be seen that most of the 14 infants who escaped infection were born prior to the mothers' illness or at least a week after the maternal rash appeared (groups 1, 4, and 5). The incubation period in the cases of congenital infection was approximately 11 days; whether the infants were born at the time of the prodromal illness or at the time of the rash in the mother, it seems probable that they were infected *in utero* as a result of maternal viremia. The effect of vaccination in this group of infants is of some interest because vaccination was recorded as "successful," yet in many instances it did not appear to prevent smallpox. Its effect on the severity of the disease is difficult to gauge, as this was, in any case, a particularly mild form of smallpox. The two infants in group I were vaccinated six to eight days after birth and did not develop smallpox. The three infants in group 5 were vaccinated with success on three separate occasions, and although it is conceivable that they had derived protection from their mothers, there is no record in the report of cutaneous lesions or scars to suggest that they had contracted smallpox *in utero*. The majority of the remaining infants in groups 2, 3, and 4 apparently were "successfully" vaccinated but contracted smallpox. Only three infants, two of whom were premature, died. Although the clinical manifestations of congenital variola have not been recorded in any detail, it has been reported that some of the lesions are often much larger than those seen in natural smallpox in the child or adult (Lynch, 1932). Similarly largesized lesions are encountered in congenital vaccinia.

Apart from spontaneous abortion and

Table 8–1. CONGENITAL AND NEONATAL SMALLPOX: DATA EXTRACTED FROM 33 PREGNANCIES SEEN IN SMALLPOX HOSPITALS IN LONDON, 1929–1934

Group*	Day of Birth in Relation to Maternal Illness	No. of Pregnancies	No. of Infants Subsequently Acquiring Smallpox	Age of Infant at Onset of Rash	Death from Smallpox
1	Before prodromal symptoms (4–7 days before rash)	2	0/2	—	—
2	During prodromal symptoms (1–4 days before rash)	9	8/9	10–15 days	1 (premature, died at 4 weeks)
3	During first week of rash (0–6 days after rash)	10†	11/12‡	6–13 days	1 (? premature)
4	After first week of rash (7–9 days after rash)	6	3/6	Birth§	1 (died on day 3)
	(11–21 days after rash)	4	0/4	—	—
5	During late convalescence (25–50 days after rash)	2‖	0/3	—	—
	Total		22/36		

*These do not refer to the groups in the original articles; they have been regrouped in relation to time of exposure.
†Two twin pregnancies.
‡One binovular twin did not contract smallpox.
§Rash in one case estimated to be 3 or 4 days old at birth.
‖One twin pregnancy.
From Marsden, J. P., and Greenfield, C. R. M.: Inherited smallpox. Arch. Dis. Child. *9*:309–314, 1934.

death in early infancy, there is no evidence of congenital defects following fetal variola, although the studies on the two fatal cases of fetal alastrim reported by Garcia (1963) suggest that if the fetuses had survived they would have suffered from severe congenital disease as a result of damage to many viscera.

CONGENITAL VACCINIA

The number of reported cases of fetal or congenital vaccinia is comparatively small, despite the widespread use of smallpox vaccine as a routine procedure before 1979. One of the reasons for this may be that until recent years routine vaccination was usually carried out in the first two years of life, so that *primary* vaccinations were rarely performed in women of childbearing age, except in the face of an imported case or a local outbreak.

One of the first cases of fetal vaccinia was reported by Lynch (1932), who described generalized vaccinial lesions in a six-month fetus born four weeks after vaccination of the mother. A distinctive feature of this case was the size of the lesions, which were similar to those reported by MacDonald and MacArthur (1953). They reported a case following primary vaccination of a young woman when she was three months pregnant. She developed a severe primary vaccinial reaction and gave birth prematurely three months later to a dead infant with generalized vaccinial lesions on the skin and throughout the viscera (Fig. 8–1). MacArthur (1952) carried out a retrospective inquiry into the effect of smallpox vaccination on pregnancy as a result of the mass vaccination program following the smallpox outbreak in Glasgow in 1950.

He found a significantly higher incidence of fetal deaths (47 per cent) in vaccinated women compared with the highest expected figure in the normal population. Forty-seven per cent of women vaccinated in the second and third months of pregnancy and 24 per cent of those vaccinated in the whole of the first trimester failed to give birth to healthy children, compared with 13 per cent in a series of normal pregnancies in Scotland. Entwistle and co-workers (1962) reported another case following primary vaccination of the mother at the nineteenth week of pregnancy. At 23 weeks she gave birth to a premature macerated infant with a similar generalized eruption. The placenta and most of the viscera were also involved. Tucker and Sibson (1962) reported a case in a 19 year old woman who received primary vaccination when she was two and a half months pregnant. After a mild vaccinial illness she recovered, but she gave birth some 10 weeks later to premature twins (Fig. 8–2), both with generalized fetal vaccinia. Vaccinia virus was isolated from the skin. A further case of special interest was observed by Bray (1975) following primary smallpox vaccination during the smallpox outbreak in South Wales in 1961, when mass vaccination was again carried out unnecessarily. The mother was vaccinated at 24 weeks, and the baby was born at 30 weeks (Fig. 8–3) with large vaccinial lesions. The baby survived and at the age of 18 months still had scars resulting from intrauterine Jennerian vaccination (Fig. 8–4). The child was at that time vaccinated without success. The patient is well at the present time but still has scars on the trunk and scalp. The fact that this infant survived suggests that he was immunologically competent to respond to the intrauterine infection, possi-

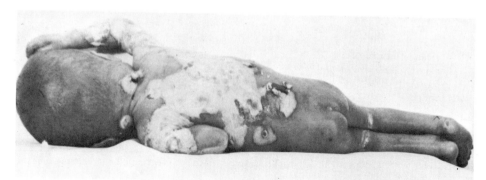

Figure 8–1. Generalized fetal vaccinia, showing diffuse cutaneous lesions, in an infant at six months' gestation. (From MacArthur, P.: Congenital vaccinia and vaccinia gravidarum. Lancet 2:1104–1106, 1952).

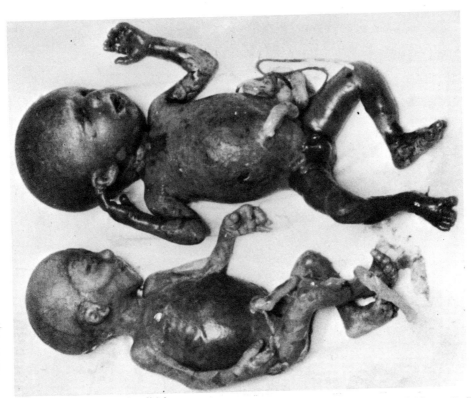

Figure 8–2. Generalized fetal vaccinia in macerated twin fetuses. (From Tucker, S. M., and Sibson, D. E.: Foetal complication of vaccination in pregnancy. Br. Med. J. 2:237–238, 1962.)

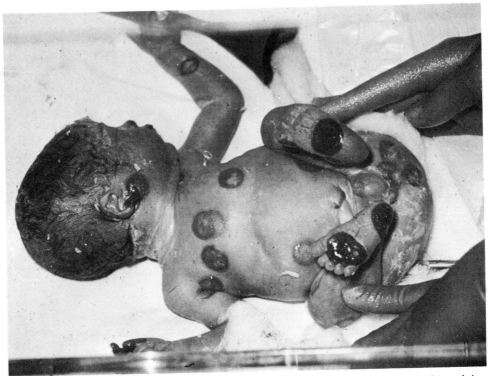

Figure 8–3. Neonate with generalized fetal vaccinia following maternal smallpox vaccination at 24 weeks' gestation, showing large cutaneous lesions.

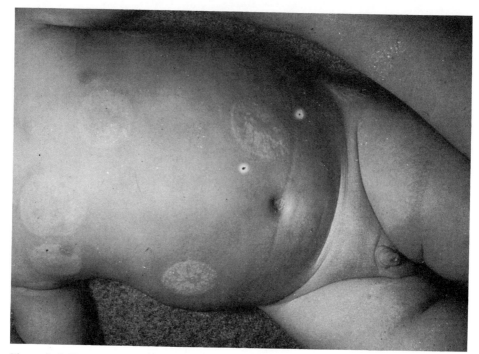

Figure 8–4. The same patient as in Figure 8–3, showing healed skin lesions at 18 months of age.

bly on account of the gestational age at which vaccination was carried out (24 weeks), which was later than those in the other cases.

Approximately 20 cases of fetal vaccinia have been reported in the literature, details of which have been summarized, together with the reasons for vaccination, by Levine and colleagues (1974) (Table 8–2) and by Wilson (1967). This is a small number in view of the very large number of vaccinations that must have been carried out as a result of mass vaccination campaigns. It can be seen from Table 8–2 that the majority of cases have followed primary vaccination of the mother; women who had been revaccinated had been vaccinated 19 to 21 years previously. The time of vaccination in relation to the stage of pregnancy ranged from the third to the twenty-fourth weeks of gestation, but the majority took place in the second trimester. Only three of the liveborn infants survived, and one of those, recorded by Harley

Table 8–2. **SUMMARY OF 20 CASES OF FETAL VACCINIA**

	No. of Cases		No. of Cases
Maternal vaccination		*Outcome of pregnancy*	
Primary	13	Products of conception	21*
Revaccination	3	Full-term infants	1
Unknown	4	Premature terminations	19
		Liveborn infants	10
Reason for vaccination		Survivors	3
Smallpox outbreak	7	Abortions and stillbirths	11
Travel	5		
Accidental vaccinia	2	*Method of diagnosis*	
Work permit	1	Virus isolation	7
Unknown	5	Histopathological method	7
Gestational age at vaccination		Immunological method	2
3rd to 12th week	7	Clinical features	4
13th to 24th week	13		

*One set of twins
From Levine, M. M., Edsall, G., and Bruce-Chwatt, L. J.: Live virus vaccines in pregnancy: risks and recommendations. Lancet 2:34–38, 1974.

and Gillespie (1972), had features of scarring similar to those reported by Bray (1975). Although other lesions were present in the case described by Harley and Gillespie (1972)—namely, destruction of the macula, choroiditis, and hypoplasia of a digit—it is difficult to be certain that these were attributable to the effect of vaccinia virus, although in view of the effect of varicella-zoster virus on the fetus, it is conceivable that they were the result of vaccinial infection.

In a retrospective survey by Greenberg and co-workers (1949) no evidence was found that vaccination had a harmful effect on the fetus. There are several objections to this study in that little or no information was available about abortions. The figures quoted by Levine and colleagues (1974) relate to 8599 vaccinated pregnant women and 11,104 controls, and there was no evidence of fetal wastage, congenital malformations, or fetal vaccinia. These authors concluded "that the cumulative experience involving several thousand women vaccinated beyond the twelfth week of pregnancy attests to the *relative* safety of the procedure. It is against this experience that the 20 cases of fetal vaccinia accumulated over 40 years must be weighed." Despite these small numbers and the almost certain lack of reporting of adverse reactions, there was a risk, albeit a remote one, which has now been removed by the discontinuence of smallpox vaccination.

Apart from a high incidence of fetal death and premature delivery, no evidence of congenital defects has been observed in infants with congenital vaccinia, although if the fetus observed by MacDonald and MacArthur (1953) had survived the probability is that the infant would have had serious damage to many organs and viscera.

Bibliography

Baxby, D.: Jenner's Smallpox Vaccine: The Riddle of Vaccinia Virus and Its Origin. London, Heinemann Educational Books, 1981.

Bray, P. T.: Personal communication, 1975.

Dixon, C. H.: Smallpox. London, J. and A. Churchill, 1962.

Dudgeon, J. A.: Development of smallpox vaccine in England in the 18th and 19th centuries. Br. Med. J. *1*:1367–1372, 1963.

Entwistle, D. M., Bray, P. T., and Laurence, K. M.: Prenatal infection with vaccinia virus. Br. Med. J. *2*:238–239, 1962.

Fenner, F.: Mousepox (infectious ectromelia of mice), a review. J. Immunol. *63*:341–373, 1949.

Garcia, A. G. P.: Fetal infection with chickenpox and alastrim with histopathological studies of the placenta. Pediatrics *32*:895–901, 1963.

Greenberg, M., Yankower, A., Krugman, S., Osborn, J. J., Ward, R. S., and Dancis, J.: Effect of smallpox vaccination during pregnancy on incidence of congenital malformations. Pediatrics *3*:456–467, 1949.

Harley, J. D., and Gillespie, A. M.: A complicated case of congenital vaccinia. Pediatrics *50*:150–153, 1972.

Jenner, E.: An Inquiry into the Causes and Effects of the Variolae Vaccinae. London, 1798.

Krugman, S., and Katz, S.: Infectious Disease of Children and Adults. 8th ed. St. Louis, C. V. Mosby Company, 1981.

Levine, M. M., Edsall, G., and Bruce-Chwatt, L. J.: Live virus vaccines in pregnancy: risks and recommendations. Lancet *2*:34–38, 1974.

Lynch, F. W.: Dermatologic conditions of the fetus. Arch. Dermatol. Syphilol. *26*:997–1019, 1932.

MacArthur, P.: Congenital vaccinia and vaccinia gravidarum. Lancet *2*:1104–1106, 1952.

MacDonald, A. M., and MacArthur, P.: Foetal vaccinia. Arch. Dis. Child. *28*:311–315, 1953.

Marsden, J. P., and Greenfield, C. R. M.: Inherited smallpox. Arch. Dis. Child. *9*:309–314, 1934.

Tucker, S. M., and Sibson, D. E.: Foetal complication of vaccination in pregnancy. Br. Med. J. *2*:237–238, 1962.

Wilson, G. S.: The Hazards of Immunization. Oxford, Oxford University Press, 1967.

World Health Organization (WHO): The achievement of global eradication of smallpox. WHO SE *79*:152, 1979.

9

Viral Hepatitis

INTRODUCTION

The history of our understanding of viral hepatitis is of special interest to those concerned with preventive medicine. The story, admirably recounted by Zuckerman (1975) and Zuckerman and Howard (1979), is full of astute clinical and epidemiological observations, made in many instances long before the etiological agents of the disease had been identified.

By the beginning of the Second World War, prevailing opinion held that jaundice was infectious in nature and existed in at least two forms. The concept of jaundice was replaced by one of hepatitis because of the inflammatory changes characteristic of the latter. During the war several outbreaks of hepatitis occurred that not only confirmed these views, but also emphasized the importance of hepatitis as a public health problem. The explosive epidemic of hepatitis in the British Eighth Army in the Western Desert in 1942 caused almost as many medical as battle casualties in some units, and there is evidence that the incidence of the disease among the opposing forces was even higher. This epidemic was almost certainly due to what is now known as hepatitis type A. In 1942 a major outbreak of hepatitis also occurred in U.S. military personnel following immunization with yellow fever vaccine. Approximately 30,000 servicemen were affected, some very severely, and 62 deaths resulted. This outbreak was almost certainly due to hepatitis type B, resulting from the then-current practice of reconstituting yellow fever vaccine in human plasma. It is of inter-

est that only a few years previously Findlay and co-workers (1939), while investigating the association between yellow fever vaccine and hepatitis, had made the following observation: "Pools of apparently normal serum should not be used for inoculation unless the medical history of all the donors can be followed over a considerable period of time, preferably for at least one month, the probable incubation period of infective hepatitis." This was a very shrewd observation, considering the state of knowledge at the time, and although it was not entirely accurate, it was not far short of the mark.

During the period from 1940 to 1960 a mass of new evidence accrued as the result of experiments on human subjects. From all these observations it became evident that at least two distinct forms of hepatitis existed. These differed in two main respects, the incubation period and the mode of transmission. MacCallum (1947) introduced the terms "hepatitis A" for infectious hepatitis and "hepatitis B" for the form associated with serum jaundice or homologous serum jaundice.

For obvious reasons, there was a limit to the amount of information that could be derived from human experimentation, and alternative methods of studying hepatitis virus diseases had to be sought. In the early 1960's much faith and hope were placed in the use of cell and tissue culture techniques, which had led to dramatic breakthroughs in the study of other virus diseases. The results were extremely disappointing, but an entirely new era opened up with a chance discovery by Blumberg and his colleagues (1965), who were working on inherited antigenic differences in human serum β-lipoproteins. These workers found that a lipoprotein antigen in human serum reacted with antisera from hemophiliacs and other multiply transfused patients. Because this lipoprotein antigen was detected in the serum of an Australian aborigine, it was referred to as the Australian (Au) antigen (Blumberg et al., 1967).

Meanwhile, Prince and his colleagues (1964) had used fluorescence techniques to describe an antigen in foci of hepatic cells from patients with hepatitis. Antibody to the antigen was detected in sera from soldiers from Korea by immunodiffusion techniques similar to those used by Blumberg. Prince (1968) was able to detect an antigen in the sera of patients with acute-phase transfusion hepatitis. It was not found in patients with short-incubation infectious hepatitis. Subsequent studies established the relationship between this serum hepatitis (SH) antigen, the Au antigen, and hepatitis B.

Many of the features of viral hepatitis, including its relevance to public health, its mode of spread, and tactics for its prevention, are reflected in the numerous names and synonyms which have, from time to time, been given to the various forms of jaundice and hepatitis. These names are listed in Table 9–1.

VIRAL HEPATITIS: THE PRESENT CONCEPT

Today, viral hepatitis presents a key problem in the control of communicable diseases. At least three distinct etiological forms are now known to exist. There may be more. They have been redesignated by the World Health Organisation (WHO) (1973) and by a WHO Working Group (Deinhardt and Gust, 1982) as follows:

Hepatitis A (HA),
Hepatitis B (HB),
Hepatitis non-A, non-B (HNANB).

Table 9–1. EARLIER NOMENCLATURE OF VIRAL HEPATITIS

Catarrhal jaundice	Homologous serum jaundice
Campaign jaundice	Serum jaundice
Epidemic jaundice	Syringe-transmitted jaundice
Infectious jaundice	Serum hepatitis
Infectious hepatitis	MS-2 long-incubation type
MS-1 short-	hepatitis
incubation type	Hepatitis B
hepatitis	
Hepatitis A	

The etiological agents of HA and HB are quite distinct and have now been fully characterized, but those of HNANB have not. All three types have been transmitted to nonhuman primates, but at present the diagnosis of HNANB, which appears to be a common form of hepatitis following transfusion, is made by exclusion of the other two types. Although HNANB constitutes a major public health problem, there is little evidence that it is an important hazard to the fetus or newborn, except with respect to fetal loss related to natural death in one epidemic (Khuroo et al., 1981).

Another form of hepatitis, associated with the Delta antigen, has recently been described (Rizzetto et al., 1977, 1981). The Delta antigen was originally detected by fluorescence in hepatocytes of patients with chronic active hepatitis. It appears to be a defective, virus-like agent that requires the presence of hepatitis B virus (HBV) for replication and transmission. Epidemiological studies have shown that it has a worldwide distribution, with an unusually high endemic focus in southern Italy. Present evidence does not suggest that it is an important problem in perinatal hepatitis infections. One instance of mother-infant transmission has been reported (Deinhardt and Gust, 1982). Nevertheless, in view of the close association between the Delta antigen and HBV and with cases of chronic active hepatitis, its contributory role in maternal-infant infections requires further study.

The proposed WHO nomenclature for the three main viral agents, their antigens, and their respective antibodies is shown in Table 9–2.

From the clinical standpoint there are few differences between the three main forms of hepatitis and the Delta-associated type. Certain features, such as clustering, may point to one form or the other, but laboratory tests should, wherever possible, be used in the investigation of cases or outbreaks. Highly sensitive tests are now available, many from commercial sources, which if used in conjunction with national reference laboratories should help to elucidate some of the outstanding problems in our understanding of viral hepatitis.

This chapter is concerned with the effect of hepatitis viruses on the fetus and newborn. It emphasizes maternal-infant transmission, especially during the perinatal period. Full details on viral hepatitis as it affects other age groups and on its pathology and epide-

Table 9–2. **THE NEW NOMENCLATURE: COMPONENTS AND CORRESPONDING ANTIBODIES OF THE HEPATITIS VIRUSES**

Virus Component or Antibody	Definition
HA	Hepatitis A
HAV	Hepatitis A virus
HAAg	Hepatitis A antigen
anti-HAV	Antibody to hepatitis A without differentiation of immunoglobulin class
anti-HAIgG	Antibody to hepatitis A of the IgG class
anti-HAIgM	Antibody to hepatitis A of the IgM class
anti-HAIgA	Antibody to hepatitis A of the IgA class
HB	Hepatitis B
HBV	Hepatitis B virus (Dane particle)
HBsAg	Hepatitis B surface antigen
HBeAg	Hepatitis B e antigen
HBcAg	Hepatitis B core antigen
anti-HBs	Antibody to hepatitis B surface antigen
anti-HBc	Antibody to hepatitis B antigen without differentiation of immunoglobulin class
anti-HBcIgM	Antibody to hepatitis B core antigen of the IgM class
anti-HBe	Antibody to hepatitis B e antigen
HNANB	Hepatitis non-A, non-B

Data from Deinhardt, F., and Gust, I.: Viral hepatitis. Bull. W.H.O. *60*:661–691, 1982.

miology can be found in monographs devoted to virus infections in general (e.g., Krugman and Katz [1981]).

HEPATITIS A

In 1973 a major breakthrough in the study of viral hepatitis was made by Feinstone and colleagues (1973). They observed virus-like particles by electron microscopy in the feces of patients with viral hepatitis induced by inoculation with MS-1 serum (see Table 9–1). The virus particles aggregated with convalescent sera from the volunteers and with sera from patients naturally infected with hepatitis A virus (HAV) but not with HBV.

The Causative Agent

HAV is an RNA virus and possesses all the features of an enterovirus. It has been classified as enterovirus type 72, a member of the Picornaviridae (Andrewes et al., 1978). The virus particles measure 27 nm in diameter, have cubic symmetry, and are made up of 32 capsomeres. HAV is more stable than the other enteroviruses, such as poliovirus.

Partial inactivation occurs at 60° C after a prolonged period of heating, but boiling for 5 minutes results in loss of infectivity. Partially purified virus is sensitive to formalin (1 in 4000) and to chlorine.

Natural History and Pathogenesis

In many respects the natural history and pathogenesis of HAV infection resemble those of poliomyelitis, the essential difference being that the target body is the hepatocyte and not the neuron. The incubation period varies from 15 to 40 days. The onset is usually acute, but anicteric infections are extremely common in children. Liver function test results are abnormal for a few days preceding the onset of jaundice, and the duration of virus excretion in the feces is relatively short. It may last for two to three weeks before the onset of the disease and persist for four to six weeks. Virus is present in the blood for a short period and does not persist as in HBV infections. Again unlike in HBV, a carrier state does not develop.

Anti-HAV—in particular, anti-HAIgM— is present at the time of onset of jaundice, reaches a peak six to eight weeks after exposure, and then declines. Anti-HAIgG persists for a prolonged period. As far as is known there is only one serotype of HAV. Long-term immunity normally follows recovery from HAV; there is no cross-immunity between HAV and HBV.

Epidemiology

HAV infection has a worldwide distribution, but major differences in the incidence of the disease, as well as in the age at which infection is acquired, have recently become apparent. In the developed countries of the world the age at which HAV is acquired is changing from childhood to adolescence. In many countries in Europe and North America notification and epidemiological data indicate a dramatic decrease in the incidence of HAV. In Europe the prevalence of anti-HAV in young adults aged 20 to 29 years varies from 3 to 5 per cent in the Scandinavian countries, to around 15 per cent in mid-Europe and the United Kingdom, to 80 to 90 per cent in Italy and Spain (Mortimer, 1980). In the developing areas of the world, where standards of hygiene and sanitation are low, the prevalence of anti-HAV as an indicator of past infection is extremely high.

The Effect on the Fetus

The effect of maternal HAV infection on the fetus and newborn has not been studied in detail. Pregnant women who, on the basis of an incubation period of 15 to 50 days and an acute but relatively transient disease course, are judged to have clinical infectious hepatitis have rarely given birth to infants with congenital malformations or acute illness of any sort. A study by Schwer and Moosa (1978) in South Africa provided no evidence that HAV infection in pregnancy posed any risk to the mother or fetus. Heiber and co-workers (1977) studied the effect of acute viral hepatitis in 50 pregnancies and concluded that neither HBV nor non–type B (not specified as to whether these were cases of HAV or HNANB) led to an increased incidence of congenital malformations, but the number of subjects in the study was small. The most common associated abnormalities are prematurity and spontaneous abortion. These are more likely if infection occurs early in the pregnancy. It is relatively rare for the infant to be born with jaundice (Zondek and Bromberg, 1947; Mickal, 1951; Hsia et al., 1952; Mansell, 1955; Siegler and Kevser, 1963; Adams and Combes, 1965).

The prospective studies on the effect of maternal virus infections on the fetus (Siegel and Fuerst, 1966; Siegel et al., 1966) referred to in Chapter 2 pointed to an increase in the frequency of premature births and abortions following several virus infections, including hepatitis (type unspecified). In the case of hepatitis the outcome was probably related to the early onset of labor resulting from the severity of the maternal illness.

Infectious hepatitis around the time of conception has been associated on epidemiological grounds with Down's syndrome by Stoller and Collmann (1965) in Australia. These investigators noted an increased prevalence of Down's syndrome, occurring nine months after peaks of viral hepatitis, at five- to six-year intervals. Pantelakis and colleagues (1970) in Athens found that mothers who had viral hepatitis prior to birth were three times more likely to deliver an infant with Down's syndrome than control mothers. Kucera (1970) in the Soviet Union observed the association of a history of viral hepatitis contact at the time of conception and the birth of an infant with Down's syndrome.

Other investigators have failed to confirm these findings (Leck, 1966; Stark and Franmeni, 1966; Ceccarelli and Torbidoni, 1967). All of these studies were done without the use of techniques to distinguish HBV from HAV. On present evidence there is nothing to substantiate an etiological relationship between HAV and Down's syndrome. Now that sensitive laboratory tests are available for the diagnosis of HAV and HBV infections, it should be possible to prove such an association if it exists.

Laboratory Aspects

The laboratory diagnosis of HAV infection is discussed in detail in Chapter 14, but a few details are mentioned here for the sake of convenience and for comparison with the subsequent section on HBV.

Virus particles of HAV can be detected in the feces by electron microscopy and by radioimmunoassay (RIA) and enzyme-linked immunosorbent assay (ELISA) during the incubation period and before the onset of symptoms. The finding of virus particles is of less diagnostic value than detection of anti-HAIgM.

The virus will replicate in a restricted number of cell culture systems, which may ultimately be of diagnostic value but are more likely to form the basis for vaccine production. HAV was initially adapted in primary cultures of marmoset liver cells (Provost and Hilleman, 1979) and in a semicontinuous line of fetal rhesus monkey kidney cells (strain FRh K6). The virus replicates in primary and continuous cell lines of primate origin, particularly at 32 and 35° C. Unlike many other viruses, HAV does not produce a cytopathic effect, and viral replication can be detected only by methods such as electron microscopy, immunofluorescence, RIA, and ELISA.

HAV can be transmitted to a number of nonhuman primates, such as marmosets, chimpanzees, and other species. The most susceptible species are chimpanzees, other apes, and marmosets (*Saguinus labiatus, S. mystax,* and *S. fuscicollis*).

HEPATITIS B

The Causative Agent

HBV is a DNA virus with unique properties. The whole virus particle, or Dane particle, has a diameter of 42 nm. This is almost certainly the infectious virus. The surface protein coat is produced in excess in the form of spherical antigen particles, 22 nm in diameter, known as the surface antigen (HBsAg). Treatment of the whole virus particle with detergents removes the surface antigen to reveal an inner core 27 nm in diameter, the core antigen (HBcAg). In addition, long, filamentous forms with the same diameter as the surface antigen can be seen in serum by electron microscopy. The viral core particle comprises the viral core antigen and genome, an unusual form of circular DNA in its fully stranded form. An additional antigen, the e antigen (HBeAg), and a DNA-dependent polymerase are also associated with the virus, probably more closely with the surface antigen. The e antigen is a soluble antigen and is closely related to infectivity.

HBV probably consists of one major antigenic type, but distinct genotype variants may exist. If they do, they are probably closely related, and, as far as prevention is concerned, it would appear that only the group antigen determinant *a* is required.

The surface antigen consists of a common specific antigen designated *a* and subdeterminants *d, w, y,* and *r.* The four major subtypes have been designated *adw, ayw, adr,* and *ayr* with minor subdeterminants of the above subtypes. These types and subtypes appear to be of little clinical significance, nor do they pose a problem as far as the antigenic composition of a vaccine is concerned, but they are of epidemiological importance in determining the geographical incidence of HBV. The same applies to minor subtypes of the e antigen, several of which have now been identified (Zuckerman and Howard, 1979; Deinhardt and Gust, 1982).

Natural History and Pathogenesis

Apart from the fact that HBV is spread by the parenteral route and that the incubation period is longer than that for HAV, little is known about the site of primary multiplication or mode of spread during the incubation period. As with HAV, the liver is the target organ and the hepatocyte the principal target cell. *Homo sapiens* appears to be the sole reservoir of infection, although nonhuman primates are susceptible to experimental infection. As far as is known, no insect vectors are involved in the transmission of the disease. Recently, however, viruses similar in nature to HBV have been identified in several animal species—the woodchuck, ground squirrel, and Peking duck (Deinhardt and Gust, 1982). These viruses have several properties in common with HBV, but they appear to be species-specific. Their relevance to HBV is not yet clear, but a study of these animal viruses of the hepadnavirus group may uncover some of the missing links in the pathogenesis of the human disease.

HBV has now been established as a major causative factor in primary hepatocellular carcinoma, an extremely common tumor in many parts of the world (Maupas and Melnick, 1981; WHO Scientific Working Groups, 1983).

Exposure to HBV may result in one of the following outcomes:

1. An acute, self-limiting infection with or without clinical hepatitis. This is the common form of HBV infection, and although infectivity may persist for somewhat longer periods than in other viral infections, it is usually lost and antibody (anti-HBc and anti-HBs) appears in the blood.

2. An acute infection followed by the development of an asymptomatic carrier state with persistence of HBsAg.

3. An acute infection followed by chronic active hepatitis and persistence of HBsAg and other stigmata of a persistent infection.

The risk of transmission of infection from a mother to the newborn—and perhaps to about 5 per cent of fetuses *in utero,* as a result of leakage of maternal blood from placental damage—exists in any of these circumstances and is likely to be greater when HBsAg and HBeAg persist for long periods. Differentiation of the three types of infection can be made by laboratory tests for the detection of the HB antigens and their respective antibodies. Possible test results and their interpretations are summarized in Table 9–3. It is helpful in understanding the mode of transmission from mother to infant to refer to the detailed stages of the pathogenesis of the three types of infection. These are shown in diagrammatic form in Figures 9–1 to 9–3 and in the publication by Deinhardt and Gust (1982) already referred to.

Epidemiology

Prevalence of the Disease

HBV is one of the major public health problems at the present time. The disease is

Table 9–3. **INTERPRETATION OF THE PRESENCE OF COMBINATIONS OF SEROLOGICAL MARKERS OF HBV**

HBsAg	HBeAg	Anti-HBe	Anti-HBc	Anti-HBs	Interpretation	Infectivity of Blood
+	+	−	−	−	Incubation period for early acute HB	High
+	+	−	+	−	Acute HB or chronic carrier	High
+	−	+	+	−	Late during HB or chronic carrier	Low
−	−	+	+	+	Convalescent from acute HB	Low
−	−	−	+	+	Recovered from past HB infection	None
−	−	−	−	+	Immunized without infection; repeated exposure to HBsAg without infection; recovered from past infection	None
−	−	−	+	−	Recovered from past HB infection with undetectable anti-HBs; early convalescent or chronic infection	Questionable

Data from Deinhardt, F., and Gust, I.: Viral hepatitis Bull. W.H.O. *60*:661–691, 1982.

endemic throughout the world. Only a rough estimate of the number of cases of HBV can be made because of lack of reporting, but it has been estimated that of the 50,000 to 60,000 new cases of hepatitis reported annually to the Centers for Disease Control in Atlanta, approximately half may be due to HBV (Deinhardt and Gust, 1982). This is in striking contrast to the epidemiology of HAV, which has shown a marked decline in many areas. A more realistic estimate, after allowing for under-reporting, would put the number of cases of HBV infection as high as 150,000 per annum in the United States. In other parts of the world the figure would be

proportionately higher. For example, Mortimer (1980) has estimated that in the United Kingdom in 1974 and 1978, when 7609 and 4603 cases of infectious hepatitis were reported to the Office of Population Census and Statistics, only 2.5 per cent and 1.9 per cent of these cases were HBsAg-positive.

More accurate data on the incidence of the carrier state are now emerging as tests for HBsAg and other markers of HBV infection become available. Deinhardt and Gust (1982) have estimated that the number of persistent carriers in the world may be 200 million or more. The risk of maternal-infant transmission has to be viewed against this background.

The prevalence of HBV throughout the world varies greatly from one region to another and among different ethnic groups. It is generally low in countries with high standards of living and high where socioeconomic

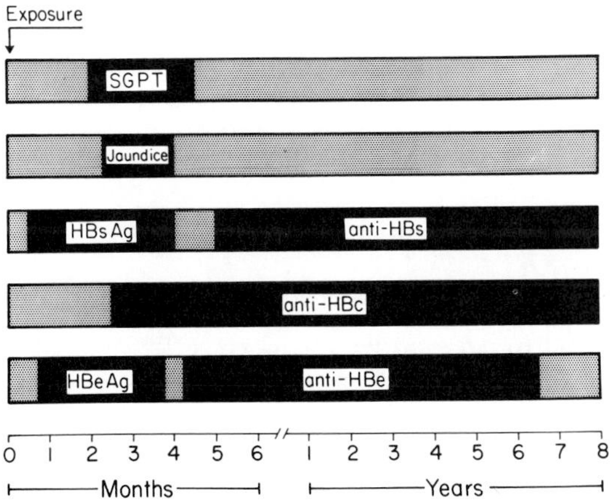

Figure 9–1. Acute viral hepatitis type B followed by recovery, showing results in one patient of serial tests over 7 years for serum aspartate aminotransferase (glutamic oxaloacetic transaminase) (SGOT), hepatitis B surface antigen (HBsAg), hepatitis B e antigen (HBeAg), antibody to hepatitis B core antigen (anti-HBc), antibody to HBeAg (anti-HBe), and antibody to HBsAg (anti-HBs). Solid black areas denote "abnormal" or "detectable" and stippled areas "normal" or "not detectable" levels. (From Krugman, S., and Katz, S. L.: *Infectious Disease of Children.* 7th ed. St. Louis, C. V. Mosby Company, 1981.)

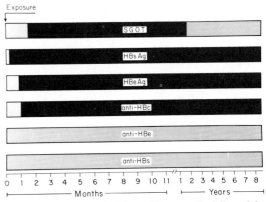

Figure 9–2. Acute viral hepatitis, type B, followed by chronic active hepatitis. Results of serial tests for SGOT, HBsAg, HBeAg, anti-HBc, and anti-HBs. See Figure 9–1 for key. (From Krugman, S., and Katz, S. L.: *Infectious Diseases of Children.* 7th ed. St. Louis, C. V. Mosby Company, 1981.

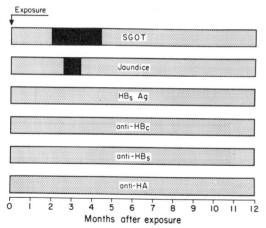

Figure 9–3. Non-A, non-B acute viral hepatitis. Results of serial tests for SGOT, jaundice, HbsAg, anti-Hbc, anti-HBs, and hepatitis A antibody (anti-HA). See Figure 9–1 for key. (From Krugman, S., and Katz, S. L.: *Infectious Diseases of Children.* 7th ed. St. Louis, C. V. Mosby Company, 1981.)

conditions are poor (see Table 9–4). In one small island in the Pacific, Rapa, it is one in two (Deinhardt and Gust, 1982). Several factors predispose to the acquisition and frequency of the carrier state:

1. The age at which infection occurs. The risk may be 5 to 10 per cent for adults but 50 per cent or more for infants.

2. The prevalence of HBV in the community and the part played by cultural, environmental, and host factors.

3. The coexistence of individuals with immunosuppressive disease, those on immunosuppressive therapy, and those with lymphoproliferative disorders, all of which predispose to the carrier state.

The pattern of HB prevalence can be broadly classified into three categories—low, intermediate, and high. Details are shown in Table 9–4.

Source of Virus

Blood and blood products are the main sources of HBV, but other body fluids and secretions, including saliva, semen, cervical secretions, and breast milk, may also contain the virus. It is not clear, however, whether this is because minute traces of blood contaminate the secretions. Similarly, fomites such as syringes, razors, toothbrushes, and other household paraphernalia may harbor the virus as a result of contamination with HBV-infected blood and thus act as a link in the chain of transmission.

Mode of Spread

Some of the ways by which HBV is transmitted are shown in Table 9–5. These can be broadly classified into two main routes: horizontal transmission, the traditional means by which infected blood or blood products lead to spread of the disease; and vertical transmission from mother to infant. The latter category is now accepted as a major route by which HBV infection is spread. Three at-risk periods have been identified in vertical or mother-to-infant transmission. These are (1) during fetal life, when intrauterine or transplacental infection may occur (the latter may account for up to 5 per cent of infections resulting from leak of maternal blood due to placental tears), (2) at parturition (from infected maternal blood and secretions), and (3) during the postnatal period.

At one time it was thought that HBV could be spread by the fecal-oral route. This now seems unlikely. It also seemed possible, in view of the prevalence of HBV in Africa, that insect vectors could be responsible for spread of the disease, but no evidence of such transmission has been forthcoming.

Transmission of HBV in Pregnancy

Acute Hepatitis in Pregnancy

Schweitzer and co-workers (1972) studied 56 mother-infant pairs in which the mothers had acquired acute viral hepatitis in pregnancy or within six months of delivery. The

Table 9–4. PATTERNS OF HB PREVALENCE

Low	Intermediate	High
HBsAg, 0.2%–0.5%	HBsAg, 2%–7%	
Anti-HBs, 4%–6%	Anti-HBs, 20%–50%	HBsAg, 8%–20%
Childhood infection infrequent	Childhood infection frequent; neonatal infection frequent	Anti-HBs, 70%–80%
		Childhood infection highly frequent; neonatal infection highly frequent
Australia, Central Europe, North America	Eastern Europe, Japan, Mediterranean, Southwest Asia, USSR	Some parts of China, southern Asia, and tropical Africa

Data from Deinhardt, F., and Gust, I.: Viral hepatitis. Bull. W.H.O. *60*;661–691, 1982.

Table 9–5. **SOURCE OF INFECTION, MODE OF SPREAD, AND AT-RISK GROUPS IN HBV INFECTIONS**

Source of Virus	Fomites	Principal Mode of Spread	Major At-Risk Groups
Blood and blood products (plasma, serum, some batches of Factor VIII)	Syringes, needles	Transfusion, contaminated abrasions, handling HBV–infected blood specimens	General population, hospital staff, health-care personnel, laboratory staff (hematology and biochemistry), drug addicts
Blood from infected or carrier mother; ingestion of maternal blood or blood-contaminated liquor	None	Vertical, perinatal, mother-infant, in utero, at birth, postnatal	Neonates
Saliva, semen, blood, cervical secretions (breast milk)	Razors, toothbrushes, towels, other household utensils	Close contact, overcrowding, sexual intercourse	Family contacts, siblings, homosexuals, drug addicts

risk of infection to the fetus was greater when maternal infection occurred late in pregnancy or after birth than when it occurred in the first or second trimesters. HBsAg was transmitted from mother to infant by 10 of the 26 mothers who were antigen-positive at the time of delivery and by eight of 17 in whom the onset of hepatitis occurred within two months of delivery. HBsAg was found in two of 19 cord blood samples. Schweitzer et al. (1972) concluded that HBsAg was probably transmitted transplacentally in three cases and that the infected babies whose mothers had had hepatitis near term were probably infected at birth. In an additional study of 31 infants, Schweitzer et al. (1973b) detected HBsAg in 17 of 31 infants; neonatal infection occurred in 16 of 21 infants (76 per cent) following infection in the third trimester or soon after birth but in only one of 10 infants (10 per cent) whose mothers had had HB in the first two trimesters. Two of the 17 infected infants who acquired a mild illness with clinical hepatitis, transient antigenemia, and a significant rise in anti-HBs recovered fully, whereas the 15 asymptomatic infants became persistent carriers of HBsAg for periods of up to 39 weeks. None of the 15 infants developed anti-HBs, and all had histopathological evidence of unresolved neonatal hepatitis and elevated transaminase levels. A further study by Schweitzer (1975) revealed that only 6 per cent of babies exposed to HBV in the first trimester became infected, compared with 69 per cent exposed during the third trimester and 70 per cent exposed in the first two months after birth.

Cossart (1973, 1974), in a review of the literature, also found that there was little or no risk of fetal infection following maternal HBV in early pregnancy but that the risk was on the order of 50 per cent when the illness occurred late in pregnancy. As further evidence of this risk, Schweitzer and colleagues

(1973a) observed three mothers who developed hepatitis and were antigen-positive at birth. The infants were antigen-negative at birth but became antigen-positive between 34 and 96 days of age. Similar findings have been reported by Merrill and co-workers (1972). Boxall (1980) also recorded a case of an infant who became antigen-positive one month after delivery following acute HBV in the mother.

Thus, it can be postulated that if HBV infection occurs early in pregnancy, the virus does not cross the placenta and there is time for the mother to recover and develop immunity before delivery. In these cases it is expected that the infant would be HBsAg-negative and antibody-positive, unless the mother had become a carrier by the end of pregnancy.

Perinatal and Neonatal Transmission from Carrier Mothers

Transmission of HBV from carrier mothers is one of the most important factors in the continued high prevalence of hepatitis in many parts of the world. There is a striking variation in the incidence of transmission from chronic carriers from one country to another. This is shown in Table 9–6. In a review of nine studies in six different countries, Boxall (1980) has shown that the incidence of HBsAg-positive infants ranged from 6 per cent in Denmark to 76.3 per cent in Hong Kong. Two fairly distinct patterns of prevalence of antigen-positive infants emerged. The incidence was low in Western Europe and North America (4.4 and 16.6 per cent) but ranged from 43 to 70 per cent in parts of Asia. It was also evident from studies in the United Kingdom that there was a marked difference in incidence among infants whose mothers were from different ethnic groups. HBsAg was found in 4.4 per

Table 9–6. **TRANSMISSION OF HBV FROM HBsAg CARRIER MOTHERS TO THEIR INFANTS**

Country	No. of Infants Studied	No. of Infants HBsAg-Positive (%)		Reference
Japan	11	8	(72)	Okada et al. (1975)
Japan	23	10	(43)	Okada et al. (1976)
Taiwan	158	63	(40.3)	Stevens et al. (1975)
Hong Kong	37	26	(70.3)	Lee et al. (1978)
Thailand	14	0	(−)	Punyagupta et al. (1973)
India	17	1	(5.9)	Aziz et al. (1973)
Denmark	28	0	(−)	Skinhoj et al. (1972)
Denmark	17	1	(5.9)	Skinhoj et al. (1976)
Greece	11	2	(18.2)	Papaevangolou (1973)
United Kingdom	90 white	4	(4.4)	Derso et al. (1978)
	13 black	4	(31)	
	14 Chinese	9	(64)	
U.S.A.	21	1	(4.7)	Schweitzer et al. (1973a)
U.S.A.	36	6	(16.6)	Schweitzer (1975)

cent of infants born to white mothers, 31 per cent of those born to black mothers, and 64 per cent of those whose mothers were of Chinese origin. According to Boxall (1980), these figures relate to the transmission of HBV from asymptomatic chronic carrier mothers, which presumably is a reflection of the persistence of HBsAg and particularly of the e antigen.

Association of the Carrier State with HBeAg

A close correlation exists between the presence of HBeAg and chronic liver disease, whereas anti-HBe is usually associated with the so-called healthy carrier state. The presence of the e antigen is a general measure of infectivity but not an absolute one. This is of special importance among different ethnic groups, particularly those of African and Chinese origin. Grady (1976), in an accident study in the United States, found that 60 per cent of individuals became infected when e antigen was detected in the initial inoculum, compared with only 31 per cent when it was not present.

If HBeAg is detected in acute-phase viral hepatitis, the risk of the infant becoming a carrier is greater than in e antigen–negative cases. Tong and co-workers (1979) described two cases of e antigen–positive mothers whose infants became chronic carriers; a baby born to an e antigen–negative mother remained antigen-free. Boxall (1980), in a review of the latest data, has concluded that, although the risk of becoming a chronic carrier is greater in infants born of e antigen–positive mothers, it is not absolute. In a study in Taiwan, Stevens and colleagues (1979)

showed that 85 per cent of babies born to e antigen–positive mothers became carriers, but 31 per cent of babies born to e antigen–negative mothers also became carriers. Reports of the risk of transmission of HBV from e antigen–positive mothers have varied from 46 per cent (Derso et al., 1978) to 80 and 85 per cent (Okada et al., 1976; Stevens et al., 1979). The figures quoted by Derso and co-workers (1978) and by Beasley and co-workers (1977) also record that between 5.5 and 9.4 per cent of e antigen–positive mothers gave birth to antigen-negative babies.

The relative roles of the surface and e antigens in determining the outcome of maternal-infant transmission are exemplified by the report of three cases made by Sinatra and colleagues (1982). They observed three infants born to carrier mothers who were HBsAg-positive but had anti-HBe. All three infants developed acute icteric HBV within three months of birth; all recovered and developed anti-HBs.

Other Forms of Perinatal and Postnatal Infection

Infection can be acquired from the mother or from an infected sibling. It has been suggested that antigen-positive mothers can infect their infants by breast-feeding. This has not been clearly established (Boxall, 1980). Beasley and co-workers (1975) found that the number of breast-fed babies who became antigen-positive was 45 of 92 (49 per cent), compared with 29 of 56 (53 per cent) bottle-fed babies. Derso and colleagues (1978), in a study in the United Kingdom, found that the incidence of antigen-positive infants was slightly higher in the bottle-fed group (23 per cent) than in the breast-fed group (12.5 per cent). Merrill and co-workers (1972) failed to detect either HBSAg or anti-HBS in the colostrum in a group of mothers, although their sera were antigen-positive. The babies became antigen-positive without being breast-fed.

Recommendations regarding breast-feeding in these circumstances require very careful case evaluation, in which the advantages of breast-feeding should be weighed against a potential, although low, risk of the infants' acquiring infection.

Postnatal Transmission within the Family

Clustering of cases of HB within families is well recognized. It is more likely to occur in households where there is overcrowding and where poor socioeconomic conditions prevail. Familial clustering of cases of Au antigen–positive hepatitis have been reported by Hadziyannis and Merikas (1970) and by Ohlayashi and colleagues (1972). The most certain evidence of familial spread was obtained by studies by Szmuness and co-workers (1973) in New York City. They observed that the incidence of familial infection was 6.7 per cent in households with HBsAg carriers, compared with 0.8 per cent in control households. Close and prolonged contact favored the spread of infection, particularly among siblings. Nonsexual transmission appeared to be the most likely mode of spread (see Table 9–5).

Summary of Mode of Spread from Mothers to Infants

Transplacental Intrauterine Infection

This appears to be an uncommon mode of transmission, particularly in the first and second trimesters of pregnancy. Infection in the third trimester undoubtedly occurs, but it is difficult to distinguish true intrauterine infection from a perinatal infection on the basis of the incubation period and the presence of HBsAg in the cord blood. Minute traces of infected maternal blood could invalidate the findings. Nevertheless, a few cases of authentic positive cord bloods have been reported, indicating that transplacental infection had taken place. Schweitzer and colleagues (1972) identified antigen in the cord blood of two of 19 infants. Cossart (1974) observed one such case. Desmyter and co-workers (1973) failed to detect antigen in the cord blood of 15 infants of antigen-positive mothers, and only one of these infants had demonstrable antibody in the cord blood. On the other hand, Bucholz and colleagues (1974) detected HBsAg in the cord blood by passive hemagglutination, and the infant, delivered by cesarean section, was antigen-positive. Schweitzer (1975) described a mother who developed clinical hepatitis in the sixth month of pregnancy; she recovered, became antigen-negative, and gave birth to an antigen-positive infant. The study by Okada and co-workers (1975) from Japan also indicated that intrauterine infection was rare.

Perinatal Infection

Infection at the time of birth seems to be most likely if the mother has acute hepatitis or is a carrier. Contaminated amniotic fluid, infected blood, and cervical secretions all provide opportunities for infection to be acquired in this way. As Krugman and Katz (1981) have observed, an infant is born "in a bath of blood," which favors infection from virus-contaminated blood. Lee and colleagues (1978) have provided convincing evidence of the risk of infection at this time. HBsAg was detected in 17 of 52 (32.7 per cent) samples of amniotic fluid extracted at 37 weeks of gestation. They also found that 61 of 64 (95.3 per cent) samples of gastric fluid aspirated from babies during resuscitation contained antigen. Oral ingestion and surface contamination provided ample opportunity for infection to occur, but despite the fact that 98.3 per cent of the infants were exposed to antigen-positive vaginal fluid, only 70.3 per cent became antigen-positive. It must be concluded that infection by the oral route requires a heavy infective dose of virus.

The Clinical Outcome for the Infected Infant

General

The majority of infants exposed and infected in the perinatal period remain clinically normal for prolonged periods despite being antigen-positive. They thrive and have no clinical evidence of hepatitis. However, some follow-up studies have revealed less encouraging results. The two studies by Schweitzer and co-workers (1972, 1973a and b) are of special significance. In the study on 56 mother-infant pairs, it was found that antigenemia persisted for four to 39 months (mean, 18 months). None of the patients examined became antigen-negative. In a more detailed study on 20 infants, it was found that two infants developed mild clinical hepatitis with anti-HBs, but the other 18 infants remained HBsAg-positive for periods of up to five years without hepatitis. All had abnormal results on liver function tests, and in 10 patients there was histological evidence of a chronic hepatitis consistent with the changes observed in neonatal hepatitis. In retrospect, it was found that there was an increased frequency of low birth weight and prematurity among these 10 infants. Both could have resulted from the severity of the maternal illness or from defects in the infants' immune mechanisms. The remaining eight infants with persistent antigenemia remained clinically normal, but two had raised transaminase levels and were subsequently found to have early portal infiltration and fibrosis on liver biopsy.

Tong and colleagues (1981) found that a group of children studied for 10 years all remained antigen-positive and had periodic increases in serum alanine aminotransferase levels. This could be explained by an intermittent release of antigen, as in other chronic or latent virus infections. Of these eight children, three developed spider angiomas, three had hepatosplenomegaly, and two had angiomas and hepatomegaly. For some reason anti-HBs rarely develops in these infants (Merrill et al., 1972), but in other latent virus infections, such as cytomegalovirus and subacute sclerosing panencephalitis, both antigen and antibody are usually present.

Relationship Between HBV and Neonatal Hepatitis

"Neonatal hepatitis" is a descriptive term for a clinical condition of diverse etiology but with a fairly consistent histopathological picture. Although HBV has been identified in association with the neonatal hepatitis syndrome, it is clearly not the major cause. Mowat and co-workers (1976) found that only six of 137 patients with neonatal hepatitis had evidence of a viral etiology, and in only two of these six was HBV considered to be the causative agent. Kattamis and colleagues (1974) carried out a study on 27 Greek infants with prolonged neonatal jaundice hepatitis. A diagnosis of HB was excluded in four cases. Of the remaining 23 children, 10 were positive for Au antigen, in three the results of the test were unclear, and in the remainder (10) other causes were identified, such as HA infection in 5 cases, and septicemia and CMV in the other five. It was also found that the infants with suspected HBV-associated neonatal hepatitis had a worse prognosis than the others. The disease was more severe and more prolonged than in the nonviral group. Eight of the 10 infants were born to carrier mothers.

Fulminant Neonatal Hepatitis

Neonatal hepatitis usually presents as a somewhat benign condition but may run a protracted course. Dupuy and co-workers (1975) reported a series of 14 cases of fulminant hepatitis from France. The subjects' ages ranged from two to five months. Eight of the 14 died, and 11 were either positive for HBsAg or showed a rise in anti-HBs. Eight of these infants had received inoculations of blood during the neonatal period and could have been infected in this way. Five of the mothers of the remaining six infants were asymptomatic carriers of HBsAg; three of the infants were also positive, and two of these (in the same family) died. Massive necrosis of liver cells was found at autopsy, and in some, in whom the illness was prolonged, periportal fibrosis was prolonged. Altogether, eight of the infants died (57 per cent) following intensive therapy with exchange transfusions and administration of hyperimmune HB immunoglobulin.

Fatal cases of neonatal hepatitis have been reported in successive pregnancies. In the study by Dupuy and colleagues (1975) just discussed, acute viral hepatitis developed in two consecutive siblings, one of whom became HGsAg-positive, at 4 and 5 months, respectively. Although there was no direct evidence of an HBsAg carrier state in the mother, it was strongly suspected. Since horizontal transmission in families is by no means uncommon, this route of infection cannot be ruled out.

Fawaz and co-workers (1975) reported maternal-fetal transmission of HB in successive pregnancies. The two infected infants each developed hepatitis at the age of three months following normal pregnancies and deliveries at term. The mother was HBsAg-positive, and an older sibling, aged six years, was both HBsAg- and anti-HBs-negative. The father was HBsAg-negative. The illness in these infected infants ran a fulminant course, and there was evidence of acute liver failure. Hyperimmune immunoglobulin was administered, but the infants died. No evidence of immune complex disease was noted.

Mollica and colleagues (1977) described a family of six children in Italy in which the first four had died in the early months of life of clinical illness compatible with neonatal hepatitis. The fifth child was born a chronic carrier of HBsAg, and the sixth child was admitted to hospital at the age of three months with HBsAg-positive hepatitis.

In a family studied at the Hospital for Sick Children in London in the early 1950's, infants born after five consecutive pregnancies had neonatal hepatitis. Four died. The histopathological picture was typical of neonatal hepatitis, but no cause could then be found.

It is interesting to speculate on the pathogenesis of HBV infection in these apparently rare familial cases. The reason why the fetus is not apparently infected at an earlier stage when the mother is a carrier for such a prolonged period is unclear. The offspring appear to become infected either late in gestation or at birth possibly as the result of a massive exposure to infection or parturition.

Relationship Between HBV and Hepatocellular Carcinoma

There is now strong epidemiological and virological evidence of a link between HBV and hepatocellular carcinoma (HCC). The geographical distribution of HCC in Africa, Senegal, Uganda, Japan, and Taiwan is closely related to a high prevalence of HBsAg and of the e antigen. A high carrier rate of HBV in mothers has also been reported. In Senegal the prevalence of HBsAg in mothers of HCC patients is four times that among the fathers (Lauroze et al., 1976). This finding does not apply to all ethnic groups. Barbara and colleagues (1978), in a study of blood donors in Britain, found that there was a male to female ratio of three to one with respect to HBsAg carriers. The e antigen was expressed in 36 per cent of male compared with 6 per cent of female blood donors. It is possible that if these were subdivided into ethnic groups it would be found that there was a higher carrier rate in individuals of Chinese and African descent. In New York City HBsAg was found in 9.3 per cent of 616 Chinese-Americans (Szmuness et al., 1978).

This figure is much higher than that for other ethnic groups in New York. Furthermore, the death rate from HCC is 10 times higher among Chinese-American adult males than among white adult males. Tabor and co-workers (1978) found that the incidence of HBsAg or anti-HBc was 70 per cent among the Chinese-American population in the United States.

It seems probable that in many parts of the world maternal-fetal transmission of HBV is a major factor in the prevalence of HCC (WHO, 1983; WHO Scientific Working Group, 1983).

HBV and Congenital Defects

There is no evidence that HBV acquired in pregnancy is capable of causing congenital defects or malformations of the fetus.

Laboratory Diagnosis

Major developments have taken place in the past few years in the laboratory tests used to detect HBV infection. Many reagents are now available on a commercial basis which, subject to cost reductions and increased experience in their use, will be of assistance to hospital laboratories. As with any diagnostic procedures there should be close cooperation between the clinician or epidemiologist and the laboratory staff. It is up to the latter to carry out the tests that are considered appropriate in a given situation and to provide an interpretation of the results whenever possible. This can be facilitated by a careful appraisal of the situation by the clinician with particular reference to the pathogenesis of HBV and the stage of the disease at which the patient is first seen (Krugman and Katz, 1981). Generally speaking, it is difficult to make a precise diagnosis with a single specimen from a patient suffering from an evolving disease process. Consequently, repeat specimens may be required to detect the presence or absence of the respective antigens and antibodies.

The main serological and other tests currently in use are shown in Table 9–7. There are, in addition, more sophisticated tests, such as those for viral DNA polymerase, Dane particles, HBcAg in serum, HBV DNA in liver biopsy material, and free DNA in serum. These latter tests are important developments, but their use is at present within the province only of highly specialized labo-

Table 9–7. **LABORATORY TESTS FOR THE DIAGNOSIS OF HB**

Serological Tests for Antigen and Antibody
 HBsAg
 HbeAg
 Anti-HBcAg, including IgM for acute-phase illness
  and up to 1 year after infection and IgG for
  evidence of immunity
 Anti-HBeAg
 Anti-HBsAg
 DNA polymerase

Liver Function Tests
 SGOT (serum glutamic oxaloacetic transaminase)
 Thymol turbidity

Direct Evidence of Liver Pathology
 Liver biopsy for histopathology and virological tests
  for HBV particles or HBcAg

ratories (Deinhardt and Gust, 1982). About 98 per cent of patients with HAV make a full recovery, but about 10 per cent of HBV patients may come to have persistent or chronic active hepatitis. Liver biopsy may be essential to the management of such cases in both parties in mother-infant infections. The tests described below are applicable to the diagnosis of infections in both the mother and the infant.

The incubation period may vary from 50 to 160 days. The time of appearance of the various antigens and antibodies is not only related to the dates of exposure and the development of clinical symptoms with jaundice, but marked variation may be encountered in their appearance and disappearance even in cases that proceed to full recovery (Mushahwar et al., 1981; Ahtone and Maynard, 1983). The sequence of events in uncomplicated acute viral hepatitis is outlined in Figure 9–1. However, the variation from case to case is marked, particularly in infants and young children. For example, the icteric phase may be considerably shorter or absent altogether in these patients.

The important markers are usually HBsAg, anti-HBc, and anti-HBs. As there is an interval between the disappearance of HBsAg and the appearance of anti-HBs, the so-called window phase, it is advisable to repeat tests if only HBsAg is detected. The presence of anti-HBs and anti-HBc, especially IgM antibody, is most certain evidence of recent infection. Wherever possible, tests for anti-HBc and anti-HBs should be carried out in parallel. Table 9–8 indicates the most likely findings in different stages of acute viral hepatitis.

The following are generally considered to be bad prognostic signs and indicate a need for further tests: (1) persistence of HBsAg and HBeAg, (2) prolonged icterus and raised levels of serum glutamic oxaloacetic transaminase (SGOT), (3) persistence of DNA polymerase, and (4) absence of anti-HBs.

In the carrier state, in the case of the asymptomatic, the persistent without symptoms, or the chronic active form of hepatitis, the essential differences are to be found in the persistence of one or both antigens and absence of anti-HBs. Some possible findings are outlined in Table 9–9. See also Figure 9–2.

A brief outline of the laboratory tests for HBV infections appears in Chapter 14.

HEPATITIS NON-A, NON-B AND DELTA AGENT

At present, these two additional forms of viral hepatitis do not appear to have been incriminated in mother-infant transmission of hepatitis except in one instance. An epidemic of HNANB occurred among women who received contaminated anti-D immunoglobulin (Deinhardt and Gust, 1982). The effect on newborn infants is unknown. One instance of perinatal transmission of Delta agent, together with HBV, has been reported (Deinhardt and Gust, 1982).

Further evidence of the severity of non-A, non-B hepatitis is indicated by a report from

Table 9–8. **RESULTS OF LABORATORY TESTS AT DIFFERENT STAGES OF ACUTE VIRAL HEPATITIS B**

Stage of Disease	Laboratory Test					
	HBsAg	HBsAg	Anti-HBcIgM	Anti-HBcIgG	Anti-HBs	Anti-HBe
Late incubation period	+	−	±	−	−	−
Early-phase hepatitis (first week)	+	+	+	−	−	−
Late-phase hepatitis (1–4 weeks)	±	+	+	−	−	−
Early convalescence (posticteric)	−	−	+	−	+	+
Late convalescence	−	−	+	−	+	+
Recovery or determination of immune state	−	−	−	+	+	−

Table 9–9. **LABORATORY FINDINGS IN THE CHRONIC CARRIER STATE OF HEPATITIS B**

Form of Carrier Stage 3 and 12 Months After Initial Exposure		Laboratory Tests						
	HBsAg	HBcAg	DNA Polymerase	SGOT	Jaundice	Anti-HBc	Anti-HBs	Anti-HBe
Asymptomatic carrier								
3 months	+	+	+	+	–	+	–	+
12 months	+	–	–	±	–	+	–	+
Chronic persistent hepatitis								
3 months	+	+	+	+	±|	+	–	–
12 months	+	+	+	+	–	+	–	–
Chronic active hepatitis								
3 months	+	+	+	+	+*	+	–	–
12 months	+	+	+	+	+*	+	–	–

*Episodes of jaundice may be intermittent.

Khuroo (1980) from India. He described an extensive and explosive epidemic of acute viral hepatitis in the Kashmir Valley in India in 1978. The nature of the epidemic pointed to a common water-borne source and the probable existence of epidemic strains of HNANB. The importance of this epidemic to maternal-infection hepatitis infections lay in the fact that many pregnant women were infected. Altogether, 275 cases of acute icteric viral hepatitis were observed in a population of 16,620 in 15 villages, an incidence of infection with jaundice of 1.65 per cent. The incidence of hepatitis in pregnant women was 17.3 per cent, compared with 2.1 per cent in nonpregnant women and 2.8 per cent in men. The incidence of the infection was higher for women in each trimester of pregnancy than in nonpregnant women, and fulminant hepatitis with hepatic encephalopathy developed in 11 patients (eight pregnant women—22.2 per cent—and three men) (Khuroo et al., 1981; Zuckerman, 1982). Fulminant hepatitis was not observed in the 71 nonpregnant women and occurred in only 2.8 per cent of the men. Fetal loss in the fatal cases of fulminant hepatitis appeared to be associated with maternal death and not with some direct effect of the disease on the fetus. Eight of the 11 cases of fulminant hepatitis occurred in the last trimester of pregnancy, and the nutritional status of these women was reported to be excellent (Khuroo et al., 1981).

Laboratory Diagnosis

The diagnosis of HNANB is made by exclusion. The results of laboratory tests, compared with those in cases of HB, reveal the elevation of SGOT, associated with a short period of icterus. All HBV markers would be negative (see Figure 9–3).

PREVENTION

The rationale for prevention of perinatal-neonatal HBV and HAV infections is discussed in detail in Chapter 15. As far as HBV infections are concerned, combined passive-active immunization of neonates born to HBsAg-positive mothers now appears to be the recommended form of treatment, but precise details of therapy, dosage, and age at which administered will depend upon the availability of these highly effective but expensive biologicals. At present, the only vaccine against HBV infection is the inactivated 22-nm surface subunit vaccine prepared from plasma of human carriers. As awareness of the importance of HBV as a public health problem increases, alternative sources of vaccine are being urgently sought. The subject is discussed in detail by Deinhardt and Gust (1982) and Zuckerman (1982).

Bibliography

Adams, R. H., and Combes, B.: Viral hepatitis during pregnancy. J.A.M.A. *192*:195–198, 1965.

Ahtone, J., and Maynard, J. E.: Laboratory diagnosis of hepatitis B. J.A.M.A. *249*:2067–2069, 1983.

Anderson, K. E., Stevens, C. E., Tsuei, J. J., Lee, W. C., Sun, S. C., and Beasley, R. P.: Hepatitis B antigen in infants born to mothers with chronic hepatitis B antigenemia in Taiwan. Am. J. Dis. Child. *129*:1389–1392, 1975.

Andrewes, C. H., Pereira, H. G., and Wildy, P.: In Viruses of Vertebrates. 4th ed. London, Bailliere Tindall, 1978.

Aziz, M. A., Khan, G., Khanum, T., and Siddiqui, A.: Transplacental and postnatal transmission of the hepatitis associated antigen. J. Infect. Dis. *127*:110–112, 1973.

Barbara, J. A. J., Mizovic, V., Cleghorn, T. E., Tedder, R. S., and Briggs, R. M.: Liver enzyme concentrations as measure of possible infectivity in chronic asymptomatic carriers of hepatitis B. Br. Med. J. *2*:1600–1602, 1978.

Barker, L. F., Shulman, N. R., Murray, R., Hirschman, R. J., Ratner, F., Diefenbach, W. C., and Geller, H. M.: Transmission of serum hepatitis. J.A.M.A. *211*:1509–1512, 1970.

Beasley, R. P., Shiao, L. S., Stevens, C. E., and Meng, H. C.: Evidence against breast feeding as a mechanism for vertical transmission of hepatitis B surface antigen. Am. J. Epidemiol. *105*:94–98, 1975.

Beasley, R. P., and Stevens, C. E.: Vertical transmission of HBV and interruption with globulin. In Vyas, G. N., and Cohen, S. N. (eds.): Viral Hepatitis. Philadelphia, Franklin Institute Press, 1978, pp. 333–345.

Beasley, R. P., Trepo, C., Stevens, C. E., and Szmuness, W.: The e antigen and vertical transmission of hepatitis B surface antigen. Am. J. Epidemiol. *105*:94–98, 1977.

Berthold, H., Mielke, G., and Merk, W.: Intrinsic interference caused by hepatitis sera. Proc. Soc. Exp. Biol. Med. *143*:698–700, 1973.

Blumberg, B. S., Alter, H. J., and Visnich, S.: A "new" antigen in leukemia sera. J.A.M.A. *191*:541–546, 1965.

Blumberg, B. S., Gerstley, B. J. S., Hungerford, D. A., London, W. T., and Sutnick, A. I.: A serum antigen (Australia antigen) in Down's syndrome, leukemia, and hepatitis. Ann. Intern. Med. *66*:924–931, 1967.

Blumberg, B. S., Sutnick, A. L., London, W. T., and Millman, I.: The discovery of Australia antigen and its relation to viral hepatitis. Perspect. Virol. *7*:223, 1971.

Boxall, E. H.: Maternal transmission of hepatitis B. In Waterson, A. P. (ed.): Recent Advances in Clinical Virology. Edinburgh, Churchill Livingstone, 1980, pp. 17–29.

Brighton, W. D., Taylor, P. E., and Zuckerman, A. J.: Changes induced by hepatitis serum in cultured liver cells. Nature, [New Biol.] *232*:57–58, 1971.

Bruguera, M., Bosch, J., and Rodes, J.: Family outbreak of hepatitis B. Letter to the editor. N. Engl. J. Med. *289*:1144, 1973.

Bucholz, H. M., Fiosner, G. G., and Ziegler, S. B.: HB$_s$Ag carrier state in infant delivered by Caesarean section. Lancet *2*:343, 1974.

Carver, D. H., and Seto, D. S. Y.: Production of hemadsorption-negative areas by serums containing Australia antigen. Science *172*:1265–1267, 1971.

Ceccarelli, G., and Torbidoni, L.: Viral hepatitis and Down's syndrome. Lancet *1*:438, 1967.

Cherubin, C. E.: Risk of post-transfusion hepatitis in recipients of blood containing S. H. antigen at Harlem Hospital. Lancet *1*:627–630, 1971.

Cossart, Y. E.: Discussion. In Intrauterine Infections. Ciba Foundation Symposium 10 (new series). Amsterdam, Associated Scientific Publishers, 1973, p. 110.

Cossart, Y. E.: Acquisition of hepatitis B antigen in the newborn period. Postgrad. Med. J. *50*:334–337, 1974.

Deinhardt, F., and Gust, I.: Viral hepatitis—on behalf of the participants of an informal WHO Meeting. Bull. W.H.O. *60*:661–691, 1982.

Derso, A., Boxall, E. H., Tarlow, M. J., and Flewett, T. H.: Transmission of HB$_s$Ag from mother to infant in four ethnic groups. Br. Med. J. *1*:949–952, 1978.

Desmyter, J., Liv, W. T., and Van Den Berghe, H.: Viral hepatitis B: studies of congenital transmission. In Intrauterine Infections. Ciba Foundation Symposium 10 (new series). Amsterdam, Associated Scientific Publishers, 1973, p. 110.

Dietzman, D. E., Matthew, E. B., Maddeh, D. L., Sever, J. L., Rostafinski, M., Bouton, S. M., and Nagler, B.: The occurrence of epidemic infectious hepatitis in chronic carriers of Australia antigen. J. Pediatr. *80*:577–582, 1972.

Dupuy, J. M., Frommel, D., and Alagillie, D.: Severe viral hepatitis type B in infancy. Lancet *1*:191–194, 1975.

Eichenwald, H. F., McCracken, G. H., and Kindberg, S. J.: Virus infections of the newborn. Prog. Med. Virol. *9*:35–104, 1967.

Fawaz, K. A., Grady, G. F., Kaplan, M. M., and Gellis, S. S.: Repetitive maternal-fetal transmission of fatal hepatitis B. N. Engl. J. Med. *293*:1357–1359, 1975.

Feinstone, A. M., Kapikian, A. Z., and Purcell, R. H.: Hepatitis A: detection by immune electronmicroscopy of a virus-like antigen associated with acute illness. Science *182*:1026–1028, 1973.

Findlay, G. M., MacCallum, F. O., and Murgatroyd, F.: Observations on epidemic catarrhal jaundice. Trans. R. Soc. Trop. Med. Hyg. *25*:7, 1939.

Giles, J. P., McCollum, R. W., Berndtson, L. W., Jr., and Krugman, S.: Viral hepatitis. Relation of Australia-SH antigen to the Willowbrook MS-2 strain. N. Engl. J. Med. *281*:119–122, 1969.

Ginsberg, A. L., Conrad, M. E., Bancroft, W. H., Ling, C. M., and Overby, L. R.: Prevention of endemic HAA-positive hepatitis with gamma globulin. Use of a simple radioimmune assay to detect HAA. N. Engl. J. Med. *286*:562–566, 1972.

Grady, G. F.: Relationship of e antigen to infectivity of HB$_s$Ag positive amongst medical personnel. Lancet *2*:492–494, 1976.

Grob, P. J., and Jemelka, H.: Faecal S. H. (Australia) antigen in acute hepatitis. Lancet *1*:206–208, 1971.

Gruber, A. E. L.: Die riesenzellige leberzirrhose des Neugeborenen. Geburtshilfe Frauenheilkd. *17*:381–387, 1957.

Hadziyannis, S. J., and Merikas, G. E.: Australia antigen in a family. Lancet *1*:1057–1058, 1970.

Heiber, J. P., Dalton, D., Shorey, J., and Combs, B.: Hepatitis and pregnancy. J. Pediatr. *91*:545–549, 1977.

Hersh, T., Melnick, J. L., Goyal, R. K., and Hollinger, F. B.: Nonparenteral transmission of viral hepatitis type B (Australia antigen–associated serum hepatitis). N. Engl. J. Med. *285*:1363–1364, 1971.

Holmes, A. W., Wolfe, L., Deinhardt, F., Capps, R. B., and Poper, H.: Studies on the transmission of human hepatitis to marmosets: further coded studies. J. Infect. Dis. *124*:520–521, 1971.

Hsia, D. Y. Y., Taylor, R. G., and Gellis, S. S.: Long-term follow-up study on infectious hepatitis during pregnancy. J. Pediatr. *41*:13–17, 1952.

Kattamis, C. A., Demetrois, D., and Matsarotis, N. S.: Australia antigen and neonatal hepatitis syndrome. Pediatrics *54*:157–164, 1974.

Khuroo, M. S.: Study on an epidemic of non-A, non-B hepatitis: possibility of another human hepatitis virus distinct from post-transfusion non-A, non-B type. Am. J. Med. *68*:818–825, 1980.

Khuroo, M. S., Teli, M. R., Skidmore, S., et al.: Incidence and severity of viral hepatitis in pregnancy. Am. J. Med. *70*:252–255, 1981.

Kohler, P. F., Dubois, R., Merrill, D. A., and Bowes, W. A.: Prevention of chronic neonatal hepatitis B virus infection with antibody to the hepatitis B surface antigen. N. Engl. J. Med. *290*:1331–1335, 1974.

Krugman, S., Friedman, H., and Lattimer, C.: Viral hepatitis, type A. Identification by specific complement fixation and immune adherence tests. N. Engl. J. Med. *292*:1141–1143, 1975.

Krugman, S., Giles, J. P., and Hammond, J.: Viral hepatitis, type B (MS-2 strain): prevention with specific hepatitis B immune serum globulin. J.A.M.A. *218*:1665–1670, 1971.

Krugman, S., and Katz, S.: Infectious Diseases of Children. 7th ed. St. Louis, C. V. Mosby Company, 1981.

Kucera, J.: Down's syndrome and infectious hepatitis. Lancet *1*:569–570, 1970.

Lauroze, B, Landen, W. T., Sanot, G., Werner, B. G., Lustraden, E. D., Payette, M., and Blumberg, B. S.: Host response to HBV infection in patients with primary hepatic carcinoma and families: a case/control study in Senegal in W. Africa. Lancet *2*:534–538, 1976.

Leck, I.: Incidence and epidemicity of Down's syndrome. Lancet *2*:457–460, 1966.

Lee, A. K. Y., Ip, H. M. H., and Wong, V. C. W.: Mechanisms of maternal-fetal transmission of hepatitis B virus. J. Infect. Dis. *138*:668–671, 1978.

MacCallum, F. O.: Homologous serum hepatitis. Lancet *2*:691–692, 1947.

Magnius, L. O., and Epsmark, J. A.: New specificities in Australia antigen positive sera distinct from the Le Bouvier determinants. J. Immunol. *109*:1017–1121, 1972.

Mansell, R. V.: Infectious hepatitis in the first trimester of pregnancy and its effect on the fetus. Am. J. Obstet. Gynecol. *69*:1136–1139, 1955.

Maugh, T. H.: Hepatitis: a new understanding emerges. Science *176*:1225–1226, 1972.

Maupas, P. S., and Melnick, J. L.: Hepatitis B virus and primary hepatocellular carcinoma. Prog. Med. Virol. *27*:1–210, 1981.

McCarthy, J. W.: Hepatitis B antigen (HB Ag)-positive chronic aggressive hepatitis and cirrhosis in an 8-month-old infant: a case report. J. Pediatr. *83*:638–639, 1973.

Merrill, D. A., Dubois, R. S., and Kohler, P. F.: Neonatal

onset of the hepatitis-associated antigen carrier state. N. Engl. J. Med. *287*:1280–1282, 1972.

Mickal, A.: Infectious hepatitis in pregnancy. Am. J. Obstet. Gynecol. *62*:409–414, 1951.

Miller, J. R., and Baird, P. A.: Some epidemiological aspects of Down's syndrome in British Columbia. Br. J. Prev. Soc. Med. *22*:81–85, 1968.

Mollica, F., Musumeci, S., and Fischer, A.: Neonatal hepatitis in five children of a hepatitis B surface antigen carrier woman. J. Pediatr. *90*:949–951, 1977.

Mortimer, P. P.: Hepatitis A and its virus. In Waterson, A. P. (ed.): Recent Advances in Clinical Virology. Edinburgh, Churchill Livingstone, 1980, pp. 1–15.

Mowat, A. P., Psacharopoulos, H. T., and Williams, R.: Extrahepatic biliary atresia versus neonatal hepatitis. Arch. Dis. Child. *51*:763–770, 1976.

Mushahwar, I. K., Dierstag, J. L., Polesky, H. S., Mc-Grath, L. C., Decca, H., and Overby, L. R.: Interpretation of various serological profiles of hepatitis B infection. Am. J. Clin. Pathol. *76*:773–777, 1981.

Ohlayashi, A., Okachi, K., and Mayumi, M.: Familial clustering of asymptomatic carriers of Australia antigen and patients with liver disease or primary liver cancer. Gastroenterology *62*:618–624, 1972.

Okada, K., Yamada, T., Miyakawa, Y., and Mayumi, M.: Hepatitis B surface antigen in the serum of infants after delivery from asymptomatic carrier mothers. J. Pediatr. *87*:360–363, 1975.

Okada, K., Kamiyama, I., Inomata, M., et al.: e antigen and anti-e in the serum of asymptomatic carrier mothers as indicators of positive and negative transmission of hepatitis B virus to their infants. N. Engl. J. Med. *294*:746–749, 1976.

Pantelakis, S. N., Chryssostomidou, O., Alexiou, D., et al.: Sex chromatin and chromosome abnormalities among 10,412 liveborn babies. Arch. Dis. Child. *45*:87–92, 1970.

Papaevangolou, G. J.: Hepatitis B in infants. N. Engl. J. Med. *288*:972–975, 1973.

Popper, H., and Mackay, I. R.: Relation between Australia antigen and autoimmune hepatitis. Lancet *1*:1161–1164, 1972.

Prince, A. M.: An antigen detected in the blood during the incubation period of serum hepatitis. Proc. Natl. Acad. Sci. U.S.A. *60*:814–821, 1968.

Prince, A. M., Fuji, H., and Gershon, R. K.: Immuno-histochemical studies on the aetiology of anicteric hepatitis in Korea. Am. J. Hyg. *79*:365, 1964.

Provost, P. J., and Hilleman, M. R.: Propagation of human hepatitis A virus in cell culture in vitro. Proc. Soc. Exp. Biol. Med. *160*:213–221, 1979.

Punyagupta, S., Olson, L. C., and Harsinatu, V.: The epidemiology of hepatitis B antigen in a high prevalence area. Am. J. Epidemiol. *97*:349–354, 1973.

Reddy, A. M., Harper, R. G., and Stern, G.: Observations on heroin and methadone withdrawal in the newborn. Pediatrics *48*:353–358, 1971.

Ricci, G., De Bac, C., Turbessi, B., and Caramia, F.: Intranuclear virus-like particles and cytoplasmic HB Ag in chronic hepatitis. Letter to the editor. N. Engl. J. Med. *289*:144–145, 1973.

Rizzetto, M., Canese, M. G., Arico, S., Crivelli, O., Trepo, O., Bonino, F., and Verne, G.: Immunofluorescence detection of new antigen antibody system associated to hepatitis B viruses in liver and in serum of HB$_s$Ag carriers. Gut *18*:997–1003, 1977.

Rizzetto, M., Canese, M. G., Arico, S., Crivelli, O., Trepo, O., Bonino, F., and Verne, G.: Delta-antigen. Evidence for a variant of hepatitis B virus or a non-A, non-B hepatitis agent. Perspect. Virol. *11*:195–217, 1981.

Schweitzer, I. L.: Vertical transmission of the hepatitis B surface antigen. Am. J. Med. Sci. *270*:287–291, 1975.

Schweitzer, I. L., Dunn, A. E. G., Peters, R. L., and Spears, R. L.: Viral hepatitis B in neonates and infants. Am. J. Med. *55*:762–771, 1973b.

Schweitzer, I. L., Edwards, V. M., and Brezina, M.: e antigen in HB$_s$AG–carrier mothers. Letter to the editor. N. Engl. J. Med. *293*:940, 1975.

Schweitzer, I. L., Mosely, J. W., and Ashcavai, M.: Factors influencing neonatal infection by hepatitis B virus. Gastroenterology *65*:227–283, 1973a.

Schweitzer, I. L., Wing, A., McPeak, C., and Spears, R. L.: Hepatitis and hepatitis-associated antigen in 56 mother-infant pairs. J.A.M.A. *220*:1092–1095, 1972.

Schwer, M., and Moosa, A.: Effects of hepatitis A and B in pregnancy on the mother and fetus. S. Afr. Med. J. *54*:1092–1095, 1978.

Sever, J. L., and White, L.: Intrauterine viral infections. Ann. Rev. Med. *19*:471–486, 1968.

Siegel, M., and Fuerst, H. T.: Low birth weight and maternal virus disease: a prospective study of rubella, measles, mumps, chickenpox and hepatitis. J.A.M.A. *197*:680–682, 1966.

Siegel, M., Fuerst, H. T., and Peress, N. G.: Comparative fetal mortality in maternal virus diseases. N. Engl. J. Med. *274*:768–771, 1966.

Siegler, A. M., and Keyser, J.: Acute hepatitis in pregnancy. A report of ten cases and review of the literature. Am. J. Obstet. Gynecol. *86*:1068–1073, 1963.

Sinatra, F., Shah, P., Weissmann, J. Y., Thomas, D. W., Merrit, R. J., and Tong, M. J.: Perinatal transmitted acute icteric hepatitis B in infants born to hepatitis B surface antigen-positive and anti-hepatitis B e positive carrier mothers. Pediatrics *70*:557–559, 1982.

Skinhoj, P., Cohen, J., and Bradbourne, A. F.: Transmission of hepatitis type B from healthy HB$_s$Ag positive mothers. Br. Med. J. *1*:10–11, 1976.

Skinhoj, P., Sandemann, H., and Cohen, J.: Hepatitis associated antigen (HAA) in pregnant women and their newborn infants. Am. J. Dis. Child. *123*:380–381, 1972.

Smithwick, E. M., Pascual, E., and Go, S. C.: Hepatitis-associated antigen: a possible relationship to premature delivery. J. Pediatr. *81*:537–540, 1972.

Stark, C. R., and Franmeni, J. E., Jr.: Viral hepatitis and Down's syndrome. Lancet *1*:1036, 1966.

Stevens, C. E., Beasley, R. P., Tsui, J., and Lew, W. L.: Vertical transmission of hepatitis B antigen in Taiwan. N. Engl. J. Med. *292*:771–774, 1975.

Stevens, C. E., Neurath, R. A., Beasley, R. P., and Szmuness, W.: HB$_e$Ag and anti HB$_e$ detection by radio-immunoassay—correlation with vertical transmission of HBV in Taiwan. J. Med. Virol. *3*:237–241, 1979.

Stokes, J., Jr., Wolman, J. J., Blanchard, M. C., and Farquhar, J. D.: Viral hepatitis in the newborn: clinical features, epidemiology and pathology. Am. J. Dis. Child. *82*:213–1951.

Stoller, A., and Collmann, R. D.: Incidence of infective hepatitis followed by Down's syndrome nine months later. Lancet *2*:1221–1223, 1965.

Szmuness, W., Prince, A. M., Hirsch, R. L., and Brotman, B.: Familial clustering of hepatitis B infection. N. Engl. J. Med. *289*:1160–1162, 1973.

Szmuness, W., Stevens, C. E., Ikram, H., Much, I. M., Harley, E. J., and Hollinger, B.: Prevalence of hepatitis B virus infection and hepatocellular carcinoma in Chinese-Americans. J. Infect. Dis. *137*:822–829, 1978.

Tabor, E., Geraty, R. J., and Dietses, J. A.: Transmission

of non-A, non-B hepatitis from man to chimpanzee. Lancet *1*:463–466, 1978.

Tong, M. J., McPeak, C. M., Thursby, M. W., Schweitzer, I. L., Henneman, C. E., and Ledger, W. J.: Failure of immune serum globulin to prevent hepatitis B infection in infants born to HB$_s$Ag positive mothers. Gastroenterology *76*:535–539, 1979.

Tong, M. J., Stephenson, D., and Cordon, I.: Correlation of e antigen, DNA polymerase activity and Dane particles in chronic benign and chronic active type B hepatitis infections. J. Infect. Dis. *135*:980–984, 1977.

Tong, M. J., Thursby, M. W., Patela, J., McPeak, C., Edwards, V. M., and Mosley, J. W.: Studies on maternal-infant transmission of the viruses which cause acute hepatitis. Gastroenterology *80*:999–1004, 1981.

World Health Organisation: Viral hepatitis. Report of a WHO Scientific Group. Tech. Rep. Sci. No. 512. Geneva, WHO, 1973.

World Health Organisation: Prevention of hepatocellular carcinoma by immunization. Bull. W.H.O. *61*:731–744, 1983.

World Health Organisation Scientific Working Group: Prevention of primary liver cancer. Lancet *1*:463–465, 1983.

Zondek, B., and Bromberg, Y. M.: Infectious hepatitis in pregnancy. J. Mt. Sinai Hosp. N.Y. *14*:222–243, 1947.

Zuckerman, A. J.: Hepatitis-associated antigens and viruses. In Human Viral Hepatitis. Amsterdam, North-Holland Publishing Company, 1975.

Zuckerman, A. J.: In Arias, I. M., Frenkel, M., and Wilson, J. H. P. (eds.): The Liver. Amsterdam, Excerpta Medica, 1982, pp. 122–153.

Zuckerman, A. J., and Howard, C. R.: Hepatitis Viruses of Man. New York, Academic Press, 1979.

Zuckerman, A. J., Baines, P. M., and Almeida, J. D.: Australia antigen as a marker of propagation of the serum hepatitis virus in liver cultures. Nature *236*:78–81, 1972.

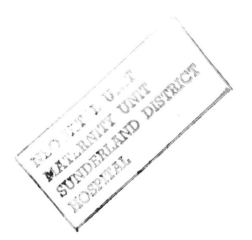

10

Other Viruses as Potential Pathogens of the Fetus and Newborn

The major viruses known to cause damage to the fetus and newborn have been discussed in detail in this volume. There remain, however, a number of viruses that have from time to time been reported as having an adverse effect on the fetus, but for which either the evidence is lacking or the effect is not proven.

INFLUENZA VIRUS

The role of influenza viruses as causes of fetal damage has long been controversial. In part, this may be explained by the difficulty of making a precise diagnosis of influenza virus infection without laboratory tests, as the result of which the term "maternal influenza" has been used somewhat loosely. Account has also to be taken of the possible pathogenic mechanism that could lead to fetal damage, since viremia does not occur in influenza or, if it does, is of very short duration—the virus has never been recovered from the blood stream, even in acute cases. If maternal influenza is causally related to fetal damage, some mechanism other than fetal infection must be postulated. Indirect toxic effects, hyperthermia, and drug therapy all have to be considered in this connection.

During pandemics or major epidemics of influenza the virulence of infection is invariably enhanced, with the result that mortality in general is increased; maternal mortality may be associated with an increase in abortions and premature births. This was evident in the 1918–1919 pandemic and in the epidemic of 1937–1938. By the 1940's two antigenic types of influenza virus had been identified: type A was isolated by Smith and co-workers (1933) and type B independently by Francis (1940) and Magill (1940). Thus, it became theoretically possible to establish a diagnosis of influenza in pregnancy and consequently, the chance of proving a causal relation between maternal influenza and congenital defects increased. Since influenza virus was first isolated in 1933, major changes have taken place in the antigenic composition of the influenza A strains (Stuart-Harris and

Schild, 1976). This problem of antigenic variation, whether it consists of a major change ("antigenic shift") or a minor change ("antigenic drift"), is of special concern in relation to prevention, but it may also have a bearing on the effect these virus strains have on the fetus if infection occurs in pregnancy.

It is evident from a perusal of the literature that the congenital defects that have been reported in association with maternal influenza do not constitute a specific syndrome like those found in congenital rubella and cytomegalovirus (CMV) infections. Defects of the neural tube and the alimentary and genitourinary systems that have been reported after maternal influenza are commonly encountered in the general population. If there is a causal relationship between maternal influenza and certain specific defects, one would expect a repetitive pattern to be found in infants born after an epidemic of influenza or in a locality where there was known to be a high prevalence of the disease.

Many of the reports concerning influenza and congenital defects relate to the effect of influenza contracted during the Asian influenza epidemic of 1957 to 1958. Two reports of epidemics earlier in the 1950's will first be examined in some detail. Reference has already been made to the study by Manson and her colleagues (1960) on the effect of rubella and other virus infections in pregnancy during the period from 1950 to 1952 in the United Kingdom. Some of the findings are pertinent to this particular topic, as both influenza and rubella were epidemic in the United Kingdom at that time. Influenza was not initially included in this study, but between 1950 and 1951 an epidemic of virus

influenza occurred. It was particularly severe in the northeast of England, where a variant of influenza A-prime virus was isolated from many patients during this epidemic. The diagnosis of influenza was made on clinical grounds by a physician, and the study by Manson and co-workers included cases confined to bed for at least 24 hours with a diagnosis of "influenza." One hundred sixty-six pregnancies associated with maternal influenza were reported; in 99—more than half—infection occurred between the thirteenth and twenty-eighth weeks. The outcome of the pregnancies did not differ very much from those of controls, as shown in Tables 10–1 and 10–2. However, one unusual sequence was noted. There were six infant deaths, five of which occurred following maternal rubella between the thirteenth and twenty-eighth weeks. These five deaths, among 97 liveborn children, resulted from a variety of unremarkable causes. Only two or three deaths would have been expected. Among the 163 liveborn children (see Table 10–2), there were six major defects. These consisted of one case each of hydrocephalus, spina bifida, and talipes (the child died before two years), cleft palate and harelip, achondroplasia, absence of left forearm and hand, mental retardation, and imperforate vagina. There were, in addition, two "suspicious" defects of delayed speech.

Coffey and Jessop (1955) reported an increase in congenital abnormalities in a study involving 12,552 total births in three maternity units in Dublin. As soon as possible after giving birth, the mothers with abnormal infants were asked to fill out a questionnaire about details of their pregnancies including

Table 10–1. **OUTCOME TO INFANT IN PREGNANCIES IN VIRUS SERIES, ACCORDING TO THE STAGE OF PREGNANCY WHEN THE INFECTION OCCURRED, COMPARED WITH THE EXPECTED OUTCOME CALCULATED FROM THE EXPERIENCE OF STANDARDIZED CONTROL GROUPS**

Stage of Pregnancy at Which Influenza Occurred	No. of Cases		Aborted		Stillborn		Born Alive but Dead at 2 Years		Alive at 2 Years	
			No.	%	No.	%	No.	%	No.	%
Total to 12th week	42	Observed	1	2.4	0	—	1	2.4	40	95.2
		Expected	1.1	2.6	1.2	2.9	1.0	2.4	38.7	92.1
Total in 13th–28th weeks	99	Observed	0	—	2	2.6	5	5.0	92	93.0
		Expected	0.5	0.5	2.7	2.7	2.6	2.6	93.2	94.2
Total in 29th week or beyond	25	Observed	—	—	0	—	0	—	25	100
		Expected	—	—	0.6	2.4	0.6	2.4	23.8	95.2
All influenza cases	166	Observed	1	0.6	2	2.1	6	3.7	157	94.6
		Expected	1.6	1.0	4.5	2.7	4.2	2.5	155.7	93.8

Data from Manson, M. M., Logan, W. P. D., and Loy, R. M.: Rubella and other virus infections during pregnancy. Rep. Public Health Med. Subj. No. 101. London, Her Majesty's Stationery Office, 1960, table G.

Table 10–2. THE NUMBER AND PERCENTAGE OF INFANTS WITH AND WITHOUT MAJOR MALFORMATIONS IN THE CONTROL SERIES AND VIRUS SERIES ACCORDING TO THE STAGE OF PREGNANCY WHEN INFECTION OCCURRED: INFLUENZA GROUP*

| | All Infants | | | | | All Liveborn Infants | | | | | Infants Born Alive but Dying Before 2 Years | | | | |
| | | Without Major Malformations | | With Major Malformations | | | Without Major Malformations | | With Major Malformations | | | Without Major Malformations | | With Major Malformations | |
Type of Case	No. of Cases	No.	%	No.	%	No. of Cases	No.	%	No.	%	No. of Cases	No.	%	No.	%
Control series	5611	5431	96.8	156	2.8	5455	5326	97.6	128	2.3	140	92	65.7	47	33.6
Influenza up to 12th week	41	41	100.0	0	–	41	41	100.0	0	–	1	1	–	0	–
Influenza in 13th–28th weeks	99	92	92.9	7	7.4	97	91	93.8	6	6.2	5	4	80.0	1	20.0
Influenza in 29th–40th weeks	25	25	100.0	0	–	25	25	100.0	0	–	0	0	–	0	–
All influenza cases	165	158	95.8	7	4.2	163	157	96.3	6	3.7	6	5	83.3	1	16.7

*Controls as described in Table 10–1, but cases delivered up to the date week of pregnancy, i.e., abortions, are excluded.
Data from Manson, M. M., Logan, W. P. D., and Loy, R. M.: Rubella and other virus infections during pregnancy. Rep. Public Health Med. Subj. No. 101. London, Her Majesty's Stationery Office, 1960, table L.

infectious diseases they might have had. Questionnaires were completed for approximately the same number of mothers with normal infants selected at random from the postnatal wards. A history of influenza in pregnancy, based on the mothers' memory, was obtained for 18.4 per cent of 204 infants with major congenital defects, compared with 3.6 per cent of the controls. Anencephaly was the predominant abnormality. As this was a retrospective study and no epidemiological or laboratory evaluation was made at the time of the maternal illness, the precise significance of the findings could not be established.

An opportunity for further study of the effect of influenza in pregnancy arose following the Asian influenza pandemic of 1957–1958. The strain responsible for this epidemic, the A1 strain, was antigenically different from the A-prime strain prevalent in the early 1950's. Coffey and Jessop (1959) were able to carry out a prospective study in Dublin during 1957 in anticipation of an influenza epidemic. Between October 1957 and October 1958, all women who attended the antenatal clinics at three hospitals in Dublin were asked, "Have you had influenza during this pregnancy?" The patient's answer was recorded, along with the date of the attack if applicable, and for each "influenza" case a control subject at about the same stage of pregnancy who had not been infected was selected. Although no serological tests were carried out, it is known that influenza virus was prevalent at the time, since Meenan (quoted by Coffey and Jessop [1959]) was isolating virus regularly from patients with influenza in Dublin and surrounding areas.

A total of 669 patients, 663 of whom were available for analysis, reported that they had had influenza. The incidence of congenital deformities in the offspring of mothers who had had influenza and the controls is shown in Table 10–3. The overall incidence of defects among the former was 2.4 times that in the offspring of controls; this was significant at the 2 per cent level. As there was a close similarity in age and number of pregnancies between the influenza patients and the controls, it appeared that some other factor had contributed to the result. It is possible that the influenza patients, as opposed to the controls, may have received medication that could have influenced the outcome. The possible adverse effect of drug therapy in pregnant women with influenza has been commented upon by Hakasolo and Saxen (1971) in Finland.

The distribution of the various defects showed that they were almost entirely confined to the central nervous system. Among 24 malformed newborns in the influenza group there were 10 cases of anencephaly, four of spina bifida, three of meningomyelocele, one of hydrocephaly, and two of Down's syndrome, along with four other defects (multiple defects were recorded under the most serious). Similar defects were encountered in the 10 control cases, and the proportion of anencephaly to other abnormalities among the maternal influenza group was similar to that among the controls and also to that seen in the 1955 study.

The distribution of defects according to the week of pregnancy when infection occurred was considered, but the numbers were

Table 10–3. **INCIDENCE OF CONGENITAL DEFORMITIES IN OFFSPRING OF MOTHERS WHO HAD HAD INFLUENZA DURING PREGNANCY AND IN OFFSPRING OF CONTROLS: DUBLIN SERIES, 1959**

Subjects	Hospital 1	Hospital 2	Hospital 3	Total
Mothers who had influenza:				
Normal births	214	295	130	669
Malformed births	6	12	6	24
Total	220	307	136	663
Malformed births as % of total	2.7	3.9	4.4	3.6
Controls:				
Normal births	214	304	135	653
Malformed births	6	3	1	10
Total	220	307	136	663
Malformed births as % of total	2.7	1.0	0.7	1.5
Previous survey (Coffey and Jessop, 1955):				
Malformed births as % of total	1.41	1.86	1.57	1.63

Data from Coffey, V. P., and Jessop, W. J.: Maternal influenza and congenital deformities. A prospective study. Lancet 2:935–938, 1959.

too small for analysis. However, when considered in relation to the month of pregnancy, the risk of a defect was found to be greater in the first trimester (7.4 per cent) than in the second (4.3 per cent) and third (2 per cent) trimesters. The incidence of stillbirths in both the influenza and the control groups was almost identical, as was the incidence of prematurity, but when congenitally deformed infants were considered separately, the incidence of prematurity was very high in the influenza group. It was concluded that the incidence of defects in the influenza group was approximately 2.4 times greater than that in the control group, but the distribution of abnormalities in the influenza and control groups was not greatly different. The influence of the infection was not apparently directed toward any specific deformity. If it is postulated that virus influenza is causally related to neural tube and other central nervous system defects, the occurrence of such defects in the control group could be explained on the basis of subclinical infection; if this is so, any such defect was unrelated to the severity of the disease.

A follow-up study of 476 of the 663 children in the influenza-exposed group and 504 of the 663 in the control group was carried out three to four years later (Coffey and Jessop, 1963). The incidence of abnormalities in the influenza group had increased from 3.6 per cent to 15.2 per cent; that in the control group had increased from 1.5 per cent to 10.1 per cent. These included cases of hearing loss, congenital heart disease, cleft lip and palate, atresia, and other defects, as might be expected. Most of the additional defects were evenly distributed between the two groups. Eye defects were most common, constituting 40 per cent of all abnormalities. They were mostly of a very minor nature, such as blocked tear ducts. Although the number of defective children in the influenza group was much higher in 1961–1962 (80, compared with 24 in 1957–1958), the preponderance in the influenza group had diminished from 2.4 times that of the controls to 1.5 times. Nevertheless, the preponderance in central nervous system defects was still apparent (26 in the influenza group and nine in the controls).

Several other studies on the effect of influenza in pregnancy were reported as a result of the Asian influenza epidemic. Walker and McKee (1959) encountered a 100 per cent rate of infection with influenza among 398 pregnant women. Serological tests were used to identify influenza infection; approximately half of these women had no symptoms. Thirteen children with congenital defects were identified (six of 214 following first-trimester influenza and seven of 184 after second-trimester illness). Ten of the children had major defects. Wilson and co-workers (1959) reported a small trial also based on serological tests for influenza. Two anomalies were found in the influenza-positive groups; both children had anencephaly, and their mothers had had a febrile "cold" in the third month of pregnancy.

Another serological study was reported by Hardy and her colleagues (1961). Serological and clinical studies on 671 patients revealed an 85 per cent infection rate; 39 per cent of these subjects had inapparent infections. The incidence of abortions, stillbirths, prematurity, and congenital malformations was higher among those with clinical infections and those with serologically proven influenza who were not apparently infected than among the uninfected (no illness, serologically negative). The incidence of malformations was 3.0 per cent in the clinical influenza group (332 cases), 5.9 per cent in the inapparent infection group (206 cases), and 1.3 per cent in the "no illness" group (73 cases). The defects encountered were all of a nonspecific nature. No neural tube defects were reported. The overall adverse effect to the fetus appeared to be greater after first-trimester influenza but was apparently unrelated to the severity of the disease.

A study by Pleydell (1960) that included observations on 43 women who had had influenza during pregnancy revealed a higher incidence of defects in the influenza group than among 1040 noninfected control subjects who were pregnant at the same time. The risk of defects did not appear to be related to the stage of pregnancy at which infection occurred.

Doll and his colleagues (1960) could detect no definite hazard to the fetus even when the attack of influenza occurred during the early stages of pregnancy. They suggested that anencephaly may be produced if the mother contracts Asian influenza during the first trimester of pregnancy and when other circumstances are suitable (e.g., in an area where the incidence of anencephaly is normally high, as in Scotland and Ireland).

Leck (1963), in an extensive review of the incidence of malformations following influenza epidemics throughout the world, concluded that although the findings in a number of the reports were suggestive of a causal relationship, they were not conclusive. He emphasized that many of the malformations were of a nonspecific nature and included those with a relatively high incidence in all births—anencephaly, congenital heart disease, hypospadias, syndactyly, and talipes. Leck also noted that the incidence of defects in infants whose mothers had had influenza either before conception or after the first trimester was higher than that among infants whose mothers had no history of influenza during pregnancy.

An opportunity to study this matter further arose in Birmingham, England, after influenza epidemics in 1957, 1959, and 1961 (Leck, 1963; Leck and Millar, 1963). No increase in cases of anencephaly or spina bifida was encountered in a study involving 22,698 births, but significant increases in esophageal atresia, cleft lip, anal atresia, and exophthalmos were demonstrated. Cases of all four malformations were considerably increased after the 1961 epidemic. Leck (1963) then reviewed the data from Scotland on stillbirths and deaths for the period from 1950 to 1960, examining cause and month of registration. This included three epidemic periods of influenza: January and February 1951, September through November 1957, and February and March 1959. When the incidence of stillbirths due to malformations was analyzed, it was found that neither specific neural tube defects nor other defects were more common in a six- to nine-month period after each epidemic. Indeed, the rates after 12 to 14 months were higher than those after the six- to nine-month period. This analysis included the data previously reviewed by Doll and co-workers (1960). If there had been a causal relationship, the reverse would have been expected.

It can only be concluded from the evidence available to date that a causal relationship between maternal influenza and congenital malformations, particularly those of the neural tube, is at present not proven. In his review article, Leck (1963) suggested three requirements that should be met to establish a causal relationship between influenza and congenital defects. They were: (1) a period of study long enough to include two or more epidemics, in order to permit comparisons between them; (2) details of the type of malformations present in each affected child; and (3) a population large enough to make it practicable to study each type of malformation separately.

In view of our current understanding of the epidemiology of influenza and greatly improved methods of diagnosis, it should be possible to mount a sufficiently large-scale prospective study to answer the important question of causation. Other factors to be taken into consideration in any such study are the effects of changes of temperature and drug therapy. Hyperthermia in early pregnancy has been suggested as a causal factor in congenital defects of a specific type (Smith et al., 1978; Fleet et al., 1981). Such observations illustrate the complex nature of the factors that can influence fetal growth and development. Wherever possible in a case-controlled study an attempt should be made to record the type of medication prescribed, in view of the observations of Hakasolo and Saxen (1971) in Finland.

MEASLES VIRUS

In the era that preceded large-scale immunization against measles, fewer than 10 per cent of women reached childbearing age without having had this infection. In the Collaborative Perinatal Research Study, 11 of 30,000 (0.3 per 1000) women had measles during pregnancy (Sever and White, 1968).

When measles occurs in the pregnant woman, there is suggestive evidence that uterine contractions may begin in some persons, particularly if the illness occurs late in pregnancy. There have been at least nine studies of the outcome of pregnancies complicated by measles (Stevenson, 1973). Although a variety of abnormalities have been seen in 14 of the 277 reported cases, they are so varied in type that it is unlikely that measles virus acted as an intrauterine pathogen. The abnormalities include Down's syndrome, cleft lip and palate, hydrocephalus, mental retardation, deafness, and various congenital heart defects.

In the 1950–1951 study in the United Kingdom (Manson et al., 1960) 103 pregnancies were reported to have been complicated by measles. The proportion of abortions and stillbirths differed little from those in control subjects, but the infant death rate was higher, and fewer infants survived to two years of age. The increase in deaths occurred among the 36 infants, six of whom died, whose mothers had had measles in the first 12 weeks of pregnancy. There were only two infant deaths from the 65 pregnancies in which measles had occurred after the twelfth week.

A simple percentage comparison of the outcome of the measles and control pregnancies is shown in Table 10–4.

A higher number of malformed children was encountered in addition to the higher infant death rate. A total of eight cases of malformations were recorded (one stillbirth with anencephaly), seven in liveborn infants (Table 10–5). This rate of 7 per cent, compared with 2.3 per cent in the controls, was higher than was expected; the incidence of malformations was slightly higher following measles in the first trimester (11.4 per cent) than in the second trimester (4.5 per cent), although the number of subjects in the study was so small that the significance of this finding is unclear. Whether these findings were spurious is difficult to say, since the defects were few in number and generally of a nonspecific nature (i.e., epilepsy, hydrocephalus, congenital dislocation of the hip, pyloric stenosis, talipes, and two cases of congenital heart disease). There may have been a confusion in diagnosis in one of the latter cases, because one child had bilateral corneal opacities that could have resulted from congenital rubella.

On this evidence, it appears that measles in pregnancy can have a harmful effect on the fetus, but the effect is less striking and certainly less specific than that seen in rubella. Rarely, when maternal measles is acquired late in pregnancy, the infant may be born with evidence of infection or may acquire measles in the form of a severe respiratory disease associated with a rash during the first 12 days of life.

This is not entirely a theoretical matter, since one effect of the control of measles by vaccination in the United States has been the occurrence of the disease in young adults (Krause et al., 1970; Gremillion and Crawford, 1981). Unless vaccination campaigns result in a total elimination of measles, the disease might be expected to occur in young adults and thereby cause a *potential* hazard to the fetus if contracted in pregnancy.

MUMPS VIRUS

In the study in the United Kingdom already referred to (Manson et al., 1960), a total of 501 cases of mumps in pregnancy were reported. Detailed information was available in 496 cases. Nothing unusual was noted in the incidence of abortions or stillbirths. Congenital abnormalities were noted in five of 12 children who died (41.7 per cent), three of whom had evidence of congenital heart disease, compared with 34 per cent of control children who died. No evidence of an excessive number of major malformations was found in the 487 liveborn children. Similar findings were reported by Connelly and co-workers (1964). Other reports, smaller in scope and, frequently, retrospective in nature, have indicated that mumps may have an adverse effect on the infant, particularly when the infection occurs in the first trimester. Fetal death is usually limited to maternal mumps occurring in the first three months of pregnancy. Fetal death followed by abortion characteristically occurs within a two-week period after maternal mumps. It has not been established that fetal death results from fetal viral infection. Usually the maternal infection is no more severe in the pregnant woman than in other persons. Siegel and colleagues (1966) have postulated that fetal death and termination of pregnancy are due to the effect of mumps virus on ovarian endocrine function in early pregnancy.

Table 10–4. **PERCENTAGE COMPARISON OF THE OUTCOME TO THE FETUS OF MATERNAL MEASLES AND CONTROL PREGNANCIES***

Subjects	No. of Cases	Abortions	Stillbirths	Liveborn Infants	Infant Deaths Before 2 Years	Infants Alive at 2 Years
All measles pregnancies	103	1.9	1.9	96.2	7.8	88.4
Controls	–	1.0	2.7	96.3	2.3	94.0
Measles within first 12 weeks	37	2.7	2.7	94.6	16.2	78.4
Controls	–	1.9	2.7	95.4	2.4	93.0

*The comparison was made with the expected outcome calculated from the experience of standardized control groups.

Data from Manson, M. M., Logan, W. P. D., and Loy, R. M.: Rubella and other virus infections during pregnancy. Rep. Public Health Med. Subj. No. 101. London, Her Majesty's Stationery Office, 1960, tables 11 and G.

Table 10–5. THE NUMBER AND PERCENTAGE OF INFANTS WITH AND WITHOUT MAJOR MALFORMATIONS IN THE CONTROL AND VIRUS SERIES ACCORDING TO THE STAGE OF PREGNANCY WHEN INFECTION OCCURRED: MEASLES GROUP*

Type of Case	All Infants					All Liveborn Infants					Infants Born Alive but Dying Before 2 Years				
	No. of Cases	Without Major Malformations		With Major Malformations		No. of Cases	Without Major Malformations		With Major Malformations		No. of Cases	Without Major Malformations		With Major Malformations	
		No.	%	No.	%		No.	%	No.	%		No.	%	No.	%
Control series	5611	5431	96.8	156	2.8	5455	5326	97.6	128	2.3	140	92	65.7	47	33.6
Measles up to 12th week	36	31	86.1	4	11.1	35	31	88.6	4	11.4	6	3	50.0	3	50.0
Measles in 13th–28th weeks	45	42	93.3	3	6.7	44	42	95.5	2	4.5	0	0	–	0	–
Measles in 29th–40th weeks	20	19	95.0	1	5.0	20	19	95.0	1	5.0	2	1	–	1	–
All measles cases	101	92	91.1	8	7.9	99	92	92.9	7	7.1	8	4	50.0	4	50.0

*Controls as described in Table 10–1, but cases delivered up to the date week of pregnancy, i.e., abortions, are excluded. Total numbers of cases are not always identical.

Data from Manson, M. M., Logan, W. P. D., and Loy, R. M.: Rubella and other virus infections during pregnancy. Rep. Public Health Med. Subj. No. 101. London, Her Majesty's Stationery Office, 1960, table L.

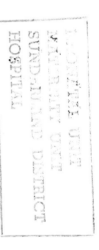

There are many case reports in the literature associating maternal mumps infection with a wide variety of congenital anomalies. These reports, taken *in toto,* do not constitute convincing evidence that mumps virus is a fetal pathogen. The largest, most carefully designed studies do not support the thesis that mumps virus is capable of producing a fetal malformation. The special, complex relationship that mumps infection has to chronic cardiomyopathy and endocardial fibroelastosis is of considerable interest and deserves further discussion.

Endocardial Fibroelastosis and Chronic Cardiomyopathy

In 1963, Noren and co-workers reported skin test reactivity to mumps antigen in patients with endocardial fibroelastosis. This finding was confirmed by Vosburgh and colleagues (1965), Shone and colleagues (1966), and St. Geme and colleagues (1966). However, Gersony and co-workers (1966) found that only five of 14 patients tested had 10 mm of erythema within 48 hours of intradermal inoculation with mumps antigen.

St. Geme and colleagues (1966) found delayed cutaneous hypersensitivity to mumps virus in 13 of 14 patients with endocardial fibroelastosis. Only two of these children had mumps neutralizing antibody. In addition, mumps virus could not be recovered from the oropharynx of the affected children or from the heart tissue of those few patients who had died. St. Geme et al. postulated that the transient nature of the viral infection contributed to a partial or "split" immunological response, that is, T-cell–mediated cellular immunity without humoral (B-cell) immunity. This had been shown to be conceptually possible by the work of Salvin and Smith (1960), which demonstrated that minimal amounts of antigen evoked only delayed hypersensitivity in the guinea pig, whereas larger amounts of antigen stimulated both cellular and humoral immunity.

It has also been noted that mothers of infants with endocardial fibroelastosis have both a higher mean geometric titer of mumps antibody and a higher prevalence of mumps infection or exposure during pregnancy. St. Geme and co-workers (1966) postulated that endocardial fibroelastosis represented the sequelae of fetal myocardial mumps infection and that the nature of the split immunological response suggests that cellular immunity

is the more primitive phylogenetic and ontogenetic response to a foreign antigen. This phenomenon has been demonstrated in the rhesus monkey by St. Geme et al. (1972).

Aase and colleagues (1972) studied the immunological response of children born to mothers exposed to mumps during an epidemic that occurred on remote St. Lawrence Island off the coast of Alaska. They found that the progeny of women exposed to mumps in pregnancy possessed delayed hypersensitivity to mumps virus but no antibody. This was in contrast to children who were infants and toddlers when the epidemic occurred. The latter group developed both cellular and humoral immunity to mumps virus.

There seems to be little doubt that mumps virus is able to infect the placenta (Aase et al., 1972) and the fetus. Mumps virus has been isolated from the tissues of a 10-week old fetus spontaneously aborted four days after an attack of clinical mumps in the mother (Kurtz et al., 1982). Specimens of fetal tissues were pooled for virus isolation and chromosomal studies, but no specific changes were noted. It is estimated that the risk of endocardial fibroelastosis in the offspring of a woman who has contracted mumps during pregnancy is approximately 2 per cent (Mitchell et al., 1966; St. Geme et al., 1971). The probability is that most fetuses with myocarditis go on to complete healing. Hutchins and Vie (1972) suggested that interstitial myocarditis may produce persistent left ventricular dilatation, relative mitral valvular insufficiency, increasing endocardial tension, and compensatory hypertrophy. These, they postulate, ultimately lead to the accumulation of the thick layer of collagen and elastic tissue beneath the endocardial lining that is characteristic of endocardial fibroelastosis.

Mumps in late pregnancy may result in infection and disease in the infant, although this must be a very rare event. Jones and co-workers (1980) have described cases that were benign in three mother-infant pairs; one infant had bilateral parotitis.

ARBOVIRUS INFECTIONS

Western Equine Encephalitis Virus

Shinefield and Townsend (1953) reported western equine encephalitis (WEE) virus infection in twins born to a mother who manifested encephalitis three days prior to term. The infants became symptomatic five days after birth with the onset of fever, twitching, lethargy, anorexia, and seizures. The spinal fluid was abnormal, with more than 500 white blood cells per cubic milliliter and elevation of cerebrospinal fluid protein. The diagnosis was confirmed by rising titers to WEE antigen during the first three weeks of life.

Other Arboviruses

Little systematic study has been made of the role of the many other arboviruses during pregnancy. The obvious reason for this is that they occur most often in countries where other health problems are too serious for the arboviruses to warrant much attention. That infections with a number of these viruses in pregnancy could cause fetal infection, and therefore the potential for damage, cannot be discounted. This is illustrated by the observations of Aaskov and his colleagues (1981) on the transmission of Ross River virus to the fetus during an epidemic in Fiji in 1979.

EPSTEIN-BARR VIRUS

Epstein-Barr (EB) virus is one of the herpes group of viruses and shares with the other members the property of latency. However, unlike CMV, herpes simplex virus, and varicella-zoster viruses, EB virus cannot be isolated directly and is identified by the capacity to transform cord blood lymphocytes from normal infants. Most clinically recognized episodes of disease are expressed as the syndrome of infectious mononucleosis. There is no seasonal variation in infection, which is generally of low transmissibility. Spread probably occurs by the saliva; intimate oral contact is required for spread among adults. Clinical disease is most frequent in the age group between 15 and 25 years. However, many primary EB virus infections—between 50 and 72 per cent in studies in young adults—are subclinical (Chang, 1980).

The epidemiology of EB virus infections gives considerable opportunity in many populations for infection to be acquired during pregnancy. The incidence of infection in young adults in several serological studies indicated a rate of up to 10 to 25 per 100 per year (Evans, 1981). Socioeconomic factors are important, because the risk of acquiring infection is much higher in individuals of low socioeconomic status. The prevalence of antibody to EB virus is very similar to that of antibody to CMV in childhood. In Barbados, Uganda, Indonesia, and Mexico, 80 per cent or more of children are seropositive by six years of age, whereas in France, Sweden, England, and the United States, only 30 to 40 per cent possess antibody. Surveys in pregnant women in France (Icart et al., 1981), Canada (Gervais and Joncas, 1979), Philadelphia (Fleisher and Bolognese, 1982), and Sacramento (Le et al., 1983) have shown that 3, 4.2, 3.1, and 3.4 per cent, respectively, were susceptible.

In spite of the opportunity for infection during the age of childbearing, there is a paucity of data on infection of the fetus or the newborn by EB virus, and there is no evidence that it has a role in the causation of congenital defects. Several studies have investigated the frequency of congenital infection using the technique of transformation of cord blood lymphocytes. Chang and Blankenship (1973) found only one infected infant among 696 cases studied. This infant was clinically normal at birth and when reexamined at two years of age. A subsequent study of 2000 infants failed to detect any infections (Chang and Seto, 1979). Visintine and co-workers (1976) reported details of one infant whose pharyngeal secretions transformed cord blood lymphocytes. This child had transient hepatomegaly in infancy, but at two years of age no abnormalities were found.

Serological studies of pregnant women to determine the occurrence of infection and reports on the outcome of the pregnancies in which infection occurred are shown in Table 10–6. There is no evidence to indicate a particular constellation of effects.

Two infants with dual congenital EB virus and CMV infections have been reported by Joncas and colleagues (1977, 1981). Both had multiple defects (hepatosplenomegaly, periventricular calcification, and microcephaly) consistent with CMV infection. Goldberg and colleagues (1981) described an infant with thrombocytopenic monocytosis, metaphysitis, hypotonia, micrognathia, cataracts, and cryptorchidism whose mother had had a nonspecific febrile illness at two months' gestation. Serological tests and prolonged cultures of peripheral lymphocytes were suggestive of active EB virus infection at birth.

Reactivation of latent infection in sero-

Table 10–6. **OUTCOME OF EB VIRUS INFECTION IN PREGNANCY: SEROLOGICAL STUDIES**

No. of Pregnancies	No. of Primary Infections*	No. in Whom Outcome Was Determined	Findings	Reference
2752	6	6	2 normal infants 2 premature infants 1 multiple defect 1 abortion at 25 weeks	Icart et al. (1981)
1939	35	24	12 normal infants 1 spontaneous abortion 4 premature deliveries 2 small for gestational age 4 hyperbilirubinemia 1 hypospadias	Fleisher and Bolognese (1982)
1729	1	1	Normal twins	Le et al. (1983)

*IgM VCA antibody positive or early antigen positive.

positive pregnant women was studied by Fleisher and Bolognese (1983). Reactivation was suggested by the presence of antibody to early antigen (anti-EA). This occurred more frequently in the 200 pregnant women (55 per cent) than in controls (22 to 32 per cent) and was usually detected early in the pregnancy. In spite of these reactivations, the infants of these women did not differ with respect to birth weight, congenital abnormalities, or neonatal jaundice from the infants of women in whom reactivation was not detected. Thus, these findings did not confirm those of Icart and Didier (1981), who reported that 21 per cent of mothers (115 of 715) with anti-EA had an adverse outcome, compared with only 7 per cent of the 607 women who did not have anti-EA.

EB virus has not been detected in cervical secretions (Chang and Seto, 1979) and if confirmed would suggest that perinatal EB virus infection is unlikely.

LYMPHOCYTIC CHORIOMENINGITIS VIRUS

Although lymphocytic choriomeningitis (LCM) has long been used as a model for the study of congenital viral infection, this virus has not been shown to be a major fetal pathogen in humans. Komrower and co-workers (1955) have presented evidence that the virus can cross the placenta in humans. Recently, a marked increase in the number of human LCM infections has been reported in the United States following exposure to infected hamsters. No cases, however, have been reported in the United Kingdom for many years. Ackermann and colleagues have reported two cases of probable congenital

LCM infection. The mother in each instance had been in contact with golden hamsters in the second half of pregnancy. Both infants had internal hydrocephalus and chorioretinitis. One also had marked myopia, the other severe hyperbilirubinemia. After cerebrospinal fluid drainage, the hydrocephalus receded. Developmental retardation and marked visual impairment occurred in both children. Neutralizing and complement-fixing LCM antibodies were demonstrated in both mother-infant pairs. The neutralizing antibody persisted, whereas the complement-fixing antibody declined during the first year of life. It is probable that the source of infection was the hamster, since this animal is known to be a major carrier of LCM. It is quite likely that, with recent evidence of increasing LCM disease in hamster owners, more cases of suspected congenital LCM infection will be reported. The phenomenon of immune tolerance that occurs in rodents infected *in utero* with LCM has not been demonstrated in humans.

Bibliography

Aase, J. M., Noren, G. R., Reddy, D. V., and St. Geme, J. W., Jr.: Mumps-virus infection in pregnant women and the immunologic response of their offspring. N. Engl. J. Med., 286:1379–1382, 1972.

Aaskov, J. G., Nair, L., Lawrence, G. W., Dalglish, D. A., and Tucker, M: Evidence for transplacental transmission of Ross River virus in humans. Med. J. Aust. 1:20–21, 1981.

Ackermann, R., Köver, G., Turss, R., et al.: Pränatale Infektion mit dem Virus der lymphozytarer Choriomeningitis: Bericht über zwer Fälle. Dtsch. Med. Wochenschr. 99:629–632, 1974.

Chang, R. S.: In Infectious Mononucleosis. Boston, G. K. Hall, 1980.

Chang, R. S., and Blankenship, W.: Spontaneous in vitro

transformation of leukocytes from a neonate. Proc. Soc. Exp. Biol. Med. *144*:337–339, 1973.

Coffey, V. P., and Jessop, W. J. E.: Congenital abnormalities. Ir. J. Med. Sci. *349*:30–48, 1955.

Coffey, V. P., and Jessop, W. J. E.: Maternal influenza and congenital deformities. A prospective study. Lancet *2*:935–938, 1959.

Coffey, V. P., and Jessop, W. J. E.: Maternal influenza and congenital deformities. A follow-up study. Lancet *1*:748–751, 1963.

Connelly, J. P., Reynolds, S., and Crawford, J. D.: Viral and drug hazards in pregnancy. Clin. Pediatr. *3*:587–597, 1964.

Doll, R., Hill, A. B., and Jakula, J.: Asian influenza in pregnancy and congenital defects. Br. J. Prev. Soc. Med. *14*:167–172, 1960.

Evans, A. S.: Epidemiology of Epstein-Barr virus infections. In Nahmias, A. K., Dowdle, W. R., and Schinazi, R. F. (eds.): The Human Herpesvirus. New York, Elsevier, 1981, pp. 172–183.

Fleet, H., Graham, J. M., and Smith, D. W.: Central nervous system and facial defects associated with maternal hyperthermia at 4–14 weeks gestation. Pediatrics. *67*:785–789, 1981.

Fleisher, G. R., and Bolognese, R.: Seroepidemiology of Epstein-Barr virus in pregnant women. J. Infect. Dis. *145*:537–541, 1982.

Fleisher, G. R., and Bolognese, R.: Persistent Epstein-Barr virus infection and frequency. J. Infect. Dis. *147*:982–986, 1983.

Francis, T., Jr.: A new type of virus from epidemic influenza. Science *92*:405–408, 1940.

Gersony, W. M., Katz, S. L., and Nadas, A. S.: Endocardial fibroelastosis and mumps virus. Pediatrics *37*:430–434, 1966.

Gervais, T., and Joncas, J. H.: Epstein-Barr virus infection: seroepidemiology in various population groups in the greater Montreal area. Comp. Immunol. Microbiol. Infect. Dis. *2*:207–212, 1979.

Goldberg, G. N., Fulginiti, V. A., Ray, G. G., Ferry, P., Jones, J. E., Cross, H., and Minnich, L.: In utero Epstein-Barr virus (infectious mononucleosis) infection. J.A.M.A. *246*:1579–1581, 1981.

Gremillion, D. H., and Crawford, G. E.: Measles pneumonia in young adults. Am. J. Med. *71*:539–542, 1981.

Hakasolo, J., and Saxen, L.: Influenza epidemic and congenital defects. Lancet *11*:1346–1347, 1971.

Hardy, J. B., Azarowicz, E. N., Mannini, A., Medearis, D. N., Jr., and Cooke, R. E.: The effect of Asian influenza on the outcome of pregnancy. Baltimore, 1957–1958. Am. J. Public Health *51*:1182–1188, 1961.

Hutchins, G. M., and Vie, S. A.: The progression of interstitial myocarditis to idiopathic endocardial fibroelastosis. Am. J. Pathol. *66*:483–496, 1972.

Icart, J., and Didier, J.: Infections due to Epstein-Barr virus during pregnancy. J. Infect. Dis. *143*:499, 1981.

Icart, J., Didier, J., Dalens, M., Chabanon, G., and Boucays, A.: Prospective study of Epstein-Barr virus infection during pregnancy. Biomedicine *34*:160–163, 1981.

Joncas, J. H., Aflieri, C., Willis, M., Jasmin, G., Brochu, P., Bolgough, I., and Huang, E.: Dual congenital infection with Esptein-Barr virus (EBV) and cytomegalovirus (CMV). N. Engl. J. Med. *304*:1399–1403, 1981.

Joncas, J. H., Wills, A., and McLaughlin, B.: Congenital infection with cytomegalovirus and Epstein-Barr virus. Can. Med. Assoc. J. *113*:1417–1418, 1977.

Jones, J. F., Kay, G. R., and Fulginiti, V. A.: Perinatal mumps infection. J. Pediatr. *96*:912–919, 1980.

Komrower, G.: Lymphocytic choriomeningitis in newborns: probable transplacental infection. Lancet *1*:697–698, 1955.

Krause, P. J., Cherry, J. D., Deseda-Tous, J., Champion, J. G., Strassburg, M., Sullivan, C., Spencer, M., Bryson, Y. J., Welliver, R. C., and Boyer, K. M.: Epidemic measles in young adults. Ann. Intern. Med. *90*:873–876, 1979.

Kurtz, J. B., Tomlinson, A. H., and Pearson, J.: Mumps virus isolated from a fetus. Br. Med. J. *284*:421, 1982.

Le, C. T., Chang, R. S., and Lipson, M. H.: Epstein-Barr virus infections during pregnancy. Am. J. Dis. Child. *137*:466–468, 1983.

Leck, I.: The incidence of malformations following influenza epidemics. Br. J. Prev. Soc. Med. *17*:70–80, 1963.

Leck, I., and Millar, E. L. M.: Short-term changes in the incidence of malformations. Br. J. Prev. Soc. Med. *17*:1–12, 1963.

Magill, T. P.: A virus from cases of influenza-like upper respiratory infection. Proc. Soc. Exp. Biol. Med. *45*:162–164, 1940.

Manson, M. M., Logan, W. P. D., and Loy, R. M.: Rubella and other virus infections during pregnancy. Rep. Public Health Med. Subj. No. 101. London, Her Majesty's Stationery Office, 1960.

Mitchell, S. C., Froelich, L. A., Banas, J. S., Jr., and Gilkerson, M. R.: An epidemiologic assessment of primary endocardial fibroelastosis. Am. J. Cardiol. *18*:859–866, 1966.

Noren, G. R., Adams, P., Jr., and Anderson, R. C.: Positive skin test reactivity to mumps virus antigen in endocardial fibroelastosis. J. Pediatr. *62*:604–606, 1963.

Pleydell, M. J.: Anencephaly and other congenital abnormalities. Br. Med. J. *1*:309–315, 1960.

Salvin, S. B., and Smith, R. F.: Delayed hypersensitivity and anamnestic response. J. Immunol., *84*:449–457, 1960.

Sever, J. L., and White, L. R.: Virus infections in pregnancy. Collaborative Perinatal Research Study. Am. Rev. Med. *19*:471–486, 1968.

Shinefield, H. R., and Townsend, T. E.: Transplacental transmission of western equine encephalitis. J. Pediatr. *42*:21–25, 1953.

Shone, J. D., Munoz, A. S., Manning, J. A., and Keith, J. D.: The mumps antigen skin test in endocardial fibroelastosis. Pediatrics *37*:423–429, 1966.

Siegel, M., Fuerst, H. T., and Peress, N. S.: Comparative fetal mortality in maternal virus diseases. A prospective study on rubella, measles, mumps, chicken pox and hepatitis. N. Engl. J. Med. *274*:768–771, 1966.

Smith, D. W., Clarren, S. K., Harvey, M. A. S.: Hyperthermia as a possible teratogenic agent. J. Pediatr. *92*:878–883, 1978.

Smith, W., Andrews, C. H., and Laidlaw, P. P.: A virus obtained from influenza patients. Lancet *2*:66–68, 1933.

Stevenson, R. E.: The Fetus and the Newly Born Infant: Influences of the Prenatal Environment. St. Louis, C. V. Mosby Company, 1973.

St. Geme, J. W., Jr., Noren, G. R., and Adams, P., Jr.: Proposed embryopathic relation between mumps virus and primary endocardial fibroelastosis. N. Engl. J. Med. *275*:339–347, 1966.

St. Geme, J. W., Jr., Peralta, H., and Van Pelt, L. F.: Intrauterine infection of the rhesus monkey with mumps virus: abbreviated viral replication in the immature fetus as an explanation for split immunologic recognition after birth. J. Infect. Dis. *126*:249–256, 1972.

St. Geme, J. W., Jr., Wanker, J. J., Jr., Arce, M. A., and

Van Pelt, L. F.: The effect of repeated mumps skin tests on the induction of antibody. Pediatrics *48*:445–447, 1971.

Stuart-Harris, C. H., and Schild, G. C.: Influenza. 1st ed. London, Edward Arnold, 1976.

Visintine, A. M., Gerber, P., and Nahmias, A. J.: Leukocyte transforming agent (Epstein-Barr virus) in newborn infants and older individuals. J. Pediatr. *89*:571–575, 1976.

Vosburgh, J. B., Diehl, A. M., Liu, C., Lauer, R. M., and

Kabisi, A.: Relationship of mumps to endocardial fibroelastosis. Am. J. Dis. Child. *109*:73, 1965.

Walker, W. M., and McKee, A. M.: 633 women with Asian flu antibodies. No congenital malformations (retrospective study). Obstet. Gynecol. *13*:394–398, 1959.

Wilson, M. G., Heins, H. L., Imagawa, D. T., and Adams, J. L.: Teratogenic effects of influenza. J.A.M.A. *171*:638–641, 1959.

Pathology of the Placenta and Cord in Some Viral Infections

The placenta and the umbilical cord may be affected by infection with herpesviruses (cytomegalovirus [CMV], herpes simplex virus, and varicella virus), poxviruses (variola virus and vaccinia virus), and rubella virus. These viral lesions have been the subjects of case reports collated and illustrated in several textbooks (Benirschke and Driscoll, 1967; Philippe, 1974; Potter and Craig, 1975) and reviews (Altshuler, 1975; Blanc, 1980, 1981). Although many placentae with rubella infection have been studied carefully (45 cases by Ornoy et al. [1973]), the largest group of placentae with CMV infection reported in detail included only five cases (Benirschke et al., 1974). Many essential questions about pathogenesis and prognostic significance remain unanswered because of the dearth of data available to individual observers. The material from Babies Hospital, New York, New York, collected over 20 years, is limited to 15 placentae affected by CMV, four by rubella, three by herpes simplex, and one each by varicella and vaccinia. This lack of material may be related to the fact that few spontaneous abortions were referred.

Our knowledge of the placental pathology in viral infections is fragmentary for several reasons. The placenta remains an organ neglected by obstetricians, pediatricians, and pathologists alike, even though it provides us with a large "biopsy specimen" of fetal and maternal tissues. Therapeutic abortions mostly provide data on early rubella infection of immature placentae. Because it is impractical and costly to examine all delivered placentae, even interested neonatologists will submit only those of stillborn or critically ill newborn infants. This explains the paucity of information about the placenta in two fairly common viral infections: in rubella, most babies survive the neonatal period and few term placentae are examined; and in CMV disease most infections are inapparent. Hence, as in herpetic or pox infections, chances are that the only placentae submitted to the pathologist will be those in cases of acute, fatal disease or chronic disease, representing the two ends of the spectrum.

The histopathological changes in the placenta may provide clues to the natural history of viral disease, and they may also be of prognostic importance for the newborn infant. The performance of placental biopsy, which was suggested by Ornoy and co-workers (1973), does not appear justifiable until the correlation between placental and fetal lesions is fully understood.

It is likely that placental disease, like fetal disease, varies with (1) the route of infection; (2) the strain, pathogenicity, and size of the inoculum; (3) the presence of partial immunity; and (4) the ability of the mother and fetus to mount a swift response. To assess properly the significance of histopathological changes, we should be able to put them in the full context of clinical and laboratory information, including, at least, prospective studies of pregnant women to determine the timing of seroconversion, virological investigations of the body fluids and of the cervix, antibody levels at birth in both mother and child, and isolation and quantitation of the virus from the mother, the child, and the placenta. Identification of the virus by immunofluorescence or transmission electron microscopy could be done. This has not been possible in most instances until recently.

The prognostic significance for the baby of a given alteration in the placenta cannot be fully evaluated as yet. We need to know more about the natural history of the placental lesions that are induced at various times during the course of pregnancy and about the modulation of disease by the maturing fetal inflammatory response and by fetal and maternal immunity.

CMV INFECTION

In cases of CMV infection, the cord shows no distinctive macroscopic or microscopic features. Macroscopically, the placenta frequently seems normal in the delivery room. Although it may be small in growth-retarded newborns, it is slightly larger than normal in some anemic infants and looks like the pallid, edematous placenta seen in mild Rh disease. No adequate information is available about fetoplacental weight ratio and other gross features in clinically silent infection; in two such cases we examined, there were no macroscopic clues. In severe CMV villitis, multiple small infarct-like areas that correspond to the agglutination of necrotic villi may be seen.

The histological changes can be divided into three categories: specific changes (i.e., cytomegalic cells), nonspecific placental responses to fetal anemia (i.e., hyperplasia, edema), and nonspecific but highly suggestive inflammatory changes (i.e., acute necrosis of cells and ground substance with karyor-

rhexis and necrotizing vasculitis, followed by obliteration of vessels, fibrosis of villi, and infiltration with dense lymphoplasmocytic aggregates).

Early Lesions

The earliest histological lesion in the young fetus is multifocal coagulation necrosis of the villi, which was observed in a 14-week abortus without remarkable macroscopic features.* The endothelial cells of villous capillaries and of larger vessels in stem villi show typical cytomegalic changes: they become acidophilic and glassy, and they may desquamate (Fig. 11–1). The vessel wall and the villous stroma become edematous, and adjacent Hofbauer cells increase in size and show typical nuclear and cytoplasmic inclusions before undergoing necrosis. A whole small villus or a segment of stem villus may undergo coagulation necrosis; fetal vessels may become unidentifiable at this stage. Only then does the trophoblastic epithelium become necrotic (Fig. 11–2), without having shown inclusion cells, and adjacent villi become agglutinated within fibrin deposits, into which maternal polymorphonuclear leukocytes migrate (Fig. 11–3). Some discrete lesions consist only of patchy stromal necrosis, with karyorrhexis of Hofbauer cells resulting in a scattering of nuclear dust within glossy ground substance, a fairly typical feature of acute viral necrosis. Similar changes were seen by Altshuler (1973). The absence of an acute inflammatory fetal response is due to the early age. Thus, from light microscopic examination of the rare early case, it appears that the virus passes through intact trophoblastic epithelium and either multiplies in stromal and vascular cells or gains access to the fetal circulation to be redistributed by viremia, thereby affecting villous vessels and adjacent stroma. The fact that necrosis was absent even though the fetal parenchymas contained many cytomegalic cells, suggests either a prolonged and severe placental involvement, with delayed, recent extension to the fetus, or a relative resistance of somatic fetal tissues.

In contrast, in a premature stillborn infant, scattered endothelial cytomegalic cells sometimes apparently free-floating in the vascular lumen, are found in placental villi and fetal

---

*Courtesy of Dr. Peter Tang, St. Luke's Hospital, Cleveland, Ohio.

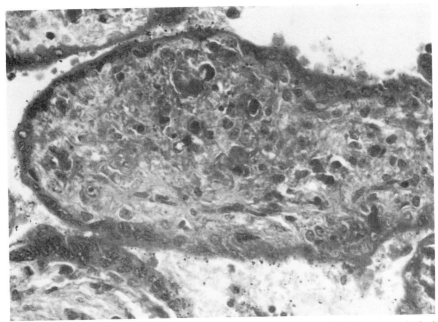

Figure 11–1. CMV infection in a young fetus, showing intact trophoblastic epithelium, many inclusion cells, and early necrosis of villous stroma. ×375. (Photograph by Ida Nathan.)

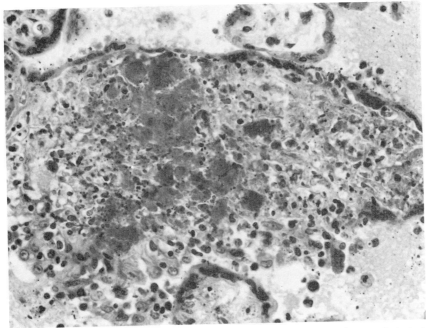

Figure 11–2. CMV infection (same case as in Fig. 11–1). Massive necrosis in which the rounded, darker "ghosts" of inclusion cells are present, surrounded by a fine dust of nuclear debris. Now the trophoblast is degenerated on the lower side, and some maternal polymorphs migrate into the villus from the intervillous space. ×325. (Photograph by Ida Nathan.)

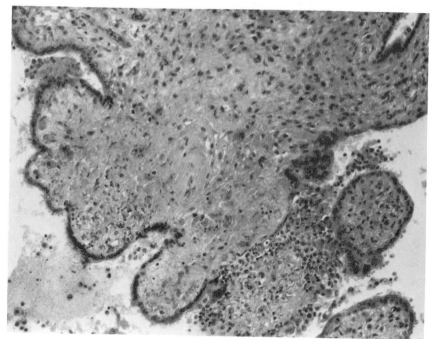

Figure 11–3. CMV infection (same case as in Fig. 11–1). Patchy necrosis in a stem villus with agglutination of villi (lower right). × 176. (Photograph by Ida Nathan.)

tissues. There are very rare cytomegalic cells in renal tubules, but a number are found in lung epithelium (Fig. 11–4). A few fresh microglial nodules are found in the brain, one around an inclusion cell. Minimal necrotizing vasculitis affects the chorionic and villous vessels. The large number of cytomegalic cells in the pulmonary epithelium, in contrast to the few affected vascular cells, may be related to infection by aspiration: whether the amnionic fluid was contaminated by fetal urine after transplacental hematogenous spread or by direct extension from an infected cervix is a matter of speculation. Of special interest is the distinct possibility that CMV may spread through infected desquamated cells of the vascular endothelium, as has been suggested to be the case with rubella (Töndury and Smith, 1966; Ornoy et al., 1973).

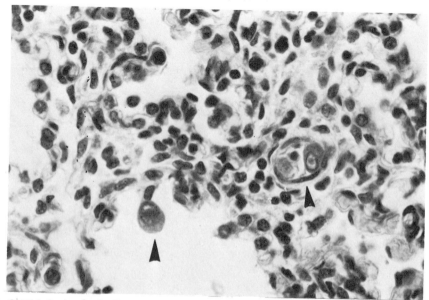

Figure 11–4. CMV infection in the lung of a premature (800-gm) stillborn infant. Two inclusion cells in the small vessel (right arrow), one inclusion cell in the air space (left arrow). ×600. (Photograph by Ida Nathan.)

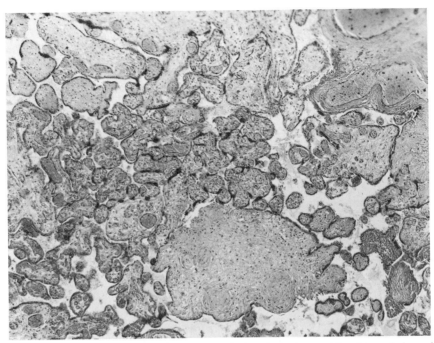

Figure 11–5. CMV infection in a jaundiced premature (1730-gm) newborn with microcephaly and intracranial calcifications. Large edematous villi (along right and upper margins) and avascular stem villus (center of lower margin). ×63. (Photograph by Ida Nathan.)

Late Lesions

In older lesions, the affected vessels are obliterated or disappear completely in affected villi or stem villi (Figs. 11–5 and 11–6), but this is not a process affecting all vessels diffusely. Rarely, damage to the vascular wall results in irregular fibrosis and thinning of the media. Hemosiderin deposits, presumably related to small hemorrhages or the resorption of blood in small thromboses, are common, as are intravillous, rounded calcifi-

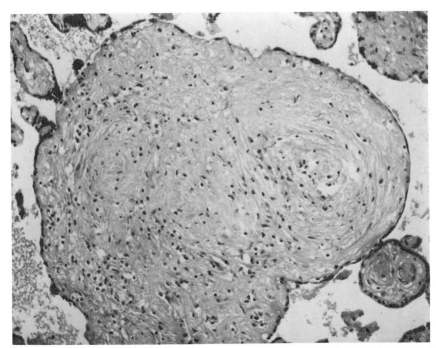

Figure 11–6. CMV infection (same case as in Fig. 11–5). The vaguely circular shape of three completely fibrosed vessels can still be made out. A few lymphocytes are scattered in the stroma. ×160. (Photograph by Ida Nathan.)

cations. The latter may result from the dystrophic calcification of the stroma, but they frequently appear to be intravascular and may be calcified thrombi. Siderocalcic impregnation of the basement membrane of villi is seen on occasion.

Most striking are aggregates of plasmocytes and lymphocytes located both in peripheral villi and around vessels in stem villi (Fig. 11–7). Large infiltrates are usually seen in avascular fibrotic villi that have lost their trophoblast and are coated with fibrin. The plasma cells are active, and their production of immunoglobulins can be demonstrated by immunofluorescent staining of frozen (Blanc, 1969) or paraffin-embedded tissue. IgM was found in a few cells, and IgG and IgA in others. Although these cells were clearly intravillous, sometimes within vessel walls, or clearly perivascular and not concentrated at the most peripheral portion of villi, their exclusive fetal origin is still not established. Our attempts to stain, by fluorescent techniques, the Y chromosome in plasma cells found in placentae of male babies were not successful. It is worth noting the persistence of active infection in the face of a good local immune response in those placentae showing side-by-side acute necrosis (with or without typical inclusion cells) and chronic infiltrates.

In view of the constant involvement of the kidneys and the probable frequent shedding of the virus in the amnionic fluid, one would expect to find specific alterations of the cord, as well as some form of chronic viral chorioamnionitis. We have not recognized such a lesion in our cases, nor have we seen inclusions in the amnionic epithelium. Thus, if inclusion cells are detected in fluid collected by amniocentesis, their origin is likely to be the fetal lungs or kidneys. Since cervical infection is not rare, the virus could spread either to the endometrium and the intervillous space of the placenta (ultimately producing a hematogenous infection) or directly through the membranes to the amnionic fluid. Shearer and colleagues' case (1972), in which only one twin was infected, suggests the latter route.

Focal decidual necrosis was found in several cases, but it also exists in many placentae free of villitis; its significance is not clear. Massive plasmocytic infiltrates in the decidua, unusual in routine material, were found only once. No inclusion cells were found in the decidual tissue in our series, including the abortus.

Placental hyperplasia occurs in response to fetal anemia. The changes resemble those seen in isoimmunization and consist of excessive formation of peripheral villi, relative immaturity, an increase in stromal cells (see Fig. 11–5) and capillaries, and erythroblastosis. An alteration of unknown origin, non-

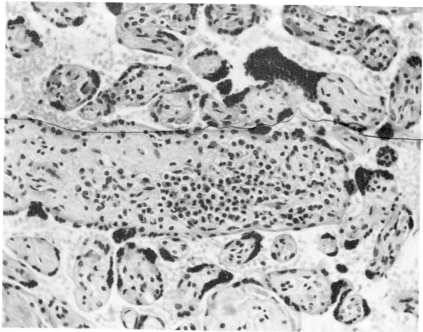

Figure 11–7. CMV infection in a 1480-gm term infant with jaundice, disseminated intravascular clotting, and microcephaly. Massive plasmocytic infiltrate in a large villus. ×350. (Photograph by Ida Nathan.)

specific but highly suggestive of chronic fetal infection, is a diffuse increase in Hofbauer cells within plump but otherwise mature villi—the "proliferative villitis" of Altshuler and Russel (1975).

The Placenta in Apparent and Inapparent Clinical Infection of the Newborn

Marked lymphoplasmocytic villitis was present in 10 of 14 premature or term infants with CMV disease. Seven were stillborn or died in the neonatal period, and all had severe CMV infection. Central nervous system involvement was found in the six patients whose brains were examined. The other three had clinical disease at birth: one is microcephalic, and one is growth-retarded, deaf, hyperactive, and probably mentally retarded at six years of age; the third (Case 2 of Feldman [1969]) was followed only to six months of age. CMV disease was actually diagnosed in the child with microcephaly by placental examination, and the diagnosis was confirmed by urine sediment examination. Mild villitis existed in an additional case in which there were very small collections of mononuclear cells with few plasma cells, some hemosiderin, and two cytomegalic cells in capillaries. This patient with distinctive but minimal villitis had a petechial rash of the head and trunk and transient hepatosplenomegaly; this child was also followed only to the age of six months (Case 4 of Feldman [1969]).

Of the three remaining cases, one was in the premature infant described earlier, who had an apparent viremic phase and endothelial cytomegalia. Both placental and fetal lesions were minimal. The last two patients, those in Cases 1 and 3 from Feldman's (1969) series, were clinically normal. A nonspecific but suspicious increase in stromal cells was present in the patient in Case 4 and in the patient in Case 3, in whom it was the only anomaly. The latter showed a few vessels with minimal fibrinoid necrosis. These two patients were also normal at six months of age. It appears that there is a fairly good correlation between the severity of lesions in the placenta and those in the newborn, a conclusion that supports those of Altshuler and Russel (1975) and Benirschke and co-workers (1974). It is noteworthy that all of Feldman's cases were presumably infected in the second trimester of pregnancy and yet presented with a spectrum of placental lesions ranging from inconspicuous to severe. It would be of interest to check the predictive value of placental histopathology by following up a large series of cases of inapparent infection with CMV. Finally, placental histology could be used to differentiate prenatal from postnatal infection (Whitley et al., 1976) and, possibly, transplacental from ascending infection.

Diagnosis

The finding of multiple plasmocytic infiltrates with proliferative villitis, focal necrosis, some obliterated vessels in stem villi or villi, and focal hemosiderin deposits suggests a diagnosis of CMV infection and indicates the need for a diligent search for typical inclusion cells. The differential diagnosis should consider all other forms of chronic villitis. In rubella, chronic inflammatory infiltrates are not prominent, hypoplasia of peripheral villi is striking, and vascular changes (total disappearance of stem villi vessels and hypoplastic vessels) are marked. Chronic villitis is not known as yet in herpes, at least in the absence of chronic chorioamnionitis. The pox lesions are granulomatous. The diagnoses of toxoplasmosis, Chagas' disease, and syphilis may be difficult if the agents are not looked for and identified, since all the placental features described in these three diseases and in CMV are nonspecific and related to the chronicity of the process. Very similar forms of villitis also occur in which a search for an agent is unsuccessful; these are diagnosed by exclusion as "villitides of unknown etiology." In these, plasma cells are less prominent, the pattern of lymphocytic infiltration may suggest a maternal origin of the lymphocytes, and the diffuse increase in Hofbauer cells is commonly impressive.

Conclusion

In CMV infection, the histopathological study of a number of placentae has conclusively demonstrated acute and chronic placental lesions presumably secondary to maternal viremia and hematogenous spread. Transcervical amnionic infection is not unequivocally proved, nor is intranatal infection from an infected maternal genital tract. Whether hematogenous fetal contamination may result from viral endometritis as well as from maternal viremia is not clear. Also, as happens in one pathway of Listeria infection (Seeliger, 1961), the villitis may indeed result from fetal viremia rather than being the initial lesion at the site of contamination.

HERPES SIMPLEX

Although extensive clinical and virological reviews are available (Nahmias et al., 1970), only four cases of herpetic lesions of the placenta have been described or briefly cited: in Case 1 there was necrotizing villitis in the placenta from a newborn with disseminated herpes (Witzleben and Driscoll, 1965); the placenta in Case 2 had chronic herpetic funisitis and chorioamnionitis (Blanc, 1969); that in Case 3 had intrapartum acute herpetic vasculitis (Blanc, 1969); and the placenta in Case 4 had herpetic chorioamnionitis (Altshuler, 1974). We have also observed a fifth case, with acute disseminated herpes, severe acute herpetic chorioamnionitis, and necrotizing villitis.

Hematogenous Lesions

The early lesion first described by Witzleben and Driscoll (1965) is a multifocal coagulative necrosis of villi (Fig. 11–8), with secondary agglutination and a minimal or absent inflammatory response similar to that observed in other tissues. One of our patients (Case 3), who died of disseminated herpes at four days of age, was thought to have a normal placenta and, since the mother had cervical herpes, was considered to have been contaminated at birth. In fact, immunofluorescent staining of the placenta showed large amounts of antigen in the villi, in capillary walls, and around capillaries. A review of the microscopic slides revealed multifocal early necrotizing endovasculitis, a rare inclusion cell, and early fibrinoid necrosis with edema of the media. The findings indicate a very early stage of transplacental disease: The acute endothelial necrosis with resulting disseminated intravascular clotting is a feature of several viral infections; it is particularly striking in herpes. In our recent case (Case 5) of severe herpetic chorioamnionitis, there was extensive multifocal necrosis in all fetal tissues but only a few foci of minimal villitis in the placenta. There were no identifiable foci of fibrosis in agglutinated villi, which would suggest healed placentitis. The fetus was very macerated, and the placental vessels showed only the usual obliterative changes seen after fetal death, without evidence of medial destruction. These features suggest that a primary amnionic infection resulted in massive disseminated fetal disease, with only minimal and late placental involvement. Thus, both primary and secondary viremia may occur.

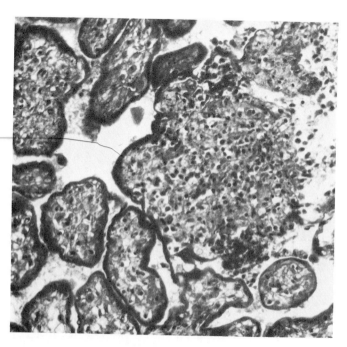

Figure 11–8. Disseminated herpes with acute necrotizing villitis in a macerated stillborn infant. Coagulation necrosis and mononuclear cell infiltrates (center right). ×240. (Photograph by Ida Nathan.)

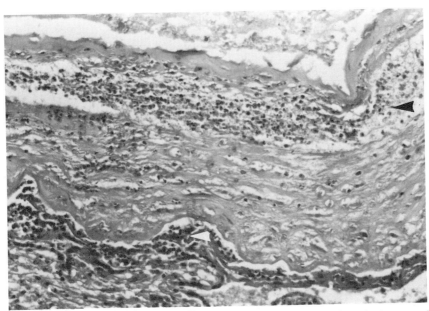

Figure 11–9. Herpetic chorioamnionitis in a fetus stillborn at 22 weeks. The amnionic cavity is on top. The amnionic epithelium has desquamated; a few necrotic cells remain. The space between amnion and chorion is infiltrated with necrotic cells (arrow). The chorion is edematous. A few cells are lined up in the intervillous space under the chorion. ×208. (Photograph by Ida Nathan.)

Transcervical Herpetic Infection

The pathological condition of transcervical herpetic infection is exemplified in its acute form by Case 5 and in its subacute and chronic forms by Cases 4 and 2, respectively.

Macroscopically, the appearance is that of chorioamnionitis (Fig. 11–9), which is similar to that of bacterial infection: the amnionic fluid and cord surface appear cloudy. Microscopically, there is severe necrotizing inflammation of amnion and chorion (see Fig. 11–9), with coagulation necrosis of amnionic cells in which inclusions can be seen (Fig. 11–10); the chorion is edematous and infiltrated with a small number of mononuclear

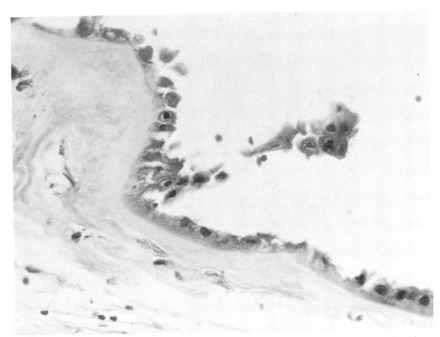

Figure 11–10. Chronic herpetic chorioamnionitis and funisitis in a 1500-gm premature infant born with several herpetic skin ulcers. Necrosis of amnionic cells and intranuclear inclusions. ×375. (Photograph by Ida Nathan.)

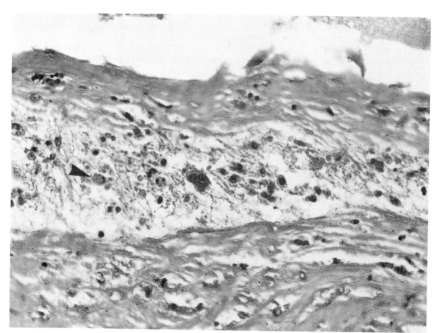

Figure 11–11. Acute herpetic chorioamnionitis (same case as in Fig. 11–9). The amniotic cavity is on top. The infiltrate is scant, made up of mononuclear cells with many dark "smudged" nuclei; the white arrow points to such dark inclusions in a binucleated cell. A more typical but less common inclusion is indicated by the black arrow: a pale (pink, in the original sections) central nuclear mass, surrounded with punctiform remnants of the nuclear membrane. ×375. (Photograph by Ida Nathan.)

cells and necrobiotic local phagocytes. The reaction is diffuse but more severe in foci. Inclusions and giant cells are present (Fig. 11–11), and in Case 5 there was minimal participation of maternal polymorphs. Acute inflammation was superimposed on Case 4, in which associated bacterial contamination was not excluded. In Case 5, we were able to demonstrate virus particles in the chorion by electron microscopy (Fig. 11–12). The cord showed a few focal amnionic lesions.

In Case 4, chronic inflammatory cells were present in the chorion and placenta and migrating from chorionic and cord vessels, and there was no villitis to suggest viremia. In Case 2, only a few chronic inflammatory

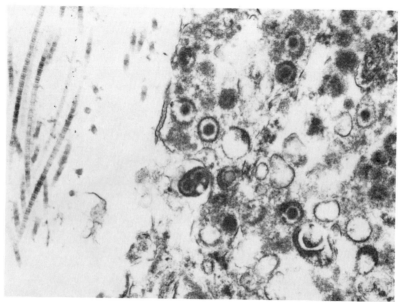

Figure 11–12. Acute herpetic chorioamnionitis (same case as in Fig. 11–9). Electron-microscopic view of an infected cell. The tissue is preserved in formalin and postfixed in Dalton's fixative. ×30,000.

cells were present in the chorionic plate, but many were found in the umbilical cord (Fig. 11–13). The media of the umbilical vessels and, to a lesser degree, of the chorionic vessels was grossly altered. It was attenuated, fibrosed and calcified in places, and combined with endothelial proliferation (Fig. 11–14). Viral particles were demonstrated in the cord,* in which fresh necroses and blurred inclusion cells were present along with the chronic infiltrates. The healed vasculitis may have resulted from chronic amnionic infection and indeed was not found in the villi, where only a few foci of chronic villitis were present. The infants in Cases 4 and 5 have both had recurrent skin herpes, and both were small for dates. Whether these infants had a mild disseminated disease *in utero* or "pure" chorioamnionitis and dermatitis is unresolved.

The diagnosis is made in acute cases by the presence of peculiar necrotizing inflammation with scant mononuclear cells and the typical inclusions. In late lesions, the plasmocytic chorionitis and funisitis is only suggestive, and electron microscopy should be used, since plasmocytic funisitis has been seen in toxoplasmosis. Electron microscopy provides confirmation.

---

*Courtesy of Dr. Rachel Morecki, Albert Einstein College of Medicine, New York, New York.

In summary, herpetic infection has two distinct morphological expressions: (1) an acute hematogenous form, characterized by acute vasculitis and villous necrosis; and (2) an acute necrotizing or chronic plasmocytic chorioamnionitis and funisitis, presumably due to ascending transcervical infection.

VARICELLA

Garcia (1963) described the placenta of a macerated fetus. It was enlarged and contained large numbers of necrotic foci made up of necrotic, agglutinated villi with some granulomatous tuberculoid lesions. We have seen one case in which gestational chickenpox was diagnosed clinically, unfortunately without viral studies. The fetal movements stopped at eight months, a few days before the rash appeared, at which time no fetal heart was heard. A month later, at term, the mother delivered a very pale, macerated stillborn infant without any necrotic lesions. The placenta showed focal plasmocytic infiltrates (Fig. 11–15) and a very peculiar fibrosis of villi, with extensive parietal and intraluminal calcifications in villous vessels, presumably resulting from dystrophic calcification of necrotic vessels (Fig. 11–16). It is tempting to speculate that acute villous vasculitis might have resulted in vascular rupture with acute

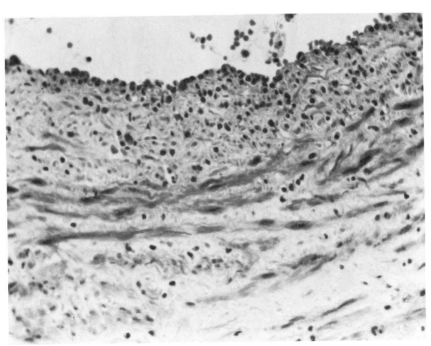

Figure 11–13. Chronic herpetic funisitis. Wall of umbilical vein with subintimal fibrosis, a few remaining strands of smooth muscle, and scattered lymphocytes. ×350. (Photograph by Ida Nathan.)

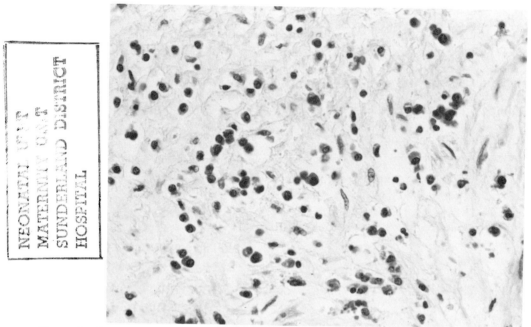

Figure 11–14. Chronic herpetic funisitis. Plasmocytic infiltrate in Wharton's jelly with scattered necrotic cells. ×375. (Photograph by Ida Nathan.)

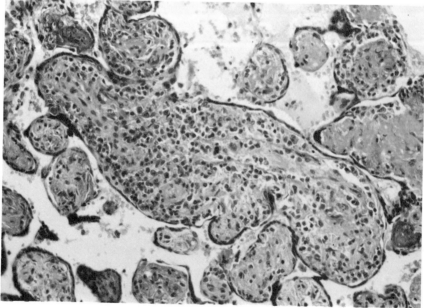

Figure 11–15. Maternal chickenpox one month before delivery of a very macerated fetus. Chronic plasmocytic villitis. ×240. (Photograph by Ida Nathan.)

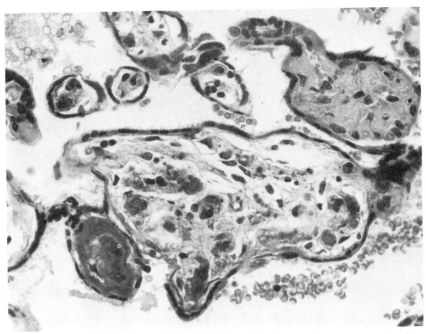

Figure 11–16. Maternal chickenpox (same case as in Fig. 11–15). Parietal and intraluminal calcifications in capillaries. Focal villous basement membrane calcification. ×375. (Photograph by Ida Nathan.)

fetomaternal bleeding, which would explain the sudden death and the severe pallor.

VARIOLA AND VACCINIA

Several cases of fatal intrauterine vaccinia have been reported. Some of these cases occurred despite the fact that vaccination had taken place in the second half of pregnancy, and two cases were the result of revaccination. Most articles, however, report abortuses. Extensive multifocal necroses were described by Benirschke and Driscoll (1967), Philippe (1974), and Green and co-workers (1966). Histologically, there is necrotizing villitis, with agglutination of villi and acute inflammation. In addition, granulomatous tuberculoid lesions are present with some inclusions.

In our case of vaccinia, the macerated fetus measured 18 cm in length, and the placenta was enlarged and pale. Numerous yellow necrotic foci were found on the skin in the fetal tissues, on the amnion, and throughout the placenta. Microscopically, there was severe granulomatous placentitis, with large necrotic areas centered by blood vessels, surrounded with palisaded epithelioid cells and giant cells with intranuclear inclusions (Figs. 11–17 and 11–18). Plasma cells were abundant. They have not been described in the

other cases. Particles identified as poxvirus were found by electron microscopy.*

Positive staining with specific antibody to vaccinia virus was obtained by Green and colleagues (1966) in inclusion cells and in the trophoblasts of their two cases.

In varicella and pox villitis, the damage results from hematogenous dissemination, and there is no histological evidence for another route of infection. Wielenga and coworkers (1961) insist on the necrosis of the trophoblast and provide evidence that it is the portal of entry. This was not seen in our case and is not commented upon by others.

RUBELLA

The changes in early placentae have been described by Töndury and Smith (1966), Driscoll (1969), and Ornoy and colleagues (1973); the later changes, those in placentae of up to six months, were described by Ornoy et al. (1973). The younger placentae displayed mononuclear perivascular infiltration, villous edema, necrosis, and fibrosis, along with occasional inclusion bodies in Hofbauer cells as well as in trophoblastic cells. Necrotic

---

*Dr. Eduardo Yunis, Children's Hospital, Pittsburgh, Pennsylvania, kindly did the electron microscopic examination.

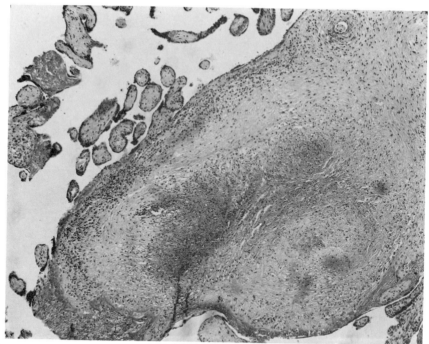

Figure 11–17. Granulomatous pox placentitis. Multiple granulomata in a stem villus with plasmocytic infiltrates at its periphery. ×63. (Photograph by Ida Nathan.)

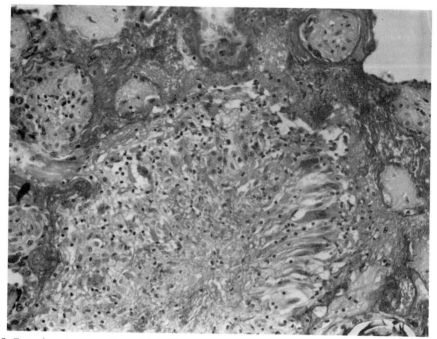

Figure 11–18. Granulomatous pox placentitis. Villi are agglutinated around a necrotic focus surrounded by palisaded epithelioid and some giant cells. ×160. (Photograph by Ida Nathan.)

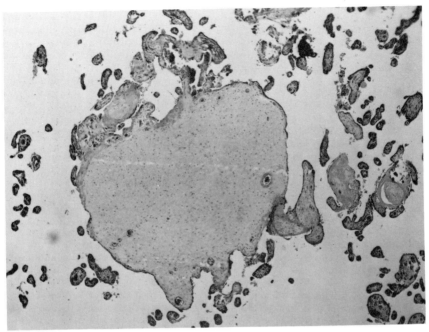

Figure 11–19. Rubella syndrome. The term placenta of a small-for-dates infant. Hypoplasia with inadequate formation of small peripheral villi. Large stem villus containing only a few tiny blood vessels. ×38. (Photograph by Ida Nathan.)

endothelial cells, presumably infected, desquamate in the lumen and may embolize to the fetus. In older placentae, necrosis becomes rare, and there is more fibrosis.

Only a few descriptions of term placentae are available. We saw only four such cases in our laboratory. Grossly, there is severe hypoplasia; the placental weight may be below 200 gm in markedly growth-retarded newborns. Histologically, the inadequate development of terminal villi is striking, and scattered stem villi show curious vascular alterations (Figs. 11–19 and 11–20). The media is irregularly atrophic, the vessels may be

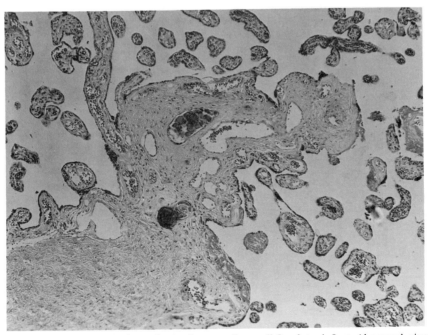

Figure 11–20. Rubella syndrome. The hypoplastic placenta of a small-for-dates infant. Abnormal, sinusoidal vessels in stem villus with two intraluminal calcifications. ×76. (Photograph by Ida Nathan.)

minute, and there are small calcified thrombi and, typically, areas of avascular villi. The corresponding stem villi may have no visible vessels or only tiny lumina. It is presumed that early vasculitis resulted in total necrosis and fibrosis. Occasionally, thick, fibrous endothelial cushions are found in chorionic vessels.

Avascular villi are seen in CMV infection, but the other vascular changes are lacking, and the massive plasmocytic infiltrates are not observed in the term rubella placenta.

As in the other viral diseases, the features of rubella placentitis, particularly the vasculitis, mirror the alterations seen in the fetus. As in CMV infection, there is a scarcity of information concerning pathological changes in the placenta in mild or inapparent rubella infection.

SUMMARY

The morphological characteristics of the placenta in the viral diseases considered in this chapter are compatible with the simultaneous involvement of the fetus and its adnexa, rather than with a progressive infection developing in the placenta and passing on to the fetus. Even though the trophoblast must, of necessity, be affected first, the changes may be too subtle for detection by light microscopy, and the earliest change, in all the cases we have personally reviewed, is observed in the vessels or in the adjacent stroma. This suggests "silent" passage through the trophoblastic layer and simultaneous dissemination to fetus and placenta. Vasculitis, ranging from endothelial necrosis to obliterative lesions or the actual disappearance of vessels, is the hallmark of viral infection.

Dissemination of the virus by infected endothelial cells may occur in CMV infection as well as in rubella. On the other hand, ascending amnionic infection is well documented only in herpes. Placental and fetal hypoplasia is frequent in rubella and occurs in CMV infection; it is likely that the extensive vascular damage, with avascular villi, contributes to fetal growth retardation. The ability of even the early fetus to mount a vigorous immune response is now well known and is demonstrated in viral placentitis.

If one considers the huge size of the placenta in relation to that of the fetal lymphoid tissues, and the extent, in some cases, of plasmocytic infiltrates, it is clear that the placental contribution to humoral fetal defense is important.

Bibliography

Altshuler, G.: Implications of two cases of human placental plasma cells. Am. J. Pathol. 70:189, 1973.

Altshuler, G.: Pathogenesis of congenital herpes virus infection. Case report including a description of the placenta. Am. J. Dis. Child. 127:427–429, 1974.

Altshuler, G., and Russel, P.: The human placental villitides: a review of chronic intrauterine infection. In Huth, F., et al. (eds.): Current Topics in Pathology Series. Berlin, Springer-Verlag, 1975, pp. 63–112.

Benirschke, K., and Driscoll, S. G.: The Pathology of the Human Placenta. Berlin, Springer-Verlag, 1967.

Benirschke, K., Mendoza, G. R., and Bazeley, P. L.: Placental and fetal manifestations of cytomegalovirus infection. Virchows Arch. (Cell Pathol.) 16:121–139, 1974.

Blanc, W. A.: The future of antepartum morphological studies. In Adamson, K. (ed.): Diagnosis and Treatment of Fetal Disorders: Proceedings. Berlin, Springer-Verlag, 1969, pp. 15–49.

Blanc, W. A.: Pathology of the placenta and cord in ascending and in hematogenous infection. In Marshall, W. C. (ed.): Perinatal Infections. CIBA Foundation Series No. 77. Amsterdam, Excerpta Medica, 1980, pp. 31–38.

Blanc, W. A.: Pathology of the Placenta, Membranes, and Umbilical Cord in Bacterial, Fungal, and Viral Infections in Man. International Academy of Pathology, Monograph No. 22. Baltimore, Williams & Wilkins Company, 1981, chap. 6.

Driscoll, S. G.: Histopathology of gestational rubella. Am. J. Dis. Child. 118:49–53, 1969.

Feldman, R. A.: Cytomegalovirus infection during pregnancy. A prospective study and report of six cases. Am. J. Dis. Child. 117:517–521, 1969.

Garcia, A. G. P.: Fetal infection in chickenpox and alastrim, with histopathologic study of the placenta. Pediatrics 32:895–901, 1963.

Green, D. M., Reid, S. M., and Rhoney, K.: Generalized vaccinia in the human foetus. Lancet 1:1296–1298, 1966.

Nahmias, A. J., Alford, A., and Korones, S. B.: Infection of the newborn with herpesvirus hominis. Advances in Pediatrics, Vol. 17. Chicago, Year Book Medical Publishers, 1970.

Ornoy, A., Segal, S., Nishmi, M., Simcha, A., and Polishuk, W. Z.: Fetal and placental pathology in gestational rubella. Am. J. Obstet. Gynecol. 116:949–956, 1973.

Philippe, E.: Histopathologie placentaire. Paris, Masson et Cie, 1974.

Potter, E. M., and Craig, J. M.: Pathology of the Fetus and the Infant. 3rd ed. Chicago, Year Book Medical Publishers, 1975.

Seeliger, H. P. R.: Listeriosis. New York, Hafner Publishing Company, 1961.

Shearer, W. T., Schreiner, R. L., Marshall, R. E., and Barton, L. L.: Cytomegalovirus infection in a newborn dizygous twin. J. Pediatr. 81:1161–1165, 1972.

Töndury, G. T., and Smith, D. W.: Fetal rubella pathology. J. Pediatr. *68*:867–879, 1966.

Whitley, R. J., Brasfield, D., Reynolds, D. W., Stagno, S., Tiller, R. E., and Alford, C. A.: Protracted pneumonitis in young infants associated with perinatally acquired cytomegaloviral infection. J. Pediatr. *89*:16, 1976.

Wielenga, G., van Tongeren, H. A. E., Ferguson, A. M., and Rijssel, T. G.: Prenatal infection with vaccinia virus. Lancet *1*:258–260, 1961.

Witzleben, C. L., and Driscoll, S. G.: Possible transplacental transmission of herpes simplex infection. Pediatrics *36*:192–199, 1965.

12

The Development of Immune Mechanisms in the Fetus and Newborn

A number of the clinical, pathological, and immunological effects of microorganisms that infect the human fetus differ from those produced when the same infection occurs in postnatal life; the most striking differences can be seen in the type and extent of damage and in the duration of the infection.

Earlier observations failed to detect an immune response to infective agents and other antigens in the young of a number of species, and, as a result, the view gradually developed that the human fetus was incapable of generating an immune response to antigens because of the immaturity or lack of development of its immune system. The fetus was thought to be in an immunologically "null" state. It was also believed, on the evidence derived from animal experiments, that "immunological tolerance" was a likely consequence of an intrauterine infection: the agent would not be eliminated because it would not be recognizable as "non-self," and the fetus would not respond immunologically to the infection. For many years lymphocytic choriomeningitis (LCM) virus infection in human fetuses and newborn mice was cited as a classic example of the phenomenon of tolerance. It has now been demonstrated that true tolerance does not occur in such LCM virus infections (Oldstone and Dixon, 1967). Although antibody was known to be present in newborns with congenital syphilis, it had not been seriously considered to be of fetal origin. The presence of increased lymphoid development and plasma cells in five- to six-month fetuses infected with *Treponema pallidum* and *Toxoplasma gondii*, however, led to the conclusion that antibody production might occur before birth (Silverstein, 1962; Silverstein and Lukes, 1962). But the paucity of information about the immune system of the human fetus and newborn contributed to the surprise that was expressed when Plotkin and co-workers (1963) and Weller and co-workers (1964) reported that children with congenital rubella possessed rubella neutralizing antibody at an age when passively acquired antibody from the mother should have disappeared. Alford (1965) then showed that rubella antibody was present in

230

IgM immunoglobulin at birth, thus providing the evidence that it had been produced by the fetus rather than passively transferred from the mother.

It is now clear that the human fetus responds immunologically to virtually all known intrauterine and perinatal infections. Furthermore, measurement of the humoral immune response plays an important role in the laboratory diagnosis of these infections. Another feature of intrauterine infections is the persistence of many of these agents for varying periods of time: the infection usually lasts throughout fetal life and can extend to several weeks after birth, and in some instances it persists for many years. Identification of the persisting agent by microscopic or by culture techniques provides an additional method of confirming the diagnosis.

Numerous mechanisms are involved in the process of resistance to infection, which extends from the prevention of invasion of the host by microorganisms to their destruction and elimination should they succeed in gaining entry. Major factors that determine which of these mechanisms are involved depend on the nature of the organism, the route of entry, and the stage of the infection. Other factors of importance are the age of the host and the existence of "memory" of previous exposure. These mechanisms seldom operate in isolation; there is very complex interaction and interdependence among the various systems.

The identification of all defense mechanisms in the mature host is still far from complete. Still less is understood of the various stages of their development and their functional capabilities in the fetus and newborn. Remarkable progress has taken place during the past decade, however, as a result of the enormous increase in technical expertise for the study of components of the immune system.

The elegant experiments on fetal lambs (Silverstein and Prendergast, 1970) have provided valuable data on the ontogeny of the immune system, but care must be taken in extrapolation of these data to humans because of such factors as differences in placentation, length of gestation, and maturity at birth of different species. The studies of various congenital immunodeficiency states have provided a greater understanding of many of the components of the immune system in humans. Some information, limited though it is, has come from the study of human fetal tissues obtained by therapeutic abortions performed for a variety of reasons, including intrauterine infections.

Defense mechanisms are customarily classified into two groups, *nonspecific* and *specific* (Table 12–1). Nonspecific mechanisms generally operate in the earlier stages of an infection and do not depend on recognition. The specific mechanisms, which are mediated by lymphoid cells, respond to a particular or, sometimes, a very closely related infectious agent or antigen. Current concepts of the interaction between some nonspecific and specific mechanisms are illustrated in Figure 12–1.

Fetal and neonatal immunity must also take into account the transfer of antibody and immune cells from the mother before birth and the consumption of antibody and other protective substances in colostrum and milk after birth.

NONSPECIFIC DEFENSE MECHANISMS

The skin and mucous membranes are important anatomical barriers to infection both before and after birth. Abrasions of the skin may occur during delivery, and some instances of perinatal infection by hepatitis B virus are thought to have occurred as a result of these abrasions. Fetoscopy and the collection of blood and other materials from the fetus for antenatal diagnosis and the sampling of blood from the scalp through the

Table 12–1. **NONSPECIFIC AND SPECIFIC HOST DEFENSE MECHANISMS**

Nonspecific	Specific

Skin and mucous membranes
Polymorphonuclear leukocytes
Macrophages
Complement
Lysozyme
Interferon
	Humoral:
	  Immunoglobulins (B-lymphocytes)
	Cellular:
	  T-lymphocytes

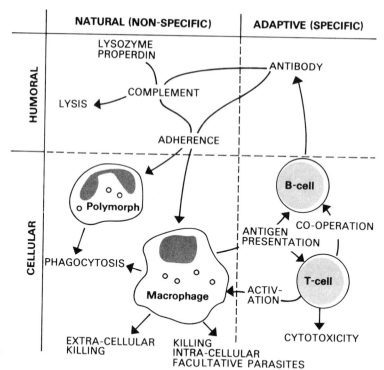

Figure 12–1. Summary of the interactions between nonspecific and adaptive immunity. (Based on Playfair, J. H. L., Br. Med. Bull. *30*:24, 1974; from Roitt, I. M.: Essential Immunology. 2nd ed. Oxford, Blackwell Scientific Publications, 1974, pp. 1–24.)

cervix during labor also breach the skin barrier.

Entry and colonization of the gut by bacteria within hours of birth is a natural event. This is usually a noninvasive process, however, and the contents of breast milk, such as lysozyme, complement, lactoferrin, and cells, as well as antibody, probably play an important role in modulating it. The normal enteric flora are usually not invasive, but some may be the cause of bacteremia and septicemia in the neonatal period. It is possible that the gastrointestinal tract of the newborn is especially permeable to these bacteria.

The role of amnionic fluid is combating certain infections is not well understood, but it contains several factors known to have antibacterial activity, including IgG immunoglobulin, lysozyme, transferrin, and B_{1A}/B_{1C} globulin. Although antibodies to parainfluenza 3 and influenza A2 were detected in amnionic fluid, hemagglutinating antibodies to *Escherichia coli* and rubella antibody were not found by Galask and Synder (1970). This inability to detect rubella antibody could explain the relative ease of isolation of rubella virus from amnionic fluid (Thompson and Tobin, 1970). Cytomegalovirus (CMV) has also been isolated from this site (Davis et al.,

1971). Amnionic fluid infections are of major importance in some tropical communities and are closely related to maternal nutrition (Ross et al., 1980). Zinc deficiency has been suggested to play an important role in the frequency and severity of these infections (Tafari et al., 1977).

Protection is afforded by the covering of fetal membranes, but following their rupture during labor an ascending infection from the maternal genital tract may occur. It is usually bacterial, but herpesvirus hominis may infect the fetus by this route. The risk of bacterial infection increases if delivery is delayed more than six hours after the membranes rupture (Gamsu, 1973).

The fetus is especially vulnerable to blood stream infection via the umbilical vessels. The role of the placenta is, therefore, of great importance (see Chapter 3). The placental barrier may be broken if there is a blood stream infection in the mother. This may lead to infection of and damage to the placenta, resulting in the entry of microorganisms into the fetal circulation, although the exact mechanism of the passage of microorganisms across the placenta to the fetus has not been elucidated (Blanc, 1961). Placentitis is believed to be an essential part of the pathogenesis of intrauterine rubella, and histological changes are also seen in CMV infection (Feldman, 1969), herpes simplex (Witzleben and Driscoll, 1965), variola (Lynch, 1932), vaccinia (Wielenga et al., 1961; Entwistle et al., 1962), and varicella (Garcia, 1963), as well as in syphilis and toxoplasmosis (Beckett and Flynn, 1953).

The placenta probably does not act solely as an anatomical barrier. Banatvala and his colleagues (1971) have shown that cells derived from the placenta produce greater amounts of interferon when infected with rubella viruses than do fetal cells. Finally, it is very likely that phagocytes and lymphoid cells present in the placenta play a role in attempting to overcome infection in this organ.

Phagocytosis

Granulocytes and other phagocytic cells play a major role in the host defense system. This role is particularly important in the early stages of bacterial infection and can greatly influence the extent and outcome of the infection. The principal cell in the circulation is the polymorphonuclear leukocyte, but other cells in the circulation, monocytes and eosinophils, have a similar function. These circulating cells also reach organisms when they lodge at various sites in the body. Their importance is well illustrated by the severe recurrent infections that are a feature of chronic granulomatous disease, a disorder in which there is a defect in the capacity of polymorphonuclear leukocytes and other phagocytes to kill certain types of bacteria following their ingestion.

The normal process of phagocytosis involves several steps: chemotaxis, opsonization, ingestion, and killing. Chemotactic factors that promote the migration of phagocytes toward pathogens may be derived from bacteria themselves, or they may be derived as a result of their interaction with complement with or without antibody. Opsonization depends very heavily on the presence of antibody, and complement is also usually involved in this process. The final stages, ingestion and killing, occur as a result of a multiplicity of enzyme and chemical reactions. Although phagocytosis is generally considered to be a nonspecific defense mechanism, there is an interaction between the phagocytes and other mechanisms, both specific and nonspecific.

Other phagocytic cells are present in the body tissues; these "fixed" phagocytes or macrophages are found in the sinusoids of the liver and spleen, lymph nodes, and pulmonary alveoli. These cells have their origin in bone marrow as monoblasts and promonoblasts. Tissue macrophages are not a static population; they are renewed regularly, and an increase in their numbers occurs during inflammation. This is due to increased production in the bone marrow and is regulated by a humoral factor (Van Furth and Sluiter, 1983). Following contact with a microorganism, these cells show an increase in size and in numbers of mitochondria and lysosomal granules. Cells that exhibit these changes have an increased capacity to kill microorganisms. The changes are induced by contact with viruses, bacteria such as *Listeria monocytogenes*, mycobacteria, and fungi. It has been suggested that these responses can be enhanced in a specific manner by the presence of lymphocytes (Mackaness, 1969). The process of enhancement is thought to be achieved by lymphokines such as macrophage migration-inhibition factor (MIF). Another important function of the macrophage is to "process" ingested microorganisms so that appropriate lymphocytes can be activated.

Macrophages play a role in the phagocytosis of viruses (Mims, 1964). The Kupffer cells in the liver are a major site for phagocytosis of some viruses, and macrophages are also capable of producing considerable amounts of the antiviral protein interferon. Allison (1970) has suggested that some viruses may persist in macrophages, as well as in the other cell types, presumably in a noninfectious form, and that the continued presence of viral antigen in these cells may offer one explanation for the long-lasting immunity that is a feature of the defense reaction against so many viral infections.

Granulocytic cells can be detected in fetal liver at about eight weeks' gestation, but subsequently the marrow takes over as the major site of production. Although very little is known of the functional capacity of fetal granulocytes, a considerable body of information has been obtained on the properties of granulocytes from newborn infants. *In vitro*, chemotactic responses are diminished (Miller, 1971) as are both bactericidal activity (Wright et al., 1975) and chemoluminescence (Strauss et al., 1980). These defects are more prominent in the presence of stress or infection (Shigeoka et al., 1979).

Very little is known of macrophage development and function in the human fetus, but it has been inferred that afferent activities, together with those associated with chemotaxis and killing, are immature in the human newborn (Albrecht and Hong, 1976). Data from animal experiments indicate that macrophage function in the rat is less mature in the neonatal than in the adult period and that immaturity of the macrophage system may be a limiting step in expression of immunocompetence to many antigenic stimuli during the neonatal period (Blaese, 1975). However, lymphocytes from newborns can produce both chemotactic and opsonic factors for macrophages (Kretschmer et al., 1976). Also, Orlowski and co-workers (1976) have demonstrated that bactericidal capacity is not significantly less than that of adult cells.

Complement System and Opsonins. It has long been recognized that there are heat-labile substances present in serum that enhance bactericidal activity. The nine components of the complement system and their sequential action are shown in Figure 12–2. During the process of activation of the complement system certain biological effects take place. For example, the fragment C3b, derived from C3, enhances phagocytosis by its opsonic activity. C3a and C5a increase vascular permeability, and the latter also promotes neutrophil chemotaxis. Although the complement system is not absolutely essential for phagocytosis, its presence greatly enhances the process.

Most complement components do not cross the placenta, and a number are synthesized early in fetal life. All components of complement are present in sera from fetuses more than 18 weeks of age (Adinolfi, 1972). C1 esterase inhibitor, C2, C3, C4, and C5 can all be detected between 8 and 14 weeks (Fireman et al., 1969; Colten, 1972; Kohler, 1973). The levels of hemolytic complement and of individual components in term and preterm infants are only approximately half those present in the adult, with correspondingly lower levels in the preterm infant (Fishel and Pearlman, 1961; Sawyer and Forman, 1971). By six months of age most components have reached adult levels (Adamkin et al., 1978).

The alternative complement pathway enables opsonization to be achieved by a method that bypasses the classical complement pathway and the need for antibody. Low levels of factor B, C3, and properdin were detected in 15 per cent of normal newborns (Stossel et al., 1973).

Interferons are glycoproteins released by cells and inhibit virus replication. Virtually all types of cells have the capacity to produce interferons, and a wide variety of substances induce synthesis of interferons. These include viruses, bacteria, rickettsial endotoxins, and double-stranded polyribonucleoids. Such interferon is called type 1. A second type of interferon, type 2 or immune interferon, is produced by lymphocytes when stimulated by specific antigens or mitogens. In comparison with many other cells, lymphocytes produce large amounts of interferon. Interferon production by lymphocytes of 8- to 14-week fetuses is quantitatively similar to that by lymphocytes of newborns, children, and adults (Cantell et al., 1968; Ray, 1970).

Interferon produced by the placenta may

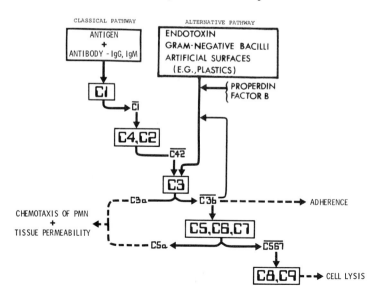

Figure 12–2. Schematic representation of activation of complement components.

play a role in preventing fetal viral infections. However, in the very early fetal life this is probably not the case with rubella, as suggested by the very high incidence of fetal infection during the first 10 to 12 weeks of gestation (Rawls et al., 1968; Thompson and Tobin, 1970).

Larsson and co-workers (1976) attempted to terminate the infection in an infant with congenital rubella by means of daily injections of interferon. This was not successful, and they concluded that the mechanism of persistence of the infection was not exclusively a defect in the endogenous interferon response. Children with congenital rubella, aged 11 to 18 months, produced interferon when inoculated with attenuated measles virus (Desmyter et al., 1967).

Emodi and Just (1974) found an interferon response by circulating lymphocytes in children with clinical manifestations of congenital CMV infection that was significantly reduced compared with that of patients with asymptomatic congenital infection. They were unable to conclude whether these findings were due to a primary defect in synthesis of interferon or were secondary to the infection. As in congenital rubella, live measles vaccine has been shown to induce an interferon response in children with congenital CMV (Glasgow et al., 1967).

Interferon may have an as yet undefined role in limiting the extent of fetal viral infections, but since there is a wide diversity in the capacity of different viruses to induce interferon, it may be effective only in certain infections.

SPECIFIC DEFENSE MECHANISMS

The method by which specific immune mechanisms operate to protect the host against viral, bacterial, fungal, and protozoal infections depends on a complex series of events. This includes the appropriate presentation of foreign material or antigens to specific lymphoid cells. Thus the cells are stimulated or activated to produce an antigen-specific reaction. This may consist of a reaction between the antibody receptors of lymphoid cells and antigen or between circulating antibody and antigen. Neither of these reactions is entirely independent in a host who possesses a competent immune system with varying degrees of previous experience.

Lymphoid cells are believed to originate from pluripotential stem cells of hematopoietic origin (Moore and Owen, 1967). These first appear in the rudimentary yolk sac but then migrate to other sites of hematopoiesis. It is not known at what stage these cells become committed to lymphoid development, but lymphocytes are found in the human fetus at seven or eight weeks (Playfair et al., 1963).

The thymus is essential for the development of competence in one population of lymphocytes. It originates from an epithelial cell outgrowth from the third and fourth pharyngeal pouches. Migration to the upper mediastinum then occurs, and from eight weeks there is a steady increase in the number of lymphocytes developing in this organ. By 10 weeks large numbers are present in the cortex. Hassall's corpuscles first appear in the thymus at 12 to 13 weeks. Thymic weight steadily increases throughout fetal life and reaches a maximum, in relation to body weight, at birth. Lymphoid cells that begin their differentiation in the thymus are called thymus-dependent or T-lymphocytes. Lymphocytes accumulate in the spleen from about the twelfth week and populate lymph nodes after 20 weeks. Germinal centers normally do not appear in these organs until after birth. Singer and co-workers (1969) have observed that there is a precocious development of germinal centers in the lymph nodes and spleen of infants with congenital rubella that is similar to the changes found in infants with other intrauterine infections (Silverstein and Lukes, 1962).

Another population of lymphoid cells, which is thought to develop independently of the thymus, become the precursors of antibody-secreting plasma cells. These are known as B- (bone marrow–derived) lymphocytes.

T- and B-lymphocytes cannot be differentiated by ordinary light microscopy. T-lymphocytes have the capacity to form rosettes with sheep red blood cells. There are several types of T-lymphocytes. Two major ones are suppressor cytotoxic T-cells and helper inducer T-cells. The numbers and ratio of these subgroups, which are indentified by monoclonal antisera, vary with age. There is a significant increase in the absolute numbers of both helper and suppressor T-lymphocytes in all newborn infants. But infants who are small for gestational age have significant deficiencies in absolute numbers of these cells, as well as in total T- and B-lymphocytes (Thomas and Linch, 1983). About 70 to 80 per cent of lymphocytes in the peripheral blood and most in the thoracic duct lymph are T-lymphocytes. They populate the paracortical areas of lymph nodes and are aggregated around the arterioles in the spleen. Besides their capacity to form rosettes, their presence can be detected by other *in vitro* tests. They undergo a blastogenic response to the plant mitogens such as phytohemagglutinin (PHA) and concanavalin A and to histocompatibility antigens in mixed lymphocyte cultures. Lymphocytes stimulated in this manner produce a number of biologically active substances called lymphokines.

PHA responsiveness has been demonstrated in fetal blood lymphocytes as early as 12 to 14 weeks (Kay et al., 1970; Stites and Pavia, 1979), and Hayward and Soothill (1972) have shown that thymic lymphocytes at 12 weeks' gestation react in mixed lymphocyte culture. They also found that in the presence of PHA, lymphocytes from 16-week fetuses are capable of cytolysis of xenogeneic cells. The blastogenic response of cord blood lymphocytes to mitogens and allogeneic cells is similar to the response to adult lymphocytes, but the former undergo a higher degree of spontaneous transformation. This could be due to stimulation *in utero* by maternal antigens (Faulk et al., 1973). A still higher degree of spontaneous activity has been observed in young infants with intrauterine rubella and CMV (Marshall et al., 1970; Gibas and Hayes, 1974).

Skin-graft rejection and graft-versus-host disease are manifestations of functioning T-cells. The capacity to reject skin grafts is well developed in newborn infants. Injection of antigens to which the subject has been previously sensitized in order to observe delayed hypersensitivity reactions in the skin is another important method for testing the competence of T-lymphocytes. For unknown reasons, delayed hypersensitivity reactions to the commonly used protein antigens are difficult to elicit in the newborn, although contact hypersensitivity to potent sensitizers such as dinitrofluorobenzene may be manifested (Uhr et al., 1960).

The importance of T-lymphocytes in recovery from viral infections is well known (Allison, 1972), and a defect in cell-mediated immunity has frequently been postulated as a cause of the persisting and chronic infection in several intrauterine viral infections, especially rubella and CMV infection. Since severe defects in cell mediated immunity are often incompatible with life, it is not surprising that prolonged suppression of all cell-mediated reactions has not been demonstrated in either congenital rubella or congenital CMV infections. In the former, lymphocyte transformation to phytohemagglutinin was reported to be defective by Olson and co-workers (1967), but others have found normal responses to PHA (Simons and Fitzgerald, 1968; White et al., 1968; Marshall et al., 1970). Buimovici-Klein and her colleagues (1979) reported a significant reduction in lymphocyte transformation and in interferon and leukocyte MIF synthesis in congenital rubella children compared with controls, but found that the impairment of these cellular immune responses was more severe in children infected in the first two months than in the later stages of gestation. Michaels (1969) found aberrations of delayed hypersensitivity reactions in newborns with congenital rubella, but in children in whom virus excretion had ceased, delayed hypersensitivity to several antigens was unimpaired. The blastogenic response of their lymphocytes was suboptimal, however (White et al., 1968).

A major factor in the investigation of this aspect of immune function has been the lack of suitable viral antigens with which to examine antigen-specific lymphocyte responsiveness and test for delayed hypersensitivity. However, Fuccillo and colleagues (1974) designed a Cr.51 lymphocytotoxicity microassay system to examine cell-mediated immunity in congenital rubella patients and found defective responses in eight of 11 children.

In a study of congenital CMV, reactivity of lymphocytes in mixed lymphocyte cultures was found to be diminished in children with symptomatic disease but not in those with asymptomatic infection (Emodi et al., 1973). By contrast, lymphocyte responsiveness to PHA, pokeweed mitogen, and concanavalin A was not impaired in either group.

Investigations of immune function in congenital rubella have sought to prove the hypothesis that virus persistence is associated with a defect in host-defense mechanisms due to either a tolerant state or an active immunosuppressive effect of the virus. However, another view is that clones of infected cells exist that, because of their limited doubling potential, eventually die out; thus, a defect in immune mechanisms need not be involved (Simons and Fitzgerald, 1968).

In summary, a conflicting picture has

emerged from the studies of cell-mediated immune function in congenital viral infections, and it is far from clear that defective immune function is the cause of the chronic infective state or that the abnormalities are the result of the continuing infection.

DEVELOPMENT OF HUMORAL IMMUNITY AND ANTIBODY IMMUNE SYSTEMS

Immunoglobulins and antibodies are synthesized and excreted by the plasma cell that is derived from a B-lymphocyte. B-lymphocytes can be identified by the presence on their surface of membrane-bound immunoglobulins. They also have surface receptors for the third component of complement (C3), the F_c fragment of IgG, and some viruses, such as Epstein-Barr virus. They are found in the outer layers of the cortices of lymph nodes and also in the medulla, and they form a major component of the primary and secondary follicles in the cortex.

It has been postulated that differentiation of the B-lymphocyte system takes place in two stages (Cooper et al., 1972). The first is the development of B-lymphocytes from stem cells, which is a normal evolutionary process believed to occur independently of stimulation by exogenous antigen. The first immunoglobulin synthesized by these cells is IgM, but some of the cells then undergo a switch from IgM to a genetic commitment to produce IgG, which is in turn followed by the development of a population of cells that produce IgA. The second stage occurs when B-lymphocytes respond to exogenous antigens and become mature antibody-producing cells with abundant cytoplasmic immunoglobulin.

Lymphocytes carrying IgM surface markers have been found in nine-week fetuses; IgG-bearing cells appeared shortly thereafter. Cells with IgA on their surfaces were not detected until later, no earlier than 11½ weeks. By the fourteenth week the proportion of IgM-, IgG-, and IgA-bearing cells was similar to that found in normal newborns (Lawton et al., 1972b).

Once a population of cells capable of synthesizing immunoglobulins relatively early in fetal life has developed, it is not unreasonable to expect that they will soon start this activity rather than remain dormant. Synthesis of immunoglobulins, which is initially most active in the spleen, takes place as early as 10½

weeks, the time when IgM can be detected. IgG and IgE synthesis begins at 12 weeks and IgA synthesis at about 30 weeks (Gitlin and Biasucci, 1969). Thus, some immunoglobulins can be produced and secreted soon after B-cell differentiation is complete. Only a small amount of the IgG in the fetal circulation is fetal in origin, however, and nearly all the IgG in cord blood is derived from the maternal circulation. IgM and IgA present in the fetus, on the other hand, are entirely of fetal origin, as these immunoglobulins do not cross the normal placenta (Alford, 1971) (Fig. 12–3). The rate of synthesis of IgM is very low during normal fetal life, and the mean levels of IgM in cord blood are only 10 ± 5 mg/dl. The rate rapidly increases after delivery, and levels comparable with those in the adult are found at approximately four years of age (Berg and Johansson, 1969).

When the fetus becomes infected, increased synthesis of IgM occurs, and cord-blood levels in excess of 20 mg/dl are common. Screening for raised levels of IgM can be a useful method for the detection of intrauterine infections (Stiehm et al., 1966; Alford, 1971). There appears to be some difference in the capacity of different types of microorganisms to stimulate prenatal synthesis of IgM. Levels of IgM in cord blood in early infancy are higher in infants with congenital syphilis than in those with congenital rubella, CMV infection, or toxoplasmosis (Alford et al., 1968).

The levels of total IgG in the cord blood are also elevated following prenatal infection, and premature synthesis is reflected in a tendency for the physiological trough of IgG to be obliterated. Synthesis of IgA along mucous surfaces commences shortly after birth, but its serum level rises more slowly than those of IgM and IgG. IgA may not even be detected in cord blood, and adult levels of serum IgA are usually not achieved until about 10 to 12 years of age. However, elevated levels of IgA may also occur in intrauterine infections (Stiehm et al., 1966), but raised levels in cord blood must be distinguished from the elevated levels that are the consequence of maternal-fetal transfusion. In the latter circumstance the IgA levels will decline rapidly after birth (Allansmith et al., 1969).

In addition to producing more immunoglobulins following an intrauterine infection, the fetus produces antibodies to the infecting agent. Detection of antibodies in IgM in cord blood provides a valuable method of diag-

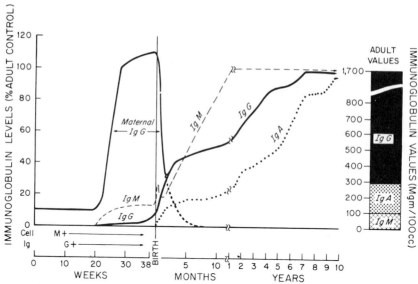

Figure 12–3. Intrauterine and extrauterine development of serum immunoglobulin levels. The line labeled "Maternal IgG" signifies serum levels thought to be derived primarily from placental transfer, whereas other lines, including those referring to IgM and IgG, indicate serum levels believed to result from the fetus's or infant's own production. (From Alford, C. A.: Immunoglobulin determinants in the diagnosis of fetal infections. Pediatr. Clin. North Am. *18*:102, 1971.)

nosis of these infections in early infancy. It has been shown in animal experiments that the capacity of the fetus to produce antibody differs with different antigens (Sterzl and Silverstein, 1967); it may be that the time of onset of fetal antibody production may vary for different infections in the human fetus, but unfortunately no information is available on this point. It is possible in some instances to determine with a certain degree of accuracy the time of fetal infection with rubella virus, and some infections occur before the capacity to produce immunoglobulins develops and even before B-cell differentiation takes place. In these cases the virus continues to replicate and, theoretically, becomes capable of evoking an immune response only when the fetal immune system develops the capacity to be stimulated. Unfortunately, very little is known of the immunological consequences of such early fetal infections: Is there a premature maturation of antibody-producing cells, or is there an opposite effect, that is, suppression of development? The observations of Alford (1965) on rubella suggest that premature maturation probably does not take place. Observations of early fetal infections with *Treponema pallidum* and *Toxoplasma gondii* suggest these agents behave in a similar manner (Silverstein and Lukes, 1962).

Soothill and co-workers (1966) reported hypogammaglobulinemia G in 18 per cent of a series of patients with congenital rubella, and a number of other reports (Plotkin et al.,

1966; South and Good, 1966; Hancock et al., 1968; Schimke et al., 1969) confirmed this phenomenon. Subsequently hypogammaglobulinemia was not observed in larger numbers of patients (Marshall, 1972). It undoubtedly is an effect of infection of the fetus with rubella, but the incidence is far less than was originally supposed. Deficiency of IgA has also been reported in congenital rubella (Lawton et al., 1972a), but this is rare. Because IgA deficiency is the most common single immunoglobulin deficiency in humans, and because of its relative infrequency in congenital rubella, it is not clear whether there is a causal relationship. However, it is of interest that Alford and colleagues (1974) have found retarded development of IgA in some cases of congenital toxoplasmosis. In one patient there were low levels of IgA in the first six months of life, following which IgA could not be detected in the serum.

South and co-workers (1975) found no immunological abnormalities in 20 children with congenital CMV other than the precocious development of immunoglobulin levels. The response to diphtheria toxoid was normal in such children (Michaels, 1972). No immunological aberrations were observed in two children following early fetal infection with herpes simplex (South et al., 1969; Montgomery et al., 1973).

In addition to fetal and neonatal synthesis of immunoglobulins, the maternal circulation is an important source of immunoglobulin for the infant. Transfer of IgG from the mother is an active process that ensures that the infant is born with levels of IgG equal to or higher than those present in the mother (Kohler and Farr, 1966).

Most of the IgG is transferred during the third trimester of pregnancy and contains whatever antibodies are present in the mother's IgG, The infant will be born with titers of antibodies of the IgG class to many infective agents similar to those present in the mother. The serum levels of these antibodies then slowly decline during the first few months of life, but they have an important protective role, especially for viral infections such as measles and rubella and for some bacterial infections. They are usually not detectable at approximately six months of age, but this will vary according to the titer of antibody present at birth. If, however, there has been synthesis of antibody by the fetus, this decline in titer of antibody does not occur. Because of the continued production of antibody by the infant, antibody can still be detected beyond the period when antibody acquired from the mother has declined. Thus persistence of antibody beyond six months of age is another method whereby the diagnosis of intrauterine infection can be established. Retrospective diagnosis of congenital rubella may be made by measuring antibody titers for up to about three years of age because of the low incidence of rubella infection in this period. Persistence of antibody occurs in congenital CMV (Stagno et al., 1975) and in early intrauterine infections with varicella-zoster virus (Gershon, 1975), but as these viral infections are more prevalent in young children than rubella, detection of antibody to these agents beyond six months of life is of little value for retrospective diagnosis. In the majority of patients with congenital rubella the titers of hemagglutination-inhibition antibody may remain stable or show only a moderate decline in the first decade of life, but a small proportion have been found to have very low or undetectable levels after several years (Cooper et al., 1971; Dudgeon et al., 1972). However, these children do not appear to be susceptible to infection with attenuated strains of rubella virus (Cooper et al., 1971).

Although it is possible to outline broadly the numerous mechanisms involved in the protection of the host from infectious agents and there is at present some understanding of the stages of development of these mechanisms in the human fetus, there remain large gaps in our knowledge of these events.

One particular aspect concerns the development and function of macrophages. The importance of these cells in the newborn is suggested by experiments in mice with herpes simplex virus: transfer of macrophages from adult animals affords some protection against the effects of infection with this virus to newborn of the species (Hirsch et al., 1970).

An important aspect of the effects of various infections on the fetus and of the persisting infection after birth concerns the interactions between the immunological responses and the agents that produce damage mediated by immunopathological mechanisms. Depending in part upon the level of immunological competence achieved by the fetus at the time of infection, there could be a wide diversity of possible adverse effects by immunopathological mechanisms (Silverstein, 1962). For example, the observations of Stagno and co-workers (1975, 1977) with respect to congenital CMV indicate that CMV antigen-antibody complexes may be responsible for vascular injury. The chronic rashes and steroid-responsive pneumonitis in late infancy in congenital rubella may similarly be caused by the effects of immunocompetent cell activation (Marshall, 1972). However, Tardieu and colleagues (1980) have drawn attention to the presence of circulating immune complexes containing rubella antigen antigen and their role in diffuse late-onset disease in congenital rubella.

Finally, mention must be made of the possible role of genetic factors in resistance or susceptibility to damage by microorganisms. As yet these are poorly understood in humans but the recent demonstration of an unusually high incidence of certain histocompatibility antigens in patients with congenital rubella (Honeyman et al., 1975) may be an important step in the investigation of this aspect of host defense.

Bibliography

Adamkin, D., Stitzel, A., Urmson, J., Fernett, M. L., Post, E., and Spitzer, R: Activity of the alternative pathway of complement in the newborn infant. J. Pediatr. 93:604–608, 1978.

Adinolfi, M.: Ontogeny of components of complement and lysozyme. In Ontogeny of Acquired Immunity. Ciba Foundation Symposium. Amsterdam, Associated Scientific Publishers, 1972, pp. 65–81.

Albrecht, R. M., and Hong, R.: Basic considerations of the monocyte-macrophage system in man. J. Pediatr. 88:751–765, 1976.

Alford, C. A.: Studies of antibody in congenital rubella infections. I. Physiochemical and immunologic investigations of rubella neutralising antibody. Am. J. Dis. Child. *110*:445–463, 1965.

Alford, C. A.: Immunoglobulin determinations in the diagnosis of fetal infection. Pediatr. Clin. North Am. *18*:99–113, 1971.

Alford, C. A., Blankenship, W. J., Straumfjord, J. V., and Cassaday, G.: The diagnostic significance of IgM-globulin elevations in newborn infants with chronic intrauterine infections. In Bergsma, D., and Krugman, S. (eds.): Intrauterine Infections. Birth Defects Original Article Series, Vol. IV, No. 7. New York, The National Foundation—March of Dimes, 1968, pp. 5–19.

Alford, C. A., Stagno, S., and Reynolds, D. W.: Congenital toxoplasmosis: clinical, laboratory and therapeutic considerations with special reference to subclinical disease. Bull. N.Y. Acad. Med., *50*:160–161, 1974.

Allansmith, M. R., McClellan, B. H., and Butterworth, M.: Individual patterns of immunoglobulin development in term infants. J. Pediatr. *75*:1231–1244, 1969.

Allison, A.: In Van Furth, R. (ed.): Mononuclear Phagocytes. Oxford, Blackwell Scientific Publications, 1970, pp. 422–440.

Allison, C. A.: Immunity and immunopathology in virus infections. Ann. Inst. Pasteur Lille *123*:585–608, 1972.

Banatvala, J. E., Potter, J. E., and Best, J. M.: Interferon response to sendai and rubella viruses in human fetal cultures, leukocytes and placental cultures. J. Gen. Virol. *13*:193–201, 1971.

Beckett, R. S., and Flynn, F. J.: Toxoplasmosis: report of two cases with a classification and with a demonstration of the organisms in the human placenta. N. Engl. J. Med. *249*:345–350, 1953.

Berg, T., and Johansson, S. G. O.: Immunoglobulin levels during childhood with special regard to IgE. Acta Paediatr. Scand. *58*:513–521, 1969.

Blaese, R. M.: Macrophages and the development of immunocompetence. In Bellanti, J. A., and Dayton, D. H. (eds.): The Phagocytic Cell in Host Resistance. New York, Raven Press, 1975, pp. 309–317.

Blanc, W. A.: Pathways of fetal and early neonatal infection, viral placentitis, bacterial and fungal chorioammionitis. J. Pediatr. *59*:473–496, 1961.

Buimovici-Klein, E., Lang, P. B., Ziring, P. R., and Cooper, L. Z.: Impaired cell-mediated immune response in patients with congenital rubella: correlation with gestational age at time of infection. Pediatrics *64*:620–626, 1979.

Cantell, K., Strander, H., Saxen, L., and Meyer, B.: Interferon response to human leukocytes during intrauterine and postnatal life. J. Immunol. *100*:1304–1309, 1968.

Colten, H. R.: Ontogeny of the human complement system: in vitro biosynthesis of individual components by fetal tissues. J. Clin. Invest. *51*:725–730, 1972.

Cooper, L. Z., Florman, A. L., Ziring, P. R., and Krugman, S.: Loss of hemagglutination inhibition antibody in congenital rubella. Am. J. Dis. Child. *122*:397–403, 1971.

Copper, M. D., Lawton, A. R., and Kincade, P. W.: A two-stage model for development of antibody-producing cells. Clin. Exp. Immunol. *11*:143–149, 1972.

Davis, L. E., Tweed, G. V., and Stewart, J. A.: Cytomegalovirus mononucleosis in a first trimester pregnant female and transmission to the fetus. Pediatrics *48*:200–306, 1971.

Desmyter, J., Rawls, W. E., Melnick, J. E., Yow, M. D., and Barrett, F. F.: Interferon in congenital rubella: response to live attenuated measles vaccine. J. Immunol. *99*:771–777, 1967.

Dudgeon, J. A., Marshall, W. C., and Peckham, C. S.: Humoral immune responses in congenital rubella. Lancet *2*:480–481, 1972.

Emodi, G., and Just, M.: Impaired interferon response of children with congenital cytomegalovirus disease. Acta Paediatr. Scand. *63*:183–187, 1974.

Emodi, G., Miggiano, A., Olafsson, A., and Just, M.: Studies of cellular immunity in congenital cytomegalovirus infection. Acta Paediatr. Scand. [Suppl.] *236*:43–44, 1973.

Entwistle, D. M., Bray, P. T., and Laurence, K. M.: Prenatal infection with vaccinia virus: report of a case. Br. Med. J. *2*:238–239, 1962.

Faulk, W. P., Goodman, J. R., Maloney, M. A., Fudenberg, H. H., and Yoffey, J. M.: Morphology and nucleoside incorporation of human neonatal lymphocytes. Cell Imunol. *8*:166–172, 1973.

Feldman, R,. A.: Cytomegalovirus infection during pregnancy: a prospective study and report of six cases. Am. J. Dis. Child. *117*:517–521, 1969.

Fireman, P., Zuchowski, D. A., and Taylor, P. M.: Development of human complement system. J. Immunol. *103*:25–31, 1969.

Fishel, C. M., and Pearlman, D. S.: Complement components of paired mother-cord sera. Proc. Soc. Exp. Biol. Med., *107*:695–699, 1961.

Fuccillo, D. A., Steele, R. W., Hensen, S. A., Vincent, M. M., Hardy, J. M., and Bellanti, J. A.: Impaired cellular immunity to rubella virus in congenital rubella. Infect. Immun. *9*:81–84, 1974.

Galask, R. P., and Snyder, I. R.: Antimicrobial factors in amniotic fluid. Am. J. Obstet. Gynecol. *106*:59–65, 1970.

Gamsu, H.: Intrauterine bacterial infections. In Intrauterine Infections. Ciba Foundation Symposium 10 (new series). Amsterdam, Associated Medical Publishers, 1973, pp. 135–146.

Garcia, A. G. P.: Fetal infection with chicken pox and alastrim with histopathologic study of the placenta. Pediatrics *32*:895–901, 1963.

Gershon, A. A.: Varicella in mother and infant: Problems old and new. In Krugman, S. and Gerson, A. A. (eds.): Infections of the Fetus and Newborn. Progress in Clinical and Biological Research, vol. 3. New York, Alan R. Liss, Inc., 1975, pp. 79–95.

Gibas, H., and Hayes, K.: In vitro activity of lymphocytes from children with prenatal cytomegalovirus infection. Aust. Paediatr. J. *10*:86–93, 1974.

Gitlin, D., and Biasucci, A.: Development of gamma G, gamma A, gamma M, beta 1C-beta 1A, C′1 esterase inhibitor, ceruloplasmin, transferrin, hemopexin, haptoglobulin, fibrinogen, plasminogen, alpha 1-antitrypsin, orosomucoid, beta-lipoprotein, alpha 2-macroglobulin and prealbumin in the human conceptus. J. Clin. Invest. *48*:1433–1446, 1969.

Glasgow, L. A., Hanshaw, J. B., Merigan, T. C., and Petralli, J. K.: Interferon and cytomegalovirus in vivo and in vitro. Proc. Soc. Exp. Biol. Med. *125*:843–849, 1967.

Hancock, M. P., Huntley, C. C., and Sever, J. L.: Congenital rubella syndrome with immunoglobulin disorder. J. Pediatr. *72*:636–645, 1968.

Hayward, A., and Soothill, J. F.: Personal communication, 1972.

Hirsch, M. S., Zisman, B., and Allison, A. C.: Macrophages and age-dependent resistance to herpes simplex virus in mice. J. Immunol. *104*:1160–1165, 1970.

Honeyman, M. C., Dorman, D. C., Menser, M. A., Forrest, J. M., Guinan, J. J., and Clark, P.: HL-A antigens in congenital rubella and the role of antigens

1 and 8 in the epidemiology of natural rubella. Tissue Antigens 5:12–18, 1975.

Kay, H. E. M., Doe, J., and Hockley, A.: Response of human foetal thymocytes to phytohaemagglutinin (PHA). Immunology 18:393–396, 1970.

Kohler, P. F.: Maturation of the human complement system. J. Clin. Invest. 52:671–677, 1973.

Kohler, P. F., and Farr, R. S.: Elevation of cord over maternal IgG immunoglobulin: evidence for an active placental IgG transport. Nature 210:1070–1071, 1966.

Kretschmer, R. R., Stewardson, P. B., Papierniak, C. P., and Getoff, S. P.: Chemotactic bactericidal capacities of human newborn monocytes. J. Immunol. 117:1303–1307, 1976.

Larsson, A., Forsgren, M., Hard A. F. Segarstad, S., Strander, H., and Cantell, K.: Administration of interferon to an infant with congenital rubella syndrome involving persistent viraemia and cutaneous vasculitis. Acta Paediatr. Scand. 65:105–110, 1976.

Lawton, A. R., Royal, S. A., Self, K. S., and Cooper, M. D.: IgA determinants on B-lymphocytes in patients with deficiency of circulating IgA. J. Lab. Clin. Med. 80:26–33, 1972a.

Lawton, A. R., Self, K. S., Royal, S. A., and Cooper, M. D.: Ontogeny of B-lymphocytes in the human fetus. Clin. Immunol. Immunopathol. 1:84–93, 1972b.

Lynch, F. W.: Dermatologic conditions of the fetus. Arch. Dermatol. Syphilol. 26:997–1019, 1932.

Mackaness, G. B.: The influence of immunologically committed lymphoid cells on macrophage activity in vivo. J. Exp. Med. 129:973–992, 1969.

Marshall, W. C.: Immunological studies of congenital rubella. Ph.D. thesis. University of London, 1972.

Marshall, W. C., Cope, W. A., Soothill, J. F., and Dudgeon, J. A.: In vitro lymphocyte response in some immune deficiency diseases and in intrauterine virus infections. Proc. R. Soc. Med. 63:351–354, 1970.

Michaels, R. H.: Immunologic aspects of congenital rubella. Pediatrics 43:339–350, 1969.

Michaels, R. H.: Suppression of antibody response in congenital rubella. J. Pediatr. 80:583–588, 1972.

Miller, M. E.: Chemotactic function in the human neonate: humoral and cellular aspects. Pediatr. Res. 5:487–492, 1971.

Mims, C. A.: Aspects of the pathogenesis of virus diseases. Bacteriol. Rev. 28:30–71, 1964.

Montgomery, J. R., Flanders, R. W., and Yow, M. D.: Congenital abnormalities and herpesvirus infection. Am. J. Dis. Child. 126:364–366, 1973.

Moore, M. A. S., and Owen, J. J. T.: Stem cell migration in developing myeloid and lymphoid systems. Lancet 2:658–659, 1967.

Oldstone, M. B. A., and Dixon, F. J.: Lymphocytic choriomeningitis: production of antibody by "tolerant" infected mice. Science 158:1193–1195, 1967.

Olson, G. B., South, M. A., and Good, R. A.: Phytohaemagglutinin unresponsiveness of lymphocytes from babies with congenital rubella. Nature 214:695–696, 1967.

Orlowski, J. P., Sieger, L., and Anthony, B. F.: Bactericidal capacity of monocytes of newborn infants. J. Pediatr. 89:797–801, 1976.

Playfair, J. H. L., Wolfendale, M. R., and Kay, H. E. M.: The leucocytes of peripheral blood in the human foetus. Br. J. Haematol. 9:336–344, 1963.

Plotkin, S. A., Dudgeon, J. A., and Ramsay, A. M.: Laboratory studies on rubella and the rubella syndrome. Br. Med. J. 2:1296–1299, 1963.

Plotkin, S. A., Klaus, R. M., and Whiteley, J. P.: Hypogammaglobulinemia in an infant with congenital rubella syndrome: failure of 1-adamantanamine to stop virus excretion. J. Pediatr. 69:1085–1091, 1966.

Rawls, W. E., Desmyter, J., and Melnick, J. L.: Serological diagnosis and fetal involvement in maternal rubella. J.A.M.A. 203:627–631, 1968.

Ray, C. G.: The ontogeny of interferon production by human leukocytes. J. Pediatr. 76:94–98, 1970.

Ross, S. M., Naeye, R. L., DuPlessis, J. P., and Visagie, M. E.: The genesis of amniotic fluid infections. In Perinatal Infections. Ciba Foundation Symposium No. 77. Amsterdam: Associated Medical Publishers, 1980, pp. 39–53.

Sawyer, M. K., and Forman, M. L.: Developmental aspects of the human complement system. Biol. Neonate 19:148–162, 1971.

Schimke, R. N., Bolano, C., and Kirkpatrick, C. H.: Immunologic deficiency in the congenital rubella syndrome. Am. J. Dis. Child. 118:626–633, 1969.

Shigeoka, A. O., Santos, J. I., and Hill, H. R.: Functional analysis of neutrophil granulocytes from healthy, infected and stressed neonates. J. Pediatr. 95:454–460, 1979.

Silverstein, A. M.: Ontogeny of the immune response. Science 144:1423–1428, 1962.

Silverstein, A. M., and Lukes, R. J.: Fetal response to antigenic stimulus. I. Plasmacellular and lymphoid reactions in the human fetus to intrauterine infection. Lab. Invest. 2:918–932, 1962.

Silverstein, A. M., and Prendergast, R. A.: Lymphogenesis, immunogenesis and the generation of immunologic diversity. In Sternbach, R. A., and Riha, I. (eds.): Developmental Aspects of Antibody Formation and Structure. New York, Academic Press, 1970, pp. 69–77.

Simons, M. J.: Congenital rubella: an immunological paradox? Lancet 2:1275–1278, 1968.

Simons, M. J., and Fitzgerald, M. G.: Rubella virus and human lymphocytes in culture. Lancet 2:937–940, 1968.

Singer, D. B., South, M. A., Montgomery, J. R., and Rawls, W. E.: Congenital rubella syndrome: lymphoid tissue and immunologic function. Am. J. Dis. Child. 118:54–61, 1969.

Soothill, J. F., Hayes, K., and Dudgeon, J. A.: The immunoglobulins in congenital rubella. Lancet 1:1385–1388, 1966.

South, M. A., and Good, R. A.: Communication to the American Pediatric Society (abstract), 1966.

South, M. A., Tompkins, W. A. F., Morris, C. R., and Rawls, W. E.: Congenital malformation of the central nervous system associated with genital type (type 2) herpesvirus. J. Pediatr. 75:13–18, 1969.

South, M. A., Montgomery, J. R., and Rawls, W. E.: Immune deficiency in congenital rubella and other viral infections. In Bergsma, D. (ed.): New Chromosomal and Malformation Syndromes. Birth Defects Original Article Series, No. 11–5. New York, The National Foundation—March of Dimes, 1975, pp. 234–238.

Stagno, S., Reynolds, D. W., Tsiantos, A., Fuccillo, D. A., Long, W., and Alford, C.: Comparative serial virologic and serologic studies of symptomatic and subclinical congenitally and natally acquired cytomegalovirus infections. J. Infect. Dis. 132:568–577, 1975.

Stagno, S., Volanakis, J. E., Reynolds, D. W., Stroud, R., and Alford, C. A.: Immune complexes in congenital and natal cytomegalovirus infections of man. J. Clin. Invest. 60:838–845, 1977.

Sterzl, J., and Silverstein, A. M.: Developmental aspects of immunity. Adv. Immunol. 6:337–459, 1967.

Stiehm, E. R., Ammann, A. J., and Cherry, J. D.: Elevated cord macroglobulins in the diagnosis of intrauterine infections. N. Engl. J. Med. *275*:971–977, 1966.

Stites, D. P., and Pavia, C. S.: Ontogeny of human T cells. Pediatrics *64*:795–802, 1979.

Stossel, T. P., Alper, C. A., and Rosen, F. S.: Opsonic activity in the newborn: role of properdin. Pediatrics *52*:134–137, 1973.

Strauss, R. G., Rosenberger, T. G., and Wallace, P. D.: Neutrophil chemiluminescence during the first month of life. Acta Haematol. *63*:326–329, 1980.

Tafari, N., Ross, S. M., Naeye, R. L., Galask, R. P., and Zaar, B.: Failure of bacterial growth inhibition of amniotic fluid. Am. J. Obstet. Gynecol. *128*:187–189, 1977.

Tardieu, M., Grospierre, G., Durandy, A., and Griscelli, C.: Circulating immune complexes containing rubella antigens in late-onset rubella syndrome. J. Pediatr. *97*:370–373, 1980.

Thomas, R. M., and Linch, D. C.: Identification of lymphocyte subsets in the newborn using a variety of monoclonal antibodies. Arch. Dis. Child. *58*:34–38, 1983.

Thompson, K. M., and Tobin, J. O. H.: Isolation of rubella virus from abortion material. Br. Med. J. *2*:264–266, 1970.

Uhr, J. W., Danois, J., and Neumann, C. G.: Delayed-type hypersensitivity in premature neonatal humans. Nature *187*:1130–1131, 1960.

Van Furth, R., and Sluiter, W.: Current views on the ontogeny of macrophages and the humoral regulation of monocytopoiesis. Trans. R. Soc. Trop. Med. Hyg. *77*:614–619, 1983.

Weller, T. H., Alford, C. A., and Neva, F. A.: Retrospective diagnosis by serological means of congenitally acquired rubella infection. N. Engl. J. Med. *270*:1039–1041, 1964.

White, L. R., Leikin, S., Villavicencio, O., Abernathy, W., Avery, G., and Sever, J. L.: Immune competence rubella. Lymphocyte transformation delayed hypersensitivity and response to vaccination. J. Pediatr. *73*:229–234, 1968.

Wielenga, G., Van Tongeren, H. A. E., Ferguson, A. H., and Van Rijssel, T. G.: Prenatal infection with vaccinia virus. Lancet *1*:258–260, 1961.

Witzleben, C. L., and Driscoll, S. G.: Possible transplacental transmission of herpes simplex infection. Pediatrics *36*:192–199, 1965.

Wright, W. C., Ank, B. J., Herbert, J., and Steihm, E. R.: Decreased bactericidal activity of leukocytes of stressed newborn infants. Pediatrics *56*:579–584, 1975.

13

Differential Diagnosis on the Basis of Physical Findings

When certain findings are present in the newborn infant, the possibility of a congenital infection must be considered in the differential diagnosis. In many instances, depending on the manifestations, the physician can suspect one specific diagnosis more strongly than another; for example, the presence of cataracts in an infant with a low birth weight and hepatosplenomegaly would point to a diagnosis of congenital rubella rather than cytomegalovirus (CMV) infection. In other circumstances, however, confirmation will depend upon the results of laboratory tests (see Chapter 14). This chapter is concerned with the differential diagnosis of those clinical manifestations that are especially suggestive of prenatal and perinatal infection. Some of the more common findings are listed in Table 13–1. It should be stated that it is often not possible to distinguish nonbacterial infections from bacterial infections that require urgent antibiotic therapy if the patient is to survive (Gotoff and Behrman, 1970). Congenital rubella, cytomegalic inclusion disease (CID), herpes simplex virus infection, Coxsackie B infection, and congenital toxoplasmosis may all mimic bacterial sepsis in the newborn. Both bacterial and nonbacterial infections of

early infancy are associated with acute illness, signs of bleeding (especially purpura), enlargement of liver and spleen, respiratory distress, fever, hypothermia, seizures, and full fontanelle. For this reason, many infants with nonbacterial infections may receive antibiotic therapy until a more definitive diagnosis can be made.

ABNORMALITIES OF THE CENTRAL NERVOUS SYSTEM

Mental Subnormality

This manifestation of congenital infection is usually not apparent during the newborn period, and, therefore, it is not an especially useful indicator to the physician evaluating a neonate with suspected congenital infection. The signs of spasticity or hypotonia may become manifest in the first month of life. The infant with "tight" muscles may tend to "scissor" the lower extremities, there may be a striking lack of muscle tone, or head control may be slow to develop. The extremes of muscle tonicity may be associated with reduced head circumference or loss of hearing.

243

Table 13–1. **SOME CLINICAL FINDINGS SUGGESTIVE OF CONGENITAL INFECTION**

NERVOUS SYSTEM	*EXTRANEURAL*
Microcephaly	Failure to thrive
Mental subnormality	Low birth weight for gestational age
Cerebral palsies	Prematurity
Seizures	Purpura
Chorioretinitis	Hepatosplenomegaly
Cataracts	Jaundice
Microphthalmus	Congenital heart disease
Cerebral calcification	Late onset disease
Sensorineural deafness	Chronic rash
Central auditory imperception	Pneumonitis

There are several variations in the neurological presentation of congenital infection in early life. Commonly there are few or no symptoms that might cause the physician or the parent to think that the child has sustained irreversible brain damage *in utero*. Even if developmental lag occurs, it is striking how seldom the possibility of a congenital infection, such as CMV infection, is considered in the differential diagnosis. This fact is brought out by our experience in testing stored cord sera several months and years after birth. One infant with a positive CMV IgM antibody titer in the cord blood had been seen by several physicians and studied extensively for marked developmental retardation. In spite of the fact that he was microcephalic, deaf, hypotonic, and retarded, with an IQ of 25, there was no mention of the possibility of congenital infection in his record, nor had any tests been done to determine if he had had a prenatal infection. The cord serum was strongly positive for CMV IgM antibody. The patient was still excreting CMV in the urine at 13 months and continued to do so into the seventh year of life.

The failure to think of congenital infection as a cause of psychomotor retardation or cerebral palsy–like syndromes is partly explained by the belief that damage caused by congenital infections is usually not restricted to the central nervous system. Yet it is clear from studies done in the past 20 years that all of the common congenital infections not only are capable of producing sequelae limited to the central nervous system, but frequently do so. These infants may be clinically indistinguishable from most other patients who present for evaluation at mental retardation clinics.

In the United States it is estimated that approximately 3 per cent of the population under 18 years of age is mentally subnormal. The great majority of these patients are never specifically diagnosed. Approximately four of every 1000 male infants and five of every 1000 female infants will at some time be admitted to a "training school" with a diagnosis of mental subnormality. These are the most severely affected children. At least 20 times this number have more subtle central nervous system abnormalities that are not recognized until the early school years.

In the United Kingdom, Catherine Peckham (1972) found that 17.3 per 1000 children are classified as educationally subnormal and 3.32 per 1000 are severely subnormal. These figures are based on a cohort of 15,438 children carefully evaluated 11 years after birth. Other findings of interest noted in this study of the frequency of abnormalities requiring special educational treatment include the following:

blindness	0.1 per 1000
partially sighted	0.4 per 1000
deaf	0.3 per 1000
partially deaf	1.1 per 1000
epileptic	0.5 per 1000
speech defect	0.3 per 1000
physically handicapped	1.7 per 1000
maladjusted	3.2 per 1000
severely subnormal	3.3 per 1000
educationally subnormal	17.3 per 1000

Thus, a total of approximately 2 per cent of British children are mentally subnormal, and an additional 0.44 per cent need special education for the conditions listed.

Although many normal, even intellectually gifted, persons may have a history of a lag in developmental motor skills, this finding occurs often enough in association with an intellectual deficit to warrant concern. In evaluating a history of motor retardation, it is particularly helpful to consider carefully the developmental progress of the siblings and parents.

In many children with mental defects no signs of gross abnormalities are detectable upon neurological examination. Certain "soft signs," such as hyperactivity, awkwardness of movement, poor coordination, persistence of infantile reflexes, increased or decreased muscle tone, and unmanageable behavior, have been associated with mental subnormality secondary to an intrauterine central nervous system infection. These children may have IQs in the "normal" range, but they are significantly lower than those of their siblings. Studies done in Rochester, New York, show that infants with congenital CMV infection detected on routine survey have mean IQs approximately 10 points below those of matched control children (Hanshaw et al., 1976).

The range of diseases capable of inducing mental subnormality is extraordinarily broad. There are many, frequently genetically determined, conditions due to metabolic abnormalities that alter amino acid, carbohydrate, lipid, purine, or mineral metabolism in such a manner as to result in suboptimal brain development. These conditions are generally rare. The most common specific abnormality known to cause moderate to severe mental deficiency is Down's syndrome. Approximately 1 in 800 to 1000 infants born in the United States and the United Kingdom is affected with this chromosomal aberration. Although the majority of Down's syndrome patients have 47 chromosomes, with a trisomy of chromosome number 21, others have a total of 46. The extra chromosome is due to nondisjunction. Patients with the normal complement of chromosomes have evidence of a translocation due to a centric fusion of two chromosomes, most commonly numbers 21 and 15. The cytogenetic disturbance in Down's syndrome has been attributed to maternal age, thyroid autoantibodies, maternal radiation, and viral infections occurring immediately prior to conception. The etiology of the cytogenetic disturbance remains unknown.

Table 13–2 lists a broad classification of conditions associated with mental subnormality. A more complete list has been compiled by Taft and Cohen (1972). It is apparent that in spite of the very large number of conditions known to be associated with mental subnormality, the great majority of patients are not specifically diagnosed. This is due in part to the difficulty in making a retrospective diagnosis of a condition in a child presenting with intellectual retardation at three or four years of age. Less than one third of patients have distinctive physical and specific laboratory findings that would permit a diagnosis at that time. A patient with microcephaly, spastic quadriplegia, and deafness could have any one of several central nervous system diseases.

Microcephaly

Microcephaly can be due to a variety of prenatal and perinatal factors as diverse as Down's syndrome, primary microcephaly, perinatal anoxia, phenylketonuria, maternal irradiation, and CID.

The finding is variable in degree among certain congenital infections. First-trimester fetal infections may result in marked diminution in brain growth, with obvious microcephaly at birth. In some instances, the head circumference is small enough to suggest a genetically determined form of microcephaly, sometimes referred to as primary microcephaly. More often, however, the diminution in brain volume is less striking, with a head circumference just below the third-percentile measurement. If other measurements—that is, length and weight—are also near the third percentile, less significance can be attributed to a small head circumference in early infancy. During the first year of life, a discrepancy may be noted between head circumference and the other indices of infantile growth. A diagnosis of microcephaly is indicated if the head measurement is less than the third percentile and the length and weight exceed those of the twenty-fifth percentile. Infants in this category have a guarded prognosis for achieving maximal intellectual and motor potential. It should be noted, however, that for inexplicable reasons, some infants with microcephaly do develop normally. Berenberg and Nankervis (1970) followed one of our original microcephalic patients with CID for more than seven years and reported that the child was not mentally retarded. It is well to remember that microcephaly and macrocephaly are statistical concepts that do not necessarily indicate that the patient will manifest cerebral dysfunction. Microcephaly is also noted in patients with congenital rubella, in whom it carries the same prognostic significance as in those with congenital CMV infection. Reduced head circumference may follow prenatal herpes simplex virus encephalitis, as well as perinatal infections. These infants are severely retarded.

Specific congenital infections and other

Table 13–2. **PATHOPHYSIOLOGICAL CLASSIFICATION OF MENTAL SUBNORMALITY**

Classification	Example
Prenatal Factors	
Chromosomal (autosomal)	Down's syndrome
Chromosomal (sex)	Klinefelter's syndrome
Metabolic	
Abnormalities of amino acid metabolism	Phenylketonuria
Abnormalities of carbohydrate metabolism	Galactosemia
Abnormalities of purine metabolism	Hyperuricemia
Abnormalities of mineral metabolism	Idiopathic hypercalcemia
Syndromes	
Skin abnormalities	Sturge-Weber syndrome
Cataracts	Marinesco-Sjögren's syndrome
Emaciation	Leprechaunism
Obesity	Laurence-Moon-Biedl syndrome
Cleft lip and cleft palate	Orofaciodigital syndrome
Facial anomalies	de Lange's syndrome
Tall stature	Cerebral gigantism
Dwarfism	Silver's syndrome
Cranial abnormalities	Apert's disease
Muscle weakness	Myotonic dystrophy
Fetal teratogens	
Chemical	Dietary inadequacies
Physical	Irradiation
Infectious agents	Cytomegalovirus
Perinatally Determined	Birth trauma, birth anoxia
Postnatally Determined	
Head trauma	Subdural hematoma
Poisoning	Lead
Infections	Herpes simplex virus encephalitis
Cerebrovascular accidents	Aneurysm
Metabolic	Hypoglycemia
Postimmunization encephalopathies	Rabies

Adapted from Taft, L. T., and Cohen, H. J.: Mental retardation. In Barnett, H. L. (ed.): Pediatrics, 15th ed. New York, Appleton-Century-Crofts, 1972, pp. 888–890.

conditions that have been associated with microcephaly are listed in Table 13–3.

Cerebral Calcifications

Three congenital infections are associated with cerebral calcifications: CMV, *Toxoplasma gondii*, and herpes simplex virus infections. It is rare to find calcifications in congenital rubella. The calcifications have distinctive features, and these differences can be helpful diagnostically.

A child with microcephaly and cerebral calcifications probably has CMV or *T. gondii* infection. The calcification patterns in the two infections are usually quite different, although there have been isolated reports of common radiological features. In general, the infant with congenital CID has periventricular calcifications, with no deposition of calcium in the brain substance (Fig. 13–1).

The degree of calcification in the periventricular area is highly variable, ranging from a short linear deposition to massive calcification outlining the entire ventricular system. In toxoplasmosis the distribution is scattered and generally discrete, with particularly heavy involvement in the parietal lobes of the cerebral cortex. Unlike that in CID patients, calcification of the brain in patients with toxoplasmosis is not necessarily associated with severe psychomotor retardation.

In both conditions calcifications are usually associated with chorioretinitis. We have observed a six month old infant with congenital toxoplasmosis who was excreting CMV in the urine. On the basis of his calcifications and the serological data, it is quite probable that the central nervous system disease was secondary to congenital toxoplasmosis and that the CMV infection was acquired during or after birth.

Whereas calcifications in CMV infection

Table 13–3. **CONDITIONS ASSOCIATED WITH MICROCEPHALY**

Present at Birth
Cytomegalovirus infection
Toxoplasmosis
Rubella
Paine's sex-linked recessive microcephaly with aminoaciduria
Chromosomal aberrations
Fetal maldevelopment of unknown origin

Normal at Birth, Apparent at One Year
Perinatal brain damage
Metabolic disorder (e.g., PKU)
Degenerative brain disease
Congenital rubella
Congenital cytomegalovirus infection
Congenital toxoplasmosis
Perinatal herpes simplex virus infection
Congenital varicella

are almost always associated with microcephaly, those in toxoplasmosis are not. More often the head is normal in circumference or enlarged owing to obstructive hydrocephalus at the level of the fourth ventricle. We have observed hydrocephalus in two patients with congenital CID. In both instances the hydrocephalus followed microcephaly, and there was extensive periventricular calcification. Both infants died in the first year of life.

Cerebral calcifications can occur with brain tumors as well as with the diseases already noted. This is unlikely to occur in early infancy, however. Tuberculous meningitis in its healing stage may be associated with the development of "silent" intracranial calcification. This disease is rare before six months of age, and calcifications are extremely rare. Tuberous sclerosis may be associated with intracranial calcifications in the region of the

Figure 13–1. Scattered calcifications in patient with congenital toxoplasmosis.

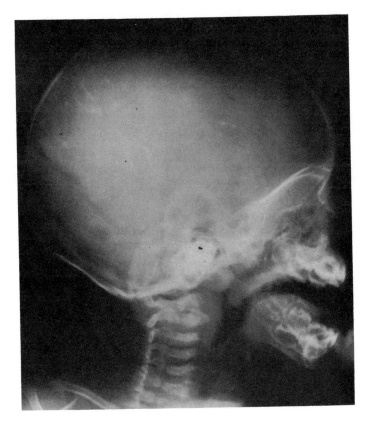

basal ganglia. In approximately 50 per cent of patients a pneumoencephalogram may show gliotic nodules projecting into the ventricle–so-called candle dripping. These patients present in a variety of ways, even those within the same family. Adenoma sebaceum, seizures, skin pigmentation, and mental retardation compose the classic symptom complex. Tuberous sclerosis should be suspected in an infant with infantile spasms and depigmented skin lesions. Although the majority of patients die by the age of 25, the disease is compatible with normal intelligence and long life. Some conditions associated with cerebral calcifications in early life are listed in Table 13–4.

Computerized tomography has been shown to be a more sensitive method of identifying calcifications than traditional skull roentgenograms (Anders et al., 1980).

Seizures

A seizure is a symptom of a central nervous system disturbance that may result from a localized or more generalized brain disturbance or from other systemic causes. Since a seizure may produce irreversible cerebral damage in an infant and the treatment is often dependent upon the diagnosis, it is particularly important to ascertain its precise cause.

In the newborn, seizures may not resemble the typical clonic-tonic convulsion seen in later life and may, therefore, go unrecognized. The infant may be having subcortical seizures manifested only by blinking, eye rolling, chewing activity, or pallor. These signs may be associated with poor feeding and apneic spells.

The major causes of seizures include hypoglycemia, hypocalcemia, hypomagnesemia, hyponatremia, hypernatremia, pyridoxine dependency, birth trauma, anoxia, and infection. It should be remembered that the diagnosis of bacterial meningitis does not rule out sodium imbalance or hypoglycemia as the explanation for the seizure.

Seizures occur in approximately 40 per cent of patients with neonatal bacterial meningitis. The percentage of patients with nonbacterial neonatal infections of the central nervous system who have seizures is significantly less, except in the case of patients with herpes simplex virus, which is often associated with convulsive activity that may be the presenting manifestation of that infection.

OCULAR MANIFESTATIONS

Chorioretinitis

The diseases commonly responsible for chorioretinitis or retinopathy in early infancy are all infectious. The agents that have been associated with these abnormalities are listed in Table 13–5. Except in rubella, the lesions are characteristically discrete and patchy, with black pigmentation interspersed with areas of depigmentation. They are variable in size and location. The retinopathy does not significantly interfere with vision unless the macular area is involved. This is less common in CMV infection than in congenital toxoplasmosis. In some patients involvement is unilateral.

It is important to differentiate toxoplasmosis and syphilis from the viral causes of chorioretinitis because of the therapeutic implications. There is preliminary but inconclusive evidence that infants with "silent" Toxoplasma infections may do better developmentally if treated with sulfadiazine and pyrimethamine (Saxon et al., 1973).

The funduscopic appearances of Toxoplasma and CMV chorioretinitis are too sim-

Table 13–4. **CONDITIONS ASSOCIATED WITH CEREBRAL CALCIFICATIONS IN EARLY LIFE**

Disease	Distinguishing Features
Toxoplasmosis	Calcifications widely distributed in cortex
Cytomegalic inclusion disease	Periventricular distribution
Herpes simplex virus infection	Periventricular and cortical with associated microcrania
Congenital rubella	Rare; small areas of calcification scattered throughout cortex
Brain tumor (craniopharyngioma, pinealoma)	Midline calcifications
Tuberous sclerosis	In basal ganglia
Calcified hematoma	Usually localized to one peripheral area
Sturge-Weber syndrome	"Trolley track" calcifications

Table 13–5. **CONDITIONS ASSOCIATED WITH RETINOPATHY IN EARLY INFANCY***

	Congenital	Acquired	Distribution
Rubella	++	−	Generalized
Toxoplasmosis	+	+	Focal
Cytomegalic inclusion disease	+	?+	Focal
Herpes simplex virus	+ (rare)	−	Focal
Varicella	+ (rare)	−	Focal
Syphilis	+	−	Focal

*Includes pigmentary retinopathy and chorioretinitis.

ilar for them to be differentiated on clinical grounds alone. Both infections may cause central or macular lesions. Whereas chorioretinitis is one of the most common features of congenital toxoplasmosis, it occurs in fewer than 10 per cent of infants with symptomatic CMV infection. Occasionally the clinical feature that draws attention to the eye is strabismus developing in the first six months of life. Funduscopic examination done on referral to an ophthalmologist may reveal an associated chorioretinitis, thereby leading to the correct diagnosis. Neither toxoplasmosis nor CID, the two most common causes of chorioretinitis in early infancy, is likely to induce cataract formation. In CID the chorioretinitis may be associated with optic atrophy. Infants with microcephaly, especially those with calcifications, usually have chorioretinitis. In toxoplasmosis, both chorioretinitis and cerebral calcification may occur in the presence of a normal head circumference.

In a newborn infant seriously suspected of congenital infection it is important that a funduscopic examination be done by an ophthalmologist because it is difficult to perform this examination in these patients.

Cataracts

Although cataracts have been described in association with CMV infection, they are very rare in any congenital infection other than rubella. The association with rubella is sufficiently strong to warrant a presumptive diagnosis of that infection provided the cataract is central and there is no family history of congenital cataracts. Rubella cataracts appear as pearly white nuclear lesions, and they are frequently associated with microphthalmus. Approximately 50 per cent are unilateral. In unilateral cataracts, a generalized retinopathy is often present in the opposite eye.

Owing to a diminution in the number of infants born with rubella in the United States, noninfectious causes of congenital cataract are now more common. These include a hereditary abnormality transmitted as a dominant trait to half of the offspring of either sex. Siblings without cataracts are not carriers.

Congenital galactosemia, an enzymatic disorder involving a structural change affecting the reactive site of the enzyme galactokinase, may cause a congenital cataract appearing as early as the second week of life. Fewer than half of patients with galactosemia manifest cataracts. Hepatomegaly, jaundice, anorexia, vomiting, and weight loss are more common findings. Mature cataracts are usually a late manifestation of the disorder. Although specific neurological abnormalities may be absent, most galactosemic infants who survive early infancy have moderate to severe mental retardation.

Cataracts are also seen in association with several other congenital defects, such as Lowe's syndrome (oculocerebrorenal syndrome), which is characterized by the triad of bilateral cataracts at birth, mental retardation, and hypotonia in a male child. A renal tubular defect appears three to six months after birth. This is associated with hyperaminoaciduria, "tubular" proteinuria, and renal tubular acidosis. Hypophosphatemic rickets occurs as a late complication. Although the majority of patients die in the first decade, a few have survived beyond adolescence. Other conditions associated with cataract formation are listed in Table 13–6. A more comprehensive list has been compiled by Kohn (1976).

Other Ocular Manifestations

Involvement of the iris and ciliary body and iridocyclitis are extremely uncommon in infants with congenital infections. Conjunctivitis in the newborn is usually chemical in nature, due to silver nitrate solution, or bacterial, due to *Nisseria gonorrhoeae, Staphylococcus aureus,* Streptococcus (group A or B), or one of several species of gram-negative organisms such as *Escherichia coli* or *Pseudomonas aeruginosa.* Occasionally inclusion blennorrhea, characterized by blue-staining granules in the cytoplasm of cells obtained from conjunctival scrapings, is seen in the newborn period after the first week of life. This infection tends to run a self-limited course of several weeks or months. There is an associated purulent exudate, and the conjunctiva has a follicular appearance. The condition can be treated with the local application of tetracycline ointment. The causative agent, *Chlamydia trachomatis,* is related to the psittacosis-lymphogranuloma venereum-trachoma group of agents. It has been associated with pneumonitis in early infancy (Beem and Saxon, 1977).

Herpes simplex virus keratoconjunctivitis is a rare infection in early infancy but should be considered in patients with vesicular lesions on the skin or other evidence of disseminated herpesvirus infection in the neonatal period. In some instances the viral infection is localized to the eye.

Glaucoma. Congenital glaucoma occurs in the rubella syndrome but is seen 10 times less often than cataract (Cooper, 1968). Glaucoma may be present at birth or may develop during infancy. It is distinguishable from hereditary infantile glaucoma. The cornea is enlarged and hazy in appearance. The anterior chamber is deep, and there is an increase in ocular tension. Glaucoma must be distinguished from the transient corneal clouding occasionally seen in rubella. Unlike glaucoma, the latter condition requires no special therapy. Infants with congenital glaucoma must undergo prompt surgical decompression of the globe to relieve the intraocular tension.

Myopia is another manifestation of the congenital rubella syndrome that may easily be missed, especially in the presence of other ocular abnormalities such a unilateral cataract.

Microphthalmus. Microphthalmus may be manifested simply as a small but functionally adequate eye. Virtually all patients have some refractive error causing hypermetropia. More often the eye is malformed as well as small. There may be associated colobomas, cataracts, chorioretinitis, or other congenital defects. The etiology is multifactorial. In some patients a hereditary pattern is apparent, with the defect appearing as an autosomal recessive. Less often the condition is autosomal dominant. Microphthalmus occurs in the intrauterine infections listed in Table 13–7. It is not an infrequent finding in the rubella syndrome and toxoplasmosis. Although it has been reported in CID, it is rare enough to make this diagnosis unlikely. When microphthalmus occurs in a patient with toxoplasmosis, the probability of associated chorioretinitis is very high. In rubella the affected as well as the opposite eye is likely to have a congenital cataract.

DEAFNESS

With the exception of rubella, congenital infection has not been extensively studied as a cause of deafness. Gumpel and co-workers (1971) found evidence of congenital rubella in 82 (59 per cent) of 139 deaf children. There are recent data to suggest that congenital CMV infection may be associated with deafness (Medearis, 1964; Reynolds et al., 1974; Hanshaw et al., 1976; Stagno et al., 1977). The importance of this agent in the overall etiology of hearing loss is not yet accurately known. Reynolds and colleagues (1974) reported significantly reduced hearing

Table 13–6. **CONDITIONS ASSOCIATED WITH CONGENITAL CATARACTS**

Disease	Common Associated Findings
Congenital rubella	Heart defects, deafness, and other lesions
Congenital galactosemia	Hepatomegaly, jaundice, and weight loss
Oculocerebrorenal syndrome (Lowe's syndrome)	Cataracts present at birth, hypotonia, mental retardation, and male sex
Oculomandibulofacial syndrome	Normal intelligence, proportionate dwarfism, and microphthalmus
Hereditary cataract	Dominant inheritance
Pierre Robin syndrome	Cleft palate, micrognathia, and glossoptosis
Hereditary nephritis and nerve deafness	Hematuria, proteinuria, sensorineural hearing loss, and family history of deafness

Table 13–7. **CONDITIONS ASSOCIATED WITH MICROPHTHALMUS**

Intrauterine infection	Toxoplasmosis
	Rubella
	Cytomegalic inclusion disease
	Herpes simplex virus infection (rare)
	Varicella (rare)
Hereditary	Autosomal recessive
	Autosomal dominant

in nine of 16 asymptomatic infants followed for two to three years after birth. Four of the affected children had unilateral involvement. Two had significant bilateral hearing loss and manifested clinically recognizable mental deficiency.

When deafness occurs in congenital rubella it may not be associated with other manifestations of that syndrome, with the exception of retinopathy. Gumpel and co-workers (1971) found isolated deafness in 60 of 139 children. As in hearing loss associated with CMV infection, involvement may be unilateral.

In both rubella and CMV infection, the deafness is usually sensorineural, without a characteristic audiometric pattern. In approximately 40 per cent of infants with congenital rubella, the audiogram demonstrates a falling pattern with increasing frequency. Although most children with rubella do well in schools for the deaf, their progress may be impaired by associated brain or ocular sequelae. Such children may have a diminished head circumference in association with hearing loss. The central nervous system status of deaf patients with CMV infections ranges from severe mental subnormality to essentially normal cerebral function. We have seen normocephalic children with severe bilateral hearing loss who had normal cerebral function. Reynolds and colleagues (1974) have also found that patients with significant hearing loss due to CMV infection do not necessarily have significant intellectual deficits. It is important, however, to follow these children into the sixth or seventh year of life before concluding that one central nervous system abnormality, such as deafness, is not associated with evidence of diminished intellectual potential.

Much needs to be done to increase our knowledge of the role of intrauterine pathogens in the pathogenesis of hearing loss. It is highly probable that the impact of congenital infection on auditory function is significantly greater than has been appreciated. Although there is no evidence that congenital mumps infection is an important cause of congenital deafness, it is a well-known, but infrequent, cause of hearing loss after birth.

Defects of hearing in congenital rubella have been shown to be caused by central auditory imperception. It is not clear how common this cause is, but it should be suspected in children who do not respond in the usual manner to tests for the detection of deafness.

EXTRANEURAL ABNORMALITIES

Failure to Thrive

Failure to thrive is usually a problem of malnutrition. It is an exceedingly comprehensive term used to refer to a common manifestation of illnesses of various etiologies. Some infants who do not thrive are adequately nourished but are of short stature. A few may have a primordial growth failure secondary to a central nervous system abnormality. Infants who have other central nervous system diseases, including congenital infections such as CMV infection or rubella, may lag not only in weight and height but also in head circumference. Table 13–8 lists some of the conditions that should be considered in the differential diagnosis. The standard pediatric measurements of weight, height, and head circumference can be used to classify infants into three general categories:

1. *Malnourished infant.* The patient is emaciated, with a weight that is low relative to his normal height and head circumference. There is often evidence of parental neglect and a dramatic response to hospitalization. Others are malnourished because of a variety of intrinsic conditions.

2. *Short stature infant.* This child's height is proportionately small compared with his

Table 13–8. **SOME CAUSES OF FAILURE TO THRIVE**

Chronic infection (usually nonbacterial)	Respiratory
Congenital cytomegalovirus infection	Cystic fibrosis
Toxoplasmosis	Chronic lung disease
Rubella	Allergies
Herpes simplex virus infection	Gastrointestinal
Acquired infection (usually bacterial)	Anomalies of the gastrointestinal tract
Pulmonary	Chronic diarrhea
Central nervous system	Defective carbohydrate absorption
Enteric	Chromosomal abnormalities
Genitourinary	Down's syndrome
Congenital malformation	D-1 trisomy
Central nervous system	E trisomy
Renal	Miscellaneous
Psychological	Placental insufficiency
Maternal deprivation	Cystinuria
Central nervous system	Diabetes mellitus
Subdural hematoma	Genetic factors
Increased intracranial pressure	Adrenal renal metabolic imbalance
Diabetes insipidus	Lead poisoning
	Galactosemia
	PKU (phenylketonuria)
	Hypercalcemia

weight and head circumference. These infants often have a family history of dwarfism.

3. *Primordial central nervous system infant.* Both height and weight of this infant are of reduced proportions. The head is usually also reduced in circumference. In most of these infants chromosomal aberrations or congenital infections cannot be specifically diagnosed.

Other possible causes of failure to thrive that should be considered are chronic intoxification, such as from lead poisoning; chronic infection of the genitourinary and respiratory tracts or other occult infection; malignant disease, including solid tumors such as Wilms' tumor or neuroblastoma; reticuloendothelial diseases; and congenital malformations. These conditions are sufficiently common to warrant special attention in the differential diagnosis of the hospitalized infant who fails to thrive.

Purpura

A petechial rash or purpura may occur in a newborn with toxoplasmosis, syphilis, rubella, herpes simplex virus infection, or, more commonly, CMV infection. The lesions are generally pinpoint and are most often seen on the head and upper trunk, perhaps because of the increased pressure on capillaries in this area during the second stage of labor. Purpura may also appear on the extremities. Applying a tourniquet or any pressure can induce capillary rupture and petechial formation. Some infants continue to have petechial rashes for weeks or months after birth. These may be occasioned by vigorous crying, coughing, or other exertion.

Characteristically, the petechial rashes associated with congenital infections (such as CMV infection, rubella, and toxoplasmosis) appear on the first day of life. The rash may be transient in character and the only abnormality noted by the physician. Purpura is a prime indication of intrauterine infection. Petechial rash due to congenital infection is not necessarily associated with a depressed platelet count. Splenomegaly, with or without associated hepatomegaly, is a relatively frequent clinical finding in infants with purpura.

Although any newborn infant with a petechial rash should be investigated for the possibility of a congenital infection, certain noninfectious conditions shown in Table 13–9 must be considered in the differential diagnosis.

A systemic approach to the diagnosis, such as that outlined by Oski and Naiman (1982), should be undertaken. It is important to question the mother regarding a history of bleeding that might suggest idiopathic thrombocytopenia, purpura, or lupus erythematosus. Other specific maternal conditions associated with neonatal purpura include previous ingestion of drugs such as quinidine, quinine, thiazide diuretics, and tolbutamide. Drug-induced purpura is less likely to be associated with hepatomegaly or splenomegaly. Inherited thrombocytopenia must also be considered: if previous infants have been affected by purpura, an immune or hereditary thrombocytopenic purpura is a possibility. A maternal platelet count will distinguish immune neonatal thrombocytopenia due to maternal disease from platelet isoimmunization; in the latter condition the mother's platelet count is normal. Other congenital diseases associated with neonatal purpura include giant hemangioma, trisomy syndromes, and absent radii. In the last condition there is deformity and shortening of the forearms, with absence of the radii, and associated amegakaryocytic thrombocytopenia. The white blood count in this syndrome may exceed 40,000 to 50,000 per cubic millimeter.

Jaundice

A useful approach to the differential diagnosis of jaundice in the newborn period emphasizes the importance of the time and onset of the syndrome as an indicator of its etiology.

Jaundice Appearing Within 24 Hours After Birth. Icterus appearing on the first day of life is usually due to a congenital infection or to a hemolytic process such as ABO disease. Jaundice in these infants is absent at birth but may become apparent four or five hours later. When jaundice does appear in the first 24 hours of life, hemolytic disease is the most probable diagnosis.

In differentiating congenital infection from hemolytic disease, special attention should be given to the presence of associated organomegaly and purpura. The latter manifestation is rare even in severe hemolytic disease, whereas it is one of the most common signs of congenital infections of nonbacterial etiology. Similarly, hepatomegaly and splenomegaly are not seen in ABO disease or in mild Rh disease. Occasionally hepatomegaly is present in more severe Rh disease. It is rare to find splenomegaly associated with Rh disease alone. Anemia occurs in both hemolytic disease and congenital infection but is usually not as severe in the latter. There is such variability in the severity of illness from congenital infection that this assessment is of limited value in the differential diagnosis. The laboratory tests of greatest use include examination of the peripheral smear for the presence of spherocytes seen in ABO disease, assessment of the number of platelets (they are rarely reduced in Rh and ABO diseases), blood-group typing of the infant's erythrocytes, and Coombs' test. Type O never occurs in an infant with ABO incompatibility. Direct and indirect Coombs' test results are usually negative in an infant with a congenital infection. Rare exceptions, in which Coombs'-positive hemolytic anemia developed in infants with congenital CMV infection, have been reported (Zuelzer et al., 1970).

The measurement of conjugated bilirubin is a useful laboratory test in differentiating hemolytic disease from congenital infection. The direct bilirubin rarely exceeds 2.0 mg/dl even in severe Rh hemolytic disease. In con-

---

Table 13–9. **SOME NONINFECTIOUS CAUSES OF NEONATAL PURPURA**

Immune disorders
  Passive
    Idiopathic thrombocytopenia, drug-induced thrombocytopenia, systemic lupus erythematosus
  Active
    Isoimmune—platelet group incompatibility
    Associated with erythroblastosis fetalis—due to the disease or to exchange transfusion
Drugs (administered to mother)
  Thiazide diuretics, tolbutamide
Congenital leukemia
Disseminated intravascular coagulation
Inherited (chronic) thrombocytopenia including Wiskott-Aldrich syndrome, May-Hegglin anomaly
Miscellaneous
  Congenital thyrotoxicosis
  Inherited metabolic disorders
  Thrombotic thrombocytopenic purpura

From Oski, F. A., and Naiman, J. L.: Hematologic Problems in the Newborn. Philadelphia, W. B. Saunders Company, 1982.

trast, all viral, bacterial, and protozoan infections capable of producing neonatal jaundice are often associated with an increase in direct or conjugated bilirubin. This elevation may not become apparent until after the first 24 to 48 hours of life.

In addition to bilirubin determinations, the serum glutamic oxalacetic transaminase is usually elevated above 150 units in congenitally infected infants with hyperbilirubinemia. This value is normal in the newborn with hemolytic disease.

Other laboratory tests that can be helpful in excluding transplacental infection include a urine culture for CMV, a total IgM antibody determination, and specific antibody determinations for CMV infection, toxoplasmosis, rubella, and syphilis. It is probable that specific IgM antibody determinations and tests for antigen using monoclonal antibody and hybridization techniques will become more generally available in the next several years. Since CMV infection is more common than the other infections, it should be ruled out first. The examination of the urinary sediment stained with Papanicolaou, Giemsa, or hematoxylin and eosin should be done when other, more sensitive, tests are not available. Although a positive test is diagnostic, the failure to find inclusion-bearing cells does not rule out CMV infection. Inclusions are found in only half the patients with classic CID. Table 13–10 lists some causes of jaundice that becomes manifest during the first week of life.

If an infant receives one or more transfusions of blood as treatment for hyperbilirubinemia secondary to Rh or ABO disease, the possibility exists that post-transfusion hepatitis secondary to CMV infection may occur (Yeager, 1974). (For this reason it is prudent to obtain the blood from a seronegative donor.) Some reports of the so-called inspissated bile syndrome, which occasionally has followed severe hemolytic disease, might be explainable by this mechanism. Stevens and co-workers (1970) found that CMV infection, documented by fourfold increases in complement-fixing antibody, occurred in 32 per cent of patients who received multiple blood transfusions for blood loss during solid tumor surgery. In addition, other infections, including hepatitis B, toxoplasmosis, Epstein-Barr virus infection, and bacterial infections, may be transmitted in transfused blood.

Jaundice Appearing More Than 24 Hours After Birth. Physiological jaundice is the most common explanation for icterus appearing on the second or third day. Hemolytic disease of any severity rarely, if ever, presents after the second day. Jaundice occurring with congenital infections, however, is not so restricted in time. The icterus that accompanies intrauterine infection may follow one of several patterns, including the appearance of jaundice after the first week of life. If an infant has hepatomegaly, splenomegaly, or purpura or appears ill, the exclusion diagnosis of physiological jaundice cannot be invoked. It is also improbable that the jaundice is secondary to a blood-group incompatibility. Bacterial infections, especially those due to gram-negative microorganisms, may be associated with neonatal jaundice appearing after the second day. Icterus in association with group B beta-hemolytic streptococcal sepsis in the newborn has also been observed. The fact that the most severely affected infants with this infection become ill in the first few hours of life indicates that the bacterial infection reaches the fetus just prior to birth.

Hepatosplenomegaly

Congenital viral diseases may induce hypertrophy of the reticuloendothelial system with resultant hepatomegaly, splenomegaly, or a combination of both. In congenital rubella, toxoplasmosis, and CMV infection, hepatosplenomegaly is more common than enlargement of the liver alone. In cases of congenital rubella it may be due to heart failure resulting from damage to the heart muscle. Hepatosplenomegaly can occur as an isolated manifestation of fetal infection. More often it is seen in association with at least one other manifestation of congenital infection, such as a petechial rash or hyperbilirubinemia.

In evaluating the newborn infant with hepatosplenomegaly, the infections shown in Table 13–11 should be considered. Any of these conditions may occur in the absence of other findings distinctive enough to lead to the correct diagnosis. All may be associated with central nervous system symptoms, jaundice, purpura, failure to feed, and low birth weight. It is important to emphasize that the most distinctive features of a given congenital infection are not always the most common manifestations noted.

Table 13–10. **CAUSES OF JAUNDICE DURING THE FIRST WEEK OF LIFE**

Infections
    Sepsis (gram-negative and gram-positive)
    Cytomegalovirus infection
    Toxoplasma gondii infection
    Rubella
    Herpes simplex virus infection
    Syphilis
    Hepatitis B virus infection
Hemolytic diseases
    Rh or ABO incompatibility
    Red cell defects
        Hereditary spherocytosis
        Enzyme deficiencies (glucose-6-phosphate dehydrogenase, pyruvate kinase, etc.)
    Hematoma
    Metabolic disorders
        Galactosemia
        Crigler-Najjar syndrome
        Breast milk jaundice (Newman and Gross, 1963)
        Transient familial neonatal hyperbilirubinemia (Lucy, 1960)
        Cretinism
Neonatal (giant cell) hepatitis of unknown cause
Physiological jaundice

From Oski, F. A., and Naiman, J. L.: Hematologic Problems in the Newborn. Philadelphia, W. B. Saunders Company, 1982.

Congenital Heart Disease

Although many patients with congenital heart disease, especially those with other anomalies, are evaluated for congenital infection, there is only suggestive evidence that infections other than rubella are capable of inducing cardiac malformations. Although it is possible that this may change as more epidemiological data become available, it is striking that rubella appears to be almost unique in this respect. Earlier studies by Brown (1964) suggested that Coxsackie B viruses may be significant causes of a variety of cardiac malformations. This observation has not been confirmed by others. Although there are several case reports of cardiac anomalies in association with congenital·CMV infections, these are varied in type and one cannot conclude at this time that this association is significant etiologically.

Some cardiac anomalies that have been described in association with congenital infections are listed in Table 13–12.

Myocarditis has also been observed in newborn infants with Coxsackie B infections. These infants generally have multisystem disease involving the central nervous system, the liver, and the heart. In some instances the mother has a history of recent pleurodynia. The prognosis for life is variable. In early reports appearing in the 1950's many infants died. More recently, Coxsackie B and other enterovirus infections occurring in the first year of life have been associated with mild neurological impairment when children were tested at two and one-half to eight years of age (Sells et al., 1975).

It is noteworthy that the cardiac malformations associated with the rubella syndrome generally follow a pattern involving the ductus arteriosus (PDA) or the pulmonary artery

Table 13–11. **INFECTIONS OF THE NEWBORN ASSOCIATED WITH HEPATOSPLENOMEGALY**

Infectious Agent or Disease	Most Distinctive Associated Features*
Cytomegalovirus	Periventricular calcifications, petechial rash
Rubella	Cataracts, congenital heart disease
Toxoplasmosis	Microphthalmus, scattered cerebral calcifications, chorioretinitis
Herpes simplex virus	Vesicular skin lesions, encephalitis
Syphilis	Bone changes, osteochondritis
Coxsackie B	Myocarditis, meningoencephalitis
Bacterial sepsis	Toxicity, fever, pneumonia

*Not necessarily the most common features.

Table 13–12. **HEART DEFECTS ASSOCIATED WITH CONGENITAL INFECTIONS**

Rubella (causation established)
  Persistent ductus arteriosus (PDA)
  Peripheral pulmonary artery stenosis (PPAS)
  Pulmonary valvular stenosis (PVS)
  Combinations of the above
  Ventricular septal defect
  ? Atrial septal defects
  ? Fallot's tetralogy
  Myocardial damage due to muscle necrosis

Rubella (causation reported but not clearly established)
  Coarctation of the aorta
  Truncus arteriosus
  Transposition of the great vessels
  Aortic stenosis

Congenital Cytomegalovirus Infection (CMV) (causation reported but not established)
  Atrial septal defect
  Congenital mitral stenosis
  Ventricular septal defect
  Anomalous venous drainage
  Enlarged ductus

Mumps (causation reported but not established)
  Primary endocardial fibroelastosis (EFE)

(pulmonary stenosis or multiple stenosis of the peripheral branches of the pulmonary artery). Of 12 rubella patients studied by Starkova and Ebrahim (1973), nine had PDA, three had pulmonary valvular stenosis, two had a ventricular septal defect, and two had peripheral pulmonary artery stenosis.

In congenital rubella the structural cardiac defect may be present at birth and there may be rapid onset of heart failure (Marshall, 1973). The patient may make a complete recovery following suitable treatment for heart failure. Heart failure may also occur in the absence of a cardiac defect in patients with active rubella myocarditis.

Bibliography

Anders, B. J., Lauer, B. A., and Foley, L. C.: Computerized tomography to define CNS involvement in congenital cytomegalovirus infection Am. J. Dis. Child., *134*:795–797, 1980.

Beem, M. O., and Saxon, E. M.: Respiratory tract colonization and a distinctive pneumonia syndrome in infants infected with *Chlamydia trachomatis*. N. Engl. J. Med., *296*:306–310, 1977.

Berenberg, W., and Nankervis G.: Long-term follow-up of cytomegalic inclusion disease of infancy. Pediatrics, *46*:403–410, 1970.

Brown, G. C.: Recent advances in the viral etiology of congenital anomalies. Adv. Teratol., *1*:55–81, 1964.

Cooper, L. Z.: Congenital rubella in the United States. In Bergsma, D., and Krugman, S. (eds.): Intrauterine Infections. Birth Defects Original Article Series, Vol.

IV, No. 7. New York, The National Foundation—March of Dimes, 1968, pp. 23–35.

Gotoff, S. P., and Behrman, R. E.: Neonatal septicemia. J. Pediatr. *76*:142–153, 1970.

Gumpel, S. M., Hayes, K., and Dudgeon, J. A.: Congenital perceptive deafness: role of intrauterine rubella. Br. Med. J. *2*:300–304, 1971.

Hanshaw, J. B., Scheiner, A. P., Moxley, A. W., et al.: School failure and deafness after silent congenital cytomegalovirus infection. N. Engl. J. Med., *295*:468–470, 1976.

Kohn, B. A.: The differential diagnosis of cataracts in infancy and childhood. Am J. Dis. Child. *130*:184–192, 1976.

Lucey, J. F.: Hyperbilirubinemia of prematurity. Pediatrics *25*:690–710, 1960.

Marshall, W. C.: The clinical impact of congenital rubella. In Intrauterine Infections. Ciba Foundation Symposium 10 (new series). Amsterdam, Associated Scientific Publishers, 1973, pp. 3–22.

Medearis, D. N., Jr.: Observations concerning human cytomegalovirus infection and disease. Bull. Johns Hopkins Hosp. *114*:181–211, 1964.

Melish, M. E., and Hanshaw, J. B.: Congenital cytomegalovirus infection: developmental progress of infants detected by routine screening. Am. J. Dis. Child. *126*:190–194, 1973.

Newman, A. J., and Gross, S.: Hyperbilirubinemia in breast-fed infants. Pediatrics *32*:995–1001, 1963.

Oski, F. A., and Naiman, J. L.: Hematologic Problems in the Newborn. Philadelphia, W. B. Saunders Company, 1982.

Peckham, C. S.: Personal communication, 1972.

Reynolds, D. W., Stagno, S., Stubbs, K. G., Dahle, A. J., Saxon, S. S., and Alford, C. A.: Inapparent congenital cytomegalovirus infection: causal relationship with auditory and mental deficiency. N. Engl. J. Med. *209*:291–296, 1974.

Saxon, S. A., Knight, W., Reynolds, D. W., et al.:

Intellectual deficits in childen born with subclinical congenital toxoplasmosis: a preliminary report. J. Pediatr. *82*:792–797, 1973.

Sells, C. J., Carpenter, R. L., and Ray, C. G.: Sequelae of central nervous system enterovirus infection. N. Engl. J. Med. *293*:1–4, 1975.

Stagno, S., Reynolds, D. W., Amos, C. S., Dahle, A. J., McCollister, F. P., Mohindra, O. D., Ermocilla, R., and Alford, C. A.: Auditory and visual defects resulting from symptomatic and subclinical congenital cytomegaloviral and *Toxoplasma* infections. Pediatrics *59*:669–678, 1977.

Starkova, O., and Ebrahim, S.: Personal communication. Cited in Marshall, W. C.: The clinical impact of congenital rubella. In Intrauterine Infections. Ciba Foundation Symposium 10 (new series). Amsterdam, Associated Scientific Publishers, 1973, pp. 3–22.

Stevens, D. P., Barker, L. F., Ketcham, A. S., et al.: Asymptomatic cytomegalovirus infection following blood transfusion in tumor surgery. J.A.M.A. *211*:1341–1344, 1970.

Taft, L. T., and Cohen, H. J.: Mental retardation. In Barnett, H. L. (ed.): Pediatrics. 15th ed. New York, Appleton-Century-Crofts, 1972, pp. 888–890.

Weller, T. H., and Hanshaw, J. B.: Virologic and clinical observations on cytomegalic inclusion disease. N. Engl. J. Med. *266*:1233–1244, 1962.

Yeager, A.: Transfusion acquired CMV infection in newborn infants. Am. J. Dis. Child. *128*:478–483, 1974.

Zuelzer, W. W., Mastrangelo, R., Stulberg, C. S., Povlik, M. D., Page, R. H., and Thompson, R. I.: Autoimmune hemolytic anemia: natural history and viral-immunologic interactions in childhood. Am. J. Med., *49*:80–94, 1970.

14

Laboratory Diagnosis

This chapter is concerned with principles of diagnosis rather than with details. What detail there is has been included to give the clinician some insight into the availability of laboratory tests that will enable him or her to make a precise diagnosis in a given situation. Increasingly, however, with the rapid development of new techniques, the responsibility for deciding what laboratory tests are appropriate will rest with the virologist. This is why close liaison between the clinician and the virologist is so important. Furthermore, as medical progress continues, early treatment with antiviral drugs will assume greater importance than in the past. No longer is the clinician concerned with a precise diagnosis solely for purposes of record keeping. It is useful for the physician to know that a case of sensorineural deafness is due either to congenital rubella or to cytomegalovirus (CMV) rather than to a genetic cause, because it will help in advising parents as to the likelihood of the same event occurring in a subsequent pregnancy. Early treatment requires early and accurate diagnosis. Just as rapid diagnosis is vital in bacterial meningitis so that appropriate chemotherapy can be started promptly, it is also important in neonatal herpes simplex virus (HSV) and varicella-zoster (V-Z) infections. The decision to protect a newborn infant against hepatitis B virus (HBV) infection, as well, requires a prompt diagnosis if immunization—active, passive, or both—is to be started.

Liaison between clinician and virologist im-plies that these practitioners understand each other's problems. The clinician wants a diagnosis, and the virologist needs information. A working diagnosis, the date of birth of the patient, and the stage of the disease process are key items that the virologist should know.

Some of the virus infections described in this book are associated with symptoms sufficiently distinctive for a provisional diagnosis to be made on clinical grounds. This is often true of congenital rubella, but occasions do arise when it is difficult or even impossible to distinguish congenital rubella, CMV, and toxoplasmosis without laboratory tests. Differentiation between neonatal HSV and V-Z infections can be equally difficult without assistance from the laboratory. The investigation of intrauterine growth retardation and of infants who are small for their gestational age but have no other obvious symptoms may also require aid from the virus laboratory.

Basically, the laboratory diagnosis of virus infections of the fetus and newborn rests on the principles that govern the diagnosis of these infections when they occur in childhood and adult life. There are, however, two differences that should be borne in mind. In postnatal infections one is most often concerned with the individual, except, for example, in epidemiological surveys; but in intrauterine and neonatal infections the mother and infant should be considered as one. It is generally prudent to carry out tests on mother and infant at the same time, bearing in mind the way in which the fetus or newborn has become infected. The key to many aspects of these infections lies in the pathogenesis. Thus, the selection of laboratory tests is affected by the stage at which infection took place and how the diagnosis can best be established. For example, the traditional method of virus isolation and examination of paired sera for a rise in antibody titer is of less practical value in intrauterine than in postnatal infections.

Progress in the diagnosis of microbial disease has advanced at an unprecedented pace in the past three decades, and the availability of tests for diagnosis of virus infections has caught up with that of tests for bacterial infections. Information on the availability of tests can be found in several publications (Gardner and McQuillin, 1974; Lennette and Schmidt, 1979; Zuckerman and Howard, 1979; Almeida, 1980; Kapikian et al., 1980; Gershon et al., 1981; World Health Organization (WHO), 1981; Enders, 1982; Field, 1982; Pattison, 1982; Booth, 1983; Schmidt, 1983; Smith, 1983).

One of the most significant changes that has taken place since the first edition of this book was published is the introduction of new techniques to identify infectious agents. Traditionally, this was done by virus culture, but many of the agents (e.g., HBV) could not

be detected by such means or could be detected only with great difficulty (e.g., hepatitis A virus [HAV]). Some diagnostic procedures were beyond the scope of many laboratories. The change that has taken place (new methods are outlined in Table 14–1) has been towards diagnosis by noncultural methods, with the emphasis on electronmicroscopy (EM) and immunological and immunoassay techniques. Many of these new techniques are highly sensitive and are applicable to the diagnosis of virus infections in neonates, but some are difficult to perform and require considerable laboratory resources. These points must be emphasized in distinguishing between what is practicable and what is feasible (Almeida, 1980).

OUTLINE OF LABORATORY PROCEDURES

The main diagnostic methods currently available are summarized in Table 14–1. They can be considered under two main headings: (1) tests for the direct detection of virus particles or viral antigen by microscopic, immunological, and other means or by isolation of the causative virus; and (2) immunological tests for the detection of specific

Table 14–1. **OUTLINE OF PROCEDURES FOR DIAGNOSIS OF VIRAL INFECTIONS OF THE FETUS AND NEWBORN***

Procedure	Methods	Examples
Detection of virus particles, viral antigen, cytopathic changes	1. Microscopy a. EM	HSV, V-Z, CMV, HBV, variola-vaccinia
	b. Light microscopy of stained smears	HSV, V-Z

	2. Immunological
	   a. IEM
	   b. IF
	   c. EIA
	   d. ELISA
	   e. RIA
	   f. PHA
	   g. RPHA
		HBV, HAV
		HSV, CMV, HBcAg
		CMV
		CMV, HBsAg, HBcAg
		HBsAg, HBeAg, HBcAg
		HBsAg
		HBsAg

Isolation of virus	3. Cell culture cytopathic changes	Rubella, CMV, HSV, V-Z, enteroviruses
	4. Liver biopsy	HBcAg, chronic HBV, neonatal hepatitis
Immunological	1. Persistence of antibody beyond the age of normal decline of maternal antibody	Rubella, CMV, V-Z, HBV
	2. IgM-specific antibody	Rubella, CMV, V-Z, HBV

*EM = electron microscopy; IEM = immunoelectron microscopy; IF = immunofluorescence; EIA = enzyme immunoassay; ELISA = enzyme-linked immunosorbent assay; RIA = radioimmunoassay; PHA = passive hemagglutination; RPHA = reverse passive hemagglutination. See also the Appendix.

antibody and immunoglobulin, particularly specific IgM.

It should be emphasized that, although a large variety of tests now exist and the number is increasing, they vary greatly in their sensitivity. Many that were in general use, such as complement-fixation (CF) and immunodiffusion (ID) techniques for HBV infections, have now been largely replaced by other tests, some of which are as much as 1000 times more sensitive than their predecessors. On the other hand, the equipment and the reagents needed in many instances are available only in specialized laboratories geared to handling large numbers of specimens and with sufficient financial resources.

Commerical reagents now available make it possible for many tests to be carried out that were hitherto outside the scope of routine virus laboratories. Now that these are available and are generally improved in their sensitivity and specificity, they can be used by laboratories that previously had to rely on locally produced reagents. One of the outcomes of these developments is a plethora of diagnostic techniques, some new and others modified to enhance the sensitivity of previously used methods. A short glossary of tests now available appears in the Appendix.

Collection of Material

As so much depends upon the collection of the appropriate material from the correct source at the right time and under the correct conditions, a few salient points have been summarized here for guidance. *It cannot be emphasized too strongly that special precautions should be taken in handling specimens designated as high-risk pathogens and that appropriate local and national safety precautions should be complied with, as well as the regulations of postal authorities if specimens are to be sent by mail.* A summary of the specimens that should be collected for the diagnosis of intrauterine and perinatal infections is shown in Table 14–2.

Material for Direct Detection of Viral Particles and Antigen. As EM, immunofluorescence (IF), and associated techniques have largely replaced light microscopy, the laboratory should be consulted as the collection of the appropriate specimens.

Smears or skin scrapings for multinucleate cells should be placed on clean glass slides and allowed to dry. Scrapings are best taken from the base of a vesicle or pustule with a flat sterile needle.

Material for Virus Culture. Most viruses are quickly inactivated if they are subjected to drying or held for any length of time at the ambient temperature. Virus particles or viral antigen is generally present in tissues or secretions in the acute phase of illness and rapidly disappears thereafter, except in the chronic infective states in congenital infections such as rubella and CMV. In order to minimize the risk of loss of virus infectivity, virus-containing material from the patient, such as urine, nasopharyngeal washings, vesicle fluid, and scrapings, should be placed directly in transport medium and kept at a constant low temperature ($4°$ C) in a thermos with wet ice ($4°$ C) until its arrival at the virus laboratory. In order to maintain the specimens at the correct low temperature, it is advisable to consult the laboratory as to whether the specimen should be packed in ice ($4°$ C) or frozen solid by packing with dry ice ($-70°$ C). Once received by the laboratory, specimens should be held at an appropriate low temperature.

Collection of Serum Samples. Approximately 1 or 2 ml of blood is required for most antibody and immunoglobulin estimations, except for cell-mediated immune responses, for which larger volumes are often required. The blood should be allowed to clot, and the serum should be removed for dispatch to the laboratory in a sterile container. Unless specific reasons are stated to the contrary, most serum specimens can be sent by first-class mail. When received in the laboratory, they should be stored in a deep-freeze container. If two specimens are required in order to detect a change in antibody titer for the diagnosis of intrauterine and perinatal infection, the first should be collected as soon as possible after birth, unless the cord blood is available, and the second three to six months later. It is an additional help in the study of intrauterine infections to collect a specimen of serum from the mother at the same time as from the child, so that the titers in mother and child can be compared.

It may be difficult to collect a sample of venous blood, in which case capillary blood can be obtained by finger prick or heel stab. This method has been found useful as a screening test for rubella hemagglutination-inhibiting (HI) antibodies in the Rubella Surveillance Programme in the United Kingdom (Dudgeon et al., 1973), but it cannot be used for CF tests. It is also difficult to read low antibody titers by this technique.

Table 14–2. COLLECTION OF SPECIMENS FOR DIAGNOSIS

Suspected Viral Cause	Material for Detection of Viral Antigen or Culture										Immunological Tests		
	Throat Swab/ Washings	Skin Swab	Feces/Rectal Swab	Urine	Lens, eye	Cerebrospinal Fluid	Brain	Vesicle Fluid	Liver Biopsy*	Microscopy‡	Routine Serology for Persistence of Antibody	Specific IgM	CMI/†
Rubella	√√	–	–	√√	√	√	√	–	√	–	√√	√√	√
CMV	√√	–	–	√√	–	√	√	–	√	√	√√	√√	–
HSV	–	√√	√	–	√	√	√	√√	√	–	√√	–	√
V-Z	√	√√	–	–	–	√	√	√	√	–	√√	√	–
Enteroviruses	√	–	√√	–	–	√√	√	–	–	–	√	√	–
Mumps	√	–	–	–	–	√√	√	–	–	–	√	√	–
HBV	–	–	–	–	–	–	–	–	–	√√	√√	√√	–
HAV	–	–	√	–	–	–	–	–	–	√√	√√	–	–
HNANB	–	–	–	–	–	–	–	–	–	–	√	–	–
EBV	–	–	–	–	–	–	–	–	–	–	√	√	–

*Liver biopsy is indicated only in special circumstances, such as chronic-active hepatitis or neonatal hepatitis.
†CMI = cell-mediated immune response.
‡Microscopy, including EM for virus particles.
Symbols: √√ indicates most practicable; √ indicates feasible but not as sensitive as √√; – indicates not detectable by this procedure.

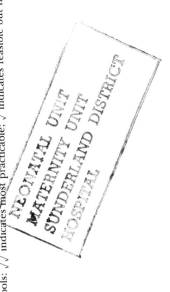

DESCRIPTION OF THE TESTS

Direct Detection of Virus Particles and Antigen

Electron Microscopy (EM). As can be seen from Table 14–1, EM and immunoelectron microscopy (IEM) have become basic tools in virological diagnosis and are still being rapidly developed (Almeida, 1980; Field, 1982). Electron microscopes have become more generally available in recent years, but they are still expensive and require skilled personnel for their use and maintenance. The use of EM with negative staining is helpful in the diagnosis of HSV and V-Z infections, although the two viruses cannot be distinguished from one another by this means. EM has played a leading role in the detection of HBV and HAV virus particles, but in nearly all instances a considerable amount of virus material must be present to be detected by this method unless some concentration procedure is utilized.

Immunological Methods. These are now being used on an increasing scale to detect virus in secretions and tissues by refined antigen-antibody techniques. Their usefulness depends on the presence of sufficient viral antigen in the material and the availability of the appropriate antisera.

Immunodiffusion (ID) and Immunoprecipitation. Viral antigen can be detected by immunoprecipitation tests such as the Ouchterlony technique, which was widely used in the rapid diagnosis of variola-vaccinia infections. The reaction between antigen and antibody causes the appearance of a "line" in an agar gel as a result of precipitation. The material being tested, usually vesicle or pustular fluid or crusts, is placed in wells cut into the agar; antisera and control materials are placed in surrounding wells. In all tests of this type, carefully selected control material is essential. Counterimmunoelectrophoresis had the advantage over standard gel diffusion of producing a more rapid result but has now been superseded by more reliable methods.

Immunoelectron Microscopy (IEM). In this technique, which combines immunological and electron microscopic procedures, the scope of EM is enhanced by the action of specific antibody, which causes clumping of the viral particles and thus aids in their detection. Virus particles in fecal specimens from cases of HAV were first detected in this way. The technique, reviewed by Kapikian and co-workers (1980), offers considerable promise for the future.

Immunoassays. Specific viral antibodies can be tagged by means of a dye, such as fluorochrome, an enzyme, or a radioisotope. All three can be utilized to detect viral antigen in body fluids, secretions, and tissues.

Immunofluorescence (IF). Viral antibody tagged with fluorescein isothiocyanate has long been used by virologists to detect viral antigen (or, in reverse, viral antibody) by means of ultraviolet light. Several methods can be used—the direct, indirect, and anticomplement techniques. Provided the pitfalls due to nonspecific staining are taken into account, the procedure is of great practical value.

Enzyme Immunoassay (EIA) and Enzyme-Linked Immunoabsorbent Assay (ELISA). In these techniques the antibody is labeled with an enzyme so that, when it comes into contact with the appropriate antigen, a color reaction takes place that is detectable by various means. Both direct and indirect methods can be used, as with IF.

Radioimmunoassays (RIA). Antibodies labeled with a radioisotope (usually ^{125}I) can be used to detect viral antigens in plasma, tissues, and secretions by either direct or indirect means. The sensitivity of the test, which can be very great, depends on the availability of non–antibody-bound antigen (the reverse for detecting antibody) and the degree of antigen-antibody reaction.

Passive Hemagglutination (PHA) and Reverse Passive Hemagglutination (RPHA) Techniques. These techniques are of special value, as is RIA, in detecting HBsAg (Zuckerman and Howard, 1979). Red cells coated with purified HBsAg or with purified anti-HBs (in RPHA) can be used to detect HBV surface antigen by hemagglutination. RPHA appears to be more sensitive and is less likely to give nonspecific results.

Examination of Smears. Infection with HSV and V-Z viruses leads to the formation of multinucleate giant cells in the epidermal cells. They can readily be seen by light microscopy (Fig. 14–1) and are not found in variola-vaccinia or with other virus infections in which cutaneous lesions are encountered (e.g., enteroviral exanthemata).

Virus Isolation. Virus isolation techniques are still used in the diagnosis of congenital infections, especially in the case of CMV.

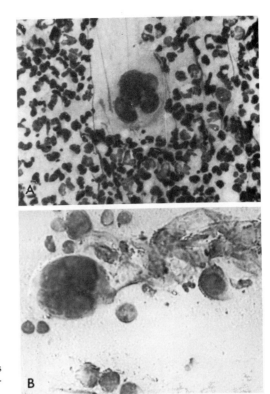

Figure 14–1. Multinucleate giant cells from epithelial smears stained with Giemsa. A, Herpes simplex virus. B, Varicella-zoster virus. Both × 250.

It can be seen that, with the exception of HBV, most of the viruses listed in Table 14–3 will grow in some form of cell culture; moreover, the cytopathic effect (CPE) they produce is in most cases sufficiently distinctive for a provisional identification of the virus to be made. This can be seen in Figures 14–2 and 14–3.

Immunological Tests

Prenatal viral infections stimulate an antibody response in much the same way as postnatal infections, but there are both quantitative and qualitative differences that are of special significance.

Fetal infection with rubella or CMV leads to an antibody response that usually persists in the newborn after the age at which maternally transmitted antibody in the uninfected newborn has disappeared—that is to say, after about six months of age. The same is true in the few cases of congenital varicella that have been examined (see Chapter 7).

Examination of two blood samples, one taken at birth (or from cord blood) or soon thereafter and another at about six months of age, should reveal any antibody persistence. IgM-specific antibody can also be detected in most infections and is a particularly useful method of diagnosis in the early months of life. The total IgM is raised beyond the normal limits for age, in many cases, in both congenital rubella and CMV, but this is a nonspecific finding that is also seen in bacteriological and protozoal infections. Testing for total IgM has largely been discontinued because of the development of sensitive techniques for IgM-specific antibody.

A wide range of immunological tests are now available for the diagnosis of viral infections of the fetus and newborn. These are set out in summary form in Table 14–4 and in the Appendix. It should be emphasized that not all of these tests are equally applicable to each infection: some are more sensitive than others, and some are technically more difficult to perform. In other infections, the development of a suitable test is awaited.

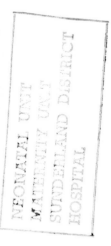

Table 14–3. **ISOLATION OF VIRUS BY CELL CULTURE AND OTHER TECHNIQUES‡**

| Virus | Cell Cultures* | | | | Chick Embryo (Chorioallantoic Inoculation) | Newborn Mice (Intracerebral Inoculation, Subcutaneous Inoculation) |
	Rabbit Kidney, Primary (RK13), Rabbit Cornea (SIRC)	Human Embryo Lung (HEL)	Monkey Kidney (AGMK, VERO, RMK)	Primary or Continuous Human (PHA, HeLa, Hep 2)		
Rubella	++	-	++	+	-	-
CMV	-	++	-	-	-	-
HSV types 1 and 2	++	++	+	++	++	++
V-Z	-	++	-	++	-	-
HBV	-	-	-	+	-	-
HAV†	-	-	+	-	-	-
Enteroviruses (Coxsackie A and B viruses)	-	++	++	+	-	+
Mumps	-	+	+	+	+	
Vaccinia	++	+	+	+	++	±

*This term includes primary cell cultures and continuous cell strains and cell lines. The term 'cell lines' is used to denote those cells that can be propagated indefinitely by repeated cell cultures, whereas the term 'cell strains' is used to denote those cells, also capable of being propagated by repeated subculture, that need limited propagation to retain their normal karyotype.

†HAV can be cultured with difficulty in special cell lines of fetal rhesus monkey kidney, unless incubated at a temperature of 32 to 35° C.

‡Key: ++ = most practical and sensitive; + = feasible but not as sensitive; − = not detectable by this procedure.

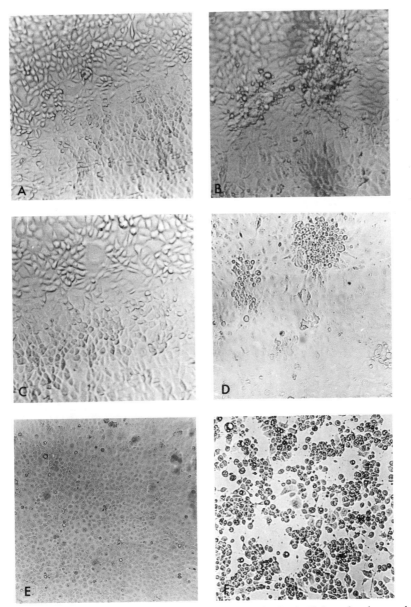

Figure 14–2. Cytopathic effect of viruses in RK13 cell cultures (unstained). A, Uninoculated control. B, Rubella. C, Cytomegalovirus. D, Herpes simplex. E, Varicella-zoster. F, Vaccinia. All × 60.

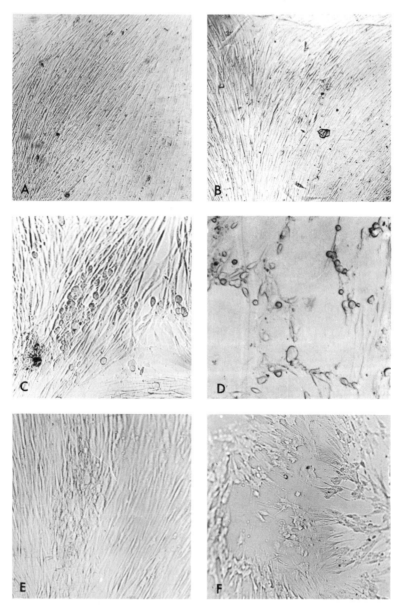

Figure 14–3. Cytopathic effect of viruses in HEL cell cultures (unstained). A, Uninoculated control. B, Rubella. C, Cytomegalovirus. D, Herpes simplex. E, Varicella-zoster. F, Vaccinia. All × 60.

Table 14–4. IMMUNOLOGICAL TESTS USED IN DIAGNOSIS OF VIRAL INFECTIONS OF THE FETUS AND NEWBORN*‡

Viral Cause	VN	HI	CF	EIA	ELISA	FAMA	ID	IF	RIA	PHA	RPHA	IA	ELISA†	RIA†	IF†
Rubella	±	+	±	−	+	−	−	−	+	−	−	−	+	+	
CMV	±	−	+	+	+	−	−	+	+	−	−	−	+	+	
HSV	±	−	+	+	+	+	−	+	−	−	−	+	+		
V-Z	±	−	+	−	+	+	−	+	+	−	−	−	+		+
HBV															
HBsAg	−	−	±	−	+	−	+	−	+	+	+	−			
Anti-HBs	−	−	±	−	+	−	−	−	+	+	+	−		+	
HBeAg	−	−	±	−	+	−	−	−	+	+	−	−			
Anti-HBe	−	−	±	−	+	−	−	−	+	−	−	+		+	
Anti-HBc	−	−	+	−	−	−	+	−	+	−	−	+			

*VN = virus neutralization; HI = hemagglutination inhibition; CF = complement fixation; EIA = enzyme immunoassay; ELISA = enzyme-linked immunosorbent assay; FAMA = fluorescent antigen membrane antibody; ID = immunodiffusion; IF = immunofluorescence; RIA = radioimmunoassay; PHA = passive hemagglutination; RPHA = reverse passive hemagglutination; IA = immune adherence.
†Test for specific IgM.
‡Key: + = most practical and sensitive; ± = feasible but not as practical; − = not detectable by this procedure.

Principal Tests Used in the Diagnosis of Viral Diseases: A Glossary of Terms

LABORATORY TESTS FOR DETECTION OF VIRAL PARTICLES OR ANTIGEN

EM: Electron microscopy. This technique is used to detect virus particles. The virus must be present in comparatively large concentrations (about 1×10^6 particles/ml) to be visualized, depending upon the circumstances. Various procedures can be used to enhance the sensitivity of this valuable and rapid diagnostic procedure (Almeida, 1980).

IEM: Immunoelectron microscopy. In this procedure viral antigen and antibody are allowed to react before negative staining and electron microscopic examination. Specific antibody tends to concentrate the virus particles by aggregation. The causative agent of HAV was first detected by this method, which has a number of useful applications in the study of viral diseases in which the agent, or suspected agent, cannot be cultured by standard procedures.

IF: Immunofluorescence. Viral antibodies can be "tagged" with a fluorochrome dye, an enzyme, or a radioisotope so that the viral antigen-antibody combination can be visualized or otherwise detected. The direct, indirect, and anticomplement immunofluorescent techniques are all based on the principle that the conjugate of antigen and fluorescein-tagged antibody can be detected by fluorescent microscopy. The variations among the alternative methods have been introduced to increase specificity.

EIA: Enzyme immunoassay. An enzyme is used instead of a fluorescein dye. Enzyme-labeled antibodies bound to virus or antigen-antibody complexes are detected by the addition of a substrate that produces a color reaction in the presence of the enzyme.

ELISA: Enzyme-linked immunosorbent assay. Both direct and indirect methods have been developed; both detect the presence of antigen and antibody by a color or fluorescent reaction.

RIA: Radioimmunoassay. Antibodies labeled with a radioisotope (usually tritiated iodine) can be used to detect viral antigen or antibody, or both, in clinical material. The principle is the same as for the fluorescein or enzyme labeling of antibody.

PHA: Passive hemagglutination. Red cells of certain species coated with purified antigen can be agglutinated by small amounts of antibody. Nonspecific results may be encountered. Inhibition of passive hemagglutination by test sera can be detected by antibody preparations of known specificity.

RPHA: Reverse passive hemagglutination. Purified antibody is attached to formalin-fixed red cells of varying species and the antibody being tested is added to the test serum.

IA: Immune adherence. This antigen-antibody test is complement-dependent and is somewhat difficult to perform.

ID: Immunodiffusion techniques are based on the principle that antigen-antibody reaction can be detected by a precipitation line. The original Ouchterlony techniques for microbiological diagnosis have been used and developed further over many years. Although their sensitivity has been increased, they have for the most part been replaced by more rapid and sensitive techniques.

IMMUNOLOGICAL TECHNIQUES

VN: Virus neutralization antibody test. This is the most reliable indicator of the presence of virus neutralizing antibody but is time consuming to perform. In addition, it is applicable only when the viral agent has been isolated in culture. VN is a useful procedure that should be reserved for special circumstances where results of other tests are in doubt.

HI: Hemagglutination-inhibition test. This is based on the capacity of several viruses to cause agglutination of red blood cells of various species. Antigen and test antibody are first mixed together in varying dilutions, and red cells are later added. The presence of antibody and its titer can be measured by the level at which hemagglutination is inhibited. Test sera must be pretreated by various means to remove nonspecific inhibitors; some of these procedures may remove small traces of specific antibody (Pattison, 1982).

CF: Complement fixation. A traditional test in microbiological diagnostic procedures, CF is now less commonly used because of its lack of sensitivity and the persistence of complement-fixing antibody.

RH or SRH: Radial hemolysis or single radial hemolysis. This test is based on the principle that lysis by antibody of antigen-coated red blood cells will occur in the presence of complement. The test is now widely used as a routine procedure for estimation of rubella antibody but is not applicable for the diagnosis of fetal infections.

FA: Fluorescent antigen-antibody test. The object of the test is to detect the presence of antigen-antibody complexes by immunofluorescence. Monolayer cell cultures are grown either in test tubes or on coverslips and then infected with virus. After incubation, virus-infected cells are removed, placed on slides fixed in acetone, and stored at a low temperature (—70° C); the coverslip preparations are fixed with acetone and also stored at —70°. When required for use, the slides or coverslips are removed from storage and incubated with volumes of diluted test sera. After washing, a fluorescein-labeled conjugated antibody is prepared from goat or other animal sera to which human globulin is added. The preparations are examined for the presence of fluorescence and, provided that adequate controls are included and close attention is paid to detail, the reaction between antibody in the serum under test and viral antigen in the cell cultures is a reliable method of antibody titration.

FAMA: Fluorescent antigen membrane antibody technique. A test used mainly to detect V-Z antibody (Williams et al., 1974), this has now largely replaced the ELISA (Gershon et al., 1981; Enders, 1982; Pattison, 1982; Booth, 1983).

IAHA: Immune adherence hemagglutination technique. IAHA is an alternative and possibly more sensitive method of detecting V-Z antigen or antibody (Gershon et al., 1976). Cells from virus-infected monolayer cell cultures are mixed together in equal proportions so that antigen and antibody can react. Complement is then added, followed by, after a further interval, a suspension of group O human red blood cells, which cause agglutination of V-Z infected cultures. This technique, like the FAMA technique, is feasible only in laboratories capable of carrying out a large number of tests, as the control tests necessary are as numerous as they are essential.

Tests for Specific IgM Antibody

In the majority of intrauterine infections, antibody of the IgM class is produced as a direct result of fetal infection. It can be detected from approximately the sixteenth week of gestation, is invariably present at birth, and usually persists for three to six months after birth depending on the individual infection. Several methods can be used to detect IgM-specific antibody. They vary in their sensitivity and their applicability to particular virus infections. For example, in the case of rubella the following tests can be employed: 2-mercaptoethanol, gel filtration, sucrose density gradient centrifugation, staphylococcal protein A method, IF, RIA, ELISA, and M-antibody capture radioim-

munoassay (MACRIA). In general, the last three are the most sensitive (Cradock-Watson et al., 1979; Mortimer et al., 1981; Pattison 1982).

Tests for IgM-specific antibody for other viruses, such as CMV, HSV, V-Z, and HBV, depend in the main on the availability of the antigen in suitable concentration for the test to be carried out. These tests are listed in Table 14–4. The references listed on page 259 contain useful details about these techniques and their applicability to the diagnosis of virus diseases in general, as well as to the specific problem of intrauterine and perinatal infections.

Bibliography

Almeida, J. D.: Practical aspects for diagnostic electron microscopy. Yale J. Biol. Med. *53*:5–18, 1980.

Booth, J. C.: The use of the enzyme-linked immunoabsorbent assay (ELISA) technique in clinical virology. In Waterson, A. P. (ed.): Recent Advances in Clinical Virology. No. 3. Edinburgh, Churchill Livingstone, 1983, pp. 73–98.

Cradock-Watson, J. E., Ridehalgh, M. K. S., Pattison, J. R., Anderson, M. J., and Kangro, H. O.: Comparison of immunofluorescence and radioimmunoassay for detecting IgM antibody in infants with congenital rubella sundrome. J. Hyg. *83*:413–423, 1979.

Dudgeon, J. A., Peckham, C. S., Marshall, W. C., Smithells, R. W., and Sheppard, S.: National Congenital Rubella Surveillance Programme. Health Trends 5:75–79, 1973.

Enders, G.: Prenatal, perinatal and early postnatal infections: laboratory diagnosis by classical and new techniques. WHO Symposium on Prenatal and Perinatal Infections, Graz, May 1982.

Field, A. M.: Diagnostic virology using electron microscopy techniques. Adv. Virus Res. *27*:2–55, 1982.

Gardner, P. S., and McQuillin, J.: Rapid Virus Diagnosis. Application of Immune Immunofluorescence. London, Butterworth & Company, 1974.

Gershon, A., Kalter, Z. G., and Kalter, S.: Detection of antibody to varicella-zoster virus by immune adherence hemagglutination. Proc. Soc. Exp. Biol. Med. *153*:762–763, 1976.

Gerson, A., Frey, H. M., Steinberg, S. P., Seeman, M. P., Bidwell, S. D., and Voller, A.: Determination of immunity to varicella using an enzyme-linked-absorbent-immuno-assay. Arch. Virol. *70*:169–172, 1981.

Kapikian, A. Z., Dienstag, J. L., and Purcell, R. H.: Immune-electron-microscopy as a method for the detection, identification and characterisation of agents not cultivable in an in vitro system. In Rose, N. R., and Friedman, H. (eds.): Manual of Clinical Immunology. 2nd edition. Washington, D.C., American Society for Microbiology, 1980, pp. 70–83.

Lennette, E. H., and Schmidt, N. J. (eds): Diagnostic Procedures for Viral, Rickettsial and Chlamydial Infections. 5th ed. Washington, D.C., American Public Health Association, 1979.

Mortimer, P. P., Tedder, R. S., Hambling, M. H., Shofi, M. S., Burkhardt, F., and Schilt, V.: Antibody capture radioimmunoassay for anti-rubella IgM (MACRIA). J. Hyg. *86*:139–153, 1981.

Pattison, J. R. (ed.): Public Health Laboratory Service: Laboratory Diagnosis of Rubella. Monograph Series No. 16, London, Her Majesty's Stationery Office, 1982.

Schmidt, N. J.: Rapid viral diagnosis. Med. Clin. North Am. *67*:953–972, 1983.

Smith, T. F.: Clinical uses of the diagnostic virology laboratory. Med. Clin. North Am. *67*:935–951, 1983.

Williams, V., Gershon, A., and Brunell, P.: Serologic response to varicella-zoster membrane antigens measured by direct immunofluorescence. J. Infect. Dis. *130*:669–672, 1974.

World Health Organisation. Report of a Scientific Group. Technical Report Series No. 661. Geneva, WHO, 1981.

Zuckerman, A. J., and Howard, C. R.: Hepatitis Viruses of Man. London, Academic Press, 1979.

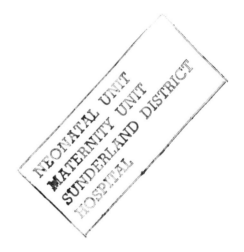

Prevention and Treatment

15

Prophylactic and therapeutic measures for the control of virus infections in the fetus and newborn require somewhat different considerations than the same procedures used to combat infections acquired after birth. During intrauterine life the embryo or fetus is relatively secure within the amniotic sac and thus is normally protected from exposure to external environmental factors such as infectious agents. The relative security of this physiological state can be breached when infections occur in the mother, especially during the early stages of fetal development, and the infectious agent passes from the maternal blood stream via the placenta to infect the fetus. Exposure to infection may also occur late in pregnancy, at parturition, or in the early weeks of postnatal life. Account must therefore be taken not only of the immune status of the mother prior to exposure and of the gestational age at which infection occurs, but of the biological properties of the virus. Marked variations may be encountered in the pathogenicity or virulence of the virus and in the immuno-responsiveness of the fetus or infant according to age. In essence, the value of any prophylactic measure, such as immunization, is to afford protection *before* the event occurs—that is, before exposure to infection—whereas therapeutic measures are of necessity used at the time infection is first suspected or immediately afterwards. The normal procedure for protecting children and adults is direct immunization of the individual, but protection of the fetus can be achieved only indirectly, by immunization of mothers-to-be at some stage before a pregnancy begins.

At present, important progress is taking place in the development of viral vaccines and antiviral chemotherapy that may ultimately be very useful in the prevention of virus infections of the fetus and newborn. Some of the factors that must be taken into consideration in the use of both established licensed products and those yet to be developed are listed in Table 15–1. These relate mainly to prevention by immunization, but the basic principles apply equally well for the development and use of antiviral chemotherapy where preventive measures are not feasible.

PREVENTION

The need for prevention is a prerequisite for the development of prophylactic measures. This need can be assessed in terms of morbidity, in both the short- and the long-term, or mortality, or both. The impact of fetal damage resulting from congenital rubella and cytomegalovirus (CMV) infections provides a useful yardstick against which the seriousness of the other viruses mentioned in this book can be gauged. For example, general prophylaxis is indicated for the control of congenital rubella, whereas for fetal or neonatal infection with varicella-zoster (V-Z) and hepatitis B (HBV) viruses, which present

Table 15–1. **FACTORS TO BE CONSIDERED IN THE DEVELOPMENT OF ANY IMMUNOLOGICAL PRODUCT, WITH SPECIAL REFERENCE TO THE PREVENTION OF INFECTIONS OF THE FETUS AND NEWBORN**

1. The need for the product, based on the morbidity and mortality associated with the disease
2. The natural history of the disease
3. The biological properties of the virus
4. The choice between active immunization with a live attenuated or killed inactivated vaccine and passive immunization
5. The cell substrate used for vaccine production
6. Methods of testing for safety and potency

less of a problem in absolute numbers, prophylactic or other preventive measures are best undertaken on an individual basis.

Consideration of the natural history of each infection is relevant to the means of prevention. There are three main routes or mechanisms of infection: maternal-fetal blood stream infection (e.g., rubella, CMV, and V-Z); ascending cervical-amniotic infection (particularly important in bacterial infec-

tions) or infection at parturition or in the newborn period (e.g., herpes simplex virus [HSV], V-Z, and HBV); and indirect damage by a toxic reaction or drug therapy (e.g., influenza). In theory, immunization is more likely to be effective in preventing those infections in which the fetus is damaged by viremic spread than those caused by exposure to infection, possibly with an overwhelming amount of infectious material, at parturition. In the latter circumstance, some rapid-acting form of prophylaxis—passive immunization in the case of exposure to HBV, or antiviral chemotherapy in neonatal HSV infections—may be effective. The likelihood that immunization, either active or passive, will be successful is enhanced when infection is caused by an agent with a single antigenic serotype or closely related subtypes. Some of these additional factors are summarized in Table 15–2.

These theoretical considerations are being confirmed in practice in the case of congenital rubella and could also apply to the prevention of fetal damage by CMV. Primary CMV infection, associated with viremia, with

Table 15–2. **SUMMARY OF FACTORS CONCERNED WITH INFECTIONS OF THE FETUS AND NEONATE***

| Virus | Serological Subtypes | Nucleic Acid | Mode of Spread from Mother to Fetus | Effect of Maternal Immune Status on Risk of Infection | | |
				Primary Infection	Reinfection	Reactivation
Rubella	1	RNA	Viremia	+ +	±	−
CMV	3†	DNA	Viremia	+ +	+	+
			Ascending cervical-amniotic	±		
HSV	2†	DNA	Viremia	+	−	−
			Cervical-amniotic	+ +	−	+
			At birth	+	−	−
V-Z	1	DNA	Viremia, perinatal	+ +	−	+
			Viremia, prenatal	+		± −
HBV	1	DNA	Antigenemia	+ +		
			At parturition—perinatal	+ +		
			Postnatal	+		
			Prenatal	±		
HAV	1	RNA	? Viremia	?	−	−
Variola-vaccinia	1	DNA	Viremia	+ +	+	−
Enteroviruses			Viremia			
Poliovirus	3†			+ +		
Coxsackie B	6†	RNA				
Coxsackie A	Numerous			+ +	−	−
ECHO	Numerous					

*+ + = major risk; + = moderate risk; ± = possible risk; − = no risk.
†Closely related.

closely related antigenic strains of virus would, in theory, suggest that prevention can be achieved. That reactivation infection occurs with CMV is not necessarily a stumbling block to the development of a CMV vaccine, as most reactivation infections that have been reported have resulted in fetal infection without fetal damage. One of the obstacles at present is the fact that many DNA viruses of the herpesvirus group, CMV, V-Z, and HSV result in latent infections, and the question naturally arises whether latent infection could result from the use of a live vaccine. Potential oncogenicity has been suggested to be an additional obstacle to the use of a live attenuated CMV vaccine, but why this should be a greater problem with CMV than with other DNA viruses, V-Z, or HSV infections is unclear.

The actual method of immunization presents the theoretical choice of active or passive immunization, or both. In practice, the choice may well be determined by the availability of the product. Active immunization with a vaccine, whether it be a live attenuated or a killed inactivated product, is likely to lead to long-term protection. The object is to render a woman immune at some stage before she becomes pregnant, so that if exposure occurs during pregnancy the fetus is protected. It must be remembered that all live vaccines are contraindicated in pregnancy; this reinforces the need for their use beforehand. On the other hand, killed vaccines are not contraindicated during pregnancy, so that if it were considered desirable, for example, to protect a pregnant woman against influenza in the face of an epidemic, an inactivated influenza vaccine could be used. Passive immunization with normal pooled or hyperimmune immunoglobulin confers only temporary protection lasting six to eight weeks. It can, therefore, be used only in special circumstances, but nevertheless has a special role to play in diseases for which a vaccine is not yet available or when rapid protection is required, as, for example, in HBV or V-Z infections.

The development of every new vaccine carries with it an element of risk that has to be accepted if progress is to continue. Nevertheless, experience has shown that damage or untoward effects that have occurred in the past following the use of vaccines could often have been prevented by forethought and attention to methods of vaccine production. And so it is that the selection of seed viruses and cell substrates is now of paramount importance. Vaccines should consist of a pure culture of the agent used for vaccine production. The culture cannot be pure if the seed virus and the cell substrate are already contaminated with extraneous agents, either bacterial or viral. This was certainly the case with some of the early batches of inactivated poliovaccines; as a result, major improvements in vaccine production and control of vaccines were introduced. Considerable skill and expertise are now required in vaccine production (World Health Organisation [WHO], 1966; Perkins, 1972; Dudgeon, 1973, 1976). The main areas of concern can be summarized in three questions: "Has the seed virus been shown to be safe and immunogenic in man?" "What laboratory tests can be used to ensure that the vaccine virus does not differ in any way from the seed virus?" "Where was this vaccine produced and by whom?" (Perkins, 1972). These are important issues; understanding them makes it possible to define what can be regarded as proof of efficacy and safety before viral vaccines are accepted for general use.

The present status of methods of immunization and the availability of immunological products is summarized in Table 15–3.

Rubella

Background

The first attempts to prevent rubella by active immunization with a live attenuated vaccine were made by Parkman and colleagues (1966) and Meyer and colleagues (1967). They showed that several passages of a strain of rubella-virus in monkey kidney cell cultures led to a modification of its biological properties. The HPV-77* strain was found to be immunogenic in rhesus monkeys and failed to infect the fetuses of pregnant monkeys, whereas the virulent low-passage virus did. When this vaccine was tested in a number of seronegative children, very few reactions were encountered, and all developed a satisfactory antibody response. However, 75 per cent of the susceptible vaccinees were found to excrete virus in the nasopharynx between the seventh and twenty-first days after vaccination, although quantitatively the titer of virus was considerably lower

---

*High-passage virus—passaged 77 times.

Table 15–3. **SUMMARY OF IMMUNOLOGICAL PRODUCTS AVAILABLE OR UNDER DEVELOPMENT***

| | Active Immunization | | Passive Immunization | | |
Virus	Killed Vaccine	Live Vaccine	Normal IG	Hyperimmune Ig	Comments
Rubella	−	Licensed products freely available for general prophylaxis	+	+	See text for schedules and usage
CMV	−	For clinical trials only in special groups, e.g., renal transplant patients	−	−	Use impractical
HSV	−	—	−	−	Efficacy of IG not established
V-Z	−	For clinical trials only for patients with leukemia and certain malignancies	+	+ + (ZIG)	See text for use of vaccine and ZIG
HBV	+	—	−	+	See text for usage

*IG = immunoglobulin; ZIG = zoster immune globulin.

in the vaccinees than in patients with natural rubella. Nevertheless, the presence of vaccine virus in the throat indicated that a vaccinee was potentially contagious and might have restricted the use of the vaccine in the general population. Concern was also expressed about the use of monkey kidney cultures as cell substrates for seed virus and vaccine production, so alternative means of development of a rubella vaccine were sought, with regard to both the seed virus and the cell substrate (International Symposium on Rubella Vaccines, 1969).

An obvious alternative to a live vaccine, if transmissibility was to prove a problem, was a killed inactivated product. Preliminary attempts to produce such vaccines by formalin inactivation had been unsuccessful, as they were only weakly immunogenic (Sever, et al., 1963) and did not confer protection against infection (Buynak et al., 1968). Failure to confer protection was due to a combination of low potency and lack of antigenicity. By 1969 many of these problems had been resolved. Pools of seed virus were prepared by propagation in cell cultures other than monkey kidney, and cell substrates that were generally considered safer for human use than monkey kidney cell cultures were selected. By 1969 extensive clinical trials had been carried out with four widely used vaccines, details of which are to be found in Chapter 3. These trials (International Symposium on Rubella Vaccines, 1969) answered three important questions. First, the vaccines appeared to be safe: clinical reactions were few and generally mild, except in the case of

one vaccine prepared in dog kidney cell cultures, which was subsequently withdrawn. Second, seroconversion occurred in at least 95 per cent of susceptible individuals. Third, no conclusive evidence of transmissibility was found among the many thousands of individuals who received the vaccines. This meant that in practice there was no bar to the use of rubella vaccine in children of school age and that the risk of children transmitting infection to their mothers was negligible. Current vaccination programs are based on this assumption.

Rubella Vaccines

Details concerning currently licensed rubella vaccines are shown in Table 15–4. The group includes four monovalent live attenuated rubella vaccines, each requiring a single dose of 0.5 ml that contains not less than 1000 tissue culture infective doses (1000 $TCID_{50}$) for effective immunization. In addition, two combined vaccines are available, one consisting of live measles-rubella (MR) vaccine and the other of measles-mumps-rubella (MMR) vaccine. The doses for the combined vaccines are the same as those for the monovalent vaccines.

The details about rubella vaccines described here are abstracted from information prepared by the manufacturers and licensing authorities. In all cases, the full instructions of the manufacturer should be strictly adhered to in order to obtain maximum effect and reduce complications.

Description. Live attenuated rubella vac-

Table 15–4. **DETAILS OF RUBELLA VACCINES LICENSED FOR ROUTINE IMMUNIZATION**

Name of Vaccine	Vaccine Strain	Type of Cell Culture	Vaccine Dose and Route of Administration
Cendevax	Cendehill	Primary rabbit kidney	0.5 ml, by subcutaneous or intramuscular route*
Meruvax	HPV-77 DE5	Duck embryo	As above
Almevax	RA 27/3	Human diploid	As above
Meruvax II	RA 27/3	Human diploid	As above
Attenuvax (measles-mumps-rubella [MMR])	HPV-77	Duck embryo	As above

*As specified in the manufacturer's instructions.

cines are presented as lyophilized preparations together with a suitable diluent for reconstitution.

Usage. The vaccines are used for immunization against rubella to prevent congenital infection and for concomitant immunization against measles and mumps when combined vaccines are used.

Dosage and Administration. Reconstituted vaccine (0.5 ml) should be given by the subcutaneous route (or the intramuscular route where stated by the manufacturer). Each dose consists of not less than 1000 tissue culture infective doses. The vaccine should be stored at the temperature recommended by the licensing authority and manufacturer. Details are contained in the leaflet supplied with the vaccine.

Indications. Vaccine is used for active immunization of children and susceptible adult females according to the schedules shown in Table 3–20. Since congenital rubella infection is preventable by active immunization, any individual or member of a community who is at risk should be vaccinated. This applies in particular to nursing, medical, health-care, and educational personnel.

Precautions. The vaccine should *not* be administered by the intravenous or intranasal route. Vaccines should not be given to anyone known to be sensitive to either neomycin or polymyxin B, which may be present in small quantities in one or other of the vaccines. Rubella vaccines should not be administered within one month of another live vaccine unless combined vaccines are used, nor should they be given after a blood transfusion.

Contraindications

1. Rubella vaccine should *not* be given to pregnant females, and pregnancy should be avoided for three months following vaccina-

tion. The action to be taken if vaccination is so administered is discussed later.

2. Vaccine should not be given to anyone with a febrile illness. It is important to ensure that anyone who misses a vaccination owing to illness is given another appointment and subsequently vaccinated.

3. Vaccine should not be given to any patient with an immune deficiency, on corticosteroid therapy, or receiving irradiation or other immunosuppressive therapy for malignant disease other than low maintenance dosage of antimetabolites. Individuals with blood dyscrasias, leukemia, lymphomas, and malignant conditions affecting the bone marrow should not be vaccinated.

Adverse Reactions. These are uncommon with currently licensed products and are usually mild and transient. Joint reactions, arthralgia, and arthritis may be encountered in adolescent and adult females. These may occasionally persist for a few weeks, but long-term sequelae are rare.

Effectiveness of Rubella Vaccination. Effectiveness can be assessed in two ways, by the interruption of the normal periodic cycle of natural epidemic rubella and by a decline in the reported incidence of congenital rubella defects.

The initial reports on immune responsiveness to rubella vaccines were encouraging (International Symposium on Rubella Vaccines, 1969). In many trials seroconversion rates of 100 per cent were reported, and overall the rate was of the order of 95 to 97 per cent. A more important question, however, was how long the immune effect would last. The initial reports were based on studies of three to four years' duration. Subsequent reports by Krugman (1973, 1977) showed that immunity, as measured by hemagglutination-inhibiting (HI) antibody, was still demonstrable four to seven years after vaccination, depending on the vaccine that had been used. Herrmann and co-workers (1976) and others (see Chapter 3) have also reported satisfactory rubella antibody levels, some showing virtually no decline in antibody titer, over a period of about seven years. Horstmann (1975) reported a decline in antibody in a group of children immunized five years previously with HPV-77 DE5 vaccine.

A follow-up study of nurses at two London teaching hospitals conducted six to 16 years following vaccination showed well-maintained levels of antibody. Of 123 volunteers, 89.4 per cent had antibody levels greater than the minimum; 8.9 per cent were on the borderline, and 1.6 per cent (two cases) were apparently seronegative (O'Shea et al., 1982). These serological results are encouraging, but they also emphasize the need for continued surveillance of vaccinated groups.

The duration of immunity following rubella vaccination must be measured in decades, not in years. Krugman (1980) has correctly identified the risk that may result from "vaccine failures"—that is, those who fail to respond to vaccination for one reason or another (about 4 to 5 per cent) and those who fail to be vaccinated. Vaccine failures could lead to a sizable population of susceptible adolescents; for this reason, Krugman (1980) recommends a second injection at the time of school entry. Basically, this is the rationale behind the Swedish vaccination scheme, which is referred to in Chapter 3 (Table 3–21).

Rubella Vaccine Surveillance. Any immunization program should have some form of surveillance built into it to ensure that both the vaccination policy and the vaccines in use are effective in controlling the disease. Cooper (1975) has reported that in the United States both the incidence of natural rubella in communities where vaccination has been carried out and the incidence of congenital rubella defects have shown a marked decline since rubella vaccines were licensed in the United States in 1968. This is encouraging news, but rubella nevertheless continues to occur in communities where the percentage of persons immunized falls short of the optimum of 90 to 95 per cent (Beasley, 1970; Centers for Disease Control, 1975). As far as the incidence of rubella defects is concerned, it is important to observe children exposed to intrauterine rubella for several years because defects that were not recognizable at birth may develop or become apparent later in life (Peckham, 1972).

The congenital rubella surveillance programs in the United States and the United Kingdom, both of which are based on a voluntary reporting system, are discussed in Chapter 3. Details can be found in Tables 3–25 through 3–27. Although reporting is clearly incomplete and some cases will not be diagnosed until later in life, these figures reflect a trend that should continue downward as more emphasis is placed on the need for vaccination.

In the United Kingdom there has been no obvious decline in the incidence of defects since vaccination was introduced in 1971 (Dudgeon et al., 1973; Sheppard et al., 1977), but an analysis of the more recent data indicates that almost all the cases of congenital rubella reported since 1971 have been in infants of women born prior to 1959. As rubella vaccines were not licensed until 1971, the mothers would not have been eligible for vaccination in the United Kingdom (Smithells et al., 1982).

Rubella Vaccination and Pregnancy. Pregnancy remains a major contraindication to the administration of rubella vaccine and any other live virus vaccine. However, data accumulated in the past few years suggest that rubella vaccines currently licensed are less teratogenic than was hitherto thought (see Table 3–24). Although the number of women inadvertently given rubella vaccine in early pregnancy is comparatively small, the data obtained so far indicate that a review of previous recommendations is due. Rubella vaccines can no longer be regarded as a cause of serious disability to the fetus, and as far as English law governing medical termination of pregnancy is concerned, the operative word is 'serious.' The present situation can be summarized as follows:

1. Do not vaccinate women of childbearing age unless you know their immune status, assuming that this can be determined.

2. Do not vaccinate a woman who is or who may be pregnant. A simple question should help to reduce the risk.

3. If vaccine has been given to a woman who is pregnant, or if she becomes pregnant within the prescribed period, do not routinely recommend termination of the pregnancy. Consultation with the patient on possible risks of fetal damage is recommended before a course of action is chosen.

Passive Immunization. The use of immunoglobulin (IG) for passive protection of women exposed to rubella in pregnancy has been controversial for many years. Many reports have appeared in the literature since the first documentation by Anderson and McLorinan (1953) in Australia in the 1950's. Other studies, some of them on rather small groups, reviewed by McDonald (1967) indicated that some degree of protection was afforded and that this was probably related to the dosage of the gamma globulin* used and, more especially, to the time of administration in relation to the interval after contact. One particularly important study, in which the effect of protection was monitored by serological tests for rubella neutralizing antibody, was carried out by Brody and co-workers (1965) during an epidemic of rubella in the Pribilof Islands in Alaska. The results indicated that although the clinical attack rate was reduced by 80 per cent in those receiving gamma globulin, the *infection rate* was only halved. The crux of the matter is that if IG is to be used in the prophylaxis of rubella in pregnant women in contact with the disease, it is essential to prevent *infection;* prevention of clinical disease is insufficient because the fetus can be damaged as a result of subclinical infection. Many observers, notably Lundström and his colleagues (1961; 1962, 1965) have produced evidence of a prophylactic effect of gamma globulin given to pregnant women, whereas others (Green et al., 1965) could find no evidence of protection whatsoever. On the other hand, trials with gamma globulin in pregnant women carried out in the United Kingdom by McDonald (1963) and by McDonald and Peckham (1967) showed not only a reduction in the clinical attack rate but also some evidence that there was no excess of cataracts, congenital heart disease, or deafness in the offspring of women who did *not* develop the disease. The possibility exists, therefore, that subclinical infection following the administration of IG may reduce the risk of fetal infection or damage, or both (Peckham, 1974).

Since these trials rubella vaccines have become available for routine active immunization against rubella before pregnancy. Current advice in the United States is that the value of IG in preventing rubella in pregnancy is not proved and, in the United Kingdom, that there is little evidence that IG prevents rubella infection (Public Health Laboratory Service, 1970). There are, however, situations in which a pregnant woman

exposed to rubella wishes the pregnancy to go to term. Under these conditions the following procedure, which is practiced by one of the authors (Dudgeon, 1974), can be adopted. If a woman is pregnant, or thinks she may be, (1) confirm that she is pregnant, and (2) attempt to ascertain whether the contact case, frequently a child, in fact had rubella and not some other infection (see Chapter 14). (3) Collect a sample of blood for a rubella antibody test to determine susceptibility. (4) Inject 1500 mg of normal pooled IG by the intramuscular route. If the antibody test is *positive* (the result of the test should be available in two or three days), no further action is necessary. If it is *negative*, it should be assumed that the patient is at risk, so (5) inject another dose of 1500 mg IG (or a smaller dose if a hyperimmune preparation is available), and (6) collect another blood sample 21 to 28 days after the day of contact. This interval is important to allow time for the incubation period and for antibody to develop if the patient was infected. (7) If the result of the second HI test is *negative*, reassure the patient that the fetus is not at risk because either the contact case was not rubella, infection did not take place, or the IG conferred protection. If seroconversion has taken place, advise the patient and her physician of the results and the relative risks.

Finally, it should be emphasized that each case must be dealt with on its own merits, particularly in relation to the interval between exposure and the first administration of IG. The staff in the virus laboratories should be consulted in such cases and precise clinical data provided to enable the virologist to make a proper interpretation of the results of the test and their validity.

Cytomegalovirus

The need for some preventive measure to control the number of children born with congenital CMV defects is as great as, or even greater than, in the case of congenital rubella. The difficulties in doing so can be understood when reference is made to the factors specified in Tables 15–1 and 15–2.

It is now generally accepted that the majority of cases of congenital CMV disease result from primary infection contracted at any stage in pregnancy. Reinfection or reactivation infection may lead to congenital *infection* but rarely to fetal *damage*. It follows, therefore, that prevention of primary infec-

---

*The term then used for the product. It is now referred to as normal pooled immunoglobulin (IG), or, in the United States, immune serum globulin (ISG).

tion could be achieved by immunization. Because CMV is a DNA virus, an attenuated virus strain of CMV could remain latent and lead to reactivation at a later date, but whether this would present a greater problem with an attenuated strain than with a wild strain is problematical. There is also the imponderable question of oncogenicity. It is known that certain DNA viruses of hamsters (e.g., SV40) can induce tumors in animals, but this does not mean that they will do so in humans. The crux of the problem concerning oncogenicity in relation to a CMV vaccine is that it is vastly more difficult to prove a negative than the reverse. This is where those concerned with safety of biologicals have a responsibility in relation to the development of new preparations.

At present nobody can answer the questions concerning latency, reactivation, and possible oncogenicity. It must be admitted that one reason for concern about oncogenicity stems from the report of Albrecht and Rapp (1973) that hamster embryo cells underwent transformation (a possible indication of a malignant change in the cells) when inoculated with ultraviolet-irradiated CMV. These results are difficult to interpret, but it must also be borne in mind that other DNA viruses—for example, adenovirus and SV40—also cause transformation. There is no evidence that CMV strains are oncogenic in man, although transformation of human fibroblast cells has been reported (Geder et al., 1976). To make the issue even more confusing it has been found that Marek's disease virus (a DNA herpesvirus causing tumors in chickens and turkeys) lost the power to cause transformation when it underwent serial passage and was used as a vaccine to protect flocks of chickens and turkeys.

Another question is whether it is necessary to "attenuate" a virus that is naturally attenuated. It may be more realistic to "modify" or "alter" the virus in some way so that it does not become latent. It is possible that administration of vaccine by an abnormal route, such as the subcutaneous or intramuscular route, as opposed to the natural nasopharyngeal route, may restrict the spread of a virus. For example, smallpox or BCG vaccine inoculated by the intradermal or intracutaneous route usually remains localized to the site of inoculation. At present CMV vaccines are in the experimental stages. Elek and Stern (1974) reported the development of a vaccine against mental retardation caused by CMV infection *in utero*. The immunizing material consisted of a tissue-culture preparation of human lung fibroblasts infected with CMV strain AD169 that had undergone several tissue-culture passages in cell cultures. Human subjects were inoculated with the preparation in varying strengths, which were measured by log dilutions of the original virus preparation, and their complement-fixing (CF) antibody response after vaccination was measured.

A further attempt to develop a live CMV vaccine, from the Towne strain of CMV, has been reported by Plotkin and co-workers (1979). This candidate vaccine virus strain has the advantage of having been isolated directly from the patient Towne in human embryo lung fibroblasts and passaged in the same cell substrate, which is now regarded in many countries as the most acceptable for vaccine production.

Plotkin and his colleagues (1979) have described a series of trials with the Towne strain of CMV. Cellular and humoral immunity followed the administration of the vaccine, and no untoward reactions were observed. Fleisher and co-workers (1982) administered the same vaccine to 10 pediatric nurses who were shown to be seronegative for CMV by the CF and anticomplement immunofluorescence (ACIF) tests. None of the nurses developed any systemic reactons, but all 10 complained of a sore arm and in nine erythema or edema, or both, developed at the injection site seven to 10 days post-vaccination. A similar finding had been reported by Elek and Stern (1974). CMV was not isolated from any of the patients despite exhaustive attempts to do so. CF antibodies developed in all 10 subjects within four weeks of vaccination, but in four cases this had declined to undetectable levels within one year. In the ACIF assay, antibody developed in all 10 subjects, as did neutralizing antibody. Although a decline in antibody to both tests was observed over a 12-month period, none of the subjects had lost ACIF of neutralizing antibody. A cell-mediated immune response, as measured by the lymphocyte proliferation test, was observed in all subjects to a greater or lesser degree. Thus the humoral and cellular response in immunocompetent individuals appears to be satisfactory, and the fact that no virus was isolated from the urine, pharynx, or cervical secretions is encouraging.

Killed Inactivated CMV Vaccine. No attempts have yet been made to develop an inactivated vaccine, but if the difficulties mentioned with live vaccine cannot be resolved, consideration should be given to development of a killed vaccine, possibly from a purified subunit preparation (Dudgeon, 1973). An alternative may be a purified inactivated vaccine developed by genetic engineering techniques. This is a distinct possibility for the future.

Passive Immunization. This has not been attempted and is unlikely to be of any practical value, even with a hyperimmune preparation. Since the majority of CMV infections are asymptomatic, it would be impossible to decide when to administer an immunoglobulin containing CMV antibody. Furthermore, there is no reason to think that such immunization would be protective for even a brief period.

Control Measures in the Presence of Cytomegalovirus Excretion

Questions are often raised about appropriate procedures to be adopted by nursing staff or others who may come into close contact with an infant excreting CMV in the early days or weeks of life. Despite the potential risk that a susceptible adult will acquire infection from such a source, a balance has to be struck between precautions that could be taken and those that are really necessary. The following points should be taken into account.

1. Transmission of CMV requires very close contact. Normal precautions taken in caring for sick children should be adequate to prevent or reduce the risk of cross-infection, but special attention should be paid to the need for hand-washing after handling an infected infant.

2. The wearing of rubber gloves is not considered necessary unless the nurse, doctor, or other individual has an open wound or cracked skin.

3. Routine screening of newborn infants for CMV excretion is not considered necessary, although it may be used as a means of collecting epidemiological information regarding the prevalence of CMV infection.

4. The routine screening of health-care personnel for seroimmunity to CMV is not considered worthwhile. Since no measures can be taken to confer protection, as in the case of rubella susceptibility, such screening would cause pointless alarm to those found to be susceptible. It is not practicable to redeploy staff because of the low risk of exposure.

5. The CMV seroconversion rate among health-care personnel working in newborn intensive care units is apparently not significantly different from acquisition rates among pregnant and nonpregnant women in the general population (Dworsky et al., 1983).

6. Children who are known to be excretors of CMV should *not* be prevented from attending school. They should be allowed to lead normal lives.

Herpes Simplex Virus

Active Immunization. Many attempts have been made to prevent recurrent herpes with herpesvirus antigen preparations. There is no evidence that they are effective, and on theoretical grounds it seems extremely unlikely that they would be, since all that could be expected from a vaccine would be a stimulation of herpes antibody. As these patients already have antibody and recurrences are not related to the antibody titer, the use of vaccine seems valueless.

In 1967, Hull and Peck undertook a study of the development of vaccines against the herpes group of viruses, as a result of the anxiety concerning the exposure of laboratory workers to B virus, or herpesvirus simiae. Although some apparent improvement was noted in adult patients inoculated with an inactivated HSV vaccine prepared in rabbit kidney cells, the results were equivocal. Hull and Peck suggested that any improvement that did result from the vaccine could have been due to the stimulation of herpes IgA antibody, as it is known that patients with recurrent herpes are often deficient in IgA antibody (Tokumaru, 1966). The only possible role of active immunization in preventing perinatal herpes would be to immunize the mother and thus protect the infant. Theoretically, there seem to be no grounds for taking such an approach.

Passive Immunization. It would be more logical to administer a large dose of normal pooled immunoglobulin to a newborn exposed to maternal genital herpes or who risks contracting neonatal herpes. There is no evidence, however, that this form of prophylaxis is clearly beneficial.

The Management of Herpes Simplex in Pregnant Women and Newborns

The infection rate in the United States at term may vary from one in 300 to one in 1000, with clinically recognized disease occurring in about one in 7500 deliveries. In the United Kingdom the rate is very much lower, with only 66 cases recorded between 1973 and 1980 (Marshall and Peckham, 1983). Despite this almost certain underreporting in the United Kingdom, it is important to realize that measures proposed for one country are not necessarily appropriate in another. The following recommendations, however, would probably be regarded as generally acceptable.

1. Women with active genital herpes at term should be delivered by cesarean section and not *per vaginum*.

2. The same should apply to delivery when the membranes have been ruptured for less than four hours.

3. Cesarean section is *not* indicated if there was evidence of genital herpes during the pregnancy but herpes virus cultures are negative.

4. Treatment of the neonate born to a mother with *any* evidence of genital herpes should begin immediately after delivery. This involves systemic antiviral therapy, using vidarabine (aRA-A) or acyclovir (ACV). The efficacy of this approach is not yet proven, but it is recommended because of the relatively high probability that fulminant disease will occur and because of the low toxicity of the drugs employed.

Varicella-Zoster

Passive Immunization. Passive administration of zoster immune globulin (ZIG) is recommended for neonates at risk from maternal varicella—that is, those born five days or less after the onset of varicella in the mother—and for neonates exposed to varicella or zoster whose mothers' medical histories suggest that they are susceptible. The recommended dosage is 0.6 ml/kg of body weight (Gershon et al., 1974). In a trial carried out in the United Kingdom, Evans and co-workers (1980) found that ZIG was largely ineffective. Twenty-nine nonimmune infants and children among a group of 43 high-risk contacts of chickenpox patients developed infection. In 24 instances the infection was symptomatic. The dosage employed—100 mg for those under one year, 250 mg for those one to five years, and 500 mg for those six to 10 years—was roughly equivalent to that employed by Gershon and colleagues (1974). Despite these disappointing results ZIG should be administered to high-risk individuals as soon as possible after exposure.

The dose recommended in the United Kingdom for neonates is 100 mg (approximately 1.0 ml) (Polakoff, 1983), but despite the shortage of ZIG it is advisable to administer at least the minimum recommended dose based on body weight. If ZIG is not available, pooled normal isoimmune globulin can be administered in at least twice the dose recommended for ZIG.

Active Immunization. A live attenuated varicella vaccine has been developed in Japan by Takahashi and his colleagues (1975). The OKA strain of varicella virus was isolated from a patient with varicella and, after serial passage in a variety of cell cultures, was adapted to growth in W1–38 human diploid cell cultures. It has been tested in human volunteer subjects, both children and adults, in whom it was found to give to be immunogenic (Arbeter et al., 1982, 1983; Brunell et al., 1982). It has also been found to give protection against varicella in family contacts (Asano et al., 1975) and to prevent the spread of varicella among hospitalized children (Takahashi et al., 1974).

At present varicella vaccine is undergoing clinical trials for the protection of children with leukemia and other malignancies, in whom the disease can be life threatening. The preparation has not yet been licensed for routine use in healthy individuals, but it is probable that this will occur in the near future.

Immunization involves a single subcutaneous injection of 0.5 ml of a reconstituted lyophilized vaccine. The same precautions and contraindications apply as for any other live virus vaccine.

Variola Vaccinia

The WHO eradication campaign has been so successful that infections of the fetus and newborn should very rarely be seen in the future. If they do occur in the newborn, vaccinial hyperimmune immunoglobulin (0.3 ml/kg) should be given in preference to methisazone (Marboran) or β-thiosemicarbazone, which are too toxic to use at this age.

Hepatitis B

Transmission of infection from HBV carrier mothers to their infants is one of the most important factors contributing to the high prevalence of hepatitis B in many parts of the world (see Chapter 9). Prevention of transmission and development of the infant carrier state is of the utmost importance. The risk transmission varies greatly in different parts of the world; it is at least 10 times higher in China, Southeast Asia, and tropical Africa than in Australia, Europe, and North America (Deinhardt and Gust, 1982).

The following facts must be taken into account in deciding upon preventive measures.

1. Most neonatal or early infant HBV infections result from infection at delivery rather than from intrauterine infection.

2. Prophylaxis must be started soon after birth, before antigenemia has developed.

3. The risk of mother-to-infant transmission of HBV is related to the infectivity of the maternal blood containing the surface antigen (HBsAg) and the e antigen (HBeAg), to the prevalence of these different ethnic groups, and to the actual degree of exposure at birth (Derso et al., 1978; Boxall, 1980). Blood containing e antigen is highly infective, e antigen–negative blood is of intermediate infectivity, and blood with e antibody to HBeAg is of low infectivity. Persistent carriage of HBV in the last situation is rare (Derso et al., 1978). Where facilities for passive protection are restricted, it may be advisable to restrict the use of hepatitis B immunoglobulin (HBIG) to the protection of infants of those mothers who are e antigen–positive, rather than giving it routinely to e antigen–negative infants or to infants of anti-HBe–positive carrier mothers.

4. The long-term prognosis for HBV carrier children, whether symptomatic or asymptomatic, with respect to the development of chronic hepatitis or hepatic carcinoma is not known. However remote this risk may be, it is important to prevent the carrier state from being established whenever possible.

Passive Immunization

Human Normal Immune Serum Globulin. Despite the general lack of protection afforded by pooled normal immune serum globulin (ISG) against HBV infections, compared with HAV infections, a few instances of protection have been recorded (Polakoff, 1983). The lack of protective efficacy can be ascribed in general to the absence of specific HBV antibody in pools of normal plasma. The occasional success may have been due to residual traces of HBsAg in some batches of ISG, resulting in passive-active immunization (Hoofnagle et al., 1978).

Two trials to test the protective efficacy of ISG in neonates exposed at birth to HBsAg carrier mothers gave conflicting results (Varma, 1976; Tong et al., 1981). ISG is not recommended for prophylaxis.

Hyperimmune Hepatitis B Immunoglobulin. Specific HBIG is now available, although in limited supply. Krugman and co-workers (1971) demonstrated a protective effect of HBIG in children given 0.04 ml/kg of body weight four hours after exposure to HBV-infected serum. Of 10 patients so treated, six were completely protected, one had a modified attack, and three developed clinical hepatitis after a prolonged incubation period. Although the HBIG was administered very soon after exposure, there was at the time no method of measuring the antibody content of the product.

Several trials of HBIG given to newborn infants of highly infective carrier mothers have demonstrated a marked protective effect. Beasley and Stevens (1978) found a significantly lower incidence of antigenemia in infants given HBIG within 48 hours of birth. Other studies showed little difference between treated and control groups when HBIG was given within a week of birth. In a trial in Belgium a high degree of protection was found in infants given HBIG within 48 hours of birth and at monthly intervals for six months (Reesnik et al., 1978). These results were confirmed by a large-scale trial in Taiwan. A three-dose schedule starting within 48 hours of birth and repeated at three and six months produced a 75 per cent protection rate compared with two control groups, one given a single dose of HBIG and the other a placebo inoculation of saline (Beasley et al., 1981).

Rosendahl and colleagues (1983) in Berlin studied two groups of infants: 14 born to HBeAg-positive mothers (anti-HBc–negative) and 60 born to anti-HBe–positive mothers. The 14 infants received a single dose of HBIG immediately after birth, whereas the 60 infants at lower risk did not receive HBIG. Fifty-seven of the 60 "unprotected" infants remained well and negative to HBsAg. Three infants developed antigenemia immediately after birth; two lost antigen and developed antibody, and the third lost antigen without acquiring antibody. Twelve of the 14 "treated" infants were protected by a single dose of HBIG, whereas two developed antigenemia.

In countries where the risk of mother-to-infant transmission is generally low, it is very important to bear in mind the higher risk of the carrier state in resident non-Caucasian pregnant women who acquire hepatitis late in pregnancy. In the United Kingdom (Polakoff, 1982) and elsewhere, a surveillance program is available to screen out and, where necessary, to protect the at-risk infants of such mothers.

In a study in Japan, Matsumato and co-workers (1982) studied the effect of a single dose of HBIG administered (0.16 ml/kg of body weight) on the fifth day after birth to the infants of HBsAg carrier mothers. Sixty-four infants did not receive HBIG. In the "protected" group, 15 of 169 (89 per cent) developed antigenemia compared with 13 of 64 (20.3 per cent) in the control group. The development of antigenemia in the treated group occurred several months later than in the untreated group. This report further emphasizes the need for prompt and continued prophylaxis with HBIG in order to reduce the carrier state.

As a result of these and other studies from many parts of the world, several alternative dosage schedules of HBIG are now being evaluated (Deinhardt and Gust, 1982).

1. In the United Kingdom it is recommended that HBIG be administered to infants exposed to HBsAg carrier mothers (in particular, those who are e antigen–positive). HBIG should be given immediately after delivery, if possible, and not later than 48 hours after birth in a dose of 200 mg (2.0 ml contained in 0.5 ml) followed by 100 mg at monthly intervals for six months. It is important to start prophylaxis early and not to wait until the infant becomes antigen-positive. In all instances the use of HBIG should be monitored by appropriate serological tests for HBsAg and anti-HBsAg and anti-HBcAg (Polakoff, 1983).

2. In the United States, the Report of the Committee on Infectious Diseases recommends that "infants of all HBsAg positive mothers should receive HBIG in three 0.5 ml doses of HBIG immediately after birth and at three and five months of age" (1982).

Complete protection cannot be guaranteed in these situations (Boxall, 1980), but the reasons for failure can usually be attributed either to the use of HBIG of low potency or to a delay in starting the administration of HBIG with an insufficient dosage. Even with a full course as recommended, infants exposed in the neonatal period may subsequently become antigen-positive. In this situation it may be advisable to use combined passive-active immunization with HBIG and HBV vaccine, in the same way as protection is afforded to patients exposed to rabies.

Active Immunization. Purified subunit vaccines have been prepared from HBV components (22-nm HB surface antigen particles) found in the blood of chronic carriers of HBV (Hilleman et al., 1975; Purcell and Gerin, 1975). HBV vaccines prepared in this way have now been licensed for specific prophylaxis in special at-risk groups, The definition of which depends on the epidemiological conditions prevailing in different countries (Deinhardt and Gust, 1982).

Hepatitis B Vaccine. Hepatitis B vaccine is a noninfectious inactivated subunit vaccine prepared from the surface antigen (HBsAg) of hepatitis virus. The antigen is harvested from the plasma of human carriers of HBV and purified by chemical and physical means. The vaccine is a sterile suspension formulated in alum hydroxide with thimersal (1 in 20,000) as a preservative.

Pre-exposure prophylaxis in the adult requires a minimum of three 1.0-ml doses given by the intramuscular route. Postexposure prophylaxis, as in the exposed neonate, has yet to be evaluated.

One study concerned the active immunization of two groups of children living in highly endemic areas (Maupas et al., 1981). Three doses of HBV subunit vaccine were administered at monthly intervals, with a fourth booster dose given at 12 months of age, to 335 children younger than two years. Another group of 267 children received diphtheria-tetanus-poliovaccine. After 12 months four children (1.7 per cent) in the HBV group were found to be carriers of HBsAg, compared with 14 (7.2 per cent) in the control group. A high proportion of children (94.5 per cent) who were HBsAg-negative before immunization had a specific anti-HBs response. No ill effects were observed from the vaccine, and maternal anti-HBs did not appear to interfere with the immune response to the vaccine. After 12 months' follow-up, the carrier state was reduced by 85 per cent in susceptible infants.

A subsequent study by Barin and co-workers (1982) on 26 Sengalese children confirmed the immunogenicity of this same inactivated and purified HBV vaccine containing aluminium hydroxide. The infants received three 1.0-ml doses of vaccine. The doses were administered within one month of birth and at monthly intervals at the second and third month of life. Of the 19 infants who were surface antigen– and antibody–negative, 18 (94.7 per cent) showed an anti-HBs response after the third dose. Seven of the neonates born to anti-HBs–positive mothers and who had antibody at the time of vaccination possessed antibody before the booster dose, indicating that the presence of maternal antibody had not interfered with the immune response.

The levels of antibody detected were similar to those found in older Sengalese'children and in adults. One infant whose mother had anti-HBc antibody failed to respond.

The need for early active immunization before antigenemia develops was emphasized in a further study by Barin and colleagues (1983). These investigators vaccinated 31 HBsAg-positive infants three to 24 months of age. A control group of 18 infants received diphtheria-tetanus-poliovaccine. Although the vaccine had no ill effects, it was judged to be inefficient; the carrier rate in the vaccinated group after a 12-month follow-up was markedly different from that in the control group (48.4 and 66.7 per cent respectively).

These studies indicate that the young infant will respond to active immunization regardless of whether anti-HBs is present at the time of vaccination. This suggests that either active or passive-active immunization could be carried out, depending on the circumstances.

Subunit vaccines are likely to be in short supply for some years because their production is complicated and costly. Alternative sources of HBsAg are being sought, and alternatives such as polypeptide vaccines (Zuckerman and Howard, 1979) may be developed in the future, as may HBV vaccines prepared by recombinant DNA technology. For reviews of these important developments, see Blumberg and Krugman (1981), Deinhardt and Gust (1982), and Zuckerman (1982).

Passive-Active Immunization of the Infant. As passive immunization with repeated large doses of HBIG cannot be relied upon completely to suppress HBV infection, an alternative method of passive-active immunization must be considered. This is particularly important because infants who remain susceptible after the decline in passive administration of HBIG have a high risk of acquiring postnatal infection from their carrier mothers. More than half of a group of infants (born of HBeAg mothers) who had no serological evidence of hepatitis B infection at 12 months of age acquired infection in the second and third years of life and became chronic carriers (Beasley and Hwang, 1983). A WHO study to evaluate a suitable regimen is currently in progress.

Many health authorities are now recommending the use of HBV vaccine in addition to HBIG. The precise number of doses and the age at which to begin the series have yet to be determined (Advisory Committee on Immunization Practice (ACIP), 1981; Deinhardt and Gust, 1982). HBV vaccine is not yet recommended for use in these circumstances in the United Kingdom, but if clinical trials now in progress suggest that it would be efficacious, the situation can be reviewed. Studies in Senegal by Barin and co-workers (1982) showed that infants and neonates responded well to administration of HBV vaccine, but if the start of immunization was delayed until three months of age, vaccination appeared to be inefficient in preventing development of the HBsAg carrier state.

A report by Tada and colleagues (1982) suggests that combined passive-active immunization can be accomplished. They investigated 10 babies born to asymptomtic HBsAg (e antigen–positive) mothers. Intramuscular injection of HBIG (200 IU) was given immediately after delivery and repeated at two and four months of age. Vaccination with 40 mg of purified formalin-inactivated subunit vaccine was given to nine babies at three, four, five and seven months after birth. Nine babies maintained detectable levels of anti-HBsAg with loss of anti-HBcAg over a 12-month period. One baby who may have been infected *in utero* became a persistent carrier and was not treated with HBIG or vaccine. This study carried out in Tokyo is encouraging, but the implementation of such a procedure in European and North American countries requires special consideration before it can be routinely recommended. Nevertheless, the ACIP recommended "that infants born to HBV-infected mothers should also receive HBV vaccine in addition to the three doses of HBIG in as much as these infants continue to be at risk from their mothers and other possible carriers in the household" (1982). The optimal age for starting vaccination has not yet been established; current recommendations suggest that it should begin at three months of age. However, the studies from Senegal already referred to indicate that immunization procedures should be started earlier, as close to birth as possible.

A preliminary report from Europe on passive-active immunization of neonates born to HBsAg carrier mothers also indicates that the combined procedure is effective. Eighteen children whose mothers were HBsAg-positive were immunized. All received HBIG (0.5 ml/kg of body weight) within two hours of birth and hepatitis B vaccine (10μg) either at zero, one, and two months or at three, four, and five months, together with diphtheria-tetanus poliovaccine. The results indicted that this procedure was well tolerated and caused no side effects; both regimens resulted in high concentrations of anti-HBs (Mazel et al., 1984).

It would therefore seem that the use of the vaccine in the neonate should be administered together with passive immunization, but the precise details of dosage and optimal time intervals have yet to be determined from study of a larger number of susceptible subjects.

A scheme for prevention of HBV infection in the neonate is shown in Table 15–5.

General Preventive Measures

As indicated here and Chapter 9, the main risk period for maternal-infant transmission is during birth. As Krugman and Katz (1981) have stated, the infant is born in a "bath of blood"—it may be infected by HBV-infected blood or amnionic fluid contaminated with blood or as a result of resuscitation measures performed in the delivery room. Certain facts

Table 15–5. PREVENTION OF MATERNAL-INFANT HBV INFECTION*

Type of Maternal Illness	Laboratory Markers of Maternal Infection	Management and Protection of Neonate
Acute HBV infection In early pregnancy	SGOT raised Jaundice HBsAG—anti-HBs Anti-HBc HBeAg—anti-HBe	No special precautions unless mother is antigen-positive at birth. Then immunize with HBIG and vaccine as below.
In late pregnancy	As above	If HBsAg-positive: 1. Delivery by cesarean section (see text) 2. General hygienic measures after delivery to clean skin; careful intubation, gastric aspiration, etc. 3. HBIG in delivery room; further doses as recommended. HBV vaccine if recommended (see text). 4. Breast-feeding to continue unless major contraindication

Chronic active hepatitis	Chronic, recurrent jaundice
	SGOT raised
	HBsAg and HBeAg persist
	Anti-HBc persists
	Absence of anti-HBe
		Major risk. Treat:
		1. Delivery by cesarean section.
		2. General hygienic measures after delivery to clean skin; careful intubation, gastric aspiration, etc.
		3. HBIG plus HBV vaccine
		4. Breast-feeding only if steps 1 through 3 are adopted
		5. Serological tests at 12 months
		If a. anti-HBs and anti-HBc present = successful passive-active immunity
		   b. anti-HBs only = active immunity from vaccine
		   c. HBsAg = treatment failure; infant becomes a chronic carrier

Chronic asymptomatic hepatitis	SGOT raised intermittently No jaundice HBsAg persists Anti HBc persists Temporary appearance of HBeAg Anti-HBe present	*Lower risk.* Treat selectively: 1. Delivery by cesarean section. 2. General hygienic measures after delivery to clean skin; careful intubation, gastric aspiration, etc. 3. HBIG only. 4. Continue breast-feeding.

*SGOT = serum glutamic oxaloacetic transaminase; HBsAg = HB surface antigen; anti-HBs = antibody to surface antigen; HBeAg = HB e antigen; anti-HBeAg = antibody to e antigen; anti-HBc = antibody to core antigen.

can be taken into account in determining general policies with regard to precautionary measures before and after delivery.

1. The incidence of HBsAg (and, in particular, the e antigen carrier rate). This varies from 0.5 per cent in low-prevalence areas (United States, Europe) to 20 per cent in Southeast Asia.

2. The provision of health-care and obstetrical services. These also vary greatly.

3. The cost of immunization by passive, active, or combined active-passive means.

When all these factors are considered, in areas of high prevalence it seems justifiable to conclude:

1. Every effort should be made to reduce the risk of transmission of HBV by pre-exposure and postexposure vaccination of infants, with the emphasis on infants born to e antigen–positive mothers.

2. No change in policy with regard to breast-feeding should be made, as the risk of acquiring HBV infection is no greater in breast-fed than in formula-fed infants (Boxall, 1980) (see Chapter 9). Furthermore, the advantages of breast-feeding in the developing areas of the world far outweigh the risks from contaminated artificial feeding.

3. Every effort should be made to develop HBV vaccines by alternative means at lower cost.

In areas of low prevalence:

1. Whenever resources permit, identify carriers by appropriate laboratory tests for the presence of HBsAg. HBsAg-positive women attending antenatal clinics should be identified before delivery (Chin, 1983).

2. Because infection is most often acquired at delivery, consideration should be given to delivery of infants of HBsAg carrier mothers (especially those of ethnic groups with a high risk of being e antigen–positive) by cesarean section. It must be emphasized, however, that this is a theoretical consideration based on observed facts and no more likely to offer a solution than is cesarean delivery in cases of HSV genital infections.

3. Whether the infant is delivered by cesarean section or vaginally, the medical and nursing staff should take the necessary precautions (a) to avoid contaminating themselves with infected blood and secretions and (b) to prevent HBV-infected material from remaining in close contact with the newborn's skin. The skin should be carefully washed in a suitable detergent or antiseptic, or both, to remove blood and other contaminants. When

resuscitation is necessary, special care should be taken to avoid abrasion of the mucosa by energetic handling. Gastric aspiration should be carried out.

4. Decisions about breast-feeding should be made on an individual basis. If the mother is still suffering from the effects of acute viral hepatitis, mother and infant should be separated. If this is not the case and the infant is going to receive some form of immunization, breast-feeding should be allowed to continue.

The precautions that are advocated are summarized in Table 15–5.

Hepatitis A

Although there is no concrete evidence that congenital defects result from HAV infection in pregnancy, there is evidence of increase in premature births and abortions. Pregnant women exposed to HAV should therefore be protected by administration of ISG, which is highly effective and is not contraindicated in pregnancy. The recommended dosage is 500 to 750 mg for adults immediately after contact (3.4 to 5.1 ml).

Hepatitis Non-A, Non-B

There are probably several causes of hepatitis non-A, non-B infection. Spread occurs mainly via infected blood, which should be avoided; otherwise, no specific form of prevention is indicated in pregnancy at the present time.

Enteroviral Infections

Poliomyelitis

Active Immunization. Poliomyelitis has been brought under control in many parts of the world by the use of oral poliovaccine (OPV) and in some countries, such as Sweden and the Netherlands, by means of inactivated poliovaccine.

In the developed countries, poliomyelitis is not a problem in pregnancy provided that primary immunization of infants and children is carried out and that immunity is maintained by booster doses of vaccine at recommended intervals. In this way the fetus should be protected.

There is a remote risk that a vaccinee will

acquire paralytic poliomyelitis from OPV, but the risk of vaccine-associated and recipient-associated disease is on the order of 0.3 and 0.4 per million doses of vaccine administered. A few vaccine-associated cases may be expected in babies receiving their first dose of OPV, but the risk is very small. Although there is a potential risk of contact-associated cases in unvaccinated parents of recently vaccinated infants, there have been no reports in the United Kingdom of mothers having contracted paralytic poliomyelitis from their vaccinated infants.

OPV is contraindicated in pregnancy on the general principle that all live vaccines are best avoided in pregnancy. If for any reason immunization of a pregnant woman is considered necessary, the inactivated Salk-type vaccine can be used, but nowadays, in the absence of epidemic poliomyelitis, this would occur very rarely.

Vaccines Against Other Enteroviruses

No vaccines against other enteroviruses are available. In view of the natural history of the nonpoliomyelitis infections and the multiplicity of antigenic and serological types, it seems unlikely that the development of a specific vaccine will be undertaken.

Prevention of Other Enteroviral Infections by OPV

It is a well-known phenomenon that infection of the alimentary tract by one enterovirus can be inhibited by the presence of another serologically unrelated enterovirus. The mechanism of inhibition is ascribed to interference between the two agents. This phenomenon may explain the poor "take rate" with OPV immunization in the developing countries; other agents, bacterial or viral, may be present in the intestinal tract at the time the OPV is administered. It also provides the rationale for administering three doses of OPV in succession to overcome interference between the individual vaccine strains.

Practitioners have taken advantage of this phenomenon on a number of occasions in trying to prevent the spread of Coxsackie B and ECHO 11 virus infections in nurseries by administering OPV to susceptible contacts. Farmer and Patten (1968) described an outbreak of Coxsackie B5 infection in a special care baby unit in Auckland in which OPV

was fed to unaffected infants. Fifteen cases of neonatal meningoencephalitis had occurred, but no further cases were observed after administration of the OPV (Farmer and Patten, 1968; Farmer et al., 1975). It is a matter of conjecture whether the OPV in fact resulted in control of the outbreak, but it is possible. Gardner and Cooper (1965) found that OPV interfered with ECHO 11 but not with ECHO 6 in a similar situation. Tobin and his colleagues (1984) also found that OPV probably had an effect during an outbreak of ECHO 11 in a special care baby unit in Oxford in 1978. No further cases occurred after OPV was administered, and the unit was not closed to admissions.

These three episodes require careful evaluation, and further studies must be undertaken before such a procedure can be recommended. Nevertheless, these results suggest a step that might be taken with comparative safety if for some reason the unit in which the cases are occurring cannot be closed to new admissions. This should be the first control procedure to be taken.

Other Viruses

The only other virus for which protection by immunization should be considered is influenza. Although there is no clear-cut evidence that influenza virus damages the fetus, it may be desirable to immunize pregnant women in the face of an epidemic, particularly of a new variant against which the adult population has little or no immunity. In such cases inactivated influenza vaccines should be used. Live influenza vaccines are contraindicated.

Transfer Factor

Very limited information is available on the role in viral infections of the extract of lymphocytes known as transfer factor (TF). Although it is generally held that augmentation of cell-mediated immunity occurs only with specific antigens to which the recipient is able to react (Lawrence, 1970), it has been suggested that cell-mediated immunity may be stimulated in a nonspecific manner (Dupont et al., 1974). The exact mechanism by which TF might accomplish this is far from clear at the present time.

The chronic infective states that are a feature of many intrauterine viral infections would seem to be appropriate conditions for investigation. Nevertheless, caution should be exercised before the use of TF is considered; of particular concern is the possibility of converting large numbers of lymphocytes to an antigen-reactive state, thereby causing an excessive cell-mediated immune response, which may damage vital tissues such as the brain and eye.

ANTIVIRAL CHEMOTHERAPY

There have been some remarkable advances in antiviral chemotherapeutic agents in the last 10 years. However, the possibility of toxicity or teratogenicity to the fetus has limited their application and, therefore, the information gained about their use in pregnancy. Experience with their use in the newborn is also limited. To date, only a small number of antiviral agents are applicable in treatment of viral infections of the fetus and newborn. Details of these agents are summarized here and in Table 15–6.

Vidarabine

Vidarabine (Ara-A, Vira-A) is available as both an intravenous and a topical ophthalmic preparation. It is a purine nucleoside analogue with some antiviral activity against all members of the herpesvirus group. Within cells, vidarabine is phosphorylated by cellular kinases to a triphosphate form that acts as a selective competitive inhibitor of viral DNA polymerase (Shipman et al., 1976; Muller 1979; Whitley et al., 1983). It thus acts as an inhibitor of viral DNA synthesis.

Pharmacokinetic studies have shown that, when given intravenously, vidarabine is rapidly deaminated to arabinosyl hypoxanthine (Ara-Hx), the plasma half-life of which is three to four hours (Shope et al., 1983), and the drug is principally eliminated by urinary excretion of this metabolite. Vidarabine and Ara-Hx are widely distributed in the body, with levels in the cerebrospinal fluid one third to one half those in the plasma (Whitley et al., 1983; Shope et al., 1983). Vidarabine is relatively insoluble, so administration requires a large fluid load, which poses a prob-

Table 15–6. **ANTIVIRAL AGENTS AVAILABLE FOR TREATMENT OF VIRAL INFECTIONS OF THE FETUS AND NEWBORN**

Agent	Preparation	Dosage and Administration	Indications
Vidarabine (Ara-A, Vira-A)	Intravenous, 200 mg/ml	15 mg/kg daily for 10 days; infuse over 12 hours in Dext/Saline, maximum concentration 0.5 mg/ml	Neonatal varicella,* localized or disseminated HSV Maternal HSV or varicella, disseminated life-threatening HSV or V-Z infection in immunosuppressed patients
Acyclovir (Zovirax)	Ophthalmic ointment, 3% Intravenous powder, 250 mg vial	5 times daily for 14 days 10 mg/kg every 8 hours; infuse over 1 hour in Dext/Saline, maximum concentration 5 mg/ml	Ophthalmic herpes† Neonatal varicella,* localized or disseminated HSV
		250–500 mg/m² every 8 hours;‡ infuse over 1 hour in Dext/Saline, maximum concentration 5 mg/ml	Maternal HSV or varicella, disseminated life-threatening HSV or V-Z infection in immunosuppressed patients
	Aqueous cream, 5%	Topical 5 times daily for 7 days	Primary or recurrent genital herpes
Idoxuridine (Stoxil, Idoxene, Kerecid, Ophthalmidine)	Ophthalmic ointment, 3%§ Ophthalmic ointment, 0.5%	5 times daily for 14 days 5 times daily for 14 days	Ophthalmic herpes† Ophthalmic herpes†
(Kerecid, Dendrid, Herplex)	Ophthalmic drops, 0.1%	Hourly by day, every 2 hours at night for 14 days	Ophthalmic herpes†
Trifluorothymidine (Viroptic)	Ophthalmic drops, 1%‖	1–2 hourly by day for 14 days	Ophthalmic herpes†

* See Table 15–8 for details of indications.
†Systemic therapy advised in combination with topical therapy in acute neonatal infection.
‡Dosage not yet fully evaluated.
§Not available in United States.
‖Not available in United Kingdom.

lem in patients with herpes encephalitis who have cerebral edema or renal failure. There should be a dose reduction of at least 25 per cent in patients with renal impairment. Vidarabine is relatively well tolerated by neonates at a dose of 15 mg/kg/day and is currently being used in trials at double this dosage (Whitley et al., 1980a). The most common adverse effects are gastrointestinal (nausea, vomiting, and diarrhea) and neurological (tremors, parathesia, ataxia, and seizures) (Ross et al., 1976; Sacks et al., 1979). High doses in children and adults (20 to 30 mg/kg/day) can lead to toxicity with megaloblastic anemia, leukopenia, and thrombocytopenia (Sacks et al., 1979). (There is some experimental evidence that vidarabine can be teratogenic and mutagenic, so its use in infants should be limited.) At present, neonatal HSV infections (local or systemic) and neonatal varicella are the only indications for the use of this drug in infancy. It is contraindicated in pregnancy. For details of dosage and administration, see Table 15–6. Infants born to mothers with active genital HSV and varicella could be treated expectantly in view of the high probability of neonatal infection, with its attendant morbidity and mortality, and the relatively low toxicity of vidarabine. The efficacy of this approach has not as yet been demonstrated for vidarabine or acyclovir.

Acyclovir

Acyclovir (Zovirax) is a recently licensed purine nucleoside analogue with a high degree of specificity against herpes simplex and V-Z viruses, yet with a very low cellular toxicity. The reason for this is that the drug is phosphorylated by a virus-specified thymidine kinase much more rapidly and effectively than by cellular enzymes, resulting in a 40- to 100-fold increase in acyclovir monophosphate in infected cells compared with noninfected cells. This compound is polarized and cannot readily diffuse out of the cell. Subsequent phosphorylation by cellular enzymes leads to the production of acyclovir triphosphate, a potent and selective inhibitor of herpesvirus DNA polymerase (St. Clair et al., 1980; Allaudeen et al., 1982; Schaeffer, 1982). Acyclovir triphosphate may also inhibit viral DNA synthesis by serving as a substrate for this enzyme, causing early chain termination of viral DNA (McGuirt and Furman, 1982).

Acyclovir is approximately 160 times more active than vidarabine against HSV type 1 (Schaeffer, 1982). HSV type 2 and V-Z viruses are also quite sensitive to acyclovir. Epstein-Barr virus is much less sensitive but can be inhibited by achievable plasma levels of the drug (Datta et al., 1980) despite the absence of a virus-coded thymidine kinase. Most clinical isolates of CMV are resistant (Tyms et al., 1981; Meyers et al., 1983).

Acyclovir is now available in the United Kingdom as an intravenous preparation, an aqueous cream, and an ophthalmic ointment (the last is not at present available in the United States; see Table 15–6). An oral preparation is also licensed in the United Kingdom, but it has no practical application in the neonate.

Pharmacokinetic data from studies of the intravenous preparation in adults, children, and neonates show the plasma half-life to be between two and five hours with normal renal function (Miranda et al., 1979; Hintz et al., 1982). Peak and trough levels are significantly higher in neonates 0 to 11 days of age than in infants 18 to 61 days of age when a standard 10 mg/kg/day dose (administered at intervals of eight hours) is used (Hintz et al., 1983). The drug is widely distributed, and CSF levels in neonates closely match trough plasma levels (Hintz et al., 1983). Acyclovir is eliminated primarily by urinary excretion of the unchanged drug. Renal clearance of acyclovir is usually two to three times greater than the glomerular filtration, indicating that a tubular secretory mechanism plays an important role in the drug's renal elimination. The dosage interval should be adjusted if there is renal impairment; recommendations based on creatinine clearance have been published by Miranda and Blum (1983) (see Table 15–7).

Reports of toxicity with acyclovir have been minimal. The rise in serum creatinine seen in some cases is thought to be related to a bolus injection and possible renal tubular crystallization of the drug. This can be avoided by administration in a concentration of no more than 5 mg/ml infused over one hour (Gould et al., 1982). To date, no significant neurological, gastrointestinal, or hematological toxicity has been reported at the recommended dosage. Results of studies of teratogenicity and mutagenicity in animals

Table 15–7. DOSAGE INTERVAL FOR ACYCLOVIR IN CASES OF RENAL IMPAIRMENT

Creatinine Clearance (ml/min/1.73²)	Acyclovir Dosage Interval
50	8 hourly (standard) (see Table 15–8)
25–50	12 hourly
10–25	24 hourly
0–10	½ dose 24 hourly

Data from Miranda, P., and Blum, M. R.: Acyclovir pharmacokinetics. J. Antimicrob. Chemother. *12* (Suppl. B):29–37, 1983.

have been largely negative. Although acyclovir is undoubtedly of high potency as an antiviral agent against HSV and V-Z viruses and is of proven clinical efficacy in immunosuppressed adults and children with HSV and V-Z infections, comparative double-blind trials have yet to confirm either its clinical efficacy in the neonate with V-Z or HSV infections or its superiority to vidarabine. Trials are underway, and results will be published shortly (Whitley et al., 1983). Until this time, firm recommendations for the drug's use in neonates cannot be given, although trials have confirmed its safety (Gould et al., 1982; Hintz et al., 1982; Yeager et al., 1982). and current data suggest efficacy in both neonatal HSV and V-Z infections (Gould et al., 1982; Yeager et al., 1982; Campbell et al., 1983). For details of dosage and administration, see Table 15–6.

Idoxuridine

Idoxuridine (IDU) (Stoxil, Idoxene, Kerecid, Ophthalmidine, Dendrid, Herplex) is a pyrimidine nucleoside that has a potent effect against herpesviruses by inhibiting viral DNA synthesis. It lacks the selectivity and specificity of vidarabine or acyclovir, as it also inhibits cellular DNA synthesis to some extent, which makes it too toxic for systemic use and potentially mutagenic and teratogenic. Ophthalmic preparations have been licensed for some time and are used widely in treating herpes simplex keratitis. Although IDU is of proven efficacy in the treatment of keratoconjunctivitis, there are now doubts about its use as a first line treatment for herpetic eye infections in the neonate, both because it interferes with DNA synthesis, so that prolonged therapy may slow the normal healing process, and because of the very significant risk that primary herpetic infection in the neonate may

spread to the central nervous system or become generalized. Topical trifluorothymidine (TFT), vidarabine, and acyclovir appear to be just as effective in controlled trials (Travers and Patterson, 1978; Coster et al., 1979; Pavan-Langton et al., 1981) and are safer (Pavan-Langton, 1983; Schinazi and Prusoff, 1983). Serious consideration should be given to the use of systemic therapy with vidarabine or acyclovir combined with topical therapy in all proven cases of neonatal herpetic eye infection.

Idoxuridine–Dimethyl Sulfoxide

Although this topical drug formulation has been licensed in the United Kingdom and has been found to be effective in adults in the management of cold sores, genital herpes, herpetic whitlow, and V-Z skin lesions, its use in the newborn cannot be recommended. It should be noted that the combination is teratogenic in several species (Caujolle et al., 1967; Percy and Albert, 1974). Topical acyclovir cream has been found to be equally or more effective in the treatment of genital herpes in the adult and is potentially less hazardous; therefore, it should be considered a safer product with which to treat genital herpes in pregnancy.

Trifluorothymidine (Trifluridine, Viroptic)

Like IDU, this pyrimidine nucleoside is thought to act by inhibiting herpesvirus DNA synthesis. Also like IDU, it is too toxic to be used systemically. A 1 per cent ophthalmic solution is now in widespread use for the treatment of herpetic keratitis. The drug has been licensed in this form for use in the United States. In several double-blind clinical studies in patients with herpetic eye infections, TFT was found to be equally if not more effective than IDU and vidarabine (Travers and Patterson, 1978; Coster et al., 1979). Unlike with IDU or vidarabine, hypersensitivity reactions are rare. The drug appears to be safe for topical use in the neonatal period.

Future Antiviral Agents

A number of antiviral agents active against herpes group viruses are now under trial.

These include Bromovinyldeoxyuridine, an agent very active against HSV type 1, and fluoroiodoaracytosine, which appears to be effective against HSV type 1 and CMV.

Clinical Indications

Neonatal Herpes Simplex Infection

Of all the perinatal infections, the most promising candidate for antiviral therapy is neonatal herpes, because infants usually acquire infection at the time of delivery, rather than early in gestation as in congenital rubella and CMV infection. It is thus conceivable that effective therapy can be delivered early in the course of disease, rather than long after the start of the infectious process.

The clinical presentation of the infant with HSV infection can be very variable. Approximately half will present with cutaneous vesiculation and less than half with ophthalmitis within a few days of birth. Skin manifestations may not appear for up to three weeks (Arvin et al., 1982). Infants often present with disseminated viremia, which is clinically indistinguishable from that of overwhelming bacterial sepsis, and show no evidence of mucocutaneous lesions (Arvin et al., 1982). Isolated ocular or cutaneous lesions are thought to pose as much as a 70 per cent risk of dissemination (Nahmias et al., 1975; Welch et al., 1980; Whitley et al., 1980b). Both rapid diagnosis and early institution of effective systemic therapy are therefore vital. Strong consideration should be given to initiating therapy at birth in newborns of mothers who have active genital lesions at parturition.

Recommendations

1. Immediate commencement of intravenous vidarabine or acyclovir when there is evidence of genital herpes simplex in the mother or cutaneous or ocular HSV infection in an infant within the first month of life, whether or not he or she is systemically ill.

2. Addition of a topical antiviral agent when there is evidence of ophthalmic infection.

Although the only form of systemic therapy that is of proven benefit in neonatal HSV infections is vidarabine (Whitley et al., 1980a and b), trials (Gould et al., 1982; Offit et al., 1982) have so far suggested comparable or greater efficacy with acyclovir. One case of disseminated HSV infection has been described in which failure to respond to vidar-

abine therapy was followed by prompt resolution upon the institution of acyclovir therapy (Campbell et al., 1983).

Genital Herpes in the Pregnant Woman

Both oral (Corey et al., 1983) and topical acyclovir (Fiffian et al., 1983) have proved effective in the treatment of genital herpes. The oral preparation should *not* be given in pregnancy. Trials of topical acyclovir 5 per cent cream (an aqueous preparation in propylene glycol) have proved its effectiveness in reducing viral shedding, formation of new lesions, time of healing, and duration of symptoms in both primary and recurrent genital lesions (Fiffian et al., 1983).

Recommendations

1. Topical 5% acyclovir cream for 7 days (see Table 15–6).
2. Monitor closely for recurrence of vesiculation.
3. Deliver by cesarean section rather than vaginally if active lesions are present at term.

The efficacy of long-term prophylaxis with topical acyclovir cream during pregnancy has not yet been studied.

Neonatal Varicella

The most important factor predisposing toward the severity of neonatal varicella is the time of onset of the maternal illness in relation to delivery. This is presumably related to the protection afforded by maternal antibody available by the time of delivery (see Chapter 7).

Infants at *special risk* (see Table 15–8) of viral dissemination are those born five days or less after the onset of varicella in the mother (Meyers, 1974) or born to immunodeficient mothers with varicella in the preceding 14 days. Infants born to mothers who

---

Table 15–8. **INDICATIONS FOR USE OF A SYSTEMIC ANTIVIRAL AGENT IN NEONATAL VARICELLA**

1. Infants at special risk of viral dissemination
2. Premature infants
3. Infants in whom the varicella rash is hemorrhagic or atypical
4. Infants in whom there is a prolonged course of disease, with new lesions continuing to erupt into the second week of life (Brunell, 1983)
5. Infants who appear systemically ill

have not had varicella who contract the disease in a neonatal unit are also likely to be at special risk. Such infants should be protected with ZIG. In the event that varicella develops, systemic therapy with either vidarabine or acyclovir should be commenced immediately. There are several other indications for the use of an antiviral agent; these are listed in Table 15–8.

V-Z virus is susceptible *in vitro* to both vidarabine and acyclovir. No comparative controlled trials have been published on the use of these drugs in varicella in the neonatal period. Both vidarabine and acyclovir have been tested in placebo-controlled trials for treatment of varicella in immunosuppressed patients, including children (Prober et al., 1982; Whitley et al., 1982). With both drugs, the most important effect appears to be the reduction of complications of visceral dissemination—from 55 per cent to 5 per cent with vidarabine therapy; there was a reduction from 45 per cent to 20 per cent in the development of pneumonitis when acyclovir was used. Suggested dosage regimens are outlined in Table 15–6.

Varicella or Disseminated Zoster in Pregnancy

All drugs that are potential DNA inhibitors, including vidarabine and acyclovir, should be avoided in pregnancy. There have been no published data on the effect of these drugs on the fetus. Cytosine arabinoside (ara-C) has been found to affect brain development adversely when given to newborn mice (Ashwal et al., 1974). It should also be remembered that although varicella during pregnancy may result in fetal malformation, the risk is probably relatively slight (see Chapter 7). The rare case of the immunodeficient pregnant women with life-threatening varicella of course merits consideration for systemic therapy with either drug. Theoretically, acyclovir might be expected to be less toxic to the fetus.

Congenital Cytomegalovirus Infection

Although some strains of CMV appear sensitive to high concentrations of both vidarabine and acyclovir *in vitro,* clinical trials of both drugs have proved disappointing. At best, a transient decrease in urinary virus excretion was noted with vidarabine. No clinical improvement in any treated cases has

been noted. A study of combined therapy with high-dose acyclovir and interferon in CMV-infected immunosuppressed patients (Meyers et al., 1983) has likewise proved disappointing.

Bibliography

Advisory Committee on Immunization Practices. Immune globulins for protection against viral hepatitis. Morbidity Mortality Weekly Rep. *30*:423–428, 1981.

Advisory Committee on Immunization Practices. Inactivated hepatitis B virus vaccine. Morbidity Mortality Weekly Rep. *31*:317–322, 327–328, 1982.

Albrecht, T., and Rapp, F.: Malignant transformation of hamster embryo fibroblasts following exposure to ultraviolet-irradiated human cytomegalovirus. Virology *55*:53–61, 1973.

Allaudeen, H. S., Descamps, J., and Sehgal, R. K.: Mode of action of acyclovir triphosphate on herpes viral and cellular DNA polymerases. Antiviral Res. *2*:123–133, 1982.

Anderson, S. G., and McLorinan, H.: Convalescent rubella gamma globulin as a possible prophylactic against rubella. Med. J. Aust. *2*:182–185, 1953.

Arbeter, A. M., Starr, S. E., Weibel, R. E., and Plotkin, S. A.: Live attenuated varicella vaccine: immunization of healthy children with the OKA strain. J. Pediatr. *100*:886–893, 1982.

Arbeter, A. M., Starr, S. E., Weibel, R. E., Neff, B. and Plotkin, S. A.: Live attenuated varicella vaccine. The KMcC strain in healthy children. Pediatrics *71*:307–312, 1983.

Arvin, A. M., Yeager, A. D., Bruhn, F. W., and Grossman, M.: Neonatal herpes simplex infection in the absence of mucocutaneous lesions. J. Pediatr. *100*:715–721, 1982.

Asano, Y., Takehiko, Y., Takao, M., Nakayama, H., Hirose, S., Ito, S., Tanaka, E., Isonura, S., Suzuki, S., and Takahashi, M.: Application of a live attenuated varicella vaccine to hospitalized children and its protective effect on spread of varicella infection. Biken J. *18*:35–40, 1975.

Ashwal, S., Finegold, M., Fish, I., et al.: Effect of the antiviral drug cytosine arabinoside on the developing nervous system. Pediatr. Res. *8*:945–950, 1974.

Barin, F., Denis, F., Chiron, J. P., Goudeau, A., Yvonett, B., Cousaget, P., and Diof Mar, I.: Immune responses in neonates to hepatitis B vaccine. Lancet *1*:251–253, 1982.

Barin, F., Yvonett, B., Goudeau, A., Cousaget, P., Chiron, J. P., Denis F., and Diof Mar, I.: Hepatitis B vaccine: further studies in children with previously acquired hepatitis B surface antigenemia. Infect. Immun. *41*:83–87, 1983.

Beasley, R. P.: Dilemmas presented by the attenuated rubella vaccines. Am. J. Epidemiol. *92*:158, 1970.

Beasley, R. P., and Hwang, L. V.: Postnatal infectivity of HB$_s$Ag carrier mothers. J. Infect. Dis. *147*:185–190, 1983.

Beasley, R. P., and Stevens, C. D.: Vertical transmission of HBV and interruption with globulin. In Vyas, G. N., Cohen, S. N., and Schmid, R. (eds.): Viral Hepatitis. Philadelphia, Franklin Institute Press; Tunbridge Wells, Abacus Press, 1978, pp. 335–345.

Beasley, R. P., Hwang, L. V., and Lin, C. C.: Hepatitis

B immune serum globulin (HBIG) efficacy in the interruption of perinatal transmission of hepatitis B virus carrier state. Initial report of randomized double-blind placebo controlled trial. Lancet 2:388–393, 1981.

Blumberg, B. S., and Krugman, S.: Passive and active immunization in the control of viral hepatitis. In Wolf, S., Altar, H. S., and Maynard, J. E. (eds.): The Proceedings of the Third International Symposium on Viral Hepatitis. Philadelphia, Franklin Institute Press, 1981, pp. 377–541.

Boxall, E.: Maternal transmission hepatitis B. In Waterson, A. P. (ed.): Recent Advances in Clinical Virology, No. 2. Edinburgh, Churchill Livingstone, 1980, pp. 17–41.

Brody, J. A., Sever, J. L., McAlister, R., Schiff, G. M., and Cutting, R.: Rubella epidemic on St. Paul Island in the Pribilofs. Arch. Ges. Virusforsch. 16:488–491, 1965.

Brunell, P. A.: Fetal and neonatal varicella-zoster infections. Sem. Perinatol. 7:47–56, 1983.

Brunell, P. A., Shehab, Z., Geisa, C., and Waugh, J.: Administration of live variella vaccine to children with leukaemia. Lancet 2:1069–1072, 1982.

Buynak, E. B., Hilleman, M. R., Weible, R. E., and Stokes, J.: Live attenuated rubella virus vaccines prepared in duck embryo cell culture. I. Development and clinical testing. J.A.M.A. 204:195–200, 1968.

Campbell, A. N., O'Driscoll, M. C., Robinson, D. L., and Read, S. E.: A case of neonatal herpes simplex with pneumonia. Can. Med. Assoc. J. 129:725–726, 1983.

Caujolle, F. M., Caujolle, D. H., Cros, S. B., et al.: Limits of toxic and teratogenic tolerance of dimethyl-sulfoxide. Ann. N.Y. Acad. Sci. 141:110–126, 1967.

Centers for Disease Control: Morbidity and Mortality. U.S. Dept. Health, Education & Welfare, Vol. 24, No. 13, Atlanta, Georgia 30333, April 4, 1975.

Chin, J.: Prevention of chronic hepatitis B virus infection from mothers to infants in the United States. Pediatrics 71:289–292, 1983.

Cooper, L. Z.: Congenital rubella in the United States. In Krugman, S., and Gershon, A. A. (eds.): Symposium on Infections of the Fetus and Newborn Infant. New York, Alan R. Liss, Inc., 1975, pp. 1–22.

Corey, L., Benedetti, J., Critchlow, C., Mertz, G., Douglas, J., Fife, K., Fahnlander, A., Remington, M. L., Winter, C., and Dragavon, J.: Treatment of primary first-episode genital herpes simplex virus infections with acyclovir: results of topical, intravenous and oral therapy. J. Antimicrob. Chemother. 12(Suppl. B):79–99, 1983.

Coster, D. J., Jones, B. R., and McGill, J. I.: Treatment of amoeboid herpetic ulcers with adenine arabinoside or trifluorothymidine. Br. J. Ophthalmol. 63:418–421, 1979.

Datta, A. K., Colby, B. M., Shaw, J. E., and Pagano, J. S.: Acyclovir inhibition of Epstein-Barr virus replication. Proc. Natl. Acad. Sci. U.S.A. 77:5163–5166, 1980.

Deinhardt, F., and Gust, I.: Viral hepatitis. Bull. W.H.O. 60:661–691, 1982.

Derso, A., Boxall, E., Tarlow, M. J., and Flewett, T. H.: Transmission of HBₛAg from mother to infant in four ethnic groups. Br. Med. J. 1:949–952, 1978.

Dudgeon, J. A.: Future developments in prophylaxis. In Intrauterine Infections. Ciba Foundation Symposium 10 (new series). Amsterdam, Associated Scientific Publishers, 1973, pp. 179–202.

Dudgeon, J. A.: Letter to the editor. Br. Med. J. 2:723, 1974.

Dudgeon, J. A.: Immunizing procedures in childhood. In Hull, D. (ed.): Recent Advances in Paediatrics. 5th ed. New York, Longman, Inc., 1976, pp. 169–201.

Dudgeon, J. A., Peckham, C. S., Marshall, W. C., Smithells, R. W., and Sheppard, S.: National Congenital Rubella Surveillance Programme. Health Trends 5:75–79, 1973.

Dupont, B., Ballow, M., Hansen, J. A., et al.: Effect of transfer factor therapy on mixed lymphocyte culture reactivity. Proc. Natl. Acad. Sci. U.S.A. 71:867–871, 1974.

Dworsky, M. E., Welch, K., Cassady, G., and Stagno, S.: Occupational risk for primary cytomegalovirus infection among pediatric health-care workers. N. Engl. J. Med. 309:950–953, 1983.

Elek, S. D., and Stern, H.: Development of a vaccine against mental retardation caused by cytomegalovirus infection in utero. Lancet 1:1–5, 1974.

Evans, E. B., Pollock, T. M., Cradock-Watson, J. E., and Ridehalgh, M. K. S.: Human anti-chickenpox immunoglobulin in the prevention of chickenpox. Lancet 1:354–356, 1980.

Farmer, K., and Patten, P. T.: An outbreak of Coxsackie B virus infection in a special care unit for newborn infants. N.Z. Med. J. 68:86–89, 1968.

Farmer, K., McCarthur, B. A., and Clayton, M. M.: A follow up study of 15 cases of neonatal meningo-encephalitis due to Coxsackie B virus. J. Pediatr. 87:566–571, 1975.

Fiffian, A. P., Kinghorn, G. R., Goldmeier, D., Rees, E., Rodin, P., Thin, R. N. J., and Konig, G. A. J.: Topical acyclovir in the treatment of genital herpes: a comparison with systemic therapy. J. Antimicrob. Chemother. 12(Suppl. B): 67–77, 1983.

Fleisher, G. R., Starr, S. E., Friedman, H. H., and Plotkin, S. A.: Vaccination of pediatric nurses with live attenuated cytomegalovirus vaccine. Am. J. Dis. Child. 136:294–296, 1982.

Gardner, P. S., and Cooper, C. E.: The feeding of oral poliovirus vaccine to a closed community excreting faecal virus. J. Hyg. 62:171–178, 1964.

Geder, L., Lausch, R., O'Neill, F., and Rapp, F.: Oncogenic transformation of human embryo lung cells by human cytomegalovirus. 192:1134–1137, 1976.

Gershon, A. A., Steinberg, S., and Brunell, P. A.: Zoster immune globulin: a further assessment. N. Engl. J. Med. 290:243–245, 1974.

Gould, J. M., Chessells, J. M., Marshall, W. C., and McKendrick, G. D. W.: Acyclovir in herpes virus infections in children: experience in an open study with particular reference to safety. J. Infect., 5:283–289, 1982.

Green, R. H., Balsamo, M. R., Giles, J. P., Krugman, S., and Mirick, G. S.: Studies of the natural history and prevention of rubella. Am. J. Dis. Child. 1101:348, 1965.

Hermann, K. L., Halstead, S. B., Brandling-Bennett, A. D., Witte, J. J., Wiebenga, N. H., and Eddins, D. L.: Rubella immunization: persistence of antibody four years after a large-scale field trial. J.A.M.A. 235:2201–2204, 1976.

Hilleman, M. R., Buynak, E. B., Roehm, R. R., Tytell, A. A., Bertland, A. V., and Lampson, G. P.: Purified and inactivated human hepatitis B vaccine: progress report. In Symposium on Viral Hepatitis. National Academy of Sciences, Washington, D.C., March 17–19, 1975, pp. 401–404.

Hintz, M., Connor, J. D., Spector, S. A., Blum, M. R., Keeney, R. E., and Yeager, A. S.: Neonatal acyclovir pharmacokinetics in patients with herpes virus infections. Am. J. Med. 73(Suppl. 1A):210–214, 1982.

Hintz, M., Yeager, A. D., Connor, J. D., Spector, S. A.,

de Vinney, R., and Van Dyke, R.: Acyclovir pharmacokinetics in neonates with herpes simplex virus infections. Abstract No. 569. Interscience Conference on Antimicrobial Agents and Chemotherapy, 1983.

Hoofnagle, J. H., Seiff, L. B., Bales, Z. B., Gerrety, R., and Tatos, E.: Serological responses in HB. In Vyas, G. N., Cohen, S. N., and Schmid, R. (eds.): Viral Hepatitis. Philadelphia, Franklin Institute Press; Tunbridge Wells, Abacus Press, 1978, pp. 581–587.

Horstmann, D. H.: Controlling rubella: problems and perspectives. Ann. Intern. Med. 83:412–417, 1975.

Hull, R. N., and Peck, F. B., Jr.: Vaccination against herpesvirus infections. In First International Conference on Vaccines Against Viral and Rickettsial Diseases of Man, November 7–11, 1966. WHO Scientific Publication No. 147. Washington, D.C., Pan American Health Organization, 1967, pp. 266–275.

International Conference on Rubella Immunization. National Institutes of Health, Bethesda, Maryland, February 18–20, 1969. Am. J. Dis. Child. 18:155–399, 1969.

International Symposium on Rubella Vaccines, London, 1968. Symposia Series in Immunobiological Standardization, Vol. 11. Basel, S. Karger, 1969.

Krugman, S.: Newer vaccines (measles, mumps, rubella): potential and problems. In International Symposium on Vaccination Against Communicable Diseases, Monaco 1973. Symposia Series in Immunobiological Standardization, Vol. 22. Basel, S. Karger, 1973, pp. 55–63.

Krugman, S.: Present status of measles and rubella immunization in the United States: a review article. J. Pediatr. 90:1–12, 1977.

Krugman, S.: Rubella immunization: present status and future prospectives. Pediatrics 65:1174–1176, 1980.

Krugman, S., and Katz, S.: Infectious Diseases of Children and Adults. 8th ed. St. Louis, C. V. Mosby Company, 1981.

Krugman, S., Giles, J. P., and Hammond, J.: Viral hepatitis type B (MS-2 strain): prevention with specific hepatitis B immune serum globulin. J.A.M.A. 218:1665–1670, 1971.

Lawrence, H. S.: Transfer factor and cellular immune deficiency disease. N. Engl. J. Med. 283:411–419, 1970.

Lundström, R.: Rubella during pregnancy. A follow-up study of children born after an epidemic of rubella in Sweden, 1951. With additional investigations on propylaxis and treatment of maternal rubella. Acta Paediatr. 51(Supl. 133):1–110, 1962.

Lundström, R.: Passive immunization against rubella. Arch. Ges. Virusforsch. 16:506–508, 1965.

Lundström, R., Thorén, C., and Blomquist, B.: Gamma globulin against rubella in pregnancy. I. Prevention of maternal rubella by gamma globulin and convalescent gamma globulin: a follow-up study. Acta Paediatr. 50:444–452, 1961.

Marshall, W. C., and Peckham, C.: The management of herpes simplex in pregnant women and neonates. J. Infect. 6(Suppl. 1):23–29, 1983.

Matsumato, S., Togashi, T., Kuwajima, S., Takebasashi, T., Fujimoto, S., Uzuki, K., Sugawara, T., Inogawa, A., Akino, N., and Iwasaki, K.: Prevention of neonatal hepatitis B virus infection by hepatitis N immune globulin. Acta Pediatr. Jpn. 24:289–293, 1982.

Maupas, P., Chiron, J. P., Barin, F., Cousaget, P., Goudeau, A., Perrin, J., Dennis, F., and Diof Mar, I.: Efficacy of hepatitis B vaccine in prevention of early HBsAg carrier state in children. Lancet 1:289–292, 1981.

Mazel, J. A., Schalm, S. W., de Gast, B. C., et al.: Passive-active immunization of neonates of HBsAg possible carrier mothers: preliminary observations. Br. Med. J. 288:613–515, 1984.

McDonald, J. C.: Gamma globulin for prevention of rubella in pregnancy. Br. Med. J. 2:416–418, 1963.

McDonald, J. C.: Gamma globulin prophylaxis of rubella. In First International Conferences on Vaccines Against Viral and Rickettsial Diseases of Man, November 7–11, 1966. WHO Scientific Publication No. 147. Washington, D.C., Pan American Health Organization, 1967, pp. 371–377.

McDonald, J. C., and Peckham, C. S.: Gammaglobulin in the prevention of rubella and congenital defects: a study of 30,000 pregnancies. Br. Med. J. 3:633–637, 1967.

McGuirt, P. V., and Furman, P. A.: Acyclovir inhibition of viral DNA chain elongation in herpes simplex virus–infected cells. Am. J. Med. 73(Suppl.1A)67–71, 1982.

Meyer, H. M., Parkman, P. D., Panos, T. C., Stewart, G. L., Hobbins, T. E., and Ennis, F. A.: Clinical studies with attenuated rubella virus. In First International Conference on Vaccines Against Viral and Rickettsial Diseases of Man. Pan. Am. Health Org. Scientific Publication No. 147, 1967, pp. 390–401.

Meyers, J. D., Wade, J. C., McGuffin, R. W., Springmeyer, S. C., and Thomas, E. D.: The use of acyclovir for cytomegalovirus infections in the immunocompromised host. J. Antimicrob. Chemother. 12(Suppl. B): 181–193, 1983.

Meyers, J. D.: Congenital varicella in term infants: risks reconsidered. J. Infect. Dis. 129:215–217, 1974.

Miranda, P., and Blum, M. R.: Acyclovir pharmacokinetics. J. Antimicrob. Chemother. 12(Suppl B):29–37, 1983.

Miranda, P., Whitley, R. J., Blum, M. R., et al.: Acyclovir kinetics after intravenous infusion. Clin. Pharmacol. Ther. 26:718–728, 1979.

Muller, W. E. G.: Mechanisms of action and pharmacology: chemical agents. In Galoxxo, G. J., Merigan, T. C., and Buchanan, R. A. (eds.): Antiviral Agents and Viral Diseases of Man. New York, Raven Press, 1979, pp. 77–149.

Nahmias, A. J., Visintine, A. M., Riemer, C. B., Del Buonos, I., Shore, S. L., and Starr, S. E.: Herpes simplex virus infection of the fetus and newborn. Progress in clinical and biological research. In Krugman, S., and Gershon, A. A. (eds.): Infections of the Fetus and Newborn Infant. New York, Alan R. Liss, 1975, pp. 63–77.

Offit, P. A., Starr, S. E., Zolnick, P., and Plotkin, S. A.: Acyclovir therapy in neonatal herpes simplex virus infection. Pediatr. Infect. Dis. 1:253–255, 1982.

O'Shea, S., Best, J. M., Banatvala, J. E., Marshall, W. C., and Dudgeo, J. A.: Rubella vaccination: persistence of antibodies for up to 16 years. Br. Med. J. 285:253–255, 1982.

Parkman, P. D., Meyer, H. M., Jr., Kirschstein, R. L., and Hopps, H. E.: Attenuated rubella virus. I. Development and laboratory characterization. N. Engl. J. Med. 275:569–574, 1966.

Pavan-Langton, D.: Ocular viral infections. Med. Clin. North Am. 67:973–990, 1983.

Pavan-Langton, D., Lass, J., Hettinger, M., et al.: Acyclovir and vidarabine in the treatment of ulcerative herpes simplex keratitis. Am. J. Ophthalmol. 92:829–935, 1981.

Peckham, C. S.: A clinical and laboratory study of children exposed in utero to maternal rubella. Arch. Dis. Child. 46:571–577, 1972.

Peckham, C. S.: Clinical and serological assessment of children exposed in utero to confirmed maternal rubella. Br. Med. J. *1*:259–261, 1974.

Percy, D. H., and Albert, D. M.: Developmental defects in rats treated postnatally with 5-iododeocyuridine (IUDR). Teratology *9*:275–286, 1974.

Perkins, F. T.: The preparation and control of vaccines. In Burland, W. L., and Laurance, B. H. (eds.): The Therapeutic Choice in Paediatrics. New York, Longman, Inc., 1972, pp. 139–146.

Plotkin, S. A., Farquhar, J., and Hornberger, E.: Clinical trials with the Towne 125 strain of human cytomegalovirus. J. Infect. Dis. *134*:470–475, 1979.

Polakoff, S.: Immunization of infants at high risk of hepatitis B. Br. Med. J. *285*:1294–1295, 1982.

Polakoff, S.: The use of immunoglobulins in virus infections. In Waterson, A. P. (ed.): Recent Advances in Clinical Virology, No. 3. Edinburgh, Churchill Livingstone, 1983, pp. 117–138.

Prober, C. G., Kirk, L. E., and Keeney, R. E.: Acyclovir therapy of chickenpox in mmunosuppressed children—a collaborative study. Pediatrics *101*:622–625, 1982.

Public Health Laboratory Service: Report of working party on the effect of immunoglobulin in pregnancy. Br. Med. J. *2*:497–500, 1970.

Purcell, R. H., and Gerin, L. G.: Hepatitis B subunit vaccine: a preliminary report of safety and efficacy tests in chimpanzees. In Symposium on Viral Hepatitis. National Academy of Sciences, Washington, D.C., March 17–19, 1975, pp. 395–399.

Reesnik, H. W., Reesnik-Brongers, E. E., Lafeber-Schut, B. J. Th., Kalshown-Benschop, J., and Brumnelhuis, H. G. J.: Prevention of chronic HB$_s$Ag carrier state in infants of HB$_s$Ag positive mothers by hepatitis B immunoglobulin. Lancet *1*:426–438, 1978.

Report of the Committee on Infectious Diseases (The Red Book). 19th ed. Evanston, Ill., American Academy of Pediatrics, 1982.

Rosendahl, C., Kochen, M. M., Fretschmer, R., Wegscheider, K., and Kaiser, D.: Avoidance of perinatal transmission of hepatitis B virus: is passive immunization always necessary? Lancet *1*: 1127–1129, 1983.

Ross, A. H., Julia, A., and Balakrishnan, C.: Toxicity of adenine arabinoside in humans. J. Infect. Dis. *133*(Suppl. B): 92–98, 1976.

Sacks, S. L., Smith, J. L., Pollard, R. B., et al.: Toxicity of vidarabine. J.A.M.A., *241*:28–29, 1979.

Schaeffer, H. J.: Acyclovir chemistry and spectrum of activity. Am. J. Med. *73*(Suppl. 1A):4–6, 1982.

Schinazi, R. F., and Prusoff, W. H.: Antiviral agents. Pediatr. Clin. North Am. *30*:77–92, 1983.

Sever, J. L., Schiff, G. M., and Huebner, R. J.: Inactivated rubella virus vaccine. J. Lab. Clin. Med. *62*:1015, 1963.

Sheppard, S., Smithells, R. W., Peckham, C. S., Dudgeon, J. A., and Marshall, W. C.: National Congenital Rubella Surveillance Programme, 1971–1975. Health Trends *9*:38–41, 1977.

Shipman, C., Jr., Smith, S. H., Carlson, R. H., and Drach, J. C.: Antiviral activity of arabinosyladenine and arabinosylhypoxanthine in herpes simplex virus–infected KB cells: selective inhibtion of viral deoxyribonucleic acid synthesis in synchronized suspension cultures. Antimicrob. Agents Chemother. *9*:120–127, 1976.

Smithells, R. W., Sheppard, Marshall, W. C., and Milton, A.: National Congenital Rubella Surveillance Programme, 1971–1981. Br. Med. J. *285*:1363, 1982.

St. Clair, M. H., Furman, P. A., Lubbers, C. M., and

Elion, G. B.: Inhibition of cellular and virally induced deoxyribonucleic acid and polymerases by the triphosphate of acyclovir. Antimicrob. Agents Chemother. *18*:741–745, 1980.

Tada, H., Yanagida, M., Mishina, J., Fuji, T., Baha, K., Ishikawa, S., Aikara, S., Tsuda, F., Miyakawa, Y., and Mayumi, M.: Combined passive and active immunization for preventing perinatal transmission of hepatitis B virus carrier state. Pediatrics *70*:613–619, 1982.

Takahashi, M., Otawka, T., and Otuno, Y.: Live vaccine to prevent the spread of varicella in children in hospitals. Lancet *2*:1288–1290, 1974.

Takahashi, M., Olumno, Y., Otsuka, T., Osame, J., Takamizawa, A., Sasada, T., and Fubo, T.: Development of a live attenuated varicella vaccine. Biken J. *18*:25–33, 1975.

Tobin, J.: unpublished data (1984)

Tokumaru, T.: A possible role of gamma A immunoglobulin in herpes simplex virus infection in man. J. Immunol. *97*:248–259, 1966.

Tong, M. J., Thursby, M. Rakola, J., McPeak, C., Edwards, V. M., and Moseley, J. M.: Studies on the maternal-infant transmission of the viruses which cause acute hepatitis. Gastroenterology *80*:999–1004, 1981.

Travers, J. P., and Patterson, A.: A controlled trial of adenine arabinoside and trifluorothymidine in herpetic keratitis. J. Int. Med. Res. *6*:102–104, 1978.

Tyms, A. D., Scamars, E. M., and Naim, H. M.: The in vitro activity of acyclovir and related compounds against cytomegalovirus infections. J. Antimicrob. Chemother. *8*:65–72, 1981.

Varma, R. R.: Hepatitis B surface antigen carrier state in neonates. Prophylaxis with large doses of conventional immune human serum globulin. J.A.M.A., *236*:2303–2304, 1976.

Welch, R. J., Nahmias, A. J., Visintine, A. M., Fleming, C. L., and Alford, C. A.: The natural history of herpes simplex infection of mother and newborn. Pediatrics *66*:489–494, 1980.

Whitley, R. J., Alford, C., Hess, F., and Buchanan, R.: Vidarabine: a preliminary review of its pharmacological properties and therapeutic use. Drugs *20*:267–282, 1980a.

Whitley, R. J., Nahmias, A. J., Soong, S. J., Gallasso, G. G., Fleming, C. L., and Alford, C. A.: Vidarabine therapy of neonatal herpes simplex virus infection. Pediatrics *66*:495–501, 1980b.

Whitley, R. J., Hilty, M., Haynes, R., Bryson, Y., Connor, J. D., Soong, S. J., Alford, C. A., and the National Institute of Allergy and Infectious Diseases Collaborative Antiviral Study Group. Vidarabine therapy of varicella in immunosuppressed patients. J. Pediatr. *101*:125–131, 1982.

Whitley, R. J., and the National Institute of Allergy and Infectious Diseases Collaborative Antiviral Study Group. Interim summary of mortality in herpes simplex encephalitis and neonatal herpes simplex virus infections: vidarabine versus acyclovir. J. Antimicrob. Chemother. *12*(Suppl. B):105–112, 1983.

World Health Organization. Human Viral and Rickettsial Vaccines. WHO Technical Report Series, No. 325, 1966.

Yeager, A. S.: Use of acyclovir in premature and term neonates. Am. J. Med. *73*(Suppl. 1A): 205–209, 1982.

Zuckerman, A. J.: Properties for immunization against hepatitis B. Br. Med. J. *284*:686–688, 1982.

Zuckerman, A. J., and Howard, C. R.: Hepatitis Viruses of Man. London, Academic Press, 1979.

Index

Note: Page numbers in *italics* indicate illustrations; those followed by (t) indicate tables.

Abortion
  spontaneous, and cytomegalovirus infection, 101–102
    and hepatitis A, 185
    and herpes simplex infection, 134
    and mumps, 206
    and rubella, 41–43, 42(t)
    viruses causing, 5(t)
  therapeutic, assessing risks for, 7–8
    for inadvertent rubella vaccination during pregnancy, 79
    for maternal cytomegalovirus infection, 124
Abrasions, and neonatal infection, 231
Acyclovir, 288(t), 289–290, 290(t)
  for cytomegalovirus infection, 123, 292
  for herpes simplex infection, 147–148, 288(t), 289–290, 290(t)
  for varicella-zoster infection, 288(t), 289–290, 292
  in pregnancy, 292
Adenine arabinoside. See *Arabinoside(s).*
Adrenals, in herpes simplex infection, 142–143
Alastrim, 175
Amnionic fluid
  as immune mechanism, 232
  infections of, 232
Anemia, hemolytic, in cytomegalovirus infection, 110
Anencephaly, and influenza, 203, 204
Angiitis, obliterative, in rubella, *34,* 35
Antibodies. See also under specific virus.
  fetal production of, 237–238
    effect of infection on, 238
  maternal transmission of, 239
  persistence of, and intrauterine infection diagnosis, 239
  and retrospective infection diagnosis, 239
Antibody-antigen complexes, pathological effects of, 239
Antigen(s). See also under specific virus.
  Australian, 183
  direct detection of, 262–263
    collection of material for, 260
  histocompatibility, in rubella, 62
Anti-HAIgM, 184
Anti-HBcIgG, and stage of disease, 194(t)
Anti-HBcIgM, and stage of disease, 194(t)
Anti-HBe, and stage of disease, 194(t)
Anti-HBs, and stage of disease, 194(t)
Anti-hepatitis A virus, 184
Aorta, abdominal, hypoplasia of, in rubella, 35

Arabinoside(s)
  for cytomegalovirus infection, 123
  for herpes simplex infection, 148
  teratogenicity of, 292
Arbovirus infections, 208–209
Arterial intimal proliferation, in rubella, *34,* 35
Australian antigen, 183
Autism, in rubella, 58

B-lymphocytes, 235
  differentiation of, 237
  identification methods for, 236
Bacteria, gastrointestinal, colonizing, 232
Bacterial infections, differential diagnosis of, 243
Behavioral disorders, and rubella, 58
Biliary atresia, and cytomegalovirus infection, 111
Bilirubin determinations, 253–254
Birth weight
  low, and rubella, 5(t), 53–54
    viruses causing, 5(t)
Bittner agent, 5
Blennorrhea, inclusion, 250
Blood samples, collection of, 260, 261(t)
Blood transfusions
  and jaundice, 254
  cytomegalovirus transmission via, 99–100, 124, 254
  infection transmission via, 254
Blood vessels
  hypoplasia of, in rubella, 35
  mineralization of, in rubella, 35
Bone lesions, in rubella, 38, 59
Bone marrow, in rubella, 36
Brain
  biopsy of, in herpes simplex infection, 144
  pathologic changes in, in cytomegalovirus infection, 105
  in rubella, 36–38
Brain tumors, cerebral calcifications in, 247, 248(t)
Breast milk
  and moderation of intestinal colonization, 232
  cytomegalovirus transmission via, 97
  hepatitis B transmission via, 190–191
  infection transmission via, 5
Bromovinyldeoxyuridine, 291

Calcifications, cerebral. See *Cerebral calcifications.*

Carcinoma, hepatocellular, and hepatitis B virus, 193

Cardiomyopathy, chronic, and mumps, 208

Cardiovascular abnormalities. See also *Heart disease.*
  and Coxsackie B infections, 157
  and cytomegalovirus infection, 111, 111(t)
  and rubella, *34,* 35, 49(t), 55–56

Cataracts
  conditions associated with, 250(t)
  differential diagnosis of, 249, 250(t)
  rubella, 35, *50,* 54, 249, 250(t)
    early diagnosis and treatment of, 65–66
    incidence of, and time of infection, 46(t), 47(t)

Cell-mediated immunity, stimulation of by transfer factor, 287–288

Central auditory imperception, in rubella, 57, 251. See also *Deafness.*

Cerebral calcifications
  computed tomography for, 248
  conditions associated with, 248(t)
  differential diagnosis of, 246–248, *247,* 248(t)
  in brain tumors, 247, 248(t)
  in cytomegalovirus infection, 107, 109, *109, 110,* 246–247, 248(t)
    vs. toxoplasmosis, 121
  herpes simplex infection, 138, *139,* 248(t)
  in rubella, 248(t)
  in toxoplasmosis, 246–247, *247,* 248(t)
  in tuberous meningitis, 247
  in tuberous sclerosis, 247–248, 248(t)

Cerebral dysfunction, minimal, in cytomegalovirus infection, 112

Cesarean section, for prevention of herpes simplex infection, 146–147, 148(t), 281

CF antigens, 67

Chemotaxis, phagocytic, 233

Chemotherapy, antiviral, 288–292, 288(t)

Chickenpox. See *Varicella; Varicella-zoster infection.*

Chorioretinitis. See also *Retinopathy.*
  and cerebral calcifications, 246
  and lymphocytic choriomeningitis virus, 210
  differential diagnosis of, 248–249, 249(t)
  in cytomegalovirus infection, 108, *108,* 248–249, 249(t)
    vs. toxoplasmosis, 121
  in herpes simplex infection, 143, 221–223, *221*
  in rubella, 36, *52,* 249(t)
  in toxoplasmosis, 248–249, 249(t)

Cochlea, epithelial necrosis of, in rubella, 36, *37*

Complement fixation test, 267(t), 269
  for cytomegalovirus, 117–118
  for rubella antibody, 23
  for varicella-zoster virus, 173

Complement system, 234, *234*

Computerized tomography, in cytomegalovirus infection, 116

Congenital defects
  and subclinical maternal infections, 6
  animal studies of, 4–6
  assessing risks of, 7–8
  causes of, classification of, 1

Congenital defects (*Continued*)
  defined, 2
  incidence of, 1–2, 2(t)
  prevention of, 3
  viral etiology of, criteria for, 8(t)
    evidence for, 7–11
    rubella model for, 8
    theories of, development of, 3–6

Conjunctivitis, 249–250

Cord. See *Umbilical cord.*

Corneal haze, transient in rubella, 55, 250

Coxsackie virus
  effects of, 5(t)
  properties of, 155(t)
  vaccine for, 159

Coxsackie virus infection, 155–157, 156(t)
  clinical manifestations of, 156–157, 156(t)
  epidemiology of, 156
  hepatosplenomegaly in, 254, 255(t)
  laboratory diagnosis of, 259–269. See also *Laboratory diagnosis* and specific techniques.
  myocarditis in, 255
  neurological impairment in, 255
  poliovirus vaccine for, 159, 287
  source of, 156

Cytomegalovirus(es)
  antigenic structure of, 115
  as herpesvirus, 112–113
  classification of, 112–113
  complement-fixation test for, 117–118
  excretion of, duration of, 95–96
    maternal, 95
    neonatal, precautions for, 100–101, 280
  fluorescent antibody test for, 118–119
  genetic relatedness of, 115–116
  growth of in tissue culture, 114–115
  hemagglutination inhibition test for, 119
  immunization for, 278–280
  morphology of, *104,* 113–114
  neutralization tests for, 119
  radioimmunoassay for, 119
  recovery of from amnionic fluid, 102
  replication of, 102–103
  staining reactions of, 114
  tissue samples of, 117
  transmission of, 96–101, 96(t)
    and sanitation, 96–97
    and socioeconomic group, 96–97
    between adults, 97
    during infancy and childhood, 96, 96(t)
    guidelines for nursery personnel for, 100–101, 280
    in hospital, 100
    intrapartum, 97–98
    prenatal, 96–97, 96(t)
    via breast milk, 97
    via cervix, 102–103
    via transfusions, 99–100, 124, 254

Cytomegalovirus antigen, monoclonal antibody test for, 117

Cytomegalovirus antigen-antibody complexes, and vascular injury, 239

Cytomegalovirus-IgM test, 118–119

Cytomegalovirus infection, 92–125
  acute fulminant, pathological findings in, 103–105
  antibody response in, immunological tests for, 263, 267(t), 269–270
  cardiovascular anomalies in, 111, 111(t)

Cytomegalovirus infection (*Continued*)
  cell-mediated immunity defect in, 236–237
  cerebral calcifications in, 107, 109, *109, 110,* 246–247, 248(t)
  cerebral lesions in, 105
  chemotherapy for, 123, 292
  chorioretinitis in, 108, *108,* 248–249, 249(t)
    vs. toxoplasmosis, 121
  clinical manifestations of, 92, 105–112
    late, 112
  congenital anomalies in, 111–112, 111(t)
  deafness in, 109–110, 250–251
    late-onset, 123
  dental abnormalities in, 111–112
  diagnosis of, 114–120
    clinical, 114
    difficulty of, 112
    histopathological, 119–120, *120*
    laboratory, 259–269
    serological, 115–116
    virological, 114–115
  differential diagnosis of, 120–122
    and placental findings, 219
  effects of, 5(t)
    long-term, 123
  enzyme-linked immunosorbent assay for, 119
  epidemiology of, 93–96
  extraneural lesions in, 103
  fetal infection with, pathogenesis of, 101
  fetal lesions in, 103
    histological, early, 214–216, *215, 216*
      late, 216–218, *217, 218*
  gastrointestinal abnormalities in, 111, 111(t)
  genitourinary abnormalities in, 111
  geographical distribution of, 93–94, 94(t)
  hemolytic anemia in, 110
  hepatic lesions in, 104–105
  hepatomegaly in, 105
  hepatosplenomegaly in, 254, 255(t)
  historical introduction to, 92–93
  host range for, 93
  hydrocephalus in, 109, *110,* 247
  hyperbilirubinemia in, 106
  immune complexes in, 112
  immunoglobulin levels in, 238
  in herpes simplex infection, 252–253, 253(t)
  interferon response in, 235
  laboratory aspects of, 112–116
  laboratory diagnosis of, 259–267. See also *Laboratory diagnosis* and specific techniques.
  learning disabilities in, 112
  maternal, abortion for, 124
    incidence of, 94–95, 95(t)
  mental retardation in, incidence of, 95
  microcephaly in, 107–108, *107*
  microphthalmus in, 250
  misdiagnosis of, 244
  musculoskeletal abnormalities in, 111, 111(t)
  ocular abnormalities in, 108–109, *108*
  optic atrophy in, 109
  pathogenesis of, 101–103
  pathological findings in, 103–105, *104*
  petechiae in, 106–107
  placental lesions in, 102, 214–220
    early, 214–216, *215, 216*
    histopathological findings in, 219
    late, 217–219, *217, 218*
  pneumonitis in, 110–111

Cytomegalovirus infection (*Continued*)
  prevention of, 124–125
  prognosis in, 122–123
  pulmonary lesions in, 104, *104*
    histopathology of, 216, *216*
  purpura in, 106–107, *106,* 252–253, 253(t)
  renal lesions in, 104
  retinopathy in, 248–249, 249(t)
  seasonal incidence of, 95
  silent, long-range effects of, 92
  spontaneous abortion in, 101–102
  subclinical, manifestations of, 112
  thrombocytopenia in, 106–107
  treatment of, 123–124
  urinalysis in, 116–117
  vaccination for, 124–125, 279–280
    reinfection in, 274
  vs. disseminated herpes simplex infection, 121–122
  vs. rubella, 121
  vs. sepsis of newborn, 122
  vs. syphilis, 122
  vs. toxoplasmosis, 121, 121(t)
  with Epstein-Barr virus infection, 209
  without fetal damage, 103
Cytomegalovirus vaccine, 124–125, 279–280
  oncogenicity of, 274
Cytosine arabinoside. See *Arabinoside(s).*

Deafness
  differential diagnosis of, 250–251
  in cytomegalovirus infection, 109–110, 250–251
    late-onset, 123
  in mumps, 251
  in rubella, 56–57, 250–251
    and gestational age at infection, 43–45, 44(t), 46(t), 47(t), 48
    infectious vs. genetic causes of, 4
Delayed hypersensitivity reactions, elicitation of, in newborn, 236
Delta-antigen associated hepatitis, 183, 194–196
  in cytomegalovirus infection, 111–112
Dental abnormalities
  in rubella, 38
Dermal erythropoiesis, 144
Dermatoglyphics, abnormal, in rubella, 61
Diabetes mellitus, and rubella, 61–62
Disciform macular degeneration, in rubella, 36, *52,* 54–55
Disseminated intravascular coagulation, in herpes simplex infection, 149
Down's syndrome, 245
  and hepatitis A, 185
Drugs. See also specific agents.
  antiviral, 288–292, 288(t)
  teratogenic, 4

ECHO virus(es), properties of, 155(t)
ECHO virus infection, 157–158
Eczema vaccinatum, 176
Electron microscopy, 262
  sample collection for, 260

Encephalitis
  herpetic, 142
    brain biopsy in, 144
  rubella, adult, vs. congenital rubella meningoencephalitis, 36
  chronic, 58
  western equine, 208–209
Endocardial fibroblastosis, and mumps, 11, 208
Enteroviral infections, 154–158. See also
    Coxsackie virus infection; ECHO virus infection; Poliomyelitis.
  central neurologic impairment in, 255
  congenital defects in, evidence for, 11
  diagnosis of, 158
  immunization for, 286–287
  oral poliovaccine for, 287
  prevention of, 158–159
  treatment of, 158
Enterovirus(es)
  hepatitis A virus as, 184
  immunization for, 286–287
  laboratory diagnosis of, 259–267. See also
    Laboratory diagnosis and specific techniques.
  properties of, 155(t)
Enzyme immunoassay, 262, 267(t), 268–269
Enzyme-linked immunoabsorbent assay, 262, 267(t), 269
  for cytomegalovirus, 119
Epstein-Barr virus, 209–210, 210(t)
  laboratory diagnosis of, 259–267. See also
    Laboratory diagnosis and specific techniques.
Erythropoiesis, dermal, 144
Eye. See also specific ocular disorders.
  in herpes simplex infection, 143
  in rubella, 49(t), 54–55. See also under *Rubella.*
  in viral infections, 248–250, 249(t), 250(t)

Failure to thrive, differential diagnosis of, 251–252, 252(t)
FAMA test, for varicella-zoster antibody, 173
Fetal membranes, rupture of, and risk of infection, 232
Fetal scalp monitoring, and viral transmission, 135
Fluorescent antibody test
  for cytomegalovirus, 118–119
  for herpes simplex infection, 145
Fluorescent antigen-antibody test, 269–270
Fluorescent antigen membrane antibody technique, 270
Fluoroiodoaracytosine, 291
Funisitis, herpetic, 221–223, *221, 223, 224*

Galactosemia, cataracts in, 249, 250(t)
Gamma globulin. See also *Immunoglobulin(s).*
  for rubella exposure in pregnancy, 278
Gastrointestinal tract
  abnormalities of in cytomegalovirus infection, 111, 111(t)
  colonization of, 232
Genital herpes, lesions in, 137, *138*
Genitourinary abnormalities, in cytomegalovirus infection, 111
Glaucoma
  differential diagnosis of, 250

Glaucoma (*Continued*)
  in rubella, 55, 250
    incidence of, and gestational age at infection, 47(t)
Graft-versus-host disease, 236
Granulocytes, 233–234
Granulomatous pox placentitis, 225, *226*
Great vessels, defects of, in rubella, 55–56
Growth hormone deficiency, in rubella, 62
Growth retardation
  intrauterine, and placental hypoplasia, 228
  in rubella, 53–54
    lymphocyte population in, 235–236
Gut, colonization of, 232

HA antigen, 67
Hamsters, and lymphocytic choriomeningitis virus, 210
HBcAG, 186
  and stage of disease, 194(t)
HBeAG, 186
  and carrier state, 190
HBsAG, 186
  and stage of disease, 194(t)
Heart disease. See also *Cardiovascular abnormalities.*
  congenital, and Coxsackie B infections, 157
  and mumps, 208
    differential diagnosis of, 255–256, 256(t)
  in enteroviral infection, treatment of, 158
  in rubella, 255–256, 256(t)
    incidence of, and time of infection, 46(t), 47(t)
Helper inducer T-lymphocytes, 235
Hemagglutination
  passive, 262, 267(t), 269
  reverse passive, 262, 267(t), 269
Hemagglutinin-infection rubella antibody, persistence of, 31–32
Hemagglutination inhibition test, 267(t), 269
  for cytomegalovirus, 119
  for rubella antibody, 23
Hemolysis, radial, 269
Hemolytic anemia, in cytomegalovirus infection, 110
Hemolytic disease, jaundice in, vs. congenital infections, 253–254
Hemorrhage, in herpes simplex infection, 141
Heparin, for disseminated intravascular coagulation, in herpes simplex infection, 149
Hepatitis
  viral, 182–196
    clinical outcome in, 191–192
    Delta antigen-associated, 183, 194–196
    forms of, 183
    fulminant, 192–193
    historical introduction to, 182–183
    nomenclature for, earlier, 183(t)
      new, 184(t)
    non-A, non-B, 194–196
      laboratory diagnosis of, 259–267. See
        also *Laboratory diagnosis* and specific techniques.
    prevention of, in pregnancy, 286
  persistent antigenemia in, 192
  post-transfusion, 254
  present concept of, 183–184

Hepatitis (*Continued*)
  serological markers of, interpretation of,
    187(t)
  transmission of, perinatal, 191
  type A, 184–185
    and Down's syndrome, 185
    and prematurity, 185
    and spontaneous abortion, 185
    causative agent of, 184
    effects of, 5(t), 185
    epidemiology of, 184–185
    immunization for, 286
    laboratory aspects of, 185
    laboratory diagnosis of, 185, 259–269.
      See also *Laboratory diagnosis* and spe-
      cific techniques.
    natural history of, 184
    pathogenesis of, 184
    prevention of, 196
  type B, 185–194
    and congenital defects, 193
    at-risk groups for, 189(t)
    carrier state in, and HBeAg, 190,
      190(t)
      factors predisposing to, 188
      laboratory findings in, 195(t)
    causative agent of, 185–186
    effects of, 5(t)
    epidemiology of, 186–188
    familial, 192–193
    human normal immune serum globulin
      for, 282, 284–285
    immunization for, 281–286
      active, 283–284
      passive, 282–283
      passive-active, 284
    laboratory diagnosis of, 193–194, 194(t),
      195(t), 259–267. See also *Laboratory di-
      agnosis* and specific techniques.
    maternal, time of, and risk of fetal in-
      fection, 189
    mode of spread of, 188, 189(t)
    natural history of, 186
    pathogenesis of, 186, *187, 188*
    prevalence of, 186–188, 188(t)
    prevention of, 196
      general measures for, 285–286, 285(t)
    prognosis in, and serological markers,
      194
    serological markers of, and prognosis,
      194
      laboratory tests for, 194, 194(t)
    sources of infection in, 188–191, 189(t),
      190(t)
      carrier mothers as, 189–190, 190(t)
    stage of, laboratory findings in, 194(t)
    transmission of, in pregnancy, 188–191
      transplacental, 191
      via breast milk, 190–191
      via carrier mothers, 189–190, 190(t)
      via family members, 191
Hepatitis A virus
  as cause of congenital defects, evidence for,
    9, 10(t), 11
  identification of, 185
  properties of, 184
Hepatitis B antibodies
  and stage of disease, *187,* 194(t)
  combinations of, interpretation of, 187(t)
  in carrier state, 195(t)
  laboratory tests for, 193–194, 194(t)
  nomenclature for, 184(t)

Hepatitis B antigen(s)
  and stage of disease, *187,* 194(t)
  combinations of, interpretation of, 187(t)
  core, 186
  e, 186
  in carrier state, 195(t)
  laboratory tests for, 193–194, 194(t)
  surface, 186
  test results for, interpretation of, 187(t)
  types of, 186
Hepatitis B immunoglobulin, with hepatitis B
    vaccine, 284–285
Hepatitis B vaccine(s), 283–284
  with hepatitis B immunoglobulin, 284–285
Hepatitis B virus, 192
  and hepatocellular carcinoma, 193
  properties of, 185–186
  sources of, 188, 189(t)
Hepatoadrenal necrosis, in herpes simplex in-
    fection, *136,* 142–143
Hepatocellular carcinoma, and hepatitis B vi-
    rus, 193
Hepatomegaly
  differential diagnosis of, 254, 255(t)
  in cytomegalovirus infection, 105, *106*
Hepatosplenomegaly
  differential diagnosis of, 254, 255(t)
  in rubella, 59
Herpes simplex infection, 132–159
  acyclovir for, 147–148, 288(t), 289–290,
    290(t), 291
  adenine arabinoside for, 148
  and congenital anomalies, 138, *139*
  and premature labor, 137
  and spontaneous abortion, 134
  antiviral drugs for, 147–148, 288(t),
    289–290, 290(t), 291
  asymptomatic, 132
  bacterial sepsis in, management of, 149
  bleeding in, 141
  brain biopsy in, 144
  central nervous system manifestations of,
    140, 142
  cerebral calcifications in, 138, *139,* 248(t)
    chemotherapy for, 147–148, 281, 288(t),
      289–290, 290(t), 291
  clinical manifestations of, 137–143
    and prognosis, 150, 150(t)
    intrauterine infection, 137–138, *138, 139*
    presenting, 291
  diagnosis of, 143–146
    clinical, 143–144
    cytological, 146
    electron microscopic, 146
    histopathological, 144–145, *145*
    laboratory, 259–269. See also *Laboratory di-
      agnosis* and specific techniques.
    serological, 145
    virological, 145–146, *146*
  disseminated intravascular coagulation in,
    149
  electrolyte monitoring in, 149
  epidemiology of, 132–133
  hepatoadrenal necrosis in, *136,* 142
  hepatosplenomegaly in, 254, 255(t)
  idoxuridine for, 147, 288(t), 290, 291
  immunization for, 280
  immunoglobulin for, 147, 280
  incidence of, 132–133
    in pregnancy, 132–133
  interferon inducers for, 148
  intrapartum, 138–143, *139–143*

Herpes simplex infection (*Continued*)
isoimmune globulin for, 147
keratoconjunctivitis in, 250
management of, 146–150, 148(t), 280–281
maternal, chemotherapy for, 291
clinical manifestations of, 137, *138*
management of, 280–281
prevention of infant infection in, 150
by cesarean section, 146–147, 148(t), 281
vulvovaginitis in, 137, *138*
ocular manifestations of, 143, 249(t)
nursery personnel guidelines for, 150
pathogenesis of, 133–136
pathology of, 136
placental, 220–223, *220–223*
prevention of, by cesarean section, 146–147, 148(t), 281
prognosis in, 150, 150(t)
purpura in, 252–253, 253(t)
respiratory distress in, 140–141
retinopathy in, 249(t)
seizures in, 140, 142, 248
skin lesions in, and diagnosis, 144
incidence of, 144
maternal, 137, *138*
neonatal, 138–141, *140, 141*
susceptibility to, 136–137
transcervical, 221–223, *221–223*
transmission of, antepartum, 133
intrapartum, 135
paternal, 135
postpartum, 135–136
time of, 135
venereal, 133–134
transplacental, 220, *220*
trifluorothymidine for, 288(t), 290
umbilical, 221–223, *221, 223, 224*
vaccination for, 280
vidarabine for, 148, 288–289, 288(t), 291
vs. cytomegalovirus infection, 121–122
Herpes varicellae, 173
Herpesvirus
cytomegalovirus as, 112–113
effects of, 5(t)
replication of, 185
strains of, 132
Histocompatibility antigens, in rubella, 62
HL-A antigens, in rubella, 62
Hydrocephalus
and lymphocytic choriomeningitis virus, 210
cytomegalovirus infection, 109, *110*, 247
Hyperbilirubinemia, in cytomegalovirus infection, 106
Hyperimmune hepatitis B immunoglobulin, 282–283
Hypermetropia, and microphthalmus, 250
Hypersensitivity reactions, delayed, elicitation of, in newborn, 236
Hypogammaglobulinemia, in rubella, 60, 238
Hypospadias, in cytomegalovirus infection, 111
Hypothyroidism, in rubella, 62
Hypotonia
differential diagnosis of, 243
in rubella, 58

Icterus. See *Jaundice.*
Idoxuridine, 288(t), 290, 291
for cytomegalovirus infection, 123

Idoxuridine (*Continued*)
for herpes simplex infection, 147, 288(t), 290, 291
Idoxuridine-dimethyl sulfoxide, 288(t), 290
IgA. See also *Immunoglobulin(s).*
deficiency of, in congenital infections, 238
fetal synthesis of, 237, *238*
in intrauterine infections, 237
rubella, 31
IgE. See also *Immunoglobulin(s).*
fetal synthesis of, 237, *238*
IgG. See also *Immunoglobulin(s).*
fetal synthesis of, 237, *238*
in intrauterine infections, 237
in rubella, 31
in reinfection, 23–24
maternal transmission of, 239
IgM. See also *Immunoglobulin(s).*
fetal synthesis of, 237, *238*
intrauterine infections, 237
in rubella, 23–24, 31
tests for, 263, 267(t), 269–270
IgM-specific antibody, tests for, 267(t), 270
Immune adherence, 267(t), 269
Immune adherence hemagglutination technique, 270
Immune complexes, in cytomegalovirus infection, 112
Immune mechanisms
activation of, factors in, 231
development of, 230–239
fetal, discovery of, 230–231
nonspecific, 231–235, 231(t), *232*
amnionic fluid as, 232
mucous membranes as, 231–232
opsonization as, 234–235
phagocytosis as, 233–235, *234*
placenta as, 228, 232–233
skin as, 231–232
specific, 235–237
Immunity, cell-mediated, stimulation of by transfer factor, 287–288
Immunization. See also *Vaccination; Vaccine(s).*
for enteroviral infections, 286–287
for hepatitis A, 286
for hepatitis B, 281–286
active, 283–284
passive, 282–283
passive-active, 284
for herpes simplex infections, 280
for influenza, 287
for rubella, 274–277
active, 274–277
passive, 277
for vaccinia, 281
for variola, 281
need for, factors in, 273(t)
Immunoassays, 262, 267(t), 268–269
Immunodiffusion techniques, 267(t), 269
Immunoelectron microscopy, 262, 268
sample collection for, 260, 261(t)
Immunofluorescence, 262, 267(t), 268
Immunoglobulin(s). See also specific immunoglobulins.
development of, 237–239, *238*
for cytomegalovirus infection, 280
hepatitis A, 286
hepatitis B, with hepatitis vaccine, 282, 284–285
for herpes simplex infection, 147, 280
for rubella exposure in pregnancy, 278

Immunoglobulin(s) (*Continued*)
 for rubella exposure in pregnancy, 278
 for varicella-zoster infection, 281
 human normal serum, for hepatitis B, 282
 hyperimmune, hepatitis B, 282–283
 levels of, in intrauterine infections, 237
 maternal transmission of, 239
 synthesis of, fetal, 237
  neonatal, 238
 vaccinial hyperimmune, 281
Immunological system
 competence of, genetic factors in, 239
 immunopathological mechanisms in, 239
Immunological tests, for virus, 259(t), 263,
  267(t), 269–270
Immunological tolerance, therapy of, 230
Inclusion blennorrhea, 250
Infections. See *Viral infection(s)*.
Influenza
 and outcome of pregnancy, 201(t), 202(t),
  203(t)
 as cause of congenital defects, 4, 5(t),
  200–205
  and time of infection, 202(t), 203–204
  criteria for, 205
  evidence for, 10(t), 11
  studies of, 201–205, 201(t)–203(t)
 effects of, 5(t)
 immunization for, 287
Influenza virus, 200–205
Inspissated bile syndrome, 254
Interferon
 action of, 234–235
 for cytomegalovirus infections, 123
  with acyclovir, 292
 production of, 234–235
  impaired, rubella, 32
 types of, 234
Interferon inducers, for herpes simplex infection, 148
Intestines, colonization of, 232
Iota antigen, 67
Iris, pathologic changes in, in rubella, 35, 55
Isoimmune globulin, for herpes simplex infection, 147

Jaundice
 and maternal hepatitis A, 185
 differential diagnosis of, 253–254, 255(t)
 in cytomegalovirus infection, 106

Keratoconjunctivitis, herpes simplex virus, 250
Kidney, cytomegalovirus lesions in, 104
Kupffer cells, 233

Laboratory diagnosis, 258–267
 collection of material for, 260, 261(t)
 immunological tests for, 263, 267(t),
  269–270
 procedures for, outline of, 259(t)
 virus isolation techniques for, 262–263,
  264(t), 265, 266
Learning disabilities, and cytomegalovirus infection, 112
Leukemia, congenital, animal models of, 5–6

Leukocytes, polymorphonuclear, 233
Liver
 in cytomegalovirus infection, 104–105
 in herpes simplex infection, *136*, 142–143
 in rubella, *34*, 36, 59, 254, 255(t)
Low birth weight
 and hepatitis B, 192
 and rubella, 5(t), 53–54
 viruses causing, 5(t)
Lowe's syndrome, cataracts in, 249, 250(t)
Lung
 in cytomegalovirus infection, 104, *104*
 in rubella, 36
Lymph nodes, in rubella, 36
Lymphocytes
 B, 235
 development of, 235
 suppressor cytotoxic, 235
 T, 235
Lymphocytic choriomeningitis virus, 210
Lymphokines, 233, 236

Macrophage(s), 233–234
 viral persistence in, 233
Macrophage migration inhibition factor, 233
Macular disciform degeneration, in rubella, 36,
  52, 54–55
Malnourished infant, diagnosis of, 251
Measles, 205–206(t), 207(t)
 and fetal and infant mortality, 205, 296(t)
 and pregnancy outcome, 205–206, 206(t)
 as cause of congenital defects, 206, 207(t)
  evidence for, 9, 10(t)
 effects of, 5(t)
Meningitis
 bacterial, seizures in, 248
 enteroviral 157
 in rubella, 58
 tuberous, cerebral calcifications in, 247
Meningoencephalitis, in rubella, 36–38
Mental retardation. See also *Psychomotor retardation*.
 differential diagnosis of, 243–248
 in cytomegalovirus infection, 95
 incidence of, 243
 pathophysiological classification of, 246(t)
 signs of, 244–245
Microcephaly
 conditions associated with, 247(t)
 differential diagnosis of, 245–246, 247(t)
 in cytomegalovirus infection, 107–108, *107*
 in rubella, 36
Microphthalmus
 differential diagnosis of, 250, 251(t)
 in rubella, 35, 55
Milk, breast. See *Breast milk*.
Minimal cerebral dysfunction, in cytomegalovirus infection, 112
Miscarriage. See *Abortion, spontaneous*.
Mucous membranes, as immune mechanism,
  231–232
Mumps, 206–208
 and chronic cardiomyopathy, 208
 and deafness, 251
 and endocardial fibroelastosis, 208
 and fetal death, 206
 and primary endocardial fibroblastosis, 11
 as cause of congenital defects, 5–6, 5(t)
  evidence for, 9–11, 10(t)

Musculoskeletal abnormalities, in cytomegalovirus infection, 111, 111(t)
Myocardial necrosis, in rubella, *34, 35*
Myocarditis
in Coxsackie B infection, 255
in rubella, 56, 256, 256(t)
prenatal, and mumps virus, 208
Myopia, in rubella, 250
Myxedema, in rubella, 62

Neural tube defects
and influenza, 202–205
causes of, 3
prevention of, by vitamin supplementation, 3
Neutralization tests, for cytomegalovirus, 119
Nystagmus, in rubella, 55

Ocular. See *Eye.*
Oculocerebrorenal syndrome, cataracts in, 249,
250(t)
Opsonins, 234–235
Opsonization, 234–235
Optic atrophy, in cytomegalovirus infection,
109
Osteopathy, in rubella, 38, 59

Panencephalitis, chronic progressive, in rubella, 36–38, 58
Parotitis. See *Mumps.*
Patent ductus arteriosus, in rubella, 35, 55–56,
255–256, 256(t)
Petechiae
differential diagnosis of, 252–253, 253(t)
in cytomegalovirus infections, 106–107
Phagocytosis, 233–235
cells in, 233
chemotaxis in, 233
macrophages in, 233–234
opsonization in, 234–235
steps in, 233
Phytohemagglutinin, lymphocyte response to,
236
Pigmentary retinopathy, in rubella, *51,* 54. See
also *Retinopathy.*
Placenta. See also *Villitis.*
as immune mechanism, 228, 232–233
hypoplasia of, and growth retardation, 228
in cytomegalovirus infection, 102, 214–219
histopathological lesions in, diagnostic significance of, 219
early, 214–216, *215, 216*
late, 217–219, *217, 218*
in herpes simplex infection, 220–223
in rubella, 28–29, 225–228, *227*
histopathological changes in, 34–35
in vaccinia, 225, *226*
in varicella, 223–225, *224, 225*
in variola, 225
interferon production by, 234–235
pathology of, 213–228
prognostic significance of, 214
variables in, 214
Placentitis, granulomatous pox, 225, *226*

Pneumonia, desquamative interstitial, in rubella, 60
Pneumonitis
in cytomegalovirus infection, 110–111
interstitial, in rubella, 36, 60
Poliomyelitis, 154–155
as cause of congenital defects, evidence for,
9, 10(t)
immunization for, 286–287
in pregnancy, 158, 287
Poliovirus
effects of, 5(t)
properties of, 155(t)
Poliovirus vaccine, 286–287
for Coxsackie B virus infection, 159, 287
pure culture for, 274
Polymorphonuclear leukocytes, 233
Pregnancy
acyclovir in, 292
herpes simplex infection in, incidence of,
132–133
poliomyelitis vaccination in, 158, 287
rubella exposure in, gamma globulin for,
278
rubella vaccination in, 11, 76–78, 77(t), 78(t),
276, 277
smallpox vaccination in, 11
Prematurity
and hepatitis A, 185
and hepatitis B, 192
and herpes simplex infection, 137
and maternal influenza, 204
Primordial central nervous system, diagnosis
of, 252
Progressive vaccinia gangrenosum, 176
Psychomotor retardation. See also *Mental retardation.*
and microcephaly, in cytomegalovirus infection, 107–108, *107*
differential diagnosis of, 243–245
in herpes simplex infection, 138, *139*
incidence of, 243
signs of, 244–245
Pulmonary artery stenosis, in rubella, 35,
55–56, 255–256, 256(t)
Purpura
differential diagnosis of, 252–253, 253(t)
in cytomegalovirus infection, 106–107, *106,*
252–253, 253(t)
in rubella, *51,* 59
incidence of, and time of infection, 47(t)

Radial hemolysis, 269
Radioimmunoassay, 262, 267(t), 269
for cytomegalovirus, 119
Rash
chronic rubelliform, *52.* 60
petechial, differential diagnosis of, 252–253,
253(t)
in cytomegalovirus infection, 106–107
Reissner's membrane, adherent to tectorial
membrane, 36, *37*
Renal artery stenosis, in rubella, 56
Respiratory disorders, in herpes simplex infection, 140–141
Retardation. See *Growth retardation; Mental retardation; Psychomotor retardation.*

Reticuloendothelial system, pathology of, in rubella, 36
Retinopathy. See also *Chorioretinitis.*
　differential diagnosis of, 248–249, 249(t)
　in cytomegalovirus infection, 248–249, 249(t)
　in herpes simplex infections, 249(t)
　in rubella, 35, 249(t)
　　disciform macular, 36, *52*, 54–55
　　incidence of, and time of infection, 46(t)
　　pigmentary, *51*, 54
　in toxoplasmosis, 248–249, 249(t)
　in varicella, 249(t)
Reverse passive hemagglutination, 262, 267(t), 269
RNA, double-stranded, as interferon-inducer, for herpes simplex infection, 149
Rubella, 13–84
　antibody response in, immunological tests for, 263, 267(t), 269–270
　as cause of congenital defects, investigation of, history of, 13–16, 15(t)
　as model of viral causation of congenital defects, 8
　cerebral calcifications in, 248(t)
　chorioretinitis in, 36, *52*, 249(t)
　congenital, auditory effects of, 36–37, 49(t).
　　　See also *Rubella, congenital, deafness in.*
　　autism in, 58
　　behavioral disorders in, 58
　　bone marrow in, 36
　　cardiovascular defects in, *34*, 35, 49(t), 55–56
　　cataracts in, 35, *50*, 54, 249, 250(t)
　　　early diagnosis and treatment of, 65–66
　　　incidence of, and time of infection, 46(t), 47(t)
　　cell-mediated immune response in, 32, 236–237
　　central nervous system defects in, 36–38, 47(t), 49(t), 57–58
　　　and time of infection, 47(t)
　　clinical manifestations of, 48–66, *49–53*, 49(t)
　　　developmental, 50
　　　in infancy, 59, 59(t)
　　　late-onset, 59–60, 59(t)
　　　permanent, 50
　　　transient, 49–50
　　congenital defects in, age at presentation of, 65(t)
　　　and age at infection, 28, 43–45, 44(t), 45(t), 47(t), 48
　　　incidence of, 47–48, 47(t)
　　　possible mechanisms of, 38–40, *39*, 39(t)
　　　reported but unproven, 49(t)
　　　single vs. multiple, 63–64, 64(t)
　　congenital heart disease in, 255–256, 256(t)
　　　incidence of, and time of infection, 46(t), 47(t)
　　corneal clouding in, transient, 55, 250
　　cytolytic changes in, 38
　　deafness in, 56–57, 250–251
　　　and gestational age at infection, 43–45, 44(t), 46(t), 47(t), 48
　　dental changes in, 38
　　dermatoglyphic abnormalities in, 61
　　diabetes mellitus in, 61–62
　　diagnosis of, 69–71, 71(t)

Rubella (*Continued*)
　congenital, diagnosis of, laboratory, 259–269. See also *Laboratory diagnosis* and specific diagnostic techniques.
　　retrospective, 30, 239
　　disciform macular degeneration in, 36, *52*, 54–55
　　encephalitis in, chronic, 58
　　endocrine disorders in, 61–62
　　fetal and infant mortality in, 53–54
　　glaucoma in, 55, 250
　　　incidence of, and time of infection, 47(t)
　　great vessel defects in, 55–56
　　growth hormone deficiency in, 62
　　hematological changes in, 49(t), 59
　　hepatic changes in, *34*, 36, 59, 254, 255(t)
　　hepatosplenomegaly in, 59, 254, 255(t)
　　histocompatibility antigens in, 62
　　histopathological changes in, 32–38, *34*
　　hypogammaglobulinemia in, 238
　　hypotonia in, 57–58
　　IgA deficiency in, 238
　　immunoglobulin levels in, 31
　　immunological effects of, 49(t)
　　immunopathological reactions in, 40
　　infant infectiousness in, 29–30
　　interferon production in, 32
　　interferon response in, 235
　　interstitial pneumonitis in, 60
　　iris defects in, 35, 55
　　laboratory aspects of, 66–71, 259–269
　　late-onset, 59–60 59(t)
　　　immune complexes in, 62–63, 239
　　long-term effects of, 63
　　low birth weight in, 5(t), 53–54
　　macular degeneration in, 36, *52*, 54–55
　　management of, 64–66
　　meningitis in, 58
　　microphthalmus in, 55, 250
　　mitotic depression in, 38
　　myocarditis in, 56, 256, 256(t)
　　myopia in, 250
　　nystagmus in, 55
　　ocular changes in, 35–36, 49(t), 54–55
　　osteopathy in, 38, 59
　　panencephalitis in, chronic progressive, 58
　　pathology of, 5(t), 32–38, 54–55
　　　auditory, 36, *37*, 49(t)
　　　cardiovascular, *34*, 35, 49(t), 55–56
　　　central nervous system, 36–38, 47(t), 49(t), 57–58
　　　dental, 38
　　　hepatic, *34*, 36, 59, 254, 255(t)
　　　ocular, 35–36, 49(t), 54–55
　　　osseous, 38, 59
　　　placental and chorionic, 32–35
　　　pulmonary, 36, 49(t)
　　　reticuloendothelial, 36
　　　vascular, 38
　　　visceral, 49(t)
　　persistent ductus arteriosus in, 55–56, 255–256, 256(t)
　　placenta in, 28–29, 225–228, *227*
　　prevention of, 71–84
　　psychomotor retardation in, 58
　　pulmonary artery stenosis in, 35, 55–56, 255–256, 256(t)
　　pulmonary disease in, 49(t)
　　　late-onset, 60

Rubella (*Continued*)
  congenital, purpura in, *51,* 59
    incidence of, and time of infection, 47(t)
    renal artery stenosis in, 56
    retinopathy in, 35, 249(t)
      and time of infection, 46(t)
        disciform macular, 36, *52,* 54–55
        pigmentary, *51,* 54
    rubelliform rash in, chronic, *52,* 60
    speech defects in, 57, 60
    strabsimus in, 55
    surveillance programs for, 81–84,
      81(t)–83(t)
    thymic hypoplasia in, 60
    thyroid disorders in, 62
    transient corneal haze in, 55, 250
    ventricular septal defect in, 256, 256(t)
    virus excretion in, 29, *30*
    virus persistence in, 38–40
    vs. cytomegalovirus, 121
  historical introduction to, 13–16
  immunity to, duration of, 24
    vaccine-induced, duration of, 79–81
  immunization for, active, 274–277. See also
    Rubella vaccination.
    passive, 72, 277–278
  laboratory diagnosis of, 259–267. See also
    Laboratory diagnosis and specific diagnostic
    techniques.
  maternal, diagnosis of, 68–69
  maternal exposure to, gamma globulin for,
    278
  postnatal, diagnosis of, 69, 70(t)
    epidemiology of, post-vaccination, 19–20,
      19(t), 20(t)
      pre-vaccination, 17–19, 18(t), 19(t)
    immunity in, 23–24
    incubation period in, 23
    natural history of, 16
    pathogenesis of, 22–27, *22,* 25(t), 26(t)
    reinfection in, 24–27, 25(t), 26(t)
  preconceptional, and congenital defects,
    45–47
  prenatal, after first trimester, 47
    consequences of, 40, *40*
      summarization of, 48
    diagnosis of, 69–71, 71(t)
    epidemiology of, post-vaccination, 22
      pre-vaccination, 20–22
    fetal infection in, incidence of, 28
    fetal injury in, incidence of, 28
      risk of, 40–48
        after first trimester, 47
        and gestational age, 41–45, 42(t),
          44(t), 46(t), 47(t)
        and maternal immune status, 40–41,
          273(t)
    immunogenesis in, 30–31
    natural history of, 16
    pathogenesis of, 22, 27–32
    placental-fetal infection in, 28–29
    spontaneous abortion in, 41–43, 42(t)
    stillbirth in, 41–43, 42(t)
    viremia in, in reinfection, 25
Rubella antibody
  complement-fixation, measurement of, 23
  hemagglutination-inhibition test for, 23
    persistence of, 31–32
  HI, persistence of, in congenital rubella,
    31–32

Rubella antibody (*Continued*)
  IgG, in congenital rubella, 31
    in reinfection, 23–24
  IgM, in congenital rubella, 31
    in primary infection, 23–24
  in primary vs. reinfection, 23–24
  incidence of, 17–19, 18(t), 19(t)
  level of, and risk of reinfection, 24–27
  measurement of, 23
  persistence of, in congenital rubella, 31–32,
    33
    and retrospective diagnosis, 239
  serologic tests for, for retrospective diagno-
    sis, 30
  virus neutralization test for, 23
Rubella antigens, 67
  in late-onset disease, 62–63
Rubella encephalitis, adult, vs. congenital ru-
    bella meningoencephalitis, 36
Rubella retinitis, 35
Rubella vaccination, 274–277
  effectiveness of, 276–277
  inadvertent during pregnancy, 11, 76–78,
    77(t), 78(t), 276, 277
  indications for, 19
  policies for, 74–75, 76(t)
  procedures for, 275–276
  surveillance for, 277
Rubella vaccine(s), 72–84, 274–277
  adverse reactions to, 276
  contraindications to, 276
  development of, 274–275
  dosage and administration of, 276, 276(t)
  duration of immunity after, 79–81
  effectiveness of, 276–277
  indications for, 276
  killed inactivated, 72
  live attenuated, 72–74, 73(t)
  policy for, 74–75
  precautions for, 276
  reactions to, 75
  requirements for, 72
  safety of, 81
  surveillance of, 80–81
  teratogenicity of, 11, 74–75, 76–79,
    77(t)–79(t)
  transmissibility of, 75–76
  types of, 275–276, 275(t), 276(t)
  usage of, 276
Rubella virus
  cultivation of, 67
  properties of, 66–67

Scalp monitoring, and virus transmission, 135
Seizures
  differential diagnosis of, 248
  in herpes simplex infection, 140, 142, 248
Sepsis, of newborn, vs. cytomegalovirus infec-
    tion, 122
Serum hepatitis antigen, 183
Serum samples, collection of, 260, 261(t)
Short stature infant, diagnosis of, 251–252
Single radial hemolysis, 269
Skin, as immune mechanism, 231–232
Skin-graft rejection, 236
Skin scrapings, collection of, 260
Small-for-gestational age infants, lymphocyte
    population in, 235–236

Smallpox. See *Variola.*
Smears
  examination of, 262, *263*
  sample collection for, 260, 261(t)
Spasticity, differential diagnosis of, 243
Speech defects, in rubella, 57, 60
Splenomegaly
  differential diagnosis of, 254, 255(t)
  in cytomegalovirus infection, 105–106, *106*
  in rubella, 36
Staining, of cytomegalovirus, 114
Stillbirth
  and mumps, 206
  and rubella, 41–43, 42(t)
  viruses causing, 5(t)
Strabismus
  in cytomegalovirus infection, 108–109, *108*
  in rubella, 55
Suppressor cytotoxic lymphocytes, 235
Syphilis
  hepatosplenomegaly in, 254, 255(t)
  retinopathy in, 249(t)
  vs. cytomegalovirus infection, 122

T-lymphocytes, 235
  competence tests for, 236
  helper inducer, 235
  identification methods for, 236
  suppressor cytotoxic, 235
Tectorial membrane, adherent to Reissner's
    membrane, 36, *37*
Teeth
  abnormalities of, in cytomegalovirus infec-
    tion, 111–112
  in rubella, 38
Teratogenic drugs, 3, 4
Thalidomide, 3, 4
Theta antigen, 67
Thrombocytopenia
  in cytomegalovirus infection, 106–107
  in rubella, 59
Thrombocytopenic purpura. See *Purpura.*
Thymus
  fetal, and lymphocyte production, 235
  in congenital rubella, 36, 60
Thyroid dysfunction, in rubella, 62
Toxoplasmosis
  cerebral calcifications in, 246–247, *247*,
    248(t)
  chorioretinitis in, 248–249, 249(t)
  diagnosis of, 121
  hepatosplenomegaly in, 254, 255(t)
  IgA deficiency in, 238
  microphthalmus in, 250
  purpura in, 252–253, 253(t)
  retinopathy in, 248–249, 249(t)
  vs. cytomegalovirus infection, 121, 121(t)
Transfer factor, 287–288
Tranfusions
  and jaundice, 254
  cytomegalovirus transmission via, 9–100,
    124, 254
  infection transmission via, 254
Trifluorothymidine, 288(t), 290
Tuberous meningitis, cerebral calcifications in,
    247
Tuberous sclerosis, cerebral calcifications in,
    247–248, 248(t)

Ulcer(s)
  gastrointestinal, in cytomegalovirus infection,
    111
  in maternal herpes simplex infection, 137,
    138
Umbilical cord
  herpes simplex infection of, 221–223, *221,
    223, 224*
  pathology of, 213–228
Umbilical vessels, infection transmisson via,
    232–233
Urinalysis, in cytomegalovirus diagnosis,
    116–117
Uveitis, nongranulomatous, in rubella, 35

Vaccination. See also *Immunization.*
  cost-benefit analysis for, 7
  for cytomegalovirus, 124–125, 279–280
    reinfection in, 274
  for herpes simplex virus, 280
  for poliomyelitis, 286–287
    in pregnancy, 158, 287
  for rubella, 274–284. See also *Rubella vacci-
    nation.*
  for smallpox. See also *Vaccinia.*
    during pregnancy, 11
  for varicella-zoster, 281
Vaccine(s)
  available, 275(t)
  Coxsackie virus, 159
  cytomegalovirus, 124–125, 279–280
    oncogenicity of, 274
  development of, need for, 273(t)
    precautions for, 274
  hepatitis B virus, 283–284
    with hepatitis B immune globulin,
      284–285
  herpes simplex virus, 280
  poliovirus, 286–287
    for Coxsackie B virus infection, 159, 287
  pure culture for, 274
  rubella, 275–277, 276(t). See also *Rubella vac-
    cine(s)*
    development of, 274–275
    types of, 275–276, 275(t), 276(t)
  under development, 275(t)
  varicella-zoster, 281
Vaccinia, 178–181, *178–180*, 180(t)
  clinical manifestations of, 176
  defined, 175
  effects of, 5(t)
  immunization for, 281
  placenta in, 225, *226*
  pathogenesis of, 176
Vaccinial hyperimmune immunoglobulin, 281
Varicella. See also *Varicella-zoster infection.*
  congenital, antibody response in, immuno-
      logical tests for, 263, 267(t), 269–270
    chemotherapy for, 288–289, 291–292,
      291(t)
    placental, infection in, 223–225
    retinopathy in, 249(t)
    vidarabine for, 288–289, 288(t), 292
  defined, 161
  prenatal, chemotherapy for, 292
    stillbirth in, 223–225, *224, 225*
  postnatal, epidemiology of, 162
    immunity in, 161, 163
    incubation period in, 161

Varicella (*Continued*)
  postnatal, lesions in, 161
    natural history of, 161–162
    pathogenesis of, 162
    pathology of, 162
Varicella-zoster antibody
  detection of, 173
  measurement of, 173
Varicella-zoster infection, 161–173. See also
    Varicella; Zoster.
  acyclovir for, 288(t), 289–290. 290(t), 292
  congenital, 163–165, *164*, 165(t)
    as cause of defects, 165–172, 166(t)–168(t),
      169, 170(t), 172(t)
      case reports of, 166(t)–168(t), 169–171
      evidence for, 9, 10(t)
    effects of, 5(t)
    management of, 172–173
    prevention of, 172–173
    severity of, and time of maternal illness,
      165, 165(t)
    skin lesions in, *169*, 170
  immunization for, 281
  laboratory diagnosis of, 173, 259–269. See
    also *Laboratory diagnosis* and specific diag-
    nostic techniques.
  maternal, management of, 172–173
    risk of fetal damage in, 172
  maternal exposure to, passive immunization
    for, 172
  vaccination for, 281
  vidarabine for, 288–289, 288(t), 292
  zoster immune globulin for, 281
Varicella-zoster virus, 173
  laboratory identification of, 173
Variola
  clinical manifestations of, 175
  congenital, 176–178, 177(t)
    effects of, 5(t)
    placenta in, 225
  forms of, 175
  history of, 175
  immunization for, 281
  in pregnancy, 11
  pathogenesis of, 175–176
  pathology of, 175–176
Variola major, 175
Variola minor, 175
Varioloid, 175
Ventricular septal defect, in rubella, 256,
  256(t)
Vidarabine, 288–289, 288(t), 291–292
  for cytomegalovirus infection, 292
  for herpes simplex infection, 148, 288–289,
    288(t), 291
  for varicella, 288(t), 292
  in pregnancy, 292
Villitis
  chronic, differential diagnosis of, 219
    in cytomegalovirus infection, 219

Villitis (*Continued*)
  in herpes simplex infection, 220–223,
    220–223
    necrotizing, 220, *220*
  in rubella, 225–228, *227*
  in vaccinia, 225, *226*
  in varicella, 223, *224*, 225, *225*
  in variola, 225
Viral infection(s)
  congenital, clinical findings suggestive of,
    244(t)
  intrauterine, effects of on fetus, range of,
    9(t)
  immunopathological mechanisms in, 239
  laboratory diagnosis of, 259–267. See also
    Laboratory diagnosis and specific diagnostic
    techniques.
  maternal, asymptomatic, 6
    subclinical, 6
  prevention of, 272–288
  risk of, after fetal membrane rupture, 232
  transmission of via breast milk, 5
Viremia, and effectiveness of immunization,
  273–274, 273(t)
Virus, persistence of in macrophages, 233
Virus cultures, sample collection for, 260,
  261(t)
Virus isolation, techniques, 262–263, 264(t),
  265, 266
Virus neutralization antibody test, 267(t), 269
  for rubella antibody, 23
Virus particles, direct detection of, 262–263
Vitamin supplementation, and prevention of
  neural tube defects, 3
Vulvovaginitis, maternal, in herpes simplex in-
  fection, 137, *138*

Western equine encephalitis virus, 208–209

Zinc deficiency, and amnionic fluid infections,
  232
Zoster. See also *Varicella-zoster infection.*
  defined, 161
  disseminated, in pregnancy, chemotherapy
    for, 292
  postnatal, epidemiology of, 162
    immunity in, 163
    incubation period in, 162
    lesions in, 162
    natural history of, 161–162
    pathogenesis of, 162
    pathology of, 162
Zoster immune globulin, 281
  for prevention of congenital varicella-zoster
    infection, 172
Zoster varicellosus, 162

MAJOR PROBLEMS IN CLINICAL PEDIATRICS

MAJOR PROBLEMS IN CLINICAL PEDIATRICS (MPCP)—
A series of important monographs focusing on significant topics of current interest. Unsurpassed in clarity and depth of coverage, each hardbound volume in the series covers a specific issue or disease, a recent advance in clinical therapeutics, or a newly developed diagnostic technique. A "mini-library" in itself, MPCP features concisely written, postgraduate-level information from highly-qualified authors.

Join the MPCP Subscriber Plan. You'll receive each new volume in the series upon publication—three to five titles publish each year—and you'll save postage and handling costs! Or you may order MPCP titles individually. If not completely satisfied with any volume, you may return it with the invoice within 30 days at no further obligation.

Timely, in-depth coverage you can count on . . . Enroll in the Subscriber Plan for MAJOR PROBLEMS IN CLINICAL PEDIATRICS today!

Available from your bookstore or the publisher.

Complete and Mail Today!

☑ **YES!** Enroll me in the **MAJOR PROBLEMS IN CLINICAL PEDIATRICS** Subscriber Plan so that I may receive future titles in the series immediately upon publication, and save postage and handling costs! If not completely satisfied with any volume, I may return it with the invoice within 30 days at no further obligation.

Name_____

Address_____

City_____State_____Zip_____

☐ Credit my salesman

Printed in USA.   283   PM2416D   Postage & handling additional outside USA.

BUSINESS REPLY MAIL

FIRST CLASS   PERMIT NO. 101   PHILADELPHIA, PA

postage will be paid by addressee

W.B. SAUNDERS COMPANY

west washington square
philadelphia, PA 19105

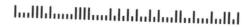